PharmFacts

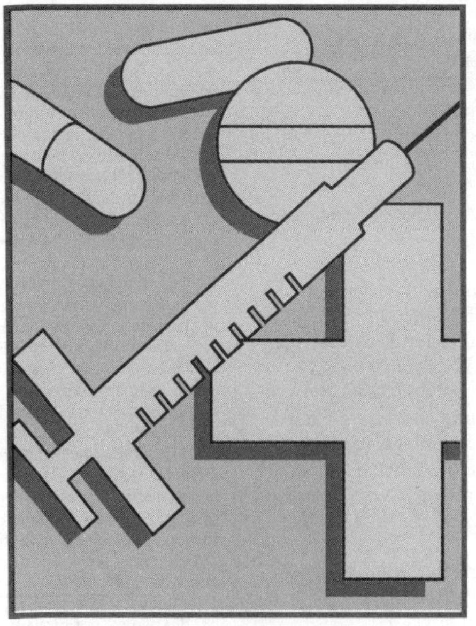

for NURSES

Springhouse Corporation
Springhouse, Pennsylvania

STAFF

Senior Publisher
Matthew Cahill

Clinical Manager
Cindy Tryniszewski, RN, MSN

Art Director
John Hubbard

Senior Editor
June Norris

Editors
Kathy Goldberg, Beth Mauro, Gale Sloan

Clinical Editors
Judith Schilling McCann, RN, BSN; Beverly Ann Tscheschlog, RN; Mary Ann Foley, RN, BSN

Copy Editors
Cynthia C. Breuninger (manager), Mary T. Durkin, Lynette D. High, Christina Ponczek, Doris Weinstock

Designers
Stephanie Peters (senior associate art director), Matie Patterson (assistant art director)

Typographers
Diane Paluba (manager), Elizabeth Bergman, Joyce Rossi Biletz, Phyllis Marron, Valerie Rosenberger

Manufacturing
Deborah Meiris (director), Pat Dorshaw (manager), T.A. Landis

Production Coordinator
Margaret A. Rastiello

Editorial Assistants
Beverly Lane, Mary Madden

Indexer
Robin Hipple

Cover
Matthew Schmidt

The clinical procedures described and recommended in this publication are based on research and consultation with medical and nursing authorities. To the best of our knowledge, these procedures reflect currently accepted clinical practice; nevertheless, they can't be considered absolute and universal recommendations. For individual application, all recommendations must be considered in light of the patient's clinical condition and, before administration of new or infrequently used drugs, in light of the latest package insert information. The authors and the publisher disclaim responsibility for any adverse effects resulting directly or indirectly from the suggested procedures, from any undetected errors, or from the reader's misunderstanding of the text.

Printed in the United States of America.
Pharmf-011295

A member of the Reed Elsevier plc group

Library of Congress Cataloging-in-Publication Data
Pharmfacts for nurses.
p. cm.
Includes index.
1. Chemotherapy — Handbooks, manuals, etc. 2. Nursing — Handbooks, manuals, etc. 3. Drugs — Handbooks, manuals, etc. I. Springhouse Corporation.
[DNLM: 1. Pharmacology — nurses' instruction. 2. Drug Therapy — nurses' instruction. QV 735 P535 1995]
RM125.P48 1995
615.5'8 — dc20
DNLM/DLC 95-36762
ISBN 0-87434-803-X CIP

CONTENTS

CONTRIBUTORS AND CONSULTANTS

Charold L. Baer, RN, PhD, CCRN, FCCM
Professor
Oregon Health Sciences University
Portland

Ellen Barker
President
Neuroscience Nursing Consultants
Greenville, Del.

Sandra Bixler, RN, MSN, CCRN
Clinical Nurse Specialist
Berks Cardiologists, Ltd.
Reading, Pa.

David J. Blanchard, BS, RPh
Pharmacist Specialist
Mary Imogene Bassett Hospital
Cooperstown, N.Y.

Betty Nash Blevins, RN, MSN, CCRN, CS
Associate Professor of Nursing
Bluefield (W.V.) State College

Kathleen C. Byington, RN, MSN, CS
Pediatric Orthopedic Clinical
Nurse Specialist and Case Manager
Vanderbilt University Medical Center
Nashville, Tenn.

Susan M. Cohen, RN, DSN, ANP
Associate Professor
University of Texas–Houston

Judith A. Crank, RN, MSN
Director, Staff Education and Training
Hahnemann University Hospital
Philadelphia

Robin Donohoe Dennison, RN, MSN, CCRN, CS
Critical Care Consultant
Winchester, Ky.

Belle Erickson, RN, MS, PhD
Assistant Professor
Villanova (Pa.) University College of Nursing

Sue Frymark, RN, BS
Manager, Clinical and Data Support Services
Legacy Good Samaritan Hospital
Portland, Ore.

Harriett W. Ferguson, RN,C, MSN, EdD
Associate Professor
Temple University Department of Nursing
Philadelphia

M. Gaedeke, RN, MSN, CCRN, CS
Clinical Nurse Specialist and Nurse Practitioner
Children's Hospital of Buffalo (N.Y.)

Julie M. Gerhart, RPh
Long-Term Care Pharmacist
Hunsicker's Pharmacy, Inc.
Long-Term Care Division
Souderton, Pa.

Mary Jo Gerlach, RN, MSNEd
Assistant Professor, Adult Nursing
Medical College of Georgia
School of Nursing
Athens

Ginny Wacker Guido, RN, MSN, JD
Professor and Chair
Department of Nursing
Eastern New Mexico University
Portales

Andrea O. Hollingsworth, RN, PhD
Associate Professor and Director
Undergraduate Program
Villanova (Pa.) University College of Nursing

Carole Kenner, RN,C, DNS, FAAN
Professor and Department Chair
Parent Child Health Nursing
University of Cincinnati (Ohio)
College of Nursing and Health

Patricia A. Keys, PharmD
Associate Professor of Clinical Pharmacy
School of Pharmacy
Duquesne University
Pittsburgh, Pa.

James J. Laub
Chief, Clinical Pharmacy Section
Carl T. Hayden V.A. Medical Center
Phoenix

Verna MacCarthy, RN
Head Nurse, I.V. Team
Hahnemann University Hospital, Philadelphia

Margo McCaffrey, RN, MS, FAAN
Nursing Consultant (Pain)
Los Angeles

Edwina A. McConnell, RN, PhD, FRCNA
Independent Nurse Consultant
Madison, Wis.

Lynn E. McGrory, RN, MSN, CCRN
Critical Care Clinical Nurse Specialist
Brandywine Hospital
Coatesville, Pa.

Melinda Mercer
Manager, Federal Government Affairs
National Association of Chain Drug Stores
Alexandria, Va.

Morgan L. Pinkerman, RN, MSN, CIC, FNPC, MLT(ASCP)
Certified Family Nurse Practitioner
Ravenswood (W.V.) Medical Center

Lori Martin Plank, RN, MSN, CS, FNP, MSPH
Assistant Professor, Adult Nurse Practitioner Program
Gwynedd Mercy College
Gwynedd Valley, Pa.

Theresa R. Prosser, PharmD, BCPS
Assistant Professor
St. Louis (Mo.) College of Pharmacy

Denise H. Rhoney, PharmD
Neurotrauma Clinical Specialist
Detroit (Mich.) Receiving Hospital and University Health Center

Joanne Farley Serembus, RN, MSN, CCRN
Instructor, Medical-Surgical and Critical Care Nursing
Roxborough Memorial Hospital School of Nursing
Philadelphia

Lynda Thomson, RPh, PharmD
Clinical Pharmacist, Infectious Diseases
Thomas Jefferson University Hospital
Philadelphia

Catherine M. Todd, RN,C, EdD
Assistant Professor
Villanova (Pa.) University College of Nursing

Bradley R. Williams, PharmD
Associate Professor
Clinical Pharmacy and Clinical Gerontology
University of Southern California
Los Angeles

ACKNOWLEDGMENT

Michael R. Cohen, MS, FASHP, president of the Institute for Safe Medication Practices, contributed the following:

FOREWORD

Clearly, administering medications and observing their effectiveness are among your most demanding responsibilities. Furthermore, in recent years your responsibilities for administering drug therapy have expanded and become significantly more sophisticated because of the rapid development of new drugs and the introduction of increasingly complex delivery systems.

As a result, learning about and implementing drug therapy is more comprehensive today than simply emphasizing the "Five Rights." And no matter whether you have prescriptive rights or a predominantly dependent role, you're still held accountable for administering safe and effective drug therapy.

To help you fulfill this responsibility, you'll find approximately 500 topics in *PharmFacts for Nurses* that are crucial to safe, effective, error-free drug therapy. Many of these topics are seldom, if ever, found in conventional drug references. A completely different kind of drug book, this reference is organized by topic (not by drug or drug class, as found in most drug references).

PharmFacts for Nurses organizes drug information into four major parts.

Part One, *Drug Essentials*, covers data, directions, and advice on issues every nurse needs to know: how to distinguish facts from fallacies, how to avoid or minimize the legal risks of drug administration, how to prevent virtually every type of medication error, and how to convert drug dosages from one form to another.

Part Two, *Drug Alerts*, stresses responding to emergencies and heeding cautions and warnings related to drug therapy. Although many handbooks delineate side effects of drugs, *PharmFacts for Nurses* identifies ways to *manage* them and describes how to *deal with* hazardous drug interactions, *prevent* drug incompatibilities, and *treat* drug overdoses.

Part Three, *Drug Administration Tips and Techniques*, provides up-to-date, step-by-step procedures for giving oral drugs, applying topical preparations, giving injections, delivering infusions, and administering drugs by many other routes (for instance, the intra-articular and intraosseous routes).

Part IV, simply called *Drug Therapy*, identifies current drug therapy for common disorders, including dosages and the relative effectiveness and importance of drug therapy in treating these disorders. Armed with this information, you can quickly assess the most commonly used drugs ordered to treat your patient's condition. Part IV also includes chapters on modifying customary drug therapy for maternal, neonatal, pediatric, and elderly patients because of changes in drug absorption, distribution, metabolism, and excretion processes in these groups.

To help you zero in on information quickly, graphic devices are used to identify special features. For example, *First-Line Drug* highlights first-line drug therapy for specific disorders. *Alert* signals dangerous signs or practices, and *Clinical Tips* pinpoints quicker, safer, more efficient ways to administer drug therapy.

Every time you give a drug, you need to follow scores of rules and precautions to protect your patient's safety — and your license. Of course, you're well aware that medication errors are the main cause of malpractice suits filed against nurses and hospitals. However, drug administration errors can be avoided, if only you have all the facts. Now you can, if you make *PharmFacts for Nurses* your primary resource for information about safe, error-free drug therapy.

Mary Jo Gerlach, RN, MSNEd
Assistant Professor, Adult Nursing
Medical College of Georgia
School of Nursing
Athens

PharmFacts for NURSES

■ PART ONE

DRUG ESSENTIALS

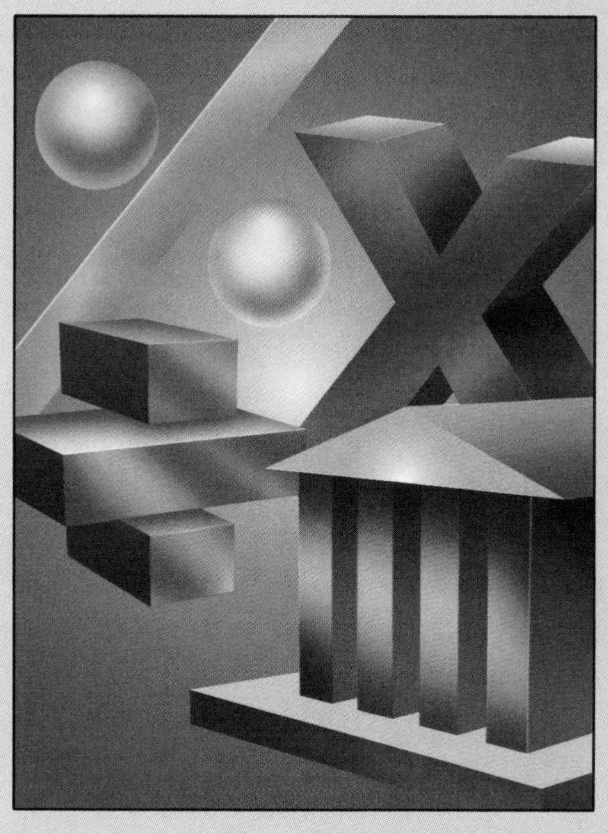

■ CHAPTER 1

DISTINGUISHING FACTS FROM FALLACIES

Dispelling myths about drug therapy

DISPELLING MYTHS ABOUT DRUG THERAPY

Antibiotic allergies

MYTH
Any patient who had an allergic reaction to an antibiotic many years ago is still sensitive today.
FACT
Years ago, impurities in drugs (rather than the drugs themselves) may have triggered many allergic reactions. A patient who had a reaction 40 years ago might be able to take today's synthetic form of the drug without problems.

MYTH
Antibiotic-sensitive patients develop allergic symptoms immediately.
FACT
Severe reactions usually occur within minutes, but symptoms can occur hours or days later. Instruct patients to report side effects to their doctor.

MYTH
A patient who developed a rash after taking ampicillin has had an allergic reaction.
FACT
Not all rashes indicate a true antibiotic allergy. A maculopapular (measleslike) rash from ampicillin, for example, isn't a true penicillin-induced allergic reaction. Urticaria, however, suggests true hypersensitivity. Ask the patient to describe the rash (including where it appeared) and to tell you about any other symptoms he had.

MYTH
Anaphylaxis is a common side effect of penicillin.
FACT
Although mild hypersensitivity reactions are common, anaphylaxis is rare: It occurs in 0.05% of all patients. Between 5% and 10% of affected patients die.

MYTH
A patient who's had an allergic reaction to penicillin can never take the drug again.
FACT
A patient can be desensitized to penicillin when no other antibiotic is appropriate, although this potentially hazardous process is rarely justified. Initially, he is prescribed a low oral or parenteral dose, which is gradually increased to a therapeutic level.

MYTH
If a patient is allergic to penicillin, the doctor may substitute a cephalosporin.
FACT
Penicillin and cephalosporin drugs, which are all beta-lactams, are chemically sim-

ilar. Consequently, cephalosporins may cause a cross-sensitivity reaction in patients who are allergic to penicillin. About 1.7% of all patients are allergic to cephalosporins, but this risk increases fivefold in patients who are allergic to penicillin. ■

Cancer

MYTH
Although chemotherapy can effectively control cancer, it isn't a cure.
FACT
Chemotherapy can cure such cancers as Hodgkin's disease, Burkitt's lymphoma, Ewing's sarcoma, neuroblastoma, and ovarian, breast, and colorectal cancers. It's also used to control advanced cancers of the prostate gland, head and neck, endometrium, bladder, breast, cervix, and stomach. ■

Cardiac conditions

MYTH
A patient gets his prescribed dose of nitroglycerin ointment when you apply it anywhere on his body.
FACT
Many factors influence nitroglycerin absorption, including the amount of hair on the person's skin. Patients have different responses to nitroglycerin when it's applied to different parts of their body. In one study, patients' responses were similar when nitroglycerin was applied to their forehead or chest, but markedly different when it was applied to their ankle.

MYTH
You won't affect the dose if you use either an occlusive plastic dressing or the manufacturer's paper applicator strip when you apply nitroglycerin ointment.
FACT
Occlusive plastic dressings slightly increase skin temperature and hydration, so more of the ointment is absorbed. Use either an occlusive dressing or the paper applicator, but stick with what you start with. Switching will deliver an inconsistent dose.

MYTH
Administer I.V. lidocaine for all wide, bizarre rhythms that resemble ventricular tachycardia (VT).
FACT
Supraventricular tachycardia (SVT) with aberrancy may resemble VT. Lidocaine may accelerate conduction of certain SVTs through the AV junction. Overall, procainamide may be the better

choice because it can correct VT and may block AV conduction in SVT with aberrancy.

MYTH
Patients with either acute or chronic digitalis toxicity will have the same side effects.

FACT
With acute digitalis toxicity, side effects are primarily cardiac: arrhythmias, sinus bradycardia, AV block, and SA exit block. If the patient has significant cardiac or pulmonary disease, he also may have ventricular arrhythmias, hyperkalemia, and GI upset.

Chronic digitalis toxicity may also cause GI upset, along with lethargy, visual disturbances, anorexia, ventricular arrhythmias, hypokalemia, and AV block.

MYTH
Sodium bicarbonate is essential to reverse cardiac arrest.

FACT
Sodium bicarbonate may actually impede resuscitation by causing side effects, such as:

- shifting the oxyhemoglobin saturation curve
- hyperosmolarity
- hypernatremia
- paradoxical acidosis from the production of carbon dioxide
- inactivating catecholamine drugs given simultaneously with sodium bicarbonate.

Use sodium bicarbonate cautiously. It may be beneficial for certain patients, such as those who have preexisting acidosis with or without hyperkalemia. When it is indicated, give 1 mEq/kg as the initial dose, then 0.5 mEq/kg every 10 minutes thereafter as needed. Before administering, check the patient's arterial pH (it should be more than 7.45) to make sure that the dose won't cause extracellular alkalosis. ■

Endocrine and metabolic conditions

MYTH
Only aqueous vasopressin can be used to manage acute or chronic diabetes insipidus.

FACT
Several drugs are used to manage these conditions, including synthetic vasopressin, vasopressin tannate in oil, desmopressin, chlorpropamide, and clofibrate. The doctor should prescribe the one that best meets the patient's needs.

MYTH
Diuretics help to eliminate third-space fluids.

FACT
Diuretics move fluid from the vascular space into the re-

nal tubules for elimination. But third-space fluid is trapped in tissue. So before the diuretic can work, the third-space fluid has to be pulled into the vascular space. To accomplish this, administer a colloid such as albumin before the diuretic.

MYTH
D_5W is an isotonic solution.
FACT
When D_5W is administered I.V., it initially is isotonic to plasma. But dextrose is quickly metabolized, leaving hypotonic free water in the vein. This free water penetrates cells and can cause edema.

MYTH
Dextrose solutions effectively correct hypovolemia.
FACT
Glucose is a powerful osmotic diuretic that may actually cause secondary hypovolemia. When infused at a rate faster than the body can metabolize, it can trigger a series of physiologic reactions: first, hyperglycemia followed by glycosuria; then, diuresis; and finally, hypovolemia.

MYTH
A patient who takes a beta-adrenergic blocker will be asymptomatic during hypoglycemic episodes.
FACT
These drugs diminish only beta-adrenergic responses such as tachycardia. Caution such patients to stay alert for other clues of hypoglycemia.

MYTH
An insulin-dependent patient must abstain from drinking alcohol.
FACT
Although alcohol interferes with glucose production in the liver, a patient may be able to drink in moderation (one to two drinks per day). But because diminished glucose production increases his risk of hypoglycemia — for up to 12 hours after his last drink — he should consult his doctor about insulin and dietary adjustments.

MYTH
Encourage patients who take diuretics to eat bananas and drink orange juice to build up their potassium levels.
FACT
The body absorbs only a small amount of the potassium in fruits, so they aren't the best choice for meeting oral potassium needs. The patient would have to eat three or four bananas daily to equal 60 to 80 mEq of potassium. Potassium-chloride preparations are more effective. Also, potassium-sparing diuretics will help prevent potassium loss. ■

Enteral and parenteral nutrition

MYTH
When diarrhea occurs during enteral therapy, the best treatment is an antidiarrheal agent, such as diphenoxylate and atropine, opium tincture, or a kaolin and pectin mixture.

FACT
Diarrhea may be a sign of bacterial contamination (food poisoning) or bacterial overgrowth from antibiotic therapy. Antidiarrheal agents may exacerbate the problem by slowing GI motility and allowing toxins to be absorbed, which could lead to sepsis.

Using aseptic technique when you prepare and administer feedings can help prevent bacterial contamination, and administering lactobacillus with antibiotics can prevent bacterial overgrowth.

MYTH
You can administer drugs by adding them directly to the enteral formula.

FACT
Drugs added directly to the enteral formula can become therapeutically ineffective, as can the formula itself. The better choice is administering the drug in a single bolus through the enteral tube. Flush the tube with water before and after administering the drug. If you're giving more than one drug, flush the tube between doses. But remember, the drugs that should be absorbed in the stomach can't be given through a nasoduodenal tube, even in a bolus dose.

MYTH
To infuse total parenteral nutrition (TPN), use the distal lumen of a multilumen catheter.

FACT
Because these catheters are designed with a separate port for each lumen and because of the distance between exit ports along the catheter, you can use any port for TPN without worrying about incompatibility.

At least one manufacturer recommends using the middle lumen for TPN infusions and reserving the 16G (or larger) distal lumen for central venous pressure readings or for infusing blood. Use the proximal lumen for other I.V. solutions or for drawing blood. Just be consistent: Always use the same port for the same purpose. ■

GI conditions

MYTH
Histamine-2 (H_2) receptor antagonists, such as cimetidine and ranitidine, are the most effective therapy for controlling gastric acid and protecting against GI bleeding.
FACT
H_2-receptor antagonists are more effective when combined with antacids. When H_2-receptor antagonists became available, doctors began to favor them over antacids. Recently, researchers concluded that the two drugs combined are the best preventive therapy.

MYTH
If patients at high risk for stress ulcers (such as those who are on ventilators) are receiving continuous enteral feeding, they should also continue taking antacids to avoid GI bleeding.
FACT
Enteral feedings decrease and neutralize gastric acid, and they're as effective as antacids or H_2-receptor antagonists in protecting against GI bleeding. So high-risk patients don't necessarily need additional antacids or H_2-receptor antagonists prophylactically.

MYTH
Antacids and H_2-receptor antagonists are the only effective antiulcer drugs.
FACT
Antibiotic therapy is effective in treating ulcers caused by *Helicobacter pylori* infection. Common regimens include bismuth subsalicylate, tetracycline, amoxicillin, or metronidazole.

MYTH
When added to lavage solutions, vasopressors (such as norepinephrine) reduce gastric bleeding through vasoconstriction.
FACT
Adding vasopressors to lavage solutions has no proven benefit. Such agents produce local ischemia, which may cause more bleeding. ■

Hormone replacement

MYTH
Women who've already gone through menopause or who don't have significant menopausal symptoms won't benefit from hormone replacement therapy (HRT).
FACT
Estrogen may protect both menopausal and postmenopausal women from cardiovascular (CV) disease. Estrogen may also decrease vaginal dryness and delay the

progress of osteoporosis, especially if therapy is started before bone demineralization occurs. Progesterone may provide protection against endometrial hyperplasia, which may lead to cancer.

MYTH
Every older woman is a candidate for HRT.
FACT
A woman may be a poor candidate for HRT if she has a history of breast cancer, unstable hypertension, thrombophlebitis, acute liver disease or chronic liver dysfunction, ocular vascular disease, or cerebrovascular accident.

MYTH
Women receiving any type of HRT are at increased risk for endometrial cancer.
FACT
Therapy with estrogen alone has been linked to endometrial cancer. However, women receiving HRT that combines estrogen and progesterone have no greater risk of developing endometrial cancer than the general population. Studies have suggested a link between progesterone and breast cancer, but this relationship hasn't been confirmed.

MYTH
All women receiving HRT should receive combination hormonal therapy.
FACT
A woman who's had a hysterectomy doesn't need progesterone, which reduces endometrial hyperplasia and the risk of endometrial cancer. These aren't concerns when the uterus is removed. Progesterone also raises cholesterol levels, increasing the risk of CV problems.

MYTH
Women receiving HRT have normal menstrual periods.
FACT
Women who are receiving HRT containing estrogen and progesterone will experience withdrawal bleeding. This occurs when estrogen levels drop, causing the endometrium to slough off. This bleeding isn't usually as heavy as a normal menstrual period, though. ■

Immune conditions

MYTH
Drug therapy is effective only for decreasing the inflammation and pain of arthritis.
FACT
Arthritis medications work in three ways: They reduce inflammation and pain, slow the disease process, and re-

duce uric acid levels in patients with gout.

MYTH
Gold salts are the treatment of last resort for patients with advanced rheumatoid arthritis.
FACT
Research shows that early use of gold salts can actually delay the disease's advancement. When second-line drugs are indicated, the patient's medication regimen may also include NSAIDs, corticosteroids, penicillamine, hydroxychloroquine (an antimalarial), and immunosuppressants. Nonpharmacologic interventions, such as rest, exercise, relaxation techniques, application of heat and cold, physical and occupational therapies, support groups, and even surgery also may help. ■

Infection

MYTH
Patients who receive the pneumonia vaccine are fully protected against this disease.
FACT
This vaccine is effective only against pneumococci, the most common cause of pneumonia acquired outside the hospital.

MYTH
Antiendotoxin monoclonal antibodies (MABs) effectively treat patients with septic shock.
FACT
In recent clinical trials with two antiendotoxin MABs (HA-1A and E5), only HA-1A lowered the mortality rate in gram-negative bacteremia and septic shock. Both products were effective against gram-negative bacteremia and sepsis that hadn't progressed to shock.

MYTH
You should give daily meatal care and use antibiotic creams and ointments to prevent urinary tract infections (UTIs).
FACT
These measures don't reduce catheter-associated bacteriuria and UTIs, researchers have found; nor does irrigating the catheter with antibacterial solutions or compounds. You should, however, clean the catheter and meatal area with soap and water as needed.

MYTH
To prevent central venous catheter (CVC) sepsis, use a polyantibiotic ointment that will kill Candida *organisms.*
FACT
Candida, a fungus, is less likely to cause CVC sepsis than *Staphylococcus epidermidis*, a bacterium normally found

on the skin. Polyantibiotic ointments are bactericidal but not fungicidal, so they can disrupt the normal balance of bacteria and fungi and allow *Candida* to flourish.

To prevent sepsis, clean the site with alcohol first, then povidone-iodine, to control skin pathogens. (Use polyantibiotic ointments on patients who are at greater risk for acquiring an infection.)

Improperly cleaning, inserting, dressing, and handling the catheter are major causes of sepsis. Use aseptic technique during insertion, and thoroughly wash your hands before dressing the site or handling the catheter. ■

Musculoskeletal conditions

MYTH

Calcium supplements help to prevent osteoporosis by increasing bone density.

FACT

Many postmenopausal women take up to 1,500 mg of calcium supplements each day. But one study found that a daily calcium intake of 1,000 to 2,000 mg won't prevent bone loss. More effective strategies include initiating postmenopausal estrogen replacement therapy, eating a well-balanced diet, and doing weight-bearing exercises such as walking.

MYTH

Calcium-based antacids are recommended for older women with ulcers because they prevent osteoporosis.

FACT

Calcium salts can increase stomach acid secretion, so calcium-based antacids aren't recommended for anyone with ulcers. Women should also avoid antacids containing aluminum hydroxide, which can contribute to osteoporosis. ■

Neurologic conditions

MYTH

Calcium channel blockers are ineffective as treatment of cerebrovascular accident (CVA).

FACT

Following a CVA, calcium channel blockers, such as nimodipine and nicardipine, increase cerebral blood flow and help reduce subsequent cerebral ischemia. They do so by slowing the influx of calcium into the smooth muscle of cerebral blood vessels. (This influx is believed to cause cerebral vasospasm.)

MYTH

The antiplatelet drug dipyridamole is the best choice for

treating patients with extracranial carotid occlusion.

FACT

Antiplatelet therapy is initiated to prevent further occlusion. But controversy exists over which antiplatelet drug to use. Aspirin remains the most popular for its effectiveness and low cost, although therapeutic dosage ranges haven't been determined yet.

MYTH

Alcohol isn't a risk factor for intracerebral or subarachnoid hemorrhage.

FACT

Moderate drinking (approximately 60 g of alcohol a day) has been associated with the risk of intracerebral and subarachnoid hemorrhage, two types of hemorrhagic CVA.

When a patient drinks that much alcohol, his liver doesn't produce enough clotting factors; he has excessive fibrinolysis, prolonged bleeding time, and impaired platelet function; and he develops hypertension. The triad of ongoing alcohol consumption, altered coagulation, and hypertension directly contributes to hemorrhagic CVA.

MYTH

Hyperosmolar agents are the treatment of choice for increased intracranial pressure (ICP).

FACT

Because you need to treat the underlying cause of increased ICP, a hyperosmolar agent like mannitol might not be right for every patient. After the cause has been determined, the treatment might include removing the mass (for example), elevating the head of the bed 30 to 40 degrees, maintaining the neck in a neutral position, hyperventilating the patient, and administering medication (hyperosmolar agents, diuretics, corticosteroids, or barbiturates). ■

Pain and fever

MYTH

Narcotics should never be given for chronic pain caused by nonmalignant disease.

FACT

Most pain specialists agree with this statement. But for some patients, narcotics are a safe alternative to surgery and are better than no treatment at all. Prolonged narcotic therapy should be used only after other reasonable attempts to relieve pain have failed and only if the patient has no history of drug abuse.

MYTH

A patient who's been taking narcotics for years to relieve pain will probably become a drug addict.

FACT

These patients almost always stop taking the drug when the pain subsides. Unlike a drug addict, who doesn't need narcotics to relieve pain, a patient in chronic pain takes narcotics legally and under a doctor's care. However, other alternatives should be tried first. Misprescribing a narcotic results in the patient misusing, but not abusing, the drug.

MYTH

Elderly patients should receive lower morphine doses than younger patients.

FACT

Regardless of age, no two patients have the same pain threshold. The morphine dose for any patient should be based on his needs, response to the drug, and tolerance. Monitor elderly patients more closely and assess their pain more frequently. Because their rates of metabolism and drug excretion have slowed, they're at greater risk for respiratory depression and drug toxicity.

MYTH

If an elderly patient becomes confused, you'll know that he's been overmedicated with an opioid.

FACT

Not necessarily — confusion can also signal uncontrolled pain. Other possible causes include hypoxia and fluid and electrolyte disturbances. To determine the reason for confusion, perform a complete physical assessment and check the patient's laboratory values and medications.

MYTH

To reduce a child's postoperative fever, give a sponge bath with isopropyl alcohol.

FACT

Never use isopropyl alcohol to reduce a child's fever. Although it isn't absorbed through the skin, its vapors are rapidly absorbed by the lungs. A child who inhales the vapors can suffer neurotoxic effects, such as headaches, confusion, apnea, coma, and death. ■

Psychiatric conditions

MYTH

If a patient takes medication for depression, he'll always have to take it.

FACT

Many depressed patients require medication only periodically for treatment of acute episodes. Other patients, once they learn new coping skills, may never need it again. ■

■ CHAPTER 2

RECOGNIZING LEGAL LIABILITIES

REVIEWING LEGISLATIVE AND PROFESSIONAL DRUG CONTROL

Defining drug control

Legally, a drug is any substance listed in an official state, provincial, or national formulary. A drug may also be defined as any substance (other than food) "intended to affect the structure or any function of the body (or) for use in the diagnosis, cure, mitigation, treatment, or prevention of disease" (New York Educational Law).

A prescription drug is any drug restricted from regular commercial purchase and sale. A state, provincial, or national government has determined that this drug is, or might be, unsafe unless used under a qualified medical practitioner's supervision.

Formal drug controls, ranging from governmental legislation to individual institutional policies help to regulate the manufacture, distribution, and use of drugs. Religious and social mores also provide informal controls on drug use. In most cases, a society's attitudes and values more strictly determine the acceptable limits of drug use than formal controls.

International controls

The United Nations, through its World Health Organization, attempts to promote international health by providing technical assistance and encouraging research for drug use. One committee has been established to cope with the problems associated with habit-forming drugs. Drug enforcement agencies in various nations cooperate, but no administrative or judicial structures enforce controls. As a result, control of the international drug trade depends largely on the voluntary cooperation of nations. ■

Reviewing federal drug laws

Two important federal laws governing the use of drugs in the United States are the Federal Food, Drug, and Cosmetic Act (FFDCA) and the Comprehensive Drug Abuse Prevention and Control Act.

The FFDCA restricts interstate shipments of drugs not approved for human use and outlines the process for testing and approving new drugs. The Comprehensive Drug Abuse Prevention and Control Act, incorporating the Controlled Substances Act, seeks to categorize drugs by how dangerous they are and regulates drugs thought to be most subject to abuse.

FFDCA

Legislative drug control in the United States began in 1906 with the passage of the FFDCA. Although the FFDCA primarily addresses the issue of food purity, it also designates the United States Pharmacopeia (USP) and the National Formulary as the official standards for drugs. (For a summary of laws and amendments adopted since 1906, see *Overview of federal drug legislation,* pages 18 and 19.)

Sherley Amendment

In 1912, the Sherley Amendment to the FFDCA increased federal involvement in drug control by prohibiting the use of fraudulent claims by drug companies. Because of less-than-rigorous enforcement of the Sherley Amendment, drug companies continue to advertise wide-ranging claims for their products.

Harrison Narcotic Act

In 1914, Congress passed the Harrison Narcotic Act. The act classifies certain drugs, such as marijuana, opium, cocaine, and their derivatives, as habit-forming narcotics. It also places regulations on the importation, manufacture, sale, and use of habit-forming narcotics. The Harrison Narcotic Act was the first narcotic control legislation passed by any nation.

1938 FFDCA Amendment

In the 1930s, the need for more stringent drug regulations became apparent when more than 100 people died from ingesting sulfanilamide, an antibacterial drug. Researchers discovered that this drug had been prepared with a previously uninvestigated toxic substance called diethylene glycol.

After the sulfanilamide incident, Congress passed the 1938 amendment to the FFDCA, which establishes regulations for approval by the federal government of all new drugs and specified requirements for drug labeling. According to the amendment, drug labels are to consist of the following elements before the products can enter interstate commerce:

- a statement accurately describing the package's contents
- the usual names of the drugs—for official drugs (preparations listed in the USP and adopted by the government as meeting pharmaceutical standards) and nonofficial drugs (those drugs not listed in the USP)
- indication of the presence, quantity, and proportion of certain drugs (such as alcohol, atropine, digitalis glyco-

Overview of federal drug legislation

Since 1906 when the U.S. Congress passed the Federal Food, Drug, and Cosmetic Act (FFDCA), the federal government has legislated the manufacture, sale, and use of drugs. The following list gives the major legislative acts and their significance.

YEAR	LEGISLATION	SIGNIFICANCE TO THE PUBLIC
1906	FFDCA	Designated official standards for drugs (United States Pharmacopeia and National Formulary)
1912	FFDCA—Sherley Amendment	Prohibited drug companies from making fraudulent claims about their products
1914	Harrison Narcotic Act	Classified certain habit-forming drugs as narcotics and regulated their importation, manufacture, sale, and use
1938	FFDCA—Amendment	Provided for governmental approval of new drugs before they enter interstate commerce; defined labeling requirements
1945	FFDCA—Amendment	Provided for certification of certain drugs through testing by the FDA
1952	FFDCA—Durham-Humphrey Amendment	Distinguished between prescription and nonprescription drugs; specified procedures for the distribution of prescription drugs

Overview of federal drug legislation *(continued)*

YEAR	LEGISLATION	SIGNIFICANCE TO THE PUBLIC
1962	FFDCA—Kefauver-Harris Amendment	Provided assurance of the safety and effectiveness of drugs and improved communication about drugs
1970	Comprehensive Drug Abuse Prevention and Control Act (Controlled Substances Act)	Outlined controls on habit-forming drugs; established governmental programs to prevent and treat drug abuse; assisted with the campaign against drug abuse by developing a classification that categorized drugs according to their abuse liability; placed drugs into schedules
1983	Orphan Drug Act	Offered substantial tax credits to companies to develop drugs that are used to treat rare diseases or that have a limited market

sides, and bromides) in the product
- a warning about habit-forming substances in the product and their effects
- the names of the manufacturer, packager, and distributor
- directions for use and warnings against unsafe use, including recommendations for dosage levels and frequency. (For more information, see *Unlabeled uses of drugs*, pages 20 and 21.)
- a statement on all new drugs not yet approved for interstate commerce, for example, *Caution: New Drug — Limited by Federal Law to Investigational Use.*

Finally, no false or misleading statements are to appear on the label.

1945 FFDCA Amendment

In 1945, the FFDCA was amended further to provide for direct governmental supervision and inspection of

Unlabeled uses of drugs

When approving a new drug, the FDA accepts it *only* for the indications for which phase II and III clinical studies have shown it to be safe and effective. These indications are approved (labeled); all others are not approved (unlabeled).

For example, the FDA may approve a new drug to treat hypertension if phase II and III studies show that it's safe and effective in patients with hypertension. If the drug also works well as an antianginal agent, the FDA can't approve it for this indication unless formal studies in patients with angina pectoris are completed successfully. Such a drug is considered unapproved for treatment of angina pectoris. Yet, it may be used for this unlabeled indication, based on empirical evidence. Here's how this may occur.

Prescribing drugs for unlabeled use

After prescribing a new drug approved to treat hypertension, a doctor may discover that it also decreases the patient's angina. Then the doctor may share this finding with colleagues in medical journals or at meetings, and they may prescribe it for unlabeled uses, too.

The FDA recognizes that a drug's labeling doesn't always contain the most current information about its usage. Therefore, after the FDA approves a drug for one indication, a doctor legally may prescribe it, a pharmacist may dispense it, and a nurse may administer it for any labeled — or unlabeled — indication.

Restricting promotion

Although clinicians are *not* prohibited from prescribing, dispensing, or administering a drug for an unlabeled use, the FDA forbids the manufacturer from promoting a drug for any unlabeled indications. That's why drug package inserts and the *Physicians' Desk Reference* (a collection of drug manufacturers' product labeling) contain no information about unlabeled uses. Furthermore, pharmaceutical sales representatives can't discuss such uses.

Unlabeled uses of drugs *(continued)*

Nevertheless, many drugs commonly are prescribed for unlabeled uses. One famous example is tretinoin (marketed as Retin-A), which is approved to treat acne — its only labeled use. However, because independent studies have shown that tretinoin helps eliminate skin wrinkles, many dermatologists prescribe it for this unlabeled use.

pharmaceutical substances during production. According to the 1945 amendment, governmental certification of certain drugs, such as antibiotics, cannot be granted until each batch of the drug produced is tested.

Durham-Humphrey Amendment

In 1952, the Durham-Humphrey Amendment to the FFDCA distinguished between prescription and nonprescription drugs. It also specified procedures for the distribution of prescription drugs.

Kefauver-Harris Amendment

In the 1960s, the public became aware of the potential dangers of drugs when 200 cases of poliomyelitis developed from hastily prepared batches of poliomyelitis vaccine. In some European countries, birth defects that were linked to thalidomide use by pregnant women also caused great public concern.

Media exposure of the poliomyelitis and thalidomide incidents and of the huge profits earned by many drug companies resulted in the 1962 passage of the Kefauver-Harris Amendment. This amendment attempts to control the safety and effectiveness of drugs and to assure the public of necessary and timely drug information. As a result, several drugs and drug combinations have been withdrawn from the market.

Controlled Substances Act

In 1970, Congress passed the Comprehensive Drug Abuse Prevention and Control Act (which included the Controlled Substances Act [CSA]), designed to contain the rapidly increasing problem of drug abuse. The CSA promotes drug education programs and research into the prevention and treatment of drug dependence. It also provides for the establishment of treatment and rehabilitation centers and strengthened drug enforcement authority. Further, the act designates categories, or schedules, that classify controlled drugs according to their abuse liability. ■

Understanding federal drug standards

The federal government establishes and enforces drug standards to ensure the uniform quality of drugs. The standards pertain to the following drug properties: purity, bioavailability, potency, efficacy, and safety and toxicity.

Purity

This property refers to the uncontaminated state of a drug containing only one active component. In reality, a drug consisting of only one active component is rare because manufacturers usually must add other ingredients to facilitate drug formation and to determine absorption rate.

Extraneous substances from the manufacturing plant also may contaminate the pure drug. As a result, standards of purity do not demand 100% pure active ingredients but specify the type and acceptable amount of extraneous material.

Bioavailability

The degree to which a drug is absorbed and transported to its target site in the body is called *bioavailability.* Factors affecting bioavailability include the particle size, crystalline structure, solubility, and polarity of the compound. The blood or tissue concentration of a drug at a specified time after administration usually determines bioavailability.

Potency

This quality refers to a drug's strength or its power to produce the desired effect. Potency standards are set by testing laboratory animals to determine the definite measurable effect of an administered drug.

Efficacy

This property refers to the effectiveness of a drug used in treatment. Objective clinical trials attempt to determine efficacy, but absolute measurement remains difficult.

Safety and toxicity

These properties are determined by the incidence and severity of reported side effects to a drug. Some harmful reactions may not appear for a considerable time. Safety and toxicity standards are being refined constantly as past experiences illuminate deficiencies in standards.

The modern laboratory testing procedure called *bioassay* significantly helps to determine drug standards and to ensure adherence to the standards. Still, much remains to be improved in testing procedures, some of which are expensive and unreliable. ■

Understanding controlled drug schedules

Schedule I
This schedule contains drugs that have a high abuse potential, have no currently accepted medical use in the United States, or pose unacceptable dangers. Clearance from the FDA is necessary to obtain schedule I drugs. Heroin is an example of a schedule I drug.

Schedule II
This schedule represents drugs with high abuse potential, but with currently acceptable therapeutic use. The use of schedule II drugs may lead to physical or psychological dependence, or both. Most common narcotics are schedule II drugs.

Schedule III
The drugs in this schedule have a lower abuse potential than those in schedule I or II. They also have currently acceptable therapeutic use in the United States. Abuse of schedule III drugs may lead to moderate or low physical or psychological dependence, or both. Some drugs in schedule III are compounds containing limited amounts of certain narcotic and nonnarcotic drugs. Schedule III also includes certain depressants and barbiturates not listed in another schedule.

Schedule IV
The drugs in this schedule have a low abuse potential compared with the drugs in schedule III. They also have acceptable therapeutic uses in the United States. Chloral hydrate is an example of a schedule IV drug.

Schedule V
This schedule includes drugs with a lower abuse potential and with currently acceptable therapeutic uses in the United States. Abuse of the drugs in schedule V leads to more limited physical or psychological dependence compared with the drugs in schedule IV. A common example of a schedule V drug is cough syrup that contains codeine. (See *Schedules of controlled drugs*, pages 24 to 29.) ■

Schedules of controlled drugs

In the United States, the Controlled Substances Act (1970) classifies drugs into categories (schedules) according to their abuse liability. In Canada, the Food and Drug Act (amended yearly) and the Narcotic Control Act (1965) provide similar classifications, although the specific drugs in each class may

UNITED STATES

Category	Examples
Schedule I No recognized medical use. High abuse potential. Research use only.	**Opiates** ▪ heroin **Hallucinogens** ▪ LSD ▪ mescaline **Depressants** ▪ methaqualone
Schedule II Written prescriptions required. No telephone renewals. In an emergency, a prescription may be renewed by telephone, but a written prescription must follow within 72 hours.	**Opiates** ▪ codeine ▪ morphine ▪ meperidine **Stimulants** ▪ amphetamines ▪ phenmetrazine **Depressants** ▪ secobarbital

differ. Health care professionals must be aware of these schedules to ensure the proper handling of controlled substances. The following list provides examples of representative controlled drugs in the United States and Canada.

CANADA

Category	Examples
Schedule H Restricted drugs. No recognized medicinal properties.	**Hallucinogens** ▪ peyote ▪ LSD ▪ mescaline
Narcotics Schedule Stringently restricted drugs. The letter *N* must appear on all labels and professional advertisements.	**Coca leaf derivatives** ▪ cocaine **Opiates and opiate derivatives** ▪ morphine ▪ codeine ▪ methadone ▪ hydromorphone ▪ meperidine **Other drugs** ▪ phencyclidine ▪ cannabis

(continued)

Schedules of controlled drugs *(continued)*

UNITED STATES	
Category	**Examples**
Schedule III Prescriptions required to be rewritten after 6 months or 5 refills. Prescriptions may be ordered by telephone.	**Opiates** ▪ codeine (less than 1.8 g/dl) ▪ opium (25 mg/ 5 ml) **Stimulants** ▪ benzphetamine ▪ mazindol **Depressants** ▪ butabarbital ▪ glutethimide ▪ methyprylon **Anabolic steroids** ▪ fluoxymesterone ▪ methyltestosterone ▪ nandrolone decanoate
Schedule IV Prescriptions required to be rewritten after 6 months or 5 refills.	**Opiates** ▪ pentazocine ▪ propoxyphene **Stimulants** ▪ fenfluramine ▪ phentermine **Depressants** ▪ benzodiazepines ▪ chloral hydrate

CANADA	
Category	**Examples**
Schedule G Controlled drugs. Prescriptions are controlled because of the abuse potential of these drugs.	**Narcotic analgesics** ▪ nalbuphine ▪ butorphanol **Stimulants** ▪ amphetamines **Barbiturates** ▪ phenobarbital ▪ amobarbital ▪ secobarbital
Schedule F Prescription drugs. Although not controlled drugs, agents in this category include some with a relatively low abuse potential. The symbol *Pr* must appear on their labels.	**Anxiolytics** ▪ benzodiazepines

(continued)

Schedules of controlled drugs *(continued)*

UNITED STATES	
Category	**Examples**
Schedule V Dispensed as any other (nonnarcotic) prescription drug. Some Schedule V drugs also may be dispensed without prescription unless additional state regulations apply.	Primarily small amounts of opiates, such as opium, dihydrocodeine, and diphenoxylate, when used as antitussives or antidiarrheals in combination products

Reviewing Canadian drug laws

Drug control in Canada falls under the direct supervision of the Department of National Health and Welfare. The 1953 Canadian Food and Drugs Act (amended yearly) provides regulations for drug manufacture and sale. In 1965, the Canadian Narcotic Control Act restricted the sale, possession, and use of narcotics. It further restricts narcotic possession to authorized personnel.

Under the law, legal possession of narcotics by a nurse is limited to occasions when the nurse administers the drug to a patient under a doctor's order, when the nurse serves as a custodian of narcotics in a health care agency, or when the nurse personally uses the narcotic as part of a prescribed treatment. (For examples of controlled substances in Canada, see *Schedules of controlled drugs*, pages 24 to 29.) ■

Reviewing state, local, and institutional controls

Although state drug controls must conform to federal laws, states usually impose additional regulations, such as those determining the legal age for drinking alcohol or those governing pharmacy practice. Local drug regulations imposed by counties

CANADA	
Category	**Examples**
Nonprescription Drug Schedule (Group 3) Drugs available only in the pharmacy and used only on the physician's recommendation. Limited public access.	**Analgesics** ▪ low-dose codeine preparations **Other drugs** ▪ insulin ▪ nitroglycerin ▪ muscle relaxants

or municipalities usually involve restrictions on the sale or use of alcohol or tobacco.

At the state and provincial (in Canada) level, pharmacy practice acts are the main laws affecting the distribution of drugs. These laws give pharmacists (in Canada, sometimes doctors as well) the sole legal authority to prepare, compound, preserve, and dispense drugs. *Dispensing* refers to taking a drug from the pharmacy supply and giving or selling it to another person. This contrasts with *administering* drugs—actually getting the drug into the patient. Your state's nurse practice act is the law that most directly affects how you administer drugs.

Nursing, medical, and pharmacy practice acts

These practice acts include:

- a definition of the tasks that belong uniquely to the profession
- a statement saying that anyone who performs such tasks without being a licensed or registered member of the defined profession is breaking the law.

In some states and provinces, certain tasks overlap. For example, both nurses and doctors can provide bedside care for the sick and, in Canada, both doctors and pharmacists can prepare medicines.

In many states, a nurse who prescribes a drug is

Court cases: The liabilities of administering drugs

Unfortunately, lawsuits involving nurses' drug errors are common. They may involve violations of state practice acts as well as errors in drug administration.

The court determines liability based on the standards of care required of nurses when administering drugs. In many instances, if the nurse had known more about the proper dose, administration route, or procedure connected with giving the drug, she might have avoided the mistake that resulted in the lawsuit.

Practice act violations

In *Stefanik v. Nursing Education Committee* (1944), a Rhode Island nurse lost her nursing license in part because she'd been practicing medicine illegally: she'd changed a doctor's drug order for a patient because she didn't agree with what had been prescribed. No one claimed she had harmed the patient. But to change a prescription is the same as writing a new prescription, and Rhode Island's nurse practice act didn't consider that part of nursing practice.

Randal v. California State Board of Pharmacy (1966) involved a state's nursing, medical, and pharmacy practice act as well as its drug-control laws. In that case, a pharmacist lost his license to practice partly because he'd taken telephone orders for controlled substances (amphetamines) from a nurse. The law in his state clearly treats telephone orders as prescriptions and, as such, requires that they be taken only from a doctor.

Drug choice errors

In *Derrick v. Portland Eye, Ear, Nose and Throat Hospital* (1922), an Oregon nurse gave a young boy a pupil-contracting drug when the doctor had ordered a pupil-dilating drug. As a result, the boy lost his sight in one eye, and the nurse and the hospital were found negligent.

A diagnostic drug can also prompt a lawsuit. In a 1967 case in Tennessee, *Gault v. Poor Sisters of St. Francis Seraph of Perpetual Adoration, Inc.*, a nurse was supposed to give a patient a saltwater gastric lavage in preparation for a gastric

Court cases: The liabilities of administering drugs *(continued)*

cytology test. Instead, she gave the patient dilute sodium hydroxide, causing severe internal injuries. The hospital lost the verdict and also an appeal.

Dosage and administration errors

Getting the dose right is also important. In a Louisiana case, *Norton v. Argonaut Insurance Co.* (1962), a nurse inadvertently gave a 3-month-old infant a digoxin overdose that resulted in the infant's death. At the malpractice trial that followed, the nurse was found liable, along with the hospital and the attending doctor.

Similarly, in *Dessauer v. Memorial General Hospital,* a 1981 New Mexico case, an emergency department doctor ordered 50 mg of lidocaine for a patient. But the nurse, who normally worked in the hospital's obstetrics ward, gave the patient 800 mg. The patient died, the family sued, and the hospital was found liable.

In *Moore v. Guthrie Hospital,* a 1968 West Virginia case, a nurse made a mistake in the administration route, giving the patient two drugs I.V. rather than I.M. The patient suffered a seizure, sued, and won.

When reviewing these cases, one point becomes clear: The courts will not permit carelessness that harms the patient.

practicing medicine without a license. If she goes into the pharmacy or drug supply cabinet, measures out doses of a drug, and puts the powder into capsules, she's practicing pharmacy without a license.

For either action, she can be prosecuted or lose her license, even if no harm results. In most states and provinces, practicing a licensed profession without a license is, at the very least, a misdemeanor. (See *Court cases: The liabilities of administering drugs.*) ■

RECOGNIZING YOUR ROLE IN DRUG CONTROL

Knowing about drugs you administer

Specifically, the law expects you to:
- know a drug's safe dosage limits, toxicity, potential side effects, and indications and contraindications for use
- refuse to accept an illegible, confusing, or otherwise unclear drug order
- seek clarification of a confusing order from the doctor and not to try to interpret it yourself
- know what the appropriate observation intervals are for a patient receiving any type of medication. Increasingly, judges and juries expect you to know this even if the doctor doesn't know or if he doesn't write an order stating how often to check on the newly medicated patient.

Consider *Brown v. State*, a 1977 New York case. After a patient was given 200 mg of chlorpromazine, the nurses on duty left him largely unobserved for several hours. When someone finally checked on the patient, he was found dead. The hospital and the nurses lost the resulting lawsuit. ■

Meeting JCAHO requirements

Your responsibilities include understanding and meeting standards established by the Joint Commission on Accreditation of Healthcare Organizations (JCAHO). To meet JCAHO standards, a hospital must have a drug side effect reporting program in place. The hospital's pharmacy and therapeutics committee is required to review "all significant untoward drug reactions" to ensure quality patient care. What constitutes a "significant" reaction? According to the JCAHO, it's one in which:
- the drug suspected of causing the reaction must be discontinued
- the patient requires treatment with another drug, such as an antihistamine, a steroid, or epinephrine
- the patient's hospital stay is prolonged—for example, because surgery had to be delayed or more diagnostic tests had to be done.

Importance of a reporting program

The quality of care improves when you know which patients are at higher risk for drug side effects and which drugs are most likely to cause these reactions. You'll be more alert for the early signs and symptoms of problems, and you'll be prepared to intervene before things get out of hand.

The hospital will save money because the lengthy stays and extra treatments associated with drug side effects will be decreased.

Reducing drug-induced injuries will decrease the number of malpractice lawsuits brought against the hospital and staff. That saves money, time, and aggravation. ■

Reporting serious drug reactions to the FDA

The law requires drug manufacturers to monitor drug side effects and report them to the FDA. The FDA also wants to hear from you when your patients experience serious reactions associated with drugs, especially drugs that have been on the market for 3 years or less.

After all, you and your colleagues are the ones most likely to see the reactions, so you can give the best clinical descriptions. But unlike the manufacturers, you aren't required by law to make a report.

What constitutes a serious reaction?

According to the FDA, it's one that:

- is life-threatening.
- causes death.
- leads to or prolongs hospitalization.
- results in permanent or severe disability.

You can submit a report to the FDA even when you aren't sure whether your patient's reaction was serious or when you suspect, but don't know for certain, that a drug caused the reaction.

Some 60,000 reports on side effects are collected annually; more than 400,000 are currently in the FDA's data base. This translates into improved patient safety because the more reports submitted, the more information the FDA will have. The agency can then alert health care professionals to these problems.

Failure to produce a therapeutic response

The FDA also wants to know about drugs that don't produce a therapeutic response. It doesn't need to hear about inappropriate drug use, prescriber errors, or administration errors. (But the United States Pharmacopeia does want to know about medication errors—especially those caused by sound-alike or look-alike drug names. See your hospital pharmacist for more information.)

How to file a report

When submitting a report to the FDA, use the MEDWATCH Form, which should be available in your pharmacy. When you fill it out, be as complete as possible. You don't have to include the patient's name or initials, but you should be able to identify the patient if the FDA requests follow-up information. ■

AVOIDING CHARTING LIABILITY

Charting complete drug information

For each medication you administer, you must document:

- the date and time of administration, name of the medication, dose, administration route and method, frequency, and your initials.
- the sites for all parenteral injections.
- your reasons for withholding a medication. If you can't reach the doctor, chart your attempts to call him and your reasons for withholding a medication.

Other critical details

If the doctor orders a medication or dose you feel is inappropriate, notify him and discuss why you're questioning the order. In your progress notes, document when you notified the doctor, what you told him, and how he responded (including any new orders he gave you).

If someone else gives the medication, make sure that this person's name and the time of administration are charted—for example, "1400 hours: Patient states that his pain was relieved after meperidine injection given by M. Medford at 1245 hours. T. Davis, RN."

Also document your evaluation of the patient's condition before and after the medication was given. ■

Charting emergencies

When charting an emergency, take care to:

- be factual
- be specific about times and interventions
- include the name of the doctor you notified, when you notified him, and what you told him
- indicate attempts to inform the patient's loved ones of his changed condition.

(See *Using a code record.*) ■

Using a code record

Use a code record to keep the progress note concise and ensure complete documentation. This special form incorporates detailed information about a code, including observations, interventions, and medications administered. The following sample shows the typical features of a code record.

CODE RECORD

Name	Body weight	Date
Sophie Harris	*178 lb*	*1/23/96*

Vital signs				**Bolus meds**					**Infused meds**			**Action**			**Blood gases**			
Time (a.m.)/p.m.	**BP**	**Heart rate**	**Heart rhythm**	**Atropine (mg)**	**Calcium chloride (ampules)**	**Epinephrine (mg)**	**Lidocaine (mg)**	**Procainamide (mg)**	**Dopamine (mg/ml)**	**Isoproterenol (mg/ml)**	**Lidocaine (g/ml)**	**Defibrillation (joules)**	**CPR**	**Airway**	**PaO_2**	**$PaCO_2$**	**HCO_3^-**	**pH**
9:20	0	0											✓	mask				
9:25	0	0	VT									200						
9:25			↓										✓					
9:26			VF									300						
9:27			│									360						
9:28			│			1	100						✓	ETT				
9:30			│									360						
9:31			│										✓					
9:31			↓								2mg	360						
9:32	90/62	94	NSR															
9:33	100/68	92	NSR															
9:35	112/64	90	↓												62	43	24	7.35

(continued)

Using a code record *(continued)*

CODE RECORD

Time	Actions
9:20	Code called, CPR initiated by N. Kanis, RN and J. Humus, RN. Ambu-bagged by J. Humus, RN
9:25	Connected to single-channel ECG, #20 Jelco inserted via Ⓛ antecubital by S. Pitts, RN.
9:28	Intubation with #9 oral ETT by M. Cirrus, anesthesiologist.
9:35	Converted to NSR, ABG via Ⓡ femoral artery drawn by L. Sennis, MD. Pressure applied x 5 min. Pt. remains unresponsive.

Time code called
9:20 p.m.

☐ Arrest witnessed
☒ Arrest unwitnessed
☒ Intubation 9:29
☒ Arrhythmia pulseless V tach
☒ Informed family
☒ Informed attending doctor M. Regis, MD

Disposition

☐ SICU
☐ MICU
☒ CCU
☐ OR
☐ Morgue
☐ Other

Status after resuscitation

BP 112/64 Heart rate 90. Bagged with 100% O_2 and transported to CCU.

Critical care nurse
Nancy Kanis, RN

Code chief
L. Sennis, MD

Charting drug errors

If you make an error in giving a drug, or if your patient reacts negatively to a properly administered drug, thorough documentation becomes even more crucial. Besides the usual drug-charting information, include information on the patient's reaction and any medical or nursing interventions taken.

When charting an incident that involves inappropriate drug administration, clearly document the facts of the situation without defending an action or placing blame. Identify what happened, the names and functions of all personnel involved, and what actions were taken to protect the patient after the error was discovered. Remember that lawyers usually have access to incident reports. ■

STEERING CLEAR OF I.V. THERAPY PITFALLS

Reviewing state and institutional standards

State laws differ concerning the practice of I.V. therapy by nurses. Some states have no specific rulings; others include policy statements in nursing practice acts or issue joint statements with state medical societies, hospital associations, and other health agencies.

No state prohibits nurses from performing I.V. therapy, but a few states specify limits. In addition, many states have specific statements regarding I.V. therapy functions performed by licensed practical nurses. For example, some facilities allow licensed practical nurses to start I.V. lines and to deliver I.V. drugs.

Increasing numbers of institutions and agencies are establishing standards of practice for I.V. therapy — detailed nursing actions based on policy. These are used as criteria for safe, competent I.V. therapy and help guarantee high-quality nursing care. For example, the Intravenous Nurses' Society's standards of practice are applied by many hospitals when formulating I.V. therapy policies and procedures. The Centers for Disease Control and Prevention also serves as a source for I.V. therapy practice recommendations. ■

Reviewing facility policies

The health care facility has the ultimate responsibility to ensure that nurses perform I.V. procedures knowledgeably and safely. A facility's written policies should cover all aspects of I.V. therapy.

Policies that vary most markedly among facilities are those involving I.V. drugs that the nurse may administer. Some facilities allow the nurse to administer any I.V. drug; others place restrictions on narcotics, antineoplastics, and emergency drugs. Before administering any I.V. drug, be sure to know the dose and effect, administration rate, incompatibilities, side effects, interactions, and contraindications.

Facility policies require nurses to fully document administration of I.V. drugs and I.V. therapy procedures. I.V. drugs are generally recorded on a preprinted medications administration record, which lists all drugs a patient receives. ■

REVIEWING YOUR LEGAL RISKS ON THE JOB

Questioning a drug order

If you question a drug order, follow your facility's policies. Usually, they'll tell you to try each of the following actions until you receive a satisfactory answer:

- Look up the answer in a reliable drug reference.
- Ask your charge nurse.
- Ask the pharmacist.
- Ask your nursing supervisor or the prescribing doctor.
- Ask the chief nursing administrator if she hasn't already become involved.
- Ask the prescribing doctor's supervisor (service chief).
- Get in touch with the hospital administration and explain your problem. ■

Using a fax machine to order medication

Although confidentiality is an issue when a fax machine is used to order medication, this device is being used more and more because it saves time and reduces errors.

Less nursing and pharmacy time

To order medication using a fax machine, a secretary or assistant takes the doctor's order, puts it into the fax machine, and transmits the order to the pharmacy. Neither the nurse nor the pharmacist is tied up unnecessarily. This process also gives the pharmacist a copy of the original order.

Furthermore, the time an order was sent and the health care facility from which it came are automatically printed by the receiver's fax machine. If a patient's identifying information is missing or unclear, the pharmacist can immediately call the right nursing unit to get the information he needs.

Less turnaround time

Orders can easily be filled on the same day, usually within 3 or 4 hours. In a hospital that doesn't use computers, orders can be faxed from the nursing unit to the pharmacy. With a fax machine, a nurse no longer has to call for someone to come to the unit, pick up the order, and take it to the pharmacy.

If an order can't be filled for some reason, the pharmacist can notify the doctor directly for clarification or a new order.

Fewer errors

Before the pharmacist dispenses a drug, he and the nurse can interpret the doctor's order. With the fax system, they can prevent errors by checking each other's work and talking with the doctor about unresolved problems. Using a fax machine also eliminates confusion over sound-alike drug names and dosages that may be misunderstood if they're given over the telephone. ■

Signing a prescription for a doctor

Never honor a doctor's request to write a prescription and sign his name. Doing so is considered by law as prescribing drugs, which is a medical practice. Of course, many states do allow nurse practitioners to write prescriptions, but they sign their own name, not the doctor's name.

If a doctor ever asks you to write a prescription and sign his name, try one of these legal alternatives:

- If your hospital's policy allows, take a verbal or telephone order for medication from the doctor, who would then have to countersign it later.
- An even safer method is to ask the doctor to have stand-

ing orders typed up for his signature. Then you can distribute the orders to his patients. Some hospitals have used this practice with discharge orders for years. Not only is this system efficient, but it can also save you from charges of practicing beyond the scope of your license. ■

Handling drug orders from nonphysicians

If a nurse practitioner or a physician's assistant writes medication orders in your hospital, are you legally bound to obey them?

In some states, nurse practitioners and physician's assistants are allowed to write medication orders. But before you comply with such an order, protect yourself from liability by taking several measures.

Review your nurse practice act

Order a copy of your nurse practice act from your state board of nursing to see what a nurse is permitted to do in your state. In most states, a physician's assistant must be directly supervised by a doctor in all of his duties, including writing medication orders.

Also, many states prohibit nurses from following a physician's assistant's order if it isn't authorized by the supervising doctor. The functions of physician's assistants are described in the state's medical practice act.

Check your hospital's policy

Practices at your hospital may not conform to your state's nurse practice act. If hospital policy says you can't take orders directly from nurse practitioners or physician's assistants, refuse to follow any such order until the attending doctor countersigns it.

If your patient's situation is life-threatening, don't wait for the attending doctor's signature. But even then, you could be liable for practicing outside the scope of your nurse practice act or for violating hospital policy.

Notify the supervising doctor

No matter what your state law or hospital policy, if you question a nurse practitioner's or physician's assistant's actions, notify the supervising doctor before carrying out the order. If state law permits autonomous nurse practitioner practice and doesn't require a supervising doctor, then you should follow the procedure for questioning a doctor's medication order.

Consult others
Discuss your concerns with your nurse-manager, director of nursing, or hospital administrator.

Get involved
Ask for assignment to your hospital's policy and procedure committee. Then help make sure that hospital policy conforms with your state's nurse practice act—and work to change the policy if it doesn't.

Become involved in your state nursing association so you can have some say about whose orders you should follow. ■

Avoiding drug dispensing

Dispensing refers to selecting a medication, then labeling or packaging it and giving it to someone else to administer. Administering refers to giving a single dose of a prescribed medication to a patient. A nurse who dispenses drugs can be charged with practicing pharmacy without a license.

Typically, state laws allow nurses to administer drugs and pharmacists to dispense them. One exception may be when a patient needs a medication that isn't stocked on your unit and a pharmacist isn't on duty. Then you're probably practicing legally if you take a single dose from the hospital pharmacy and give it to your patient yourself. That's administering, not dispensing.

How to escape liability
Follow these guidelines to avoid dispensing drugs:
- Never take a container of medication from the pharmacy after hours for use on a unit.
- Never refill an empty container.

Rarely, a nurse may have to administer a drug that isn't available on the unit. If she's working on the night or weekend shift and no pharmacist is available, she may have to dispense the drug herself. However, if a lawsuit results, the nurse can't escape liability.

Special situations
Some hospitals and nursing homes have written policies that permit a nurse under special circumstances to go into the pharmacy and dispense an emergency drug dose. In the emergency department (ED), doctors frequently write emergency orders for one to three doses, just enough to give the patient until he can go to the pharmacy himself and have his prescription filled. If no pharmacist is on duty to fill the emergency order, hospi-

tal policy may allow the nurse to obtain, package, and label the required drug.

Regardless of whether the facility has such a policy, a nurse who dispenses drugs is doing so unlawfully unless her state's pharmacy practice act specifically authorizes her actions. If she makes an error in dispensing the drug and the patient later sues, the fact that she was practicing as an unlicensed pharmacist can be used as evidence against her.

When ethics and law conflict

If you need to dispense an emergency drug dose, you may choose to disregard the laws that govern your practice for the benefit of your patient's well-being. But you do so at your own risk. And even if you don't harm your patient, you can still be prosecuted and perhaps lose your license.

When ethics and the law conflict, and you have to weigh concern for your patient's life or health against concern for your license, you must make up your own mind about what action to take.

When policies conflict

If your hospital's policy requires you to dispense emergency medications and is in clear violation of your state's nurse practice act, consider taking steps to have your hospital's policy changed. Start by approaching your nurse-manager with a copy of the nurse practice act and relevant hospital policies. Point out the inconsistencies and the professional risk nurses in the ED are taking. Then offer to accompany your nurse-manager when she approaches nursing administrators and the policy and procedure committee.

Hospital administrators may designate an ED pharmacist, hire additional pharmacy staff, or prevail upon pharmacists on staff to take greater responsibility for distribution of ED medications. ■

Refusing to administer a drug

All nurses have the legal right not to administer drugs they think will harm patients. You may choose to exercise this right in a variety of situations:

- when you think the dosage prescribed is too high.
- when you think the drug is contraindicated because of possible dangerous interactions with other drugs or with substances such as alcohol.
- because you think the patient's physical condition

contraindicates using the drug.

In limited circumstances, you may also legally refuse to administer a drug on grounds of conscience. Some states and Canadian provinces have enacted right-of-conscience laws. These laws excuse medical personnel from the requirement to participate in any abortion or sterilization procedure. Under such right-of-conscience laws, you may, for example, refuse to give any drug you believe is intended to induce abortion.

Steps to take

When you refuse to carry out a drug order, be sure you do the following:

- Notify your immediate supervisor so she can make alternative arrangements (assigning a new nurse or clarifying the order).
- Notify the prescribing doctor if your supervisor hasn't done so already.
- If your employer requires it, document that the drug wasn't given and explain why. ■

Coping with drug and alcohol abusers

A patient who abuses drugs or alcohol presents a liability to you and to the facility. If he harms himself or someone else, you may be held legally responsible for his actions. The guidelines for handling drug and alcohol abusers vary, so you should be familiar with the rules of your facility.

Your facility may require that you confiscate drugs or alcohol from the patient and that you take further steps to prevent the patient from obtaining more.

Institutional policy

If you think a patient is taking drugs but have no proof, a drug search may become necessary.

If you believe that a patient poses a threat to himself or to others, and you can document this, check your facility's policy regarding such searches. Usually, the nurse is advised not to search a patient's room and belongings, even if she believes that the patient may harm himself or others.

Most facilities have written policies that allow for such searches by security personnel (either hospital or city police) and a designated person, such as the risk manager or the nursing supervisor. This policy ensures that the patient's rights are protected and avoids placing the facility at risk for potential liability.

What can be searched

A facility's policy generally spells out what can and cannot be searched. Typically, the search includes the patient's room and his belongings, and requires confiscating illegal drugs. Alcohol should also be confiscated and returned to the patient when he is discharged from the facility.

Document the search in your notes and file an incident report. Also inform the patient's doctor. ■

Managing a patient who won't take medication

In the last few years, many medical experts, legislators, and lawyers have debated this issue. As a result, some state laws now affirm the patient's right to refuse "excessive or unnecessary" medications. However, they don't define "excessive" or "unnecessary."

You may administer medication against a patient's will if he's in danger of harming himself or others. But if he isn't, forcing drugs on a patient probably violates his rights. He'd probably be successful if he filed assault and battery charges against you.

Patient advocacy

Some patients, such as those on psychiatric units, may be so severely impaired that they can't seek counsel to protect their rights. If that's the case, you and other nurses on the unit need to be their advocates. When you believe a patient is being excessively or unnecessarily medicated, discuss the situation with other members of the health care team, including the unit manager. ■

Delegating drug administration

When units are understaffed, nurses run the risk of delegating medication administration and other tasks to subordinates who aren't qualified to perform them. This can lead to negligence lawsuits if a patient is harmed.

You're responsible for delegating medication administration only to qualified nurses. So when you delegate, make sure that the person is permitted to administer medications under your state law and hospital policy and that she's competent to do so. If she's not, you could be legally liable.

Tips for delegating medication administration safely

Here are some suggestions for avoiding liability when delegating medication administration:

- After you've delegated the task, make sure that the drug was actually given. If it wasn't, and the patient is harmed, both you and the nurse you delegated could be held liable.
- Ask your nurse-manager for periodic updating and posting of the skills and judgments nurses need for all types of medication administration.
- Ask for posted lists of who can administer medications together with reminders of related hospital policies and procedures. This list may one day help you defend a charge of negligent delegation if the name of a nurse you've delegated is on it.

Drug administration by non-critical care nurses

Imagine if you assigned I.V. lidocaine administration to a pediatric nurse unfamiliar with cardiac care unit routine. You could both be liable for negligence, especially if she administered the medication improperly and injured the patient. Also, some hospitals don't allow non–critical care nurses to administer I.V. medications.

Drug administration by LPNs and LVNs

Or suppose you asked a licensed practical nurse (LPN) to administer medications, and your state law doesn't authorize LPNs to do so. The LPN could be charged with practicing outside the scope of her nurse practice act, and you and your employer could be charged with aiding and abetting that unauthorized practice. (See *Tips for delegating medication administration safely.*)

Some states' nurse practice acts specifically permit LPNs and licensed vocational nurses (LVNs) with the appropriate educational background or on-the-job training to give drugs under the supervision of a registered nurse (RN), a doctor, or a dentist. Other nurse practice acts specify delegation of tasks to qualified practitioners after they've completed educational requirements or verified their competency to perform skills.

What constitutes appropriate training or educational background? Most courts probably would be satisfied if an LPN or LVN could prove that her supervising RN or doctor had watched her administer drugs and judged her skills to be competent.

Courts look at what a reasonable practitioner would deem necessary to ensure competency, such as correctly answering questions about the procedure or task and performing the procedure or task under supervision correctly three times. In most states, LPNs and LVNs administer all forms of medications. ■

CHAPTER 3

PREVENTING MEDICATION ERRORS

OBSERVING THE RIGHTS OF MEDICATION ADMINISTRATION

Choosing the right drug

Before you administer any medication, always compare the doctor's order with the order on the patient's medication administration record (MAR). Then mentally check off the "five rights": the right drug, right dose, right patient, right route, and right time. In addition to ensuring that the patient receives the medication properly, using this technique guards against liability.

Today, you must not only know about many drugs, you must also perform many procedures on different patients within a relatively short time span. What's more, many drug names sound similar (for example, digoxin, digitoxin, and Desoxyn) and look alike. These factors increase the risk of mistaking one drug for another.

Check drug name and spelling

To prevent errors, take your time, and check the name and spelling of every drug you're going to administer against the patient's MAR. Even unit-dose items should be checked against the MAR. Then, for every drug, check the drug name:

- when removing the drug from the drawer or the shelf
- when unwrapping and pouring the drug
- just before giving the drug to the patient.

Consult others and double-check

If you have a question about a drug, ask the pharmacist or doctor, or consult one of your colleagues. If a drug order is not clearly written, notify the doctor who wrote it.

If a patient tells you, "I never received a pink pill before," recheck the order. The order may have been transcribed onto the wrong MAR. Or you may have to explain that the drug or dosage was changed.

If a drug that appears in the MAR is not in the patient's drawer, recheck the original order. The order may have been transcribed into the wrong MAR.

If the container label is blurred or the instructions are unclear, consult the pharmacist, your colleagues, or the attending doctor. ■

Giving the right dose

Many problems associated with drug dosage have been

alleviated by unit-dose packaging and the commercial availability of a variety of prepared doses. Even so, problems still exist. Now, an even greater chance of error exists when a nurse must calculate a drug dosage because doing so is no longer common.

Calculate the dose

To avoid drug dosage errors resulting from incorrect drug calculations, develop this standard practice:

- First mentally calculate the approximate dose.
- Then calculate the actual dose in writing, using the correct formulas.
- Recheck all calculations with another nurse or the pharmacist when possible.

Many hospitals require double checks of dosage calculations for children's medications and for drugs with narrow safety margins, such as heparin and insulin. Rechecking dosage calculations is even more important than usual when you're in a hurry. Always check the dosages of drugs used during a cardiac arrest before you administer them.

Be alert for errors

Whenever your calculations call for more than one or two dosage units or for a very small percentage of the dosage unit, suspect a dosage error. Call the pharmacist and explain your problem.

Remember that anyone can easily misplace a decimal point, making a safe dose of 0.25 mg become a lethal dose of 2.5 mg. Be especially careful when you're administering drugs, such as antineoplastic agents, which have a narrow margin between a therapeutic and a lethal dose.

Also trust your instincts. If a dose seems especially high or low, it may be incorrect. Check a reliable drug source and then ask the doctor to clarify the order. ■

Identifying the right patient

This may seem a simple error to avoid, but that isn't always the case. For example, patients may have the same or similar surnames. They may be physically unable to state their name. Confused patients may get into another patient's bed, making bed labels an unreliable means of identification.

Check the ID band

The most reliable way to identify a patient is to read his identification (ID) band. Using it avoids confusion with similar sounding names and spelling variations of the same name. Check the patient's ID band every time you administer a drug. If you're unfamiliar with the patient, ask him to tell you his name after you check his ID band. If you have any doubt of the patient's answer, ask a nurse who knows the patient to confirm his identity. ■

Choosing the right time

By administering all drugs at evenly spaced intervals and at consistent times each day, you can prevent errors and accommodate the patient's daily schedule. Routine administration schedules also help the patient develop the habit of taking the drug at a regular time. As a result, the patient is less likely to forget the drug after returning home.

Check facility policy

Most facilities establish routine times for drug administration. Usually these times are found in the facility's drug policy manual. If the facility where you work doesn't have such a manual, suggest that an interdepartmental committee of representatives from nursing, medicine, and pharmacy formulate one. Every nursing unit should have a copy of this manual so that questions about drug administration times can be answered quickly and authoritatively on all three shifts.

Check other requirements

- When administering a drug for which a consistent blood level must be maintained to achieve a therapeutic effect, you must maintain consistent blood levels around the clock.
- You may also have to measure a patient's response to a therapy before administering another dose. For instance, you should check the patient's apical rate before giving digoxin, and assess his respiratory rate before giving a drug such as morphine.
- For a drug with no special requirements, you may schedule the divided doses over the patient's waking hours. Scheduling the patient's daily dose helps prevent side effects, which might be caused by a too-high concentration of the drug in the bloodstream at any given time. Sometimes, you must consider other events, such as mealtime, when administering a drug.

Avoid busy hours

Avoid scheduling drug administration at busy hours on the nursing unit, such as during a shift change. Instead of scheduling twice daily medications for 8 a.m. and 6 p.m., schedule them for 9 a.m. and 7 p.m. to avoid the busy hour after the shift change. Always follow the standard practice, and allow a half hour before and after the designated time for drug administration. In many facilities, drugs given beyond these time limits are considered errors. ■

Choosing the right route

The choice of route for drugs is determined by their chemical properties, where the drug is supposed to take effect, and the desired onset of action, among other things.

Pay careful attention to the administration route specified in the medication order and on the product label.

Check the drug's form

Some drugs must be given in certain forms to be appropriate for particular entry routes into the body. For example, never inject a solution anywhere into the body unless the label clearly indicates that the solution is for injection.

Check the dose

The route can also affect the amount of medication given. If given I.M., 10 mg of morphine sulfate, a frequently used adult dose, relieves pain. If the drug is given I.V., the equivalent dose decreases to 2 to 4 mg. To produce the same effect, an oral dose of morphine needs to be greater than 10 mg.

Check drug absorption

The procedure used to administer a drug also may affect the rate of drug absorption into the bloodstream. Some topical ointments, such as nitroglycerin paste, enter the bloodstream more rapidly and completely when spread over a large surface area and covered with plastic wrap or special paper supplied with the medication.

On the other hand, crushing enteric-coated tablets or opening sustained-release capsules and dissolving the drug in liquid will result in improper absorption of the drug into the bloodstream and, possibly, unintended effects. The patient should swallow sufficient water when he takes an oral tablet or capsule. If he doesn't, the medication may lodge in his esophagus and cause esophageal lesions. ■

GIVING DRUGS SAFELY

Taking a complete drug history

You should know all the drugs your patient is taking,

including nonprescription products. Ask the patient if he's taking any drugs prescribed by dentists and psychiatrists. Ask about alcohol intake and smoking habits too.

Note on the patient's chart if he has any allergies. Assess your patient's reactions to drugs you have administered. Any drug may cause an unpredictable reaction. Keep in mind that whenever two or more drugs are given together, their combination can enhance or diminish a drug's effect or absorption. ■

Storing and handling drugs properly

Handle and store drugs carefully to maintain their stability and strength. Temperature, air, moisture, and light may affect a drug's stability, so remember to follow drug-specific precautions such as refrigerating drugs that require cool temperatures. Keep drugs in the containers in which the pharmacy dispensed them. Cap bottles tightly and store them away from heat, light, and moisture. Most drugs are stored at room temperature, but always refrigerate drugs that require cool temperatures.

Keep in mind the following precautions:

- Always note a drug's expiration date, the date after which the original potency of the drug is believed to change. Never administer an outdated drug or one that looks or smells unusual.
- Don't administer a drug if it looks as though the manufacturer's packaging has been tampered with. Return these drugs to the pharmacy.
- After reconstituting drugs, label any unused medication with the date, time, strength, and your initials. Discard any drug that will remain stable for only a short time and will reach its expiration date before another dose is scheduled. Never administer a drug that hasn't been labeled properly after reconstitution.
- Don't give a drug from a poorly labeled or an unlabeled container. Don't attempt to label or reinforce drug labels yourself. This should be done by a pharmacist.
- Never allow your medication cart or tray out of your sight.
- Never return unwrapped or prepared drugs to stock containers. Instead, dispose of them, and notify the pharmacy. ■

Providing careful monitoring

- Make sure you have a written order for every drug given. Verbal orders should be signed by the doctor within the facility's specified time period.
- Don't open a unit-dose drug until you're at the patient's bedside. It's easy to lose or inadvertently discard the unit dose wrapper and thus the label that identifies the dose.
- Read all drugs labels three times, including once just before you administer the drug.
- Administer only the drugs that you or the pharmacist prepared. Never administer drugs prepared by another nurse.
- Stay with the patient until he takes the drug. This way you can ensure that the right patient took the drug properly.
- Never leave drug doses at the patient's bedside unless you have a specific order to do so. If you have such an order, the drug should be labeled with the patient's name, the drug's name and dose, and instructions. You're still responsible for supervising the patient whose medications are left at the bedside. ■

Documenting drug administration accurately

Accurate documentation is essential for proper patient care and for your own protection. In the patient's medication administration record, include:

- the name of the drug
- the date and time you gave it to the patient
- the dose, site, and route
- the patient's reaction to the drug
- what steps you took if the patient experienced side effects of the drug.

Also note when and why you withheld a drug, or if you discontinued administration. Remember to chart all drugs immediately after you administer them. ■

Providing thorough patient teaching

The time you invest in educating a patient usually pays off. Stress to the patient and his family the importance of taking both prescribed and nonprescription medications as directed. Explain the procedure, respond to any questions, and provide privacy.

If the patient asks about his medication or the dosage, check his medication record again. If the medication is correct, reassure him. Make sure you tell him about any changes in his medication or dosage. Instruct him, as appropriate, about possible side effects. Ask him to report anything that he feels may be a side effect. ■

USING CONTROLS AND CHECKPOINTS

Building in redundancies

Hospital policy may require another nurse to check your calculations or a drug you've drawn up. This may seem unnecessary, but it decreases the chances of making an error.

That's also true of the back-and-forth repetition with telephone orders. You may spend more time processing the order, but you're also likely to catch any errors in interpretation.

This system provides maximum protection from errors, as long as you follow it. The possibility of errors increases if you borrow a dose from one patient to give to another, take an item from the unit stock instead of waiting for the pharmacy to deliver it, or otherwise bypass the system.

Use a fax machine

A fax machine also allows for cross-checking. In the past, nurses in nursing homes had to interpret new orders and telephone the pharmacist to order new drugs. This sometimes led to medication errors, especially if the nurse wasn't familiar with a newly marketed drug or a rarely used one that had a name similar to that of an established drug. If she gave the wrong name to the pharmacist, the patient probably received the wrong drug. Now, in nearly all facilities, a form without a carbon must be used, or the nurse must fax the original order to the pharmacy so that she and the pharmacist both can interpret it.

Note product design

Product design can also prevent errors. For example, a blue box on the label of procainamide injection vials from Elkins-Sinn, Inc. once listed only the concentration, 500 mg/ml. But the vials actually contained 2 ml, or 1 g, something many nurses didn't know. The new labels clear up the mystery by including the concentration per milliliter (500 mg/ml) and per container (1 g/ 2 ml). ■

Adding a fail-safe system

A product's fail-safe system can prevent tragic errors. For example, many electronic infusion pumps use an I.V. set with a gravity control clamp that shuts off the flow of the I.V. solution. But not everyone knows that this clamp must be closed before the set is removed from the pump. And even those who do, don't always remember to close the clamp. So patients can be harmed by the accidental free flow of I.V. solution.

Automatic fail-safe system

Many manufacturers of electronic infusion pumps have recognized, or are beginning to recognize, such knowledge and performance deficiencies and produce pumps that use I.V. sets with an automatic fail-safe clamping mechanism. Unfortunately, not all facilities can afford to invest in new pumps (and administrators may not understand the dangers of unprotected devices).

Premixed I.V. drug containers

With a fail-safe system, premixed I.V. drug containers don't require activation, assembly, or preparation to deliver the dose. ■

Eliminating sources of confusion

Patients have suffered permanent brain damage or died when their nurses mistook liter containers of 5% sodium chloride solution for dextrose 5% in normal saline solution or 23.4% sodium chloride solution for normal saline solution.

Some nurses have accidentally picked up a 1- or 2-g prefilled syringe of 1% lidocaine instead of a 100-mg syringe and injected the contents of the larger-dose syringe into a patient, causing cardiac arrest and death. (The 1- and 2-g syringes are no longer available.)

These accidents could have been prevented if items unnecessary for routine patient care had been removed from unit stock. ■

Eliminating unneeded procedures

This concept applies to routine procedures as well.

Unnecessary calculations

Many calculations you may perform are unnecessary. For example, suppose you work in a critical care unit. You don't have to calculate doses in micrograms per kilogram per minute if the concentrations of many critical care drug solutions are standardized, and if charts with flow rates based on the patient's weight and desired dose are already available.

Unneeded I.V. lines

Removing unneeded I.V. lines (and labeling all lines that remain) can reduce the risk of an oral drug's being injected I.V. One patient died when a kaolin and pectin mixture that was supposed to be instilled into his nasogastric tube was attached to his I.V. catheter. Similar errors have involved tube feedings, antacids, and reconstituted psyllium powder. ■

Limiting dangerous drug use

Potassium chloride concentrate for injection is one of the most dangerous drugs on a nursing unit, and it should not be there. It's been used to reconstitute other drugs or flush I.V. catheters when nurses mistook it for look-alike vials of sterile water for injection or normal saline injection.

In another incident, a nurse injected potassium chloride into a bag of I.V. solution that was already hanging, but never removed the bag from the pole to shake it. So the drug pooled in the bag, and her patient inadvertently received a potassium chloride bolus when the I.V. was restarted.

Many hospitals secure dangerous drugs such as potassium chloride. They're available only in premixed I.V. containers through the pharmacy's I.V. admixture service, or through nursing supervisors or other experienced individuals who are permitted to obtain these drugs. ■

Limiting pharmacy access

Facilities that don't have 24-hour pharmacy coverage may not limit access to the pharmacy. Sometimes, a nurse is allowed to enter the pharmacy after hours and obtain the ordered drug (this is illegal in some states). This can be dangerous. The more prudent approach is to provide a well-designed, collaboratively developed night drug supply in a locked storage area or automated dispensing cabinet.

Certification or privileging

Facilities also may use certification or privileging. For example, only specially prepared nurses would give chemotherapy drugs, only anesthesiologists or nurse-anesthetists would administer neuromuscular blocking drugs, and only nurses who have demonstrated the ability to do so properly would take doctors' telephone orders.

Formulary control
Through formulary control, as authorized by the medical staff, your pharmacists can limit the number of doses a patient receives by enforcing automatic stop orders, performing drug use evaluation studies, and promoting drugs with longer dose intervals (for example, antibiotics that are given once a day instead of every 4 hours). The fewer doses, the fewer chances that the wrong drug will be used or that a drug will be prepared improperly or given by the wrong route, and so on. ■

Limiting access to dangerous drugs

Manufacturers could also rethink the way they package dangerous drugs. For example, such drugs should be difficult to open, requiring the nurse to read the instructions or be familiar with the package to figure out how to open it. This would put the drug into the hands of only those nurses who have correctly identified it and know how to administer it. ■

Avoiding confirmation bias

Drugs with similar names or packaging shouldn't be stored next to each other. You might take the wrong one because you tend to see what you're looking for and don't check for other, disconfirming evidence. This is called confirmation bias.

For example, hydromorphone and morphine have similar names. A nurse may only see the syllable "morph" and inadvertently administer hydromorphone instead of morphine.

In another example, potassium chloride concentrate for injection and 0.9% sodium chloride injection are both clear liquids in vials that are the same shape and available in the same volume. In the past, patients died when the two were confused because nurses relied on the shape of the vial or saw only "chloride" on the label. This error has been virtually eliminated because manufacturers of potassium chloride concentrate are now required to use black caps and vial closures imprinted with "must be diluted" in a contrasting color. This differentiates potassium chloride's appearance from 0.9% sodium chloride for injection. ■

Adopting "lock-and-key" design

You can't fit the nozzle of a kerosene fuel hose into the gasoline tank of a car that uses unleaded fuel. The same principle can be applied to prevent medication accidents.

Liquids meant for oral use, for example, shouldn't be drawn into a syringe that fits the luer-lock connection of an I.V. line. Otherwise, sooner or later, someone will try to inject the oral drug. Oral syringes for nonparenteral liquids are already available; needles and I.V. tubing can't be attached to their tips. Special catheter tips on tubing can also prevent enteral fluids from being injected I.V.

Lock-and-key designs could be useful (but don't currently exist) for other lines that are involved in medication errors, such as epidural catheters. The Association for the Advancement of Medical Instrumentation is currently developing standards that would address this issue. ■

Using tactile cues and special packaging

Remember when insulin vials had distinctive shapes: regular insulin in round glass containers, NPH in square ones, and so on? That helped diabetic patients with poor eyesight readily identify their insulin so they wouldn't use the wrong type and inject too much or too little. Unfortunately, this system was discontinued with the advent of U-100 insulin. The Diabetes Division of the National Federation of the Blind is campaigning to reinstate the old system.

Keep tactility in mind when you're trying to improve a safety system. You might place strips of adhesive tape, raised shapes, or special figures on the tops or sides of containers to help patients differentiate one drug from another. Some commercially available drug containers have similar tactile cues.

Unique packaging can help too. Some neuromuscular blockers are now packaged in oddly shaped containers. The container for atracurium, for example, is hexagonal. ■

Using hazard warnings

Manufacturers are starting to label premixed containers on both sides so that the names can be seen from all angles. They're also posting warning labels where they can be clearly seen. To add another layer of safety, auxiliary warning labels can be affixed to particularly troublesome drugs.

Some researchers believe that red is the most vivid warning because it reminds people of blood (although this has never been proved), and that certain words convey greater urgency than others: The word *danger* is preferred to the word *warning,* which is preferred to *caution,* which is preferred to *notice,* which is better than nothing at all. ■

Using alarms

Alarms on the equipment you use already warn of danger. For example, alarm systems on I.V. infusion pumps tell you that an infusion has stopped, that air is in the line, that the solution has infiltrated, and so on. Other alarms signal that someone has gained access to a restricted storage area, that the temperature of a drug storage refrigerator or freezer needs immediate adjustment, or that you've made an error when you were typing on the computer. ■

Using computers and other advances

Computers can play an important role in preventing errors. Computer-generated medication administration records, for example, greatly reduce transcription errors (the nurse and the pharmacist can check each other's interpretation of the order). Errors in interpreting handwritten drug orders are eliminated when doctors enter their orders into the computer.

For pharmacy orders, dispensing errors can be avoided by using computers that automatically screen for drug allergies, interactions, and duplicate or contraindicated drug therapies.

Other advances now being introduced in hospitals such as bar coding, voice, and handwriting-recognition systems, and bedside terminals also can help make dispensing and administering drugs more accurate. ■

Following protocols and procedures

Protocols and procedures can limit the drugs and doses that may be used, establish monitoring parameters, provide treatment guidelines in case of an error, and designate which nurses may administer certain drugs. ■

Reviewing the record

Documenting on the medication administration record helps to prevent errors. That's because you have the chance to check previous therapy, read any notes that apply to a specific patient, and see what occurred the last time the drug was given.

For example, suppose you're about to give warfarin. After checking the pattern of therapy and the patient's prothrombin level, you believe the ordered dose would constitute an overdose. You notify the doctor and learn that he wrote the order on the wrong chart. ■

Taking preventive steps

Education is an important part of preventing medication errors. Knowing your patients, the drugs they're taking, and why they need them is vital. You might chain a drug reference book to your drug cart or store it where you prepare medications.

Many hospitals are now using a computer network that allows easy access to drug information from the nursing unit's computer terminal.

You also must be aware of your facility's protocols and procedures. This is accomplished through orientation and staff-development classes. Copies of the policy and procedure manuals should be available on the nursing unit. ■

Responding to medication errors

Sometimes, medication errors occur. When they do, your goal is to limit the damage. Here are two examples.

Be cautious
Err on the side of caution. Stocking a lower concentration of a drug can prevent serious injury. Suppose the doctor orders morphine, 4 ml/hour with a 2-ml bolus dose through a patient-controlled analgesia pump. (Morphine should be ordered in milligrams, of course.) Prefilled syringe cartridges of morphine come in two concentrations:

1 mg/ml and 5 mg/ml. This pump has a default dose of 1 mg/ml.

What if the 5-mg/ml cartridge is used and you forget to reset the pump? The patient would receive morphine, 20 mg/hour with 10-mg boluses. That's too much for most patients to tolerate.

What if the pump had a default dose of 5 mg/ml instead? If a 1-mg/ml syringe were used, the patient would receive too small a dose. The damage would be limited: He would probably complain of pain, but he wouldn't suffer respiratory depression.

Reduce the amount of drug
Limit the number of capsules, tablets, ampules, or vials, or reduce the volume or amount of drug in a single container. Even if the wrong drug or container were chosen, the total amount that the patient could receive would be limited to a tolerable level.

For example, a few years ago, several patients in a dialysis unit experienced cardiac arrest when they were accidentally injected with 50 ml of lidocaine. They were supposed to receive mannitol, but lidocaine (in 50-ml vials) had been mistakenly stored in the mannitol bin and was administered instead. There is, in fact, no reason for 50-ml vials of lidocaine to be in a dialysis unit. If 5- or 10-ml vials had been available instead, the possibility of a patient's dying from such an error would have been largely eliminated. ■

Acknowledging errors

Making errors is part of human nature. If we accept this, we can work on devising error traps that will prevent some accidents, reduce the possibility that others will occur, and minimize the consequences when they do. ■

READING DRUG LABELS PRECISELY

Checking the drug name and concentration

Before you administer any drug, read the label carefully. Remember, many labels look similar, so be sure to note the drug name and concentration. To ensure accuracy and avoid errors, check the label against the patient's medication administration record (MAR). (See *Differentiating drug labels*, opposite, and *Comparing a drug order with a drug label*, pages 66 and 67.) ■

(Text continues on page 67.)

Differentiating drug labels

The following pairs of look-alikes must be read carefully to avoid errors.

Guaifenesin syrup

These two containers are the same size, but the container on the top has a 5-ml dose of 100 mg, whereas the container on the bottom has a 10-ml dose and contains 200 mg.

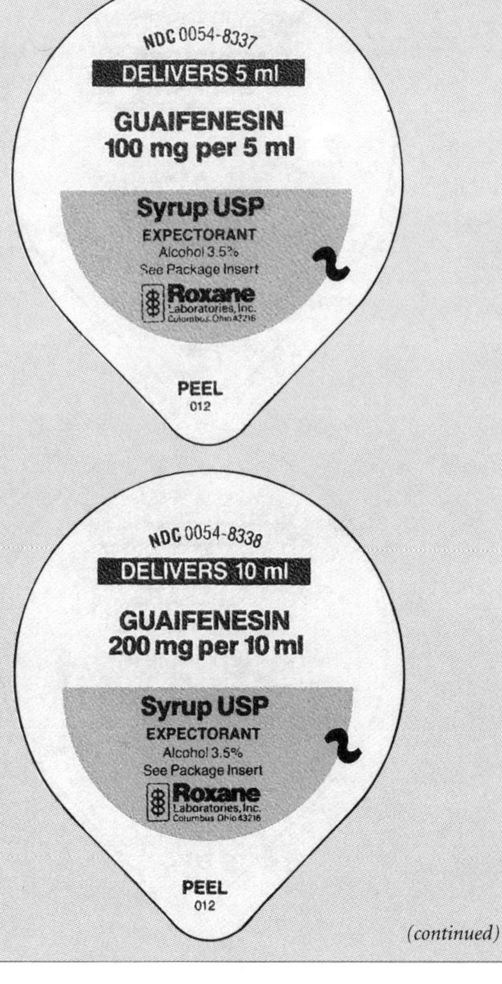

(continued)

Differentiating drug labels *(continued)*

Morphine sulfate oral solution
These two containers are the same size, and they both hold morphine sulfate in a 10-mg/5-ml concentration. Yet the one on the top contains 5 ml and the one on the bottom contains 10 ml.

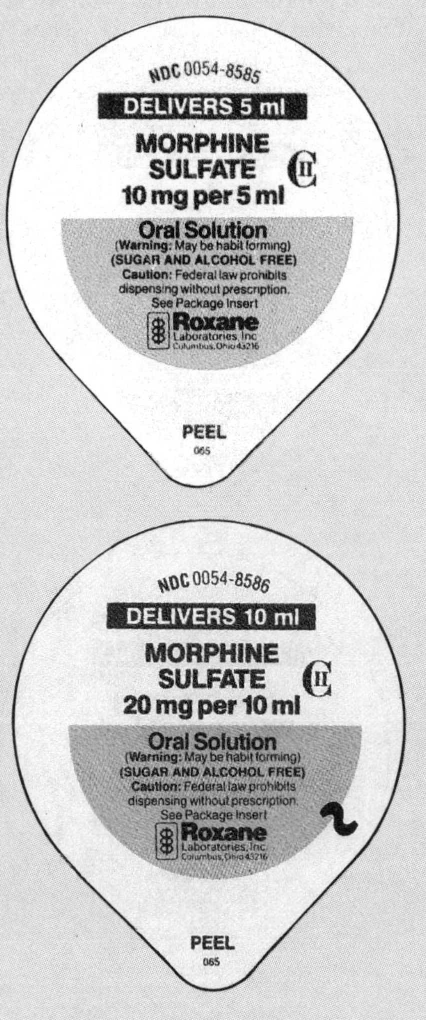

Differentiating drug labels *(continued)*

Thorazine

Although both of these bottles hold 4 oz (118 ml) of thorazine in a solution, they differ in one major way: The drug concentration in the bottle on the top is 10 mg/5 ml (2 mg/1ml); the concentration in the bottle on the bottom is 30 mg/1 ml — 15 times greater than the other bottle. If these bottles were accidentially interchanged, serious consequences could result.

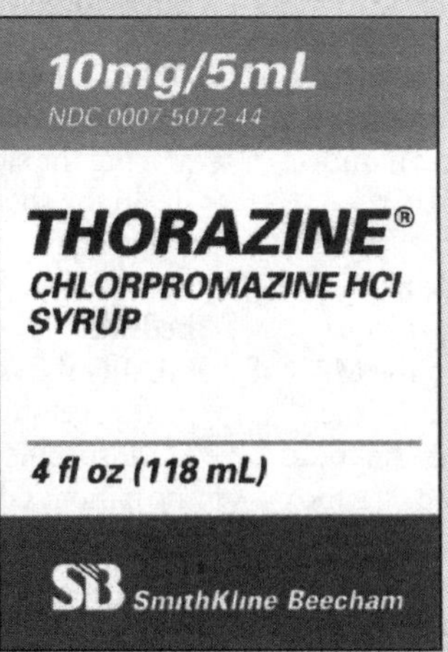

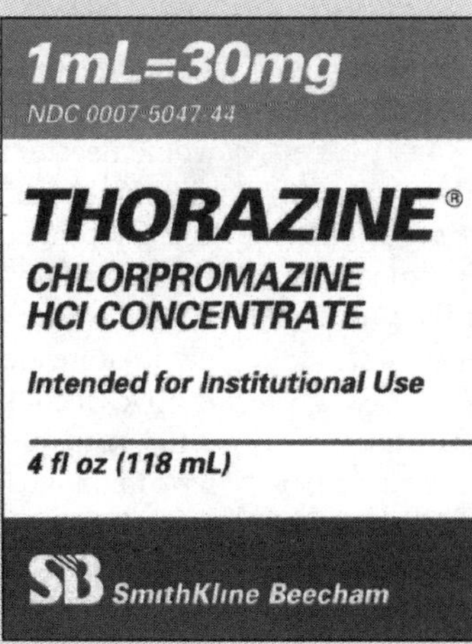

Comparing a drug order with a drug label

Before administering a drug, compare each part of the order on the medication administration record (MAR) with the drug label; hold the label next to the MAR to ensure accuracy.

Compare generic names
Read the drug's generic name on the MAR (digoxin), and compare it with the generic name on the label (digoxin).

Compare trade names
Read the trade (proprietary) name on the MAR, if present (Lanoxin), and compare it with the trade name on the label (Lanoxin).

Compare dosage
Read the dosage specified on the MAR (0.25 mg); and compare it with the dosage on the label (0.25 mg).

Compare routes
Read the route specified on the MAR (P.O.), and note the dosage form on the label (oral tablet).

Special considerations
- Note any special considerations on the MAR. (Hold the dose if the apical rate is less than 56 beats/minute, and notify the house officer.)
- Compare the MAR and drug label *three times* before administering the drug: once when obtaining the drug from floor stock or the patient's supply, a second time before placing the drug in the medication cup or other device, and a third time before either replacing the stock drug bottle on the shelf or removing the drug from the unit-dose packet at the patient's bedside.
- Using the example on the next page, suppose the MAR specified digoxin and the patient's drug packet was labeled only as Lanoxin; you would need to know that Lanoxin is the trade name for the drug digoxin.
- Suppose the drug packet was labeled digitoxin; you would need to recognize that this is a different digitalis glycoside that can't be substituted for digoxin.
- Suppose the generic names were identical, but the packet contained an 0.125-mg tablet; you would have to know that you need two tablets to administer the required dose.

Comparing a drug order with a drug label *(continued)*

MEDICATION ADMINISTRATION RECORD										
DATE ORD.	STOP DATE	MEDICATION DOSE / ROUTE FREQUENCY	R.N. INT.	HR.	DATE 8/8	8/9	8/10	8/11	8/12	8/13
8/8	8/11	digoxin (Lanoxin)	Ry	A10	X			x		d/c
		0.25 mg P.O. T.I.D. x 11 doses		2P	LB				x	p̄
		HOLD DOSE IF APICAL RATE <56/MIN AND NOTIFY HOUSE OFFICER		6P	AP-SO				x	8/11

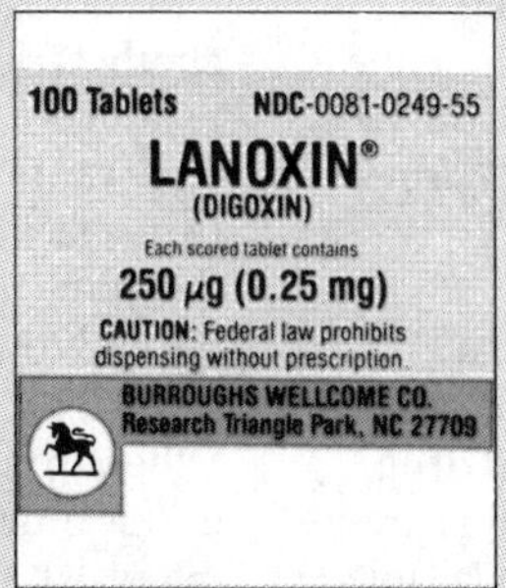

100 Tablets
NDC-0081-0249-55
LANOXIN®
(DIGOXIN)
Each scored tablet contains
250 µg (0.25 mg)
CAUTION: Federal law prohibits dispensing without prescription.
BURROUGHS WELLCOME CO.
Research Triangle Park, NC 27709

READING MEDICATION ORDERS CORRECTLY

Understanding drug orders

You're responsible for ensuring that the proper drug, strength, and dosage are transcribed onto the Kardex or medication administration record (MAR) and given to the patient. To do so, you must know how to read drug orders correctly. This includes interpreting the abbreviations doctors use when they write prescriptions, clarifying unclear or incomplete drug orders, and handling difficult orders.

These three guidelines will help you interpret drug orders:

- The generic name of a drug should appear in lowercase letters only.
- The trade, or brand, name of a drug should begin with a capital letter.
- Drug abbreviations should be avoided but, when used, should appear in all capital letters.

Unclear drug orders

Once you know how to read drug orders, you'll need to learn how to handle unclear orders. For example, many doctors develop their own abbreviations and notations for drug orders; others have illegible handwriting. In either case, you must ask the doctor for clarification. (See *Coping with difficult drug orders.*)

Dosage calculations

You'll also need to know how to handle orders for drug doses in strengths that are not commercially available. For example, phenytoin is available only in 100-mg capsules or vials. If the doctor orders phenytoin 300 mg P.O. or I.V., you'll need to calculate the number of capsules or vials required to provide the correct dose.

Incomplete drug orders

In an outpatient setting, a doctor or other individual licensed to prescribe drugs may write an order on a prescription form and give it directly to the patient. In turn, the patient gives the order to a pharmacist who dispenses the drug to the patient for home use. In a hospital, the prescriber writes the drug order on the doctors' order sheet in the patient's chart. Because this order sheet must include complete patient information, it's usually stamped with the patient's admission data plate.

Each order must include:

- the date and time of the order
- the name of the drug (generic or proprietary)
- the dosage form (in metric, apothecaries', or household measure)
- the route of administration (some facilities' policies state that if the route is not given, the oral route may be assumed)
- the administration schedule (as times per day or hour intervals)
- any restrictions or specifications related to the order
- the doctor's signature (may follow a group of orders)
- the doctor's issued registration number for controlled drugs (if applicable).

If any of this required information is missing, you must question and clarify the order before signing the transcription. A copy of the order is sent to the pharmacy, where the drug is dispensed

Coping with difficult drug orders

The combination of poor handwriting and inappropriate abbreviations on a drug order can lead to confusion and errors. For any drug order that doesn't clearly state the drug's name, amount, route of administration, and timing of administration, you should notify the doctor. The examples below illustrate drug orders that need clarification.

Each doctor has a unique handwriting style and possibly a unique way of writing medication orders. Thus, you bear a great responsibility to ensure that the proper drug, strength, and dosage form is ordered, transcribed onto the Kardex or medication administration record, and given to the patient.

Note the examples that follow.

DATE	TIME	ORDERS	DOCTOR'S SIGNATURE	NURSE'S SIGNATURE
2/14	12³⁰P	[illegible] 25/250 ī po [illegible]		
		[illegible] 1mg PO BID		
		Benadryl 25 mg PO HS		
		ROM [illegible]		
		Soft diet [illegible]		
		[illegible] MD		D Adams RN
1/29		DC [illegible]		
		DC Venogram		
		Keflin 1.0 g IV q 6h		

according to the facility's policy.

Risk of error

To limit the risk of error, make sure that only approved abbreviations are used in the order. The actual times at which the drug is administered depend on the facility's policy (for drugs given a specific number of times per day) and on the drug's nature and onset and duration of action. These actual times are recorded on the MAR; the drug should be administered within ½ hour either before or after the times specified. ■

Interpreting drug orders

The following examples illustrate how to read and interpret a wide range of drug orders.

DRUG ORDER	INTERPRETATION
Colace 100 mg P.O. b.i.d. p.c.	Give 100 mg of Colace by mouth twice a day after meals.
Vistaril 25 mg I.M. q3h p.r.n.	Give 25 mg of Vistaril intramuscularly every 3 hours, as needed.
↑ Duramorph to 6 mg I.V. q8h	Increase Duramorph to 6 mg intravenously every 8 hours.
folic acid 1 mg P.O. daily	Give 1 mg of folic acid by mouth daily.
Minipress 4 mg P.O. q6h, hold for sys BP 120	Give 4 mg of Minipress by mouth every 6 hours; withhold drug if systolic blood pressure falls below 120 mm Hg.
nifedipine 30 mg SL q4h	Give 30 mg of nifedipine sublingually every 4 hours.
Begin ASA 325 mg P.O. daily	Begin giving 325 mg of aspirin by mouth daily.
Begin Dyazide 1 cap P.O. q.a.m.	Begin giving 1 capsule of Dyazide by mouth every morning.
phenytoin 300 mg I.V. STAT	Give 300 mg of phenytoin intravenously immediately.
digoxin 0.25 mg P.O. daily	Give 0.25 mg of digoxin by mouth daily.

Interpreting drug orders *(continued)*

DRUG ORDER	INTERPRETATION
Zyloprim 100 mg P.O. b.i.d.	Give 100 mg of Zyloprim by mouth twice a day.
Benadryl 25-50 mg P.O. h.s. p.r.n. insomnia	Give 25 to 50 mg of Benadryl by mouth at bedtime, as needed, for insomnia.
Alupent inhaler 2 puffs q6h	Give 2 inhalations of Alupent every 6 hours.
Nitrostat 1½ in q.i.d. to chest	Apply 1½ inches of Nitrostat ointment to chest four times a day.
Persantine 75 mg P.O. t.i.d.	Give 75 mg of Persantine by mouth three times a day.
aspirin gr $\overline{\text{v}}$ P.O. t.i.d.	Give 5 grains of aspirin by mouth three times a day.
Vasotec 2.5 mg P.O. daily	Give 2.5 mg of Vasotec by mouth daily.
1,000 ml D_5W I.V. $\bar{c}$ KCl 20 mEq at 100 ml/hour	Give 1,000 ml of dextrose 5% in water with 20 mEq of potassium chloride intravenously at a rate of 100 ml/hour.
D/C PCN I.V., start PCN-G 800,000 U P.O. q6h	Discontinue I.V. penicillin; start 800,000 units of penicillin G by mouth every 6 hours.
diphenhydramine 25-50 mg P.O. h.s. p.r.n.	Give 25 to 50 mg of diphenhydramine by mouth at bedtime, as needed.

Reviewing common pharmacologic abbreviations

To transcribe medication orders and document drug administration accurately, review the following commonly used abbreviations for drug measurements, dosage forms, routes and times of administration, and related terms. Remember that abbreviations often are subject to misinterpretation, especially if written carelessly or quickly. If an abbreviation seems unusual or doesn't make sense to you, given your knowledge of the patient or the drug, always question the order, clarify the terms, and clearly write out the correct term in your revision and transcription.

DRUG AND SOLUTION MEASUREMENTS

cc	cubic centimeter	mEq	milliequivalent
ʒ	dram	mg	milligram
℥	ounce	ml	milliliter
G or GM	gram	Mx	minim
gal	gallon	pt	pint
gr	grain	qt	quart
gtt	drop	$\overline{ss}$	one half
kg	kilogram	Tbs	tablespoon
L	liter	tsp	teaspoon
mcg	microgram	U	unit

DRUG DOSAGE FORMS

cap	capsule	sp	spirits
DS	double-strength	supp	suppository

Reviewing common pharmacologic abbreviations

(continued)

DRUG DOSAGE FORMS *(continued)*			
elix	elixir	susp	suspension
LA	long-acting	syr	syrup
liq	liquid	tab	tablet
S.A.	sustained action	tinct or tr	tincture
S.R.	sustained release	ung or oit	ointment
sol	solution		
ROUTES OF DRUG ADMINISTRATION			
A.D.	right ear	O.S.	left eye
A.S.	left ear	O.D.	right eye
A.U.	each ear	O.U.	each eye
I.M.	intramuscular	P.O. or p.o.	by mouth
I.T.	intrathecal	R. or P.R.	by rectum
I.V.	intravenous	Ⓡ	right
IVPB	intravenous piggyback	Ⓛ	left
NGT	nasogastric tube	S.C. or SQ	subcutaneous
V or P.V.	vaginally	SL or sl	sublingual
		S&S	swish and swallow

(continued)

Reviewing common pharmacologic abbreviations
(continued)

TIMES OF DRUG ADMINISTRATION			
a.c.	before meals	q.h.	every hour
ad lib	as desired	q2h q3h and so on	every 2 hours, every 3 hours
b.i.d.	twice a day	q.i.d.	four times a day
h.s.	at bedtime	q.n.	every night
p.c.	after meals	q.o.d.	every other day
p.r.n.	as needed	STAT	immediately
q.a.m. or Q.M.	every morning	t.i.d.	three times a day
q.d. or Q.D.	every day		
MISCELLANEOUS			
AMA	against medical advice	Rx	treatment, prescription
ASAP	as soon as possible	$\bar{s}$	without
$\bar{c}$	with	TO	telephone order
D/C or dc	discontinue	VO	verbal order
HO	house officer	≈	approximately equal to
KVO	keep vein open	>	greater than
MR	may repeat	<	less than
NKA	no known allergies	↑	increase
N.P.O.	nothing by mouth	↓	decrease

Reviewing abbreviations to avoid

The Joint Commission on Accreditation of Healthcare Organizations requires every health care facility to develop a list of approved abbreviations for staff use. But certain abbreviations should be avoided, if possible, because they're easily misunderstood, especially when handwritten. Here's a list of abbreviations to avoid.

ABBREVIATION	INTENDED MEANING	MISINTERPRETATION	CORRECTION
Apothecaries' symbols			
℥	fluid ounce	Frequently misinterpreted	Use the metric equivalents.
ʒ	fluidram	Frequently misinterpreted	Use the metric equivalents.
♏	minim	Frequently misinterpreted	Use the metric equivalents.
℈	scruple	Frequently misinterpreted	Use the metric equivalents.
Drug names			
MTX	methotrexate	mustargen	Use the complete spelling for drug names.
CPZ	Compazine (prochlorperazine)	chlorpromazine	Use the complete spelling for drug names.
HCl	hydrochloric acid	potassium chloride ("H" is misinterpreted as "K")	Use the complete spelling for drug names.

(continued)

Reviewing abbreviations to avoid *(continued)*

ABBREVIATION	INTENDED MEANING	MISINTERPRETATION	CORRECTION
Drug names *(continued)*			
DIG	digoxin	digitoxin	Use the complete spelling for drug names.
MVI	multivitamins *without* fat-soluble vitamins	multivitamins *with* fat-soluble vitamins	Use the complete spelling for drug names.
HCTZ	hydrochlorothiazide	hydrocortisone (HCT)	Use the complete spelling for drug names.
ara-a	vidarabine	cytarabine (ara-C)	Use the complete spelling for drug names.
Dosage directions			
au	*auris uterque* (each ear)	Frequently misinterpreted as "OU" (*oculus uterque* — each eye)	Write it out.
μg	microgram	Frequently misinterpreted as "mg"	Use "mcg."
OD	once daily	Frequently misinterpreted as "OD" (*oculus dexter* — right eye)	Don't abbreviate "daily." Write it out.

Reviewing abbreviations to avoid *(continued)*

ABBREVIATION	INTENDED MEANING	MISINTERPRETATION	CORRECTION
Dosage directions *(continued)*			
OJ	orange juice	Frequently misinterpreted as "OD" (*oculus dexter* — right eye) or "OS" (*oculus sinister* — left eye). Medications that were meant to be diluted in orange juice and given orally have been given in a patient's right or left eye.	Write it out.
i/d	once daily	Misinterpreted as "t.i.d." (three times daily)	Write it out.
Per os	orally	The "os" is frequently misinterpreted as "OS" (*oculus sinister* — left eye).	Use "P.O." or "by mouth" or "orally."

(continued)

Reviewing abbreviations to avoid *(continued)*

ABBREVIATION	INTENDED MEANING	MISINTERPRETATION	CORRECTION
Dosage directions *(continued)*			
q.d.	every day	The period after the "q" has sometimes been misinterpreted as "i," and the drug has been given q.i.d. rather than daily.	Write it out.
qn	nightly or at bedtime	Misinterpreted as "qh" (every hour)	Use "h.s." or "nightly."
qod	every other day	Misinterpreted as "q.d." (daily) or "q.i.d."	Use "q other day" or "every other day."
subq	subcutaneous	The "q" has been misinterpreted as "every." For example, a prophylactic heparin dose meant to be given 2 hours before surgery may be given every 2 hours before surgery.	Use "subcut," or write out "subcutaneous."
u u	unit	Misinterpreted as a "0" or a "4," causing a tenfold or greater overdose.	Write it out.

MAINTAINING ACCURATE MEDICATION RECORDS

Verifying and transcribing drug orders

After the doctor writes a drug order, you must verify the order by reviewing the drug, its chemical content, the dose (which may require checking the calculations), and the dosage form ordered. If you detect a problem, notify the doctor before the drug order goes to the pharmacy. If you don't detect the problem until after the drug order has gone to the pharmacy, notify the doctor and the pharmacist.

Once the prescription has been verified, transcribe the order onto the Kardex or medication administration record (MAR). Drug order transcription requires close attention because a small error in rewriting an order can cause a serious medication error. If you're not using a computer, be sure to write legibly in ink. The information you record can serve as a legal document, if necessary, to prove that a drug dose was given.

Patient information

Record all patient information on the Kardex or MAR exactly as it appears on the patient's identification (ID) bracelet, stamping the Kardex or MAR with an addressograph plate, if possible. If this is not available, write the patient's full name, hospital ID number, unit number, and bed assignment on the Kardex or MAR. Also include all known allergies, even those that aren't drug related. If the patient has no known allergies, document this with the abbreviation NKA.

Dates

Certain dates must always appear on the Kardex or MAR: the date the order was written, the date the medication should begin (if different from the original order date), and the date the medication should be discontinued. In some facilities, the time the order should start is recorded with the date. This serves as a reference for the precise time to discontinue a drug when a limited period is indicated.

Drug information

As part of medication charting information, include the following items.

Drug name
Always record the drug's full, preferably generic, name. If the doctor orders the drug with a particular proprietary name, record this name as well. Avoid using abbreviations, chemical symbols, research names, and special facility names, which could cause errors or delays in therapy.

Drug strength
Be sure to document the actual amount of drug to be administered.

Drug dosage form
Indicate the dosage form as ordered by the doctor. When recording the drug dosage form, consider the patient's special needs and the drug's physical form. For example, suppose a patient with a nasogastric tube needs medication for COPD, and the doctor orders sustained-release theophylline. Because of the patient's special needs, the tablets would have to be crushed. But because of the drug's physical form (as a sustained-release tablet), crushing would destroy its integrity and, possibly, its therapeutic effect. In such a case, you would have to notify the doctor to discuss and resolve the problem.

Route of administration
Always specify the route of administration. This is especially important for drugs that may be given by two different routes; for example, orally or rectally, as with acetaminophen. Some parenteral medications can be given by only one correct route; for example, NPH insulin may be given S.C. but not I.V.

Time of administration
The doctor's order includes a desired administration schedule, such as "t.i.d." or "q6h." This is transcribed on the MAR and then converted into actual times based on the facility's scheduled times (t.i.d. may be 9 a.m., 1 p.m., and 5 p.m. in one facility and 10 a.m., 2 p.m., and 6 p.m. in another), the availability and characteristics of the drug, or the drug's onset and duration of action (b.i.d. may be 10 a.m. and 6 or 10 p.m.; q6h may be 10 a.m., 4 p.m, 10 p.m., and 4 a.m. or 12 a.m., 6 a.m., 12 p.m., and 6 p.m.).

Some facilities have separate MARs or specially designated areas of the MAR for recording single drug orders or special drug orders (for example, drugs given as they are needed). Other facilities include these drugs on the daily MAR; in the latter case, one must carefully distinguish these drugs from scheduled drugs.

Initials

Usually, the person who transcribes the order to the MAR from the order sheet indicates this by signing the order sheet and initialing the order on the MAR. If someone other than a nurse transcribes the order, you must cosign the order sheet and the MAR.

Before administering medications, you should read the doctor's orders to ensure that the MAR accurately reflects the orders, including any recent orders or changes in orders. Many facilities require you to initial the doctors' order sheet, on the line following the last order, to indicate that all orders have been transcribed correctly onto the MAR. ■

Documenting drug administration

After administering a drug, add the dosage, route and time of administration, and your initials to the medication administration record (MAR).

Dosage

If the dosage you administer varies in any way from the dosage strength or amount ordered, note this fact in a special area on the MAR or in the progress notes. For example, you would document whether the patient refused to take a drug, consumed only part of the drug, or vomited shortly after ingesting the drug.

Route

When administering a drug by a parenteral route, record the injection site to facilitate site rotation. Most MARs include a numbered list of recognized sites so that you can record the site by its number in the limited space available. If you administer a drug by a different route than that originally specified, you must indicate that, along with the reason and authorization for the change.

Time

Immediately after administering a drug, accurately document the time of administration to help prevent repeat administration of the same drug dose.

For scheduled drugs (those with a planned time schedule), initial the appropriate time slot for the date you're giving the drug. Scheduled drug administration is considered on time if given within ½ hour before or after the ordered time. For unscheduled drugs (single doses and emergency or as-needed drugs), indicate the exact time of administration in the appropriate time slot.

If a drug isn't given as scheduled, be sure to document the reason for the delay or omission. Some MARs have a place for this information; in others, you'll record the information in the progress notes. Your facility's policy may require you to initial and circle the particular time that was missed on the MAR to draw attention to the omitted dose.

Identifying initials

When you administer a drug, verify that the dose was given by initialing the MAR in the appropriate time slot. Make sure your initials are clearly legible and different from those of other nurses on the unit who might give drugs to this patient. (Use your middle initial for clarification if necessary.) Then, identify the initials as yours by recording them in the signature section of the MAR, along with your signature and title. Your signature and initial identification must appear on every record that you have initialed when administering drugs. Always sign your initials in the same way on every record. (See *Completing a medication record.*) ■

Documenting omitted doses

Facility policies vary greatly regarding documentation of medications that aren't administered when scheduled. In any facility, however, you must record that the medication wasn't given and must provide a reason for the omission in the progress notes or medication administration record (MAR). Some common reasons include the patient's refusal to take the medication, his NPO status, or inadequate apical pulse or blood pressure for cardiovascular drug administration.

Always fill in the time slot on the MAR; leaving it blank suggests that a medication administration error was made and that the patient did not receive the prescribed medication. ■

Documenting on other medication records

Some facilities require you to document all drugs that a patient receives on a single Kardex or medication administration record (MAR). Other facilities use separate forms for as-needed drugs, large-volume parenteral drugs, one-time-only doses, and treatment items (derma-

Completing a medication record

The medication Kardex below illustrates the kind of information required on all types of medication administration forms. Although different facilities may use different forms, the information required is basically the same: patient information, the date, drug information, time for and route of administration, and your initials after you administer the drug.

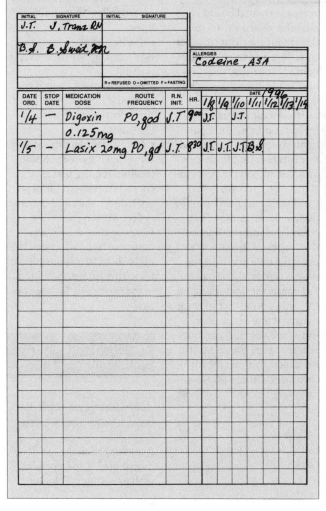

INITIAL	SIGNATURE	INITIAL	SIGNATURE
J.T.	J. Tranz RN		
B.S.	B. Sweit, RN		

R = REFUSED O = OMITTED F = FASTING

ALLERGIES
Codeine, ASA

DATE ORD.	STOP DATE	MEDICATION DOSE	ROUTE FREQUENCY	R.N. INIT.	HR.	DATE 1996 1/8	1/9	1/10	1/11	1/12	1/13	1/14
1/4	—	Digoxin 0.125mg	PO, qod	J.T	9⁰⁰	J.T.		J.T.				
1/5	-	Lasix 20mg	PO, qd	J.T.	8³⁰	J.T.	J.T.	J.T.	B.S.			

tologic and ophthalmic medications dispensed in bottles or tubes).

Perpetual inventory record
Federal and state laws regulate the dispensing, administration, and documentation of controlled substances. When a controlled substance is issued to a patient care area, a perpetual inventory record is issued with it to document the disposition of each dose and to record the name of the nurse responsible for administering each dose.

If a doctor orders a controlled substance for a patient, you must record its administration on the Kardex or MAR and on the perpetual inventory record. When the dose is removed from the double-locked storage site, record this information on the perpetual inventory record: the date and time the dose is removed, the patient's full name, the doctor's name, the drug's dose, and your signature. If any of the dose must be discarded, two nurses must verify the amount discarded and sign the form. (See *Completing a perpetual inventory record.*) ■

Avoiding transcription errors

Drug administration errors often result from mistakes made in transcribing an order from the order sheet to the medication administration record (MAR) or medication Kardex. To avoid such errors, follow these guidelines:

- Transcribe all orders in a quiet, distraction-free area, if possible.
- Before signing the order sheet and initialing the MAR, carefully review all parts of the order.
- Follow your facility's policy for reviewing orders. Some facilities require that all charts be reviewed for new orders each shift and that any orders written within 24 hours be checked. Others designate one shift (often the night shift) as responsible for reviewing all orders written in the preceding 24-hour period. ■

AVOIDING COMMON DRUG ERRORS

Confusing morphine and hydromorphone

A doctor ordered 4 mg of morphine I.V. for a patient with pneumonia. Thinking

Completing a perpetual inventory record

Federal and state laws require special documentation for administering controlled substances, usually on a form like this one.

HARRIS HOSPITAL
RECORD OF CONTROLLED SUBSTANCES DISPOSITION

DIVISION ______

COST CENTER # ______

PREPARED BY ______

DELIVERED BY ______

Demerol
50 mg/cc
Lot: 309HCl

DATE 1/18/96

NURSE SIG. S. Wilson RN

AMOUNT DELIVERED 15

REMOVE THIS FORM AND RETURN TO PHARMACY AFTER NURSE'S SIGNATURE IS OBTAINED.

DATE	TIME	PATIENT'S FULL NAME	PHYSICIAN'S NAME	NURSE'S SIGNATURE	[illegible]	[illegible]	WITNESS SIGNATURE	[illegible]
1/9	10 AM / PM	Woods, Vamin	Lingle	S. Saladaze, RN	50	—		14
1/9	11 AM / PM	Nunse, Gail	Katz	S. Saladaze, RN	25	25	B. Miller, R.N.	13
	AM / PM							
	AM / PM							
	AM / PM							
	AM / PM							
	AM / PM							
	AM / PM							
	AM / PM							
	AM / PM							
	AM / PM							
	AM / PM							
	AM / PM							
	AM / PM							
	AM / PM							
	AM / PM							
	AM / PM							
	AM / PM							
	AM / PM							
	AM / PM							

HOW TO USE THIS FORM:

1. NUMBER ON THIS FORM MUST COINCIDE WITH NUMBER ON CONTAINER
2. ALL ENTRIES MUST BE IN INDELIBLE INK
3. DOSAGE WASTED, DISCARDED, OR LOST MUST HAVE SHORT EXPLANATION AND SIGNATURE OF SECOND PERSON (WITNESS SIGNATURE)

ABOVE RECORD VERIFIED AS COMPLETE (NURSING) ______ DATE ______

ABOVE RECORD VERIFIED AS COMPLETE (PHARMACY) ______ DATE ______

that morphine was the trade name for hydromorphone (Dilaudid), a nurse obtained a 4-mg, prefilled hydromorphone syringe from unit stock. She gave the drug to her patient, who went into bradycardia and respiratory arrest; he later died.

This is one of the most common medication errors involving opioids. Many nurses make the same mistake that this nurse did.

But hydromorphone isn't a generic name for morphine; both are generic names for different drugs. Besides the problem with similar names, both drugs are available in 4-mg, prefilled syringes.

Although hydromorphone and morphine are opioids, I.V. hydromorphone is nearly six times more potent than morphine. So you can understand the danger in confusing these two drugs.

Preventive measures
To prevent confusing similar drug names, discuss these points with your nurse-manager:

- Wherever possible, eliminate hydromorphone from unit stock (or reduce the amount). That way, you'll have to obtain the drug from the pharmacy when it's prescribed, allowing the pharmacist to double-check the order.
- If you must stock both drugs, stock them in different doses; for example, 2-mg syringes of hydromorphone and 4-mg syringes of morphine.
- Place a fluorescent "not morphine" sticker on hydromorphone containers. Some label manufacturers provide these stickers. If none is available, create your own.
- Institute a nursing policy requiring another nurse to check the drug name on the syringe against the order, especially for I.V. narcotics.
- Schedule a staff-development workshop to address this potential medication error.
- Display a poster in your unit to alert staff to this frequent mix-up (it will reinforce the workshop). ■

Misreading Levoxine for Lanoxin

Here's how a doctor ordered 0.1 mg of oral levothyroxine (Levoxine) for a patient with hypothyroidism:

Lanoxin 0.1 mg
p.o. qd

The pharmacist misread the order as Lanoxin (a trade name for digoxin). However, Lanoxin isn't available as a 0.1-mg tablet: The closest strength is 0.125 mg, which has the same effect as a 0.1-mg Lanoxicaps capsule. (Lanoxicaps, another form of digoxin, is more readily absorbed, which is why the smaller amount is equal to the 0.125-mg Lanoxin tablet.) The pharmacist believed that the doctor meant Lanoxicaps, so that's what he dispensed.

This occurred late at night. The next morning, when the first dose was due, the patient's doctor was making rounds. The patient mentioned that he hadn't received his thyroid medication yet. The doctor spoke with the patient's nurse, who went to his medication drawer to obtain the drug. That's when she discovered the error. She immediately called the pharmacy; the correct drug was then dispensed.

You can understand how Levoxine and Lanoxin could be confused. If Lanoxin had been dispensed instead of Lanoxicaps, would the tablet's appearance have alerted the patient's nurse to the error? Maybe not. She might have assumed that the pharmacist had dispensed some other generic form of levothyroxine. The patient would have missed his thyroid hormone, *and* he would have received digoxin without proper monitoring.

Preventive measures
To protect patients from this error, the manufacturer of Levoxine has recently changed the name of the product to Levoxyl. ■

Not listening to your patient

A student nurse drew up 85 units of NPH insulin for a diabetic patient, as ordered on the patient's medication Kardex. But when she and her instructor approached the patient to administer the insulin, he protested that the syringe held too much. When the student explained that an order had been written for 85 units, the patient refused the injection, saying his usual dose was 10 units each morning.

Immediately, the student and instructor checked the patient's medication Kardex and the doctor's original order. Both specified 85 units. Then they called the patient's doctor, who told them the patient was correct. The doctor immediately changed the order to 10 units of NPH insulin every morning.

Hoping to get to the root of the error, the nursing instructor checked with the doctor who'd been on call the night before, when the patient was admitted. This doctor explained that he'd taken the order for 85 units from the patient's chart for his last admission—a year before. Apparently, he never asked the patient whether his insulin requirements had changed since the last admission. Nor did he check with the patient's regular doctor.

Preventive measures
By listening to the patient, these nurses prevented a dangerous medication error. Too often, a patient's questions about his medication are not taken seriously. Yet, patients are becoming more aware of the need to know what they're taking. And their knowledge has become in-

creasingly important in preventing medication errors.

So listen to your patient. If he says the dose looks too large or his usual pills are a different color, hold the dose and confirm the order with his doctor.

And take every opportunity to encourage a patient to be a careful health consumer. Teach him his drugs' names, what they're used for, what they look like, and his usual dosage of each. When you administer a drug, say something like "Here's your daily dose of NPH insulin for your diabetes — 10 units." That way, the patient will become familiar with his drugs and will be more likely to question a different tablet or a changed dose. ■

Forgetting to check the administration route

A nurse working the night shift read this medication order for a woman recovering from a cerebral vascular accident:

Mycostatin suppository, one at bedtime

The nurse prepared a Mycostatin (nystatin) vaginal tablet according to its package instructions and inserted it into the patient's vagina.

The following morning, the oncoming supervisor asked the nurse if she had given the patient her suppository vaginally. The nurse said yes, but sensing something was amiss, asked, "Is anything wrong?" The supervisor replied, "Well, the patient was supposed to dissolve the drug in her mouth. She has an *oral* yeast infection." The nurse immediately checked the patient's medication Kardex. Sure enough, next to the order were the letters "P.O." and "dissolve in mouth."

The patient suffered no ill effects from receiving the Mycostatin vaginally, although she missed out on a dose to treat her infection.

Preventive measures

So even when a drug's administration route seems obvious, check it against the medication Kardex anyway. You may prevent an error and save yourself and your patient some embarrassment. ■

Becoming complacent in using unit-dose medication

A patient was receiving I.V. antibiotics through a heparin lock every 6 hours. Every time a nurse administered an antibiotic dose, she had to follow standard procedure for flushing the lock and instilling 1 ml of a 100-units/ml solution of heparin to maintain patency.

On the 3rd day of this regimen, the evening nurse checked the unit-dose heparin syringe cartridges in the patient's supply and was surprised to find they all were labeled "heparin sodium injection — 5,000 units/ml." She realized that since one of these cartridges had been used earlier that day, the patient had received a heparin overdose.

The nurse notified the patient's doctor, who ordered an immediate activated PTT. The results were normal. The pharmacy was also notified, and the heparin cartridges were exchanged for those of the correct strength.

Preventive measures

Unit-dose Tubex cartridges and syringes go a long way in making drug administration safer and easier. But don't let their ease of use and similar appearance lure you into cutting corners. *Always* read the label before administering a drug: when pouring it, when giving it, and when discarding the empty container. ■

Confusing two patients with the same first name

Robert Brewer, age 5, was hospitalized for measles. Robert Brinson, also age 5, was admitted after he suffered a severe asthma attack. The boys were assigned to adjacent rooms on a small pediatric unit, and each boy had a nonproductive cough as a result of his condition.

During morning rounds, Robert Brewer's nurse took her patient's vital signs, then told his mother she had to get an expectorant the doctor had prescribed for his cough. When the nurse returned with the drug just 5 minutes later, the boy's mother told her Robert had already been given his medicine.

Puzzled, the nurse questioned Mrs. Brewer. She explained that another nurse had come in and asked her if the patient's name was Robert. When Mrs. Brewer answered yes, the nurse said she had the medicine for Robert's cough, and she gave it to him. Mrs. Brewer said she didn't know the name of the medicine but added that the nurse had made Robert "breathe it in through a mask."

The nurse quickly went to the nurses' station to find out

what had happened. There, she found a newly assigned nurse charting that she had given Robert Brinson his prescribed mucolytic, acetylcysteine, which is administered with a nebulizer. Robert Brewer's nurse then realized that the other nurse, who was unfamiliar with the patients on the pediatric unit, had mistakenly given the mucolytic intended for Robert Brinson to Robert Brewer.

Both nurses went immediately to Robert Brewer's room and checked his condition. The mucolytic hadn't seemed to do any harm; in fact, it actually appeared to have improved his cough. But of course, any medication mix-up is potentially serious and a cause for concern.

This mix-up began when the newly assigned nurse obtained the prescribed Mucomyst for Robert Brinson. As she was walking down the hall, she realized she was unsure of his room number. But she spotted a young boy, so she entered the room and asked if he was Robert, adding that she had the medicine for his cough.

Unfortunately, the nurse had entered Robert Brewer's room. And because Mrs. Brewer knew her son was supposed to be given some cough medicine, she assumed that Robert's nurse had asked this nurse to give it to him.

Preventive measures
This error could have been prevented if the newly assigned nurse had identified the patient correctly—by checking his identification (ID) band. Asking a patient (or family member) to confirm his name is not foolproof. A patient who is feverish, in severe pain, sedated, or preoccupied by his illness could easily misunderstand your question and give you inaccurate information. Similarly, a distraught family member may also respond inaccurately.

So always check the patient's ID band before giving medication, even if you think you know him by sight. That's the only way to confirm that you're giving medication to the right patient. ■

Neglecting to question an unusually high dose

A nurse noticed that a postpartum patient with a relatively minor infection was scheduled to receive an unusually high dose of penicillin:

Penicillin G.5 million units

Thinking that another nurse had transcribed the order incorrectly, she looked at the original on the patient's chart and discovered a dangerous misinterpretation. The doctor's sloppy handwriting made the "G" after penicillin look like a "6." And he had written the 500,000 units as ".5 million units," instead of "0.5 million units." So the order *did* look like "6.5 million units."

The nurse called the doctor, who confirmed that he really wanted his patient to have only 500,000 units every 4 hours — a total of 3,000,000 units a day.

Preventive measures
The doctor and the nurse who transcribed the order share the blame for this error. The doctor should have been more careful when he wrote the order. If he had put a zero in front of the decimal point and used the drug's proper name, penicillin G potassium, the order would have been clear.

The first nurse, however, should have realized that the apparent dose was much too high. Although it occasionally causes a serious allergic reaction, penicillin G is usually a safe drug. But because each million units contains 1.7 mEq of potassium, a mistake in the administration rate or the dose could be fatal for a child or for an adult with a serious illness. ■

Misunderstanding verbal orders

Two nurses transcribed medication orders for their patients this way:

Gentamicin 18 mg. I.V.
Inderal LA AT 1 q a.m.

Both nurses misunderstood the orders. The doctor had actually ordered 80 mg (not 18 mg) of gentamicin (Garamycin) and 80 mg (not AT) of Inderal LA (propranolol). When the pharmacist read the orders, he realized that the nurses had made transcription errors. He asked them to contact the doctors for correct doses.

Preventive measures
To avoid errors like these: Always repeat verbal orders back to the doctor to make sure you heard him correctly. This is common practice among military personnel, pilots, and air traffic controllers, and it should be among health care professionals as well. If the doctor says that he's too busy, remind him that the order involves his patient care and he'd be responsible too if something were misheard.

Of course, you should avoid taking verbal orders whenever possible. But, if you must take one, remember that numbers in the teens can easily be misunderstood. For example, the number 15 may sound like 50, 16 like 60, and so on. Enunciate these numbers clearly; then repeat them like this: "That's gentamicin one eight milligrams, correct?" "No," the doctor will say, "I meant eight zero milligrams." You'll prevent a serious error this way. ■

Giving accidental overdoses

Four children have died after being given chloral hydrate as a sedative—three from massive overdoses and one from complications of his preexisting cardiopulmonary disease (the drug exacerbated the disease effects).

Here's what happened in one case: A 5-year-old boy who was undergoing a computed tomography (CT) scan received double the intended dose of chloral hydrate. The label on the syrup correctly read "Give three teaspoons prior to CT. If needed, give two more." But the pharmacist had dispensed the drug in the wrong concentration — 500 mg/5 ml instead of 500 mg/10 ml. The boy was fine during the procedure, but when his mother took him home, she realized that he'd stopped breathing. They returned to the hospital, where the boy died.

Preventive measures

Because many clinicians believe that chloral hydrate is safe for children undergoing ambulatory procedures that require sedation, you may see orders for it. If so, keep the following points in mind:

- Chloral hydrate is available in two concentrations — 500 mg/5 ml and 500 mg/10 ml. If the ordered concentration isn't available, the pharmacist should make this clear on the drug label and tell you. And he should be involved in calculating the correct amount to be administered.
- The pediatric dose is based on the child's weight in kilograms, but keep in mind the maximum doses: For sedation, the normal dose for children is 8 mg/kg or 250 mg/m^2 orally three times a day (a maximum of 500 mg per dose). If chloral hydrate is given before an EEG, the dose is 20 to 25 mg/kg in a single dose (a maximum of 1 g per dose). And if it's given to treat insomnia, the dose is 50 mg/kg or 1.5 g/m^2 (a maximum dose of 1 g).

The dose should be written in milligrams, not just the volume of the drug or number of teaspoons. For example, the label on the medication for the 5-year-old boy would have been safer if it had read "750 mg, followed by 500 mg if needed."

- Only health care professionals who are authorized to prepare and administer medications should do so. (Unsupervised technicians who were unfamiliar with chloral hydrate dose limitations had administered the drug in three of the four cases.) Medical records detailing the patient's weight, preexisting conditions, and drug allergies must be available for them to consult.
- Monitor patients carefully after they receive chloral hydrate, and carry out necessary precautions. These actions need to be charted. ■

Failing to read container labels

An 8-year-old diabetic patient who had developed ketoacidosis was admitted to an emergency department. As one nurse drew blood for glucose levels and other laboratory tests, another nurse took an I.V. bag from a box labeled "sodium chloride injection" and started an I.V. infusion. She also administered insulin.

When the first nurse finished drawing blood, she looked up at the I.V. container and noticed that it was a dextrose solution—the last thing a diabetic patient in ketoacidosis needs. The nurse immediately clamped the line, found the correct solution, and hung it. Luckily, only a small amount of dextrose had been infused.

Preventive measures

Don't rely on the labels on boxes to identify drugs or I.V. solutions. Someone may have put the drug or solution in the wrong box. (The same goes for labeled trays, drawers, or shelves.) The only reliable way to identify a drug or solution is by reading the immediate container label. ■

Confusing similar containers

A nurse mistook a bottle of Hemoccult (5% hydrogen peroxide and 70% ethanol) for a patient's eyedrops and placed the stool developer in the patient's eye. He immediately cried out in pain, and the nurse flushed his eyes with water. The patient's eyes weren't permanently damaged. However, when this type of error has occurred in the past, some patients have developed severe, painful keratitis.

Preventive measures
To avoid this error, remember that bottles of Hemocult and Seracult, a similar developer, resemble ophthalmic containers. The best way to avoid errors is to store these developers in the utility room or the laboratory, not in patient-care areas. And, of course, always read the label before using any drug or solution. Don't let the inconvenience interfere with patient safety.

At least one manufacturer has revised the container label to minimize the risk of error. The label is white with an icon that signifies "not for the eye." ■

Interpreting ambiguous labels

A pharmacist sent a vial of ampicillin, 250 mg/2 ml, to a pediatric unit. The label read "0.40 q12h I.M., 100 mg dose."

When the nurse saw the label, she was afraid that she'd given the baby twice the prescribed dose the day before. She'd calculated the volume of the dose as 0.8 ml. Her nurse-manager agreed with her calculations and reassured her that she hadn't made an error. Together, they called the pharmacist and reported that the volume on the label was incorrect. He explained that those figures did not refer to the volume. They referred to the correct dose — 0.40 (or 40%) of the total amount of ampicillin in the vial.

Preventive measures
Such ambiguous labeling can't be tolerated. Pharmacists are supposed to help nurses administer drugs safely by clearly labeling medications. But don't assume that this information will always be accurate. Make sure you double-check labels and the pharmacist's calculations and measurements. If your information doesn't match his, withhold the drug until you clarify the situation. ■

Giving unclearly labeled drugs

A hypotensive newborn was transferred to the neonatal intensive care unit (NICU) for treatment. The NICU doctor ordered 20 ml of 0.9% sodium chloride injection to be piggybacked over 30 minutes. The nurse saw several small vials of 0.9% sodium chloride on the medication cart. But knowing that the doctor probably needed to give several doses of this solution to elevate the baby's blood volume, she bypassed the smaller vials and chose a

50-ml vial marked "sodium chloride injection."

She prepared and administered 20 ml of the solution. Later, the doctor also gave a dose from the same vial.

Shortly after this second dose, the baby became apneic and required intubation. Blood tests revealed a serum sodium level of 195 mEq/L (the normal range is 135 to 148 mEq/L). The baby's hypernatremia led to severe, permanent brain damage.

After the error, investigators found a vial labeled "14.6% sodium chloride" in the trash. They determined that this concentrated sodium chloride was injected inadvertently. The label on the vial didn't clearly warn that the solution was concentrated and had to be diluted.

Preventive measures

How can you avoid a similar error?

- Don't stock concentrated sodium chloride in the nursing unit, especially in the NICU.
- If you must keep concentrated sodium chloride in your unit, use a brand that's prominently labeled, or ask your pharmacist to provide auxiliary labels.
- If you need to prepare a solution using concentrated sodium chloride, ask your pharmacist to make it. ■

Interpreting an AZT order

A night nursing supervisor received an order for "AZT, 100 mg every 4 hours." The hospital pharmacy was closed at night, but the supervisor had a key. She entered the pharmacy, took four 50-mg tablets of azathioprine, and gave them to the patient's nurse. The nurse administered two tablets and put the other two in the patient's medication drawer for his next dose.

Unfortunately, the doctor wasn't prescribing azathioprine, an immunosuppressant. His patient, who had AIDS, was supposed to receive zidovudine, formerly known as azidothymidine. Luckily, the error was discovered and the patient wasn't harmed.

This error is occurring more often, sometimes with tragic results. Recently a hospital was sued for a similar error that led to an AIDS patient's death. In that case, the already-immunosuppressed patient received azathioprine and subsequently developed a massive infection.

Preventive measures

Never refer to azathioprine, zidovudine, or aztreonam (Azactam, an antibiotic) as AZT. And if you receive an order with that abbreviation, make sure you talk with the doctor to clarify the order. ■

Misinterpreting abbreviations

A nurse who was caring for a patient with borderline CHF received the following order from the doctor:

after 2nd unit of blood - give 20mg Lasix IVP

Because he didn't have room to write "I.V. push," the doctor abbreviated the administration method as "IVP." In her haste, the nurse interpreted "IVP" as "I.V. pyelogram."

She sent the patient to the radiology department without his chart. The radiologist performed an I.V. pyelogram, using 100 ml of ionic contrast media. This caused a shift in the patient's vascular volume, resulting in too much fluid for his already weakened heart to tolerate. The patient developed CHF, from which he eventually recovered.

Preventive measures
Some abbreviations (such as IVP) are so likely to be misinterpreted that they shouldn't be used on medical records. A list of these troublesome abbreviations should be updated as necessary and circulated to the staff.

Of course, the patient's chart should always be sent with him to other patient care areas or for diagnostic tests. That way, other health care professionals will know if they need to take any special precautions or if the treatment is even appropriate for the patient. ■

Failing to clarify incomplete orders

A 64-year-old woman was hospitalized for treatment of rheumatoid arthritis. Her doctor wrote this order for the anti-inflammatory drug piroxicam (Feldene):

Feldene 20mg PO pc

Both the patient's nurse and the hospital pharmacist interpreted the "p.c." to mean "after each meal" and that's how the drug was scheduled.

The patient was given piroxicam three times a day for more than a week. Then she began vomiting blood. Studies revealed severe anemia and a peptic ulcer. The doctor ordered several units of blood administered, then set out to find the cause of the bleeding.

His search didn't take long. As soon as he reviewed the patient's medication administration record, he saw that she was being given piroxicam three times a day, not once a day as he had intended. He was well aware that this drug can cause bleeding, even when given no more than once daily as recommended. The doctor discontinued the piroxicam and prescribed drug therapy for the patient's ulcer.

The doctor, nurse, and pharmacist all contributed to this error. The abbreviation "p.c." commonly means "after a meal." The doctor wrote an incomplete order by not specifying after *which* meal or noting that the drug was to be given only once a day. The nurse and pharmacist transcribed, filled, and carried out the order mechanically, without considering that it was incomplete. Ironically, both said later that they knew piroxicam shouldn't be given more than once daily. But they were so busy when they reviewed the order, that none of them had noticed.

Preventive measures

Don't let a hectic pace cause an error. When you're especially busy, review drug orders even more diligently. Think each order through, and clarify those that are incomplete. ■

Coining new, unapproved abbreviations

A doctor ordered I.M. injections of Demerol (meperidine), Phenergan (promethazine), and Thorazine (chlorpromazine) as premedication for an 18-month-old boy undergoing whirlpool treatments. After listing the drugs and doses, he wrote: "Please give DPT now." The nurse and pharmacist thought that he was ordering a diphtheria and tetanus toxoids and pertussis vaccine, commonly referred to as *DPT.* When the patient's nurse called the doctor, she found that he had created the abbreviation DPT to refer to the three drugs he'd ordered.

Preventive measures

As you know, unauthorized abbreviations are likely to cause problems sooner or later because no one can possibly know what everything means. That's why you and your colleagues should resist coining your own abbreviations. Any abbreviations of drug names must be approved by the hospital's pharmacy and therapeutics committee and should apppear on the hospital's approved list of medical abbreviations established by the medical records committee. ■

Failing to understand dosage differences

Patients at two nursing homes were supposed to receive 100 international units of calcitonin-salmon, a drug used to treat hypercalcemia, Paget's disease, and postmenopausal osteoporosis.

Thinking that one unit of a drug is the same as one unit of another, nurses in both nursing homes used U-100 insulin syringes to draw up what they believed was 100 international units of calcitonin-salmon. But insulin has a concentration of 100 units/ml; calcitonin, 200 international units/ml. So the nurses had drawn up 200 international units (1 ml) of calcitonin-salmon in the U-100 insulin syringes and had given their patients double doses.

Preventive measures
A U-100 insulin syringe should be used only for U-100 insulin. Calcitonin-salmon requires a syringe with a volumetric scale, such as a tuberculin syringe. ■

Failing to identify errors in doctors' orders

Esmolol is an injectable beta-adrenergic blocker used on critical care units to treat supraventricular tachycardia. This drug comes in two concentrations: 10 mg/ml in 10-ml vials (100 mg/vial) and 250 mg/ml in 10-ml ampules (2.5 g/ampule). The vials are used for direct injection of a loading dose; the ampules, to prepare infusions. Because the ampules are so concentrated, they shouldn't be used for direct injection.

A doctor ordered "an amp" of esmolol. He meant a 100-mg dose, but the nurse misunderstood him; she thought he was ordering one ampule, or 2.5 g. She administered a 2.5-g bolus. The patient suffered profound bradycardia. Esmolol's half-life is only 9 minutes, so the effect was transient. However, the patient needed vasopressors and a temporary pacemaker.

Preventive measures
The best way to prevent errors such as this is to make sure that concentrated ampules of esmolol are clearly labeled. (Of course, you should also read labels carefully and be familiar with the drugs you're administering.)

The manufacturer's label does carry a warning, but it isn't very prominent, so you could easily overlook it. If your unit stocks esmolol for emergencies, consider placing a label stating "Warning—for constant infusion after dilution only" on the neck of each ampule. And if you see a doctor ordering a drug by "ampule" instead of its concentration, remind him of the proper way to write an order. ■

Separating the patient from the MAR

A doctor ordered hydromorphone 2 mg S.C. every 3 hours for a woman who had severe back pain from metastatic cancer. She was given an injection at 1 p.m.; then, an hour later, she was sent for her daily radiation treatment.

When she returned to her room at 3:50 p.m., she complained of pain. Because her next dose of hydromorphone was scheduled for 4 p.m. and her vital signs were stable, her nurse gave the injection.

At 4:30 p.m., the patient's sister arrived to visit. Almost immediately, she called the nurse into the room, saying that her sister wouldn't respond. The nurse quickly checked the patient's vital signs and found that her respiratory rate had dropped from 18 to 10 breaths/minute and her diastolic blood pressure had dropped by 15 mm Hg.

The nurse called the doctor, explained the situation, and added that the patient had last received hydromorphone at 4 p.m. But the doctor explained that the radiology nurse had called him at 3 p.m. to say that the patient was in severe pain and couldn't tolerate further treatment. So he had ordered it given an hour early.

The doctor then ordered 1 mg of naloxone, which quickly counteracted hydromorphone's effects.

Preventive measures
This error resulted from a combination of inadequate charting and lack of communication. Although the radiology nurse had documented the 3 p.m. dose in the progress notes, she couldn't write it in the patient's medication administration record (MAR) because it wasn't in the patient's chart. But she could have alerted the patient's nurses by calling the unit or placing a note on the front of the chart. When the patient returned to her room, her nurse checked the MAR but didn't think to check the progress notes or

doctors' order sheet before giving the 4 p.m. dose.

Send a patient's MAR with him when he goes to other areas for treatment or tests. And make it a habit to read the progress notes when he returns. ■

Interrupting drug administration

A nurse on an oncology unit was preparing to flush a patient's heparin lock. A doctor approached her and said that he was going to perform a bone marrow biopsy on another patient. He requested that the nurse get a biopsy tray immediately. He told another nurse to prepare an injection of morphine 3 mg.

The first nurse stopped what she was doing and got the tray. When she brought it to the patient's room, she saw the doctor administering an injection into the patient's I.V. line. He then performed the biopsy. The second nurse came in just as he was finishing the procedure.

After they picked up the equipment and left the patient's room, the second nurse said to the doctor, "I guess you didn't want this after all." She showed him the syringe of morphine he'd told her to prepare. The doctor looked at the empty cartridge on the tray. He'd given the patient the heparin flush the first nurse had been preparing when he came to the unit. She'd set the syringe down when she went to get the biopsy tray, and the doctor had picked it up, thinking it was the morphine he had ordered.

The patient wasn't harmed by the heparin, but he suffered unnecessary pain during the biopsy. Of course, the doctor was at fault for not reading the cartridge's label before administering the medication.

Preventive measures

The first nurse shouldn't have left a medication untended. The lesson? When you're preparing medication, finish administering it, and chart what you've done—before going on to the next task. ■

Failing to check the MAR before giving a drug

A few minutes before the afternoon report, the day medication nurse gave a patient 7.5 mg of warfarin, then charted what she'd done in the medication administration record (MAR). When the evening medication nurse asked the nurse giving report if the patient had received the drug, she said she didn't know.

After report, the evening medication nurse took a dose of warfarin into the patient's room and asked him if he'd been given the drug. The patient said he'd gotten a new medication about an hour earlier, but he didn't know its name. The nurse left the warfarin on the patient's bedside table and went to check the MAR. She discovered that the patient had received the warfarin, so she went to retrieve the drug from the patient's room. But the patient had already taken it.

Preventive measures

What went wrong? First, the evening medication nurse shouldn't have tried to give the drug without checking the MAR before she went into the patient's room. Second, she shouldn't have left medication on the bedside table. Finally, if the day medication nurse had taught the patient about his new drug, he could have told the other nurse what he'd taken. ■

Allowing stress to hinder drug administration

A prisoner from a county jail was hospitalized for gallbladder surgery. During his 1st postoperative day, he developed a bad case of hiccups. His nurse tried several comfort measures to relieve the hiccups without success.

The patient soon became agitated by the constant tension on his suture line. His two assigned guards also became concerned, and the three men bombarded the nurse with constant demands for relief of the hiccups.

Yielding to their pressure, the nurse called the patient's doctor, who ordered chlorpromazine (Thorazine), 50 mg I.M., stat. She quickly obtained the drug from floor stock and administered it, planning to chart the medication order afterward.

When the nurse checked the patient a short time later, he said, "That shot really helped. What was it anyway?"

"Thorazine," the nurse told him.

"Thorazine! I'm allergic to Thorazine!" yelled the patient.

The nurse checked his chart. Sure enough, both his chart and his medication administration record (MAR) had large stickers reading "ALLERGY TO THORAZINE." Also, the patient was wearing a red bracelet with the same warning.

The nurse immediately called the doctor, who told her to watch the patient closely. Fortunately, the patient, who'd had a dystonic reaction (not really an allergy) to Thorazine in the past, had no side effect this time.

Preventive measures

A tense situation caused this nurse to panic and skip a vital step in the medication administration process: Check for allergies or a history of side effects before administering a drug. She should have checked the patient's chart, his MAR, his identification bracelet, and any other places where this information is routinely listed. She could even have asked the patient whether he'd ever had any reaction to a medication.

But this incident has still another lesson for nurses: Don't let patients, family, friends or even prison guards interfere with your nursing actions. You're responsible for your actions, and you know how they should be carried out. Don't let a tense situation make you deviate from the correct procedure. ■

■ CHAPTER 4

CARRYING OUT CONVERSIONS AND CALCULATIONS

SYSTEMS OF MEASUREMENT

Reviewing the metric system

Prescriptions can be written in a variety of measurement systems: metric, apothecary, household, and unit, among others. You may need to convert units of measure if a prescribed drug is only available in a measurement system that's different from the one the doctor ordered. Depending on how a drug is packaged, you also may need to calculate smaller or larger units of measure within the same system.

Used by most countries, the metric measurement system is based on powers of 10. This offers several advantages over other measurement systems: It eliminates common fractions, simplifies calculation of larger or smaller units, and simplifies calculation of drug dosages.

Metric terms

The metric system consists of three basic units of measurement: the meter, liter, and gram.

The *meter (m)* is the basic unit of length. The *liter (L)* is the basic unit of volume, representing one-tenth of a cubic meter. The *gram (G, Gm, or GM)* is the basic unit of weight, representing the weight of one cubic centimeter of water at 4° C. The preferred abbreviation for gram is "G." The abbreviations "gm" and "g" should not be used; they can be easily confused with gr (grain) when handwritten, which could lead to dangerous errors. "GM" is an old abbreviation for gram that still may be used by some doctors.

Multiples of the basic units

Besides the three basic units of measurement, the metric system includes other units that are multiples of the basic units. Each of these units has a prefix indicating its relationship to the basic unit and its own abbreviation for easy notation. For example, the most common subdivision of the gram is the *milli*gram *(mg)*, which represents one-thousandth, or 0.001, of a gram. The most common multiple of a gram is the *kilo*gram *(kg)*, which is 1,000 times greater than the gram.

These prefixes and others apply to meters, liters, and grams and can be used to express units of measure ranging from *kilo*meters *(km)* to *nano*grams *(ng)* to *deci*liters *(dl)*.

The metric system also includes one unusual unit of volume, the *cubic centimeter (cc)*. Because the cubic centimeter occupies the same space as one milliliter of liquid, these two units of volume are considered equal and are frequently used interchangeably. (Technically, however, cubic centimeters refer to gas volume and milliliters refer to liquid volume.)

Metric conversions
Because the metric system has a decimal basis, conversions between units of measure are fairly easy. To convert a smaller unit to a larger one, move the decimal point to the left or divide by the appropriate multiple of 10. To convert a larger unit to a smaller one, move the decimal point to the right or multiply by the appropriate multiple of 10.

Grams to milligrams
To convert from grams to milligrams (one-thousandth of a gram), multiply by 1,000, or move the decimal point three places to the right on the metric conversion scale. Likewise, to convert from milligrams to grams, divide by 1,000, or move the decimal point three places to the left.

Meters to kilometers
To convert 5 m to kilometers, first count the number of places to the right or left of "meter" to reach "kilo" on the scale. Because a kilo is three decimal places to the left of a meter (1,000 times larger), move the decimal point to the left, indicating that 5 m equals 0.005 km. Remember to place a zero in front of the decimal point.

Milligrams to micrograms
To convert 50 mg to micrograms (mcg), locate "milli" and "micro" on the scale. The Greek symbol μg sometimes is used for microgram, but it can be misread to mean milligrams (mg). Because a microgram is three decimal places to the right of milligram, or 1,000 times smaller, move the decimal point to the right, indicating that 50 mg equals 50,000 mcg.

Centiliters to liters
To convert 250 centiliters (cl) to liters, find these units on the scale. Because a liter is two places to the left of a centiliter, or 100 times larger, move the decimal point two places to the left, indicating that 250 cl equals 2.5 L.

Memorize the equivalents of commonly used measures. (See *Metric measures*, page 106.)

Practicing conversion skills
- An infant weighs 4.72 kg (10.4 lb). What's the infant's weight in grams? Knowing that 1 kg equals 1,000 G, set

Metric measures

This table shows the equivalents of some commonly used metric measures. Several less commonly used measures, such as the hectogram, are included.

LIQUIDS		
1 milliliter (ml)	=	1 cubic centimeter (cc)
1,000 ml	=	1 liter (L)
100 centiliters (cl)	=	1 L
10 deciliters (dl)	=	1 L
10 L	=	1 dekaliter (dkl)
100 L	=	1 hectoliter (hl)
1,000 L	=	1 kiloliter (kl)
SOLIDS		
1,000 micrograms (mcg)	=	1 milligram (mg)
1,000 mg	=	1 gram (G)
1,000 G	=	1 kilogram (kg)
100 centigrams (cg)	=	1 G
10 decigrams (dg)	=	1 G
10 G	=	1 dekagram (dkg)
100 G	=	1 hectogram (hg)

up the following equation:

$$X\ G = 4.72\ kg \times 1{,}000\ G/kg$$

Solving for X, the unknown factor, you find that the infant weighs 4,720 G.

- A patient received 0.5 L of I.V. fluid. How many milliliters did he receive?

First, find "liter" and then "milli" on the metric conversion scale. Because "milli" is located three places to the right of "liter," move the decimal point three places to the right, indicating that 0.5 L is equal to 500 ml. ■

Reviewing the apothecaries' system

Before the metric system became standard, doctors and pharmacists used the apothecaries' system of measurement. After the metric system was introduced, however, use of the older system began to decline. Although the apothecaries' system is being phased out, it's still used on a limited basis, which means you may see it on prescriptions and bottle labels.

The apothecaries' system traditionally uses a Roman numeral and places the unit of measurement before it. For example, grains would be written *grains v.* Some doctors and other health care professionals don't follow this traditional convention. Instead, they express apothecaries' system dosages in Arabic numbers followed by units of measurement, such as *5 grains.*

Roman numerals

A doctor who writes prescriptions in the apothecaries' system usually expresses quantities of drugs or ingredients with Roman numerals. The following letters, when used as Roman numerals, indicate these numeric values:

$\overline{\text{ss}}$ = ½	L = 50
I = 1	C = 100
V = 5	D = 500
X = 10	M = 1,000

In pharmacologic applications, Roman numerals *ss* (an abbreviation of the Latin word *semis,* meaning "half") through *X* usually are written in lower case: $\overline{ss}$, $\overline{i}$, $\overline{v}$, and $\overline{x}$, often with a line above. The dot over the *i* helps to clarify this symbol as the number one and prevents mistaking $\overline{iii}$ for $\overline{iv}$. Fractions of less than one-half ($\overline{ss}$) are written as common fractions using Arabic numbers.

Units of measurement

With the metric system, you can measure length in meters, volume in liters, and weight in grams. With the apothecaries' system, however, you can measure only volume and weight. In this system, the basic unit for measuring liquid volume is the *minim* (M_x) and that for measuring solid weight is the *grain (gr).* To visualize these standards, remember that a minim is about the size of a drop of water, which weighs about the same as a grain of

Apothecaries' measures

This table displays the relationships between measures of liquid volume and solid weight in the apothecaries' system.

LIQUID VOLUME		
60 minims (M_x)	=	1 dram (ʒ)
8 (ʒ)	=	1 ounce (℥)
16 (℥)	=	1 pint (pt)
2 pt	=	1 quart (qt)
4 qt	=	1 gallon (gal)
SOLID WEIGHT		
60 grains (gr)	=	1 (ʒ)
8 (ʒ)	=	1 (℥)
12 (℥)	=	1 pound (lb)

wheat. The following equation sums up this relationship:

1 drop = 1 minim (M_x) = 1 grain

Remember, however, that these are only approximate equivalents. For example, the size of an actual drop varies with the density and viscosity of the liquid (if other than water) and with the size and configuration of the dropper.

Other units of measure in the apothecaries' system build on these basic units. (See *Apothecaries' measures.*) Many of these units also are used as common household measures.

Practice in using conversion skills

- Part of a doctor's order is written, "Give acetaminophen gr *x* for Temp. 100° F." How many grains of the medication must you administer?

You need to convert *gr x* from Roman numerals to Arabic. *Gr* represents grains, and *x* in Roman numerals equals 10 in Arabic numbers. This means:

gr $\overline{x}$ = grains 10 = 10 grains of acetaminophen ■

Reviewing the household system

Many of the units of liquid measure in the apothecaries' system are identical to those used in the household system of measurement. Because all droppers, teaspoons, tablespoons, and glasses aren't alike, the household system of liquid measurement can be used for approximate measures only. In the hospital setting, you should *not* use the household system to measure medications; instead, use the metric or apothecaries' system.

Most people in the United States are familiar with the household system of weights and measures. In most cases, food products, recipes, nonprescription drugs, and home remedies use the household system. Although the household system is of limited use in the hospital setting, home health nurses need to be familiar with it because the patient may use this measurement system and is probably more comfortable with it.

Most liquid medications are prescribed and dispensed in the metric system. To ensure the accuracy of dosages measured in the household system, teach the patient how to use devices that ensure more accurate drug measurement. (See *Household measures*, page 110.) Also teach the patient how to convert household to metric measurements. ■

Reviewing the avoirdupois system

You should be aware of the avoirdupois system because it's used for ordering and purchasing some pharmaceutical products and for weighing patients in clinical settings.

In the avoirdupois system, the solid measures or units of weight include grains, ounces (437.5 gr), and pounds (16 oz or 7,000 gr). Note that the apothecaries' pound is 12 oz, but the avoirdupois pound is 16 oz. ■

Reviewing the unit system

Some drugs are not measured in the metric, apothecaries', or household systems. Rather, they are measured in *units,* such as United States Pharmacopeia (USP) units *(U)* or international units *(IU).*

The most common drug measured in units is insulin, which comes in 10-ml multidose vials of U-40 or U-100 strength. The U refers to the number of units of insulin

Household measures

This table shows the equivalents of the most commonly used household measures, which are used to measure liquid volume. *Note:* The abbreviations "t" (teaspoon) and "T" (tablespoon) should be avoided because they carry a high potential for error when written quickly. Always clarify a prescription that includes these symbols.

LIQUIDS		
60 drops (gtt)	=	1 teaspoon (tsp)
3 tsp	=	1 tablespoon (Tbs)
2 Tbs	=	1 ounce (oz)
8 oz	=	1 cup (c)
16 oz (2 c)	=	1 pint (pt)
2 pt	=	1 quart (qt)
4 qt	=	1 gallon (gal)

per milliliter. For example, 1 ml of U-40 insulin contains 40 units; 1 ml of U-100 insulin contains 100 units. Use of U-40 insulin has declined in recent years; the U-100 strength, which is based on metric measurement, makes measurement in a standard syringe easier.

Other drugs are also measured in units. For example, the anticoagulant heparin for parenteral use is available in liquid forms that contain 10 to 20,000 units/ml. Bacitracin, an antibiotic, is available in a topical form that contains 50 units/ml. Penicillins G and V are available in different forms that contain 400,000 units/ml (approximately equal to 250 mg) or 800,000 units/ml (approximately equal to 500 mg). The hormone calcitonin is measured in IU, as are the fat-soluble vitamins A, D, and E. Some forms of vitamins A and D also are measured in USP units.

To calculate the dose to administer when the medication is available in units, use the following proportion:

$$\frac{\text{amount of drug (ml)}}{\text{dose of drug required (units)}} = \frac{1 \text{ ml}}{\text{drug available (units)}}$$

Practice in using calculation skills

- A patient requires 24 units of insulin daily. How many milliliters of U-100 insulin should be given?

First, identify the insulin available (100 units/ml) and the dose of insulin required (24 units). Then, set up the proportion:

$$\frac{X \text{ ml}}{24 \text{ units}} = \frac{1 \text{ ml}}{100 \text{ units}}$$

Solve for X, the unknown factor:

$$X \text{ ml} \times 100 \text{ units} = 24 \text{ units} \times 1 \text{ ml}$$

$$X = \frac{24 \text{ ml}}{100}$$

$$X = 0.24 \text{ ml}$$

The patient should be given 0.24 ml of insulin.

- If only U-40 insulin is available for a patient who needs 24 units daily, how many milliliters of insulin should be given? Begin by identifying the insulin available (40 units/ml) and the dose of insulin required (24 units). Then set up the proportion:

$$\frac{X \text{ ml}}{24 \text{ units}} = \frac{1 \text{ ml}}{40 \text{ units}}$$

Solve for X:

$$X \text{ ml} \times 40 \text{ units} = 24 \text{ units} \times 1 \text{ ml}$$

$$X = \frac{24 \text{ ml}}{40}$$

$$X = 0.6 \text{ ml}$$

The patient should be given 0.6 ml of insulin.

- The doctor orders 400,000 units of penicillin G for a patient. The pharmacy has run out of vials that contain 400,000 units/ml, so they send a vial labeled "Penicillin G 800,000 units/ml." How many milliliters must be administered?

Set up the proportion:

$$\frac{X \text{ ml}}{400{,}000 \text{ units}} = \frac{1 \text{ ml}}{800{,}000 \text{ units}}$$

$$X \text{ ml} \times 800{,}000 \text{ units} = 400{,}000 \text{ units} \times 1 \text{ ml}$$

$$X = \frac{400{,}000 \text{ ml}}{800{,}000}$$

$$X = 0.5 \text{ ml}$$

The patient should be given 0.5 ml of the penicillin G solution. ■

Reviewing the milliequivalent system

You'll find that electrolytes are measured in milliequivalents (mEq). Drug manufacturers provide information about the number of metric units required to provide the prescribed number of milliequivalents. For example, the manufacturer's instructions may indicate that 1 ml equals 4 mEq.

A doctor usually orders the electrolyte potassium chloride in milliequivalents. Potassium preparations for I.V., oral, or other use are available as liquid (elixir and parenteral) and solid (powder and tablet) forms.

Practice in using conversion skills

- A patient who is receiving medications and feedings via a nasogastric tube is to receive 20 mEq of potassium chloride. You obtain the electrolyte in elixir form. The label states "Potassium chloride, 30 mEq = 30 ml." How many milliliters must be given to the patient?

Set up the proportion:

$$\frac{X\text{ ml}}{20\text{ mEq}} = \frac{30\text{ ml}}{30\text{ mEq}}$$

Solve for X, the unknown factor:

$$X\text{ ml} \times 30\text{ mEq} = 20\text{ mEq} \times 30\text{ ml}$$

$$X = \frac{600\text{ ml}}{30}$$

$$X = 20\text{ ml}$$

More simply, you may have realized that if a solution contains 30 mEq in 30 ml, it contains 1 mEq/ml. Thus, if 20 mEq is needed, 20 ml should be given to the patient. ■

Understanding equivalent measures

In practice, you may find that a doctor's order for medication is written in one system of measurement whereas the medication is available in a different system. For example, the doctor may order the medication in *grains* but the medication may be available in *milligrams.* To convert medication orders from one system to another, you must know the equivalent measures among systems of measurement.

Although references and charts that list equivalent measures among systems usually are available in the clinical setting, most nurses memorize the most frequently used equivalents. (See *Equivalent measures.*)

The plastic medication cup used for liquid preparations is also available on the nursing unit, providing a quick reference for equivalents among measures in the metric, apothecaries', and household systems. Additionally, some syringes are labeled in both the metric and apothecaries' systems and

Equivalent measures

Remember that a facility may cite a particular set of equivalents as their standard for exchanges among systems. All health care professionals prescribing, dispensing, or administering drugs under such a purview should abide by established protocols. If no protocols exist, use the equivalent measure that's easiest to manipulate in any given problem.

This chart shows some *approximate* liquid equivalents among the household, apothecaries', and metric systems.

APPROXIMATE LIQUID EQUIVALENTS

Household	Apothecaries'	Metric
1 drop (gtt)	1 minim (M_x)	0.06 milliliter (ml)
15* or 16 gtt	15* or 16 M_x	1 ml
1 teaspoon (tsp)	1 dram (ʒ)	4 or 5 ml
1 tablespoon (Tbs)	½ ounce (oz)	15 or 16 ml
2 Tbs	1 oz	30* or 32 ml
1 cup (c)	8 oz	240* or 250 ml
1 pint (pt)	16 oz	480* or 500 ml
1 quart (qt)	32 oz	960 or 1,000* ml (1 liter)
1 gallon (gal)	128 oz	3,840 or 4,000* ml

(continued)

Equivalent measures *(continued)*

The following chart shows some *approximate* solid equivalents among the avoirdupois, apothecaries, and metric systems.

APPROXIMATE SOLID EQUIVALENTS

Avoirdupois	Apothecaries'	Metric
1 grain (gr)	1 grain (gr)	0.06* or 0.065 gram (G)
15.4 gr	15 gr	1 G (1,000 mg)
1 ounce	480 gr	28.35 G
1 pound (lb)	1.33 lb	454 G
2.2 lb	2.7 lb	1 kilogram (kg)

The following chart shows some *approximate* solid equivalents between the apothecaries' and metric systems.

Apothecaries'	Metric
15 grains (gr) (4 ʒ)	1 gram (G) (1,000 mg)
10 gr	0.6* G (600 mg) or 0.65 G (650 mg)
7½ gr	0.5 G (500 mg)
5 gr	0.3* G (300 mg) or 0.325 G (325 mg)
3 gr	0.2 G (200 mg)
1½ gr	0.1 G (100 mg)
1 gr	0.06* G (60 mg) or 0.064 G (64 mg) or 0.065 G (65 mg)
¾ gr	0.05 G (50 mg)

Equivalent measures *(continued)*

Apothecaries'	Metric
½ gr	0.03* G (30 mg) or 0.032 G (32 mg)
¼ gr	0.015* G (15 mg) or 0.016 G (16 mg)
1/60 or 1/64 gr	0.001 G (1 mg) or 1/100 gr
1/120 gr	0.5 mg
1/150 gr	0.4 mg

*Indicates the most commonly used equivalent

can be used as a quick reference for liquid measures between these two systems.

Practice in using equivalent measurement skills

- A patient has been taking 30 ml of a medication while hospitalized and is to continue taking this dose at home. The patient's medication cup at home is marked in ounces. How many ounces per dose should the patient take at home?

You know that 30 ml and 1 oz are equivalent measures. Thus, the patient should take 1 oz of the medication per dose at home. To show the patient that the two measures are equivalent, you use a plastic medication cup labeled in milliliters and ounces.

- A patient who must restrict daily fluid intake has been receiving 480 ml of fluid on each of the three daily food trays. The same fluid restriction is to continue at home, where available containers are marked in ounces, pints, and quarts. How much fluid is the patient permitted at each meal?

Use the following equivalent measures:

1 pt = 16 oz = 480 ml

1 qt = 32 oz

Because the patient is allowed to have 480 ml of fluid at each meal, tell him that this is equivalent to 1 pt, 16 oz, or ½ qt of fluid. ■

Estimating body surface area in adults

Draw a straight line from the patient's height in the left-hand column to his weight in the right-hand column. The intersection of this line with the center scale reveals the body surface area. The adult nomogram is especially useful in calculating dosages for chemotherapy.

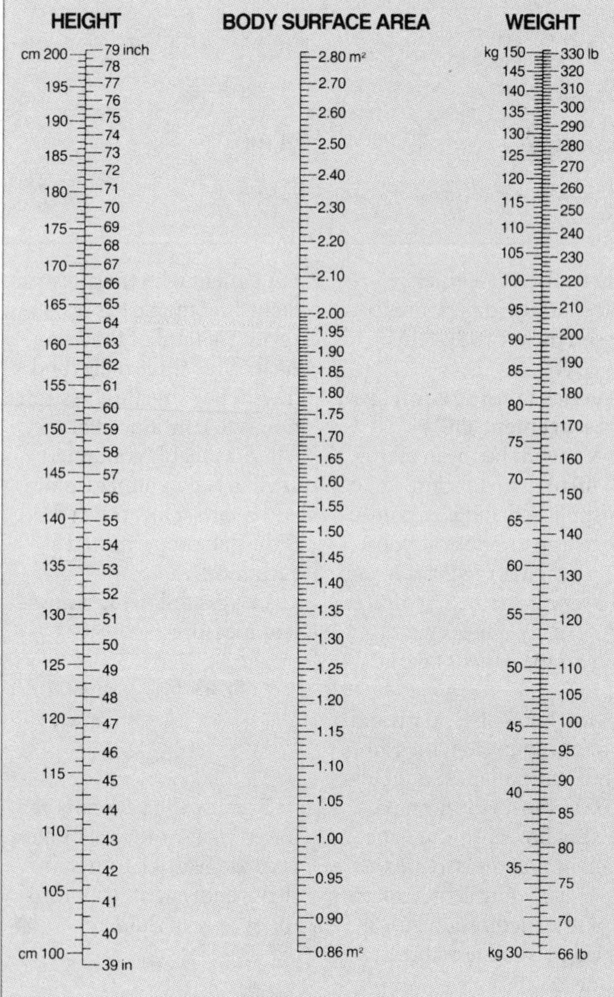

DOSAGE CALCULATIONS IN ENTERAL DRUG THERAPY

Reviewing ratios and proportions

You can easily determine the amount of tablets, capsules, or solution to administer by using a process of ratios and proportions.

A ratio is a mathematical expression of the relationship between two things. A proportion is a set of two equal ratios. A ratio may be expressed with a fraction, such as ⅓, or with a colon, such as 1:3.

When ratios are expressed as fractions in a proportion, their cross products are equal, as indicated below:
Proportion:

$$\frac{2}{4} = \frac{5}{10}$$

Cross products:

$$2 \times 10 = 4 \times 5$$

When ratios are expressed using colons in a proportion, the product of the means equals the product of the extremes:
Proportion:

means: 3:30 :: 4:40 :extremes

(means = 30 and 4; extremes = 3 and 40)

Product of means and extremes:

$$30 \times 4 = 3 \times 40$$

Whether fractions or ratios are used in a proportion, they must appear in the same order on both sides of the equal sign. When the ratios are expressed as fractions, the units in the numerators must be the same, and the units in the denominators must be the same (although they do not have to be the same as the units in the numerators). The example below demonstrates this principle:

$$\frac{\text{mg}}{\text{kg}} = \frac{\text{mg}}{\text{kg}}$$

If the ratios in a proportion are expressed with colons, the units of the first term on the left side of the equal sign must be the same as the units of the first term on the right side. In other words, the units of the mean on one side of the equal sign must match the units of the extreme on the other side, and vice versa. The example below demonstrates this principle:

mg:kg :: mg:kg ■

Simplifying dosage calculations

To help make dosage calculations simpler and avoid errors, follow these tips.

Incorporate units of measure in the calculation

This incorporation helps protect you from one of the most common dosage calculation errors — the incorrect unit of measure. When you include units of measure in the calculation, those in the numerator and the denominator cancel each other out and leave the correct unit of measure in the answer. The following example uses units of measure in calculating a drug with a usual dose of 4 mg/kg for a 55-kg (121-lb) patient:

- State the problem in a proportion:

$$4 \text{ mg:}1 \text{ kg} :: X \text{ mg:}55 \text{ kg}$$

- Solve for X, the unknown factor, by applying the principle that the product of the means equals the product of the extremes:

$$1 \text{ kg} \times X \text{ mg} = 4 \text{ mg} \times 55 \text{ kg}$$

- Divide and cancel out the units of measure that appear in the numerator and denominator:

$$X = \frac{4 \text{ mg} \times 55 \cancel{\text{kg}}}{1 \cancel{\text{kg}}}$$

$$X = 220 \text{ mg}$$

Check zeros and decimal places

Suppose you receive an order to administer 0.1 mg of epinephrine S.C., but the only epinephrine on hand is a 1-ml ampule that contains 1 mg of epinephrine. To calculate the volume for injection, use the ratio and proportion method:

- State the problem in a proportion:

$$\frac{X \text{ ml}}{0.1 \text{ mg}} = \frac{1 \text{ ml}}{1 \text{ mg}}$$

- Solve for X by applying the principle that the product of the means equals the product of the extremes:

$$1 \text{ ml} \times 0.1 \text{ mg} = 1 \text{ mg} \times X \text{ ml}$$

- Divide and cancel out the units of measure that appear in the numerator and denominator, carefully checking the decimal placement:

$$X = \frac{0.1 \cancel{\text{mg}} \times 1 \text{ ml}}{1 \cancel{\text{mg}}}$$

$$X = 0.1 \text{ ml}$$

Recheck calculations that seem unusual

If, for instance, a calculation yields an answer that suggests you administer 25 tablets, you've probably made an error and should recheck your figures carefully. If you still have doubts, review your calculations with a colleague. ■

Converting between measurement systems

In practice, you frequently see more than one system of measurement used in the same prescription. Before units such as grains and grams can be combined, however, you must convert all quantities to the same measurement system — metric, apothecaries', household, or avoirdupois.

When you convert a measurement from one system to another, you will obtain an approximate or practical equivalent, not a precise one. This is permissible because up to 10% variation between the dose ordered and the dose administered is considered acceptable in most cases.

Four-step conversion

To convert between measurement systems, follow these four basic steps:

1. Set up a ratio or fraction with the known conversion factor. Remember, when more than one conversion factor is available, use the one that fits your problem most easily. For example, gr $\bar{\text{i}}$ can equal 60 mg, 64 mg, or 65 mg.

2. Set up a ratio or fraction with X, the unknown quantity, and the quantity to be converted.

3. State these ratios or fractions in a proportion. Be sure that the units appear in the same order on both sides of the double colon or equal sign.

4. Solve for X, either by applying the principle that the product of the means equals the product of the extremes (when using the ratio method) or by cross multiplying (when using the fraction method).

Practicing conversions

By applying the four-step process, you can make conversions and determine the correct dosage to give.

Conversion between grains and milligrams

A doctor orders aspirin gr $\bar{\text{v}}$ for a patient, but the aspirin tablets are available in milligrams only. How many milligrams should you administer?

- Set up the first ratio with the conversion factor:

$$1 \text{ gr}:65 \text{ mg}$$

- Set up the second ratio with X in the appropriate position:

$$5 \text{ gr}:X \text{ mg}$$

- Use these ratios in a proportion:

1 gr:65 mg :: 5 gr:X mg

- Solve for X by applying the principle that the product of the means equals the product of the extremes:

$$65 \text{ mg} \times 5 \text{ gr} = 1 \text{ gr} \times X \text{ mg}$$

$$X = \frac{65 \text{ mg} \times 5 \cancel{\text{gr}}}{1 \cancel{\text{gr}}}$$

$$X = 325 \text{ mg}$$

Conversion between teaspoons and milliliters

A drug order calls for 2½ tsp of co-trimoxazole suspension twice daily. You must convert this to the metric system. What is the equivalent in milliliters?

To convert between teaspoons in the household system and milliliters in the metric system, you must use the conversion factor 5 ml = 1 tsp in the four-step process:

- Set up the first ratio with the conversion factor:

5 ml:1 tsp

- Set up the second ratio with the unknown metric quantity:

X ml:2.5 tsp

- Use these ratios in a proportion:

5 ml:1 tsp :: X ml:2.5 tsp

- Solve for X by applying the principle that the product of the means equals the product of the extremes:

$$1 \text{ tsp} \times X \text{ ml} = 5 \text{ ml} \times 2.5 \text{ tsp}$$

$$X = \frac{5 \text{ ml} \times 2.5 \cancel{\text{tsp}}}{1 \cancel{\text{tsp}}}$$

$$X = 12.5 \text{ ml}$$

Conversions among ounces, milliliters, and tablespoons

A drug order calls for milk of magnesia 1½ oz h.s. You must convert this to the metric system. What is the equivalent in milliliters?

To convert ounces to milliliters, you must use the conversion factor 1 oz = 30 ml in the four-step process:

- Set up the first ratio with the conversion factor:

1 oz:30 ml

- Set up the second ratio with the unknown metric quantity:

1.5 oz:X ml

- Use these ratios in a proportion:

1 oz:30 ml :: 1.5 oz:X ml

- Solve for X by applying the principle that the product of the means equals the product of the extremes:

$$30 \text{ ml} \times 1.5 \text{ oz} = 1 \text{ oz} \times X \text{ ml}$$

$$X = \frac{30 \text{ ml} \times 1.5 \cancel{\text{oz}}}{1 \cancel{\text{oz}}}$$

$$X = 45 \text{ ml}$$

To convert this dosage to tablespoons, follow the same steps, using the fraction method and the conversion factor 1 Tbs = 15 ml:

- Set up a fraction with the conversion factor:

$$\frac{1 \text{ Tbs}}{15 \text{ ml}}$$

- Set up a fraction with the unknown household quantity:

$$\frac{X \text{ Tbs}}{45 \text{ ml}}$$

- Use these fractions in a proportion:

$$\frac{X \text{ Tbs}}{45 \text{ ml}} = \frac{1 \text{ Tbs}}{15 \text{ ml}}$$

- Solve for X by cross multiplying:

$$X \text{ Tbs} \times 15 \text{ ml} = 45 \text{ ml} \times 1 \text{ Tbs}$$

$$X = \frac{4.5 \cancel{\text{ml}} \times 1 \text{ Tbs}}{15 \cancel{\text{ml}}}$$

$$X = 3 \text{ Tbs}$$

■

Determining how many tablets or capsules to give

Most tablets, capsules, and similar dosage forms are only available in a few strengths. Therefore, you'll frequently needs to administer more than 1 tablet, or one-half of a scored tablet. Breaking an unscored tablet in portions smaller than halves usually does not yield an accurate dose. Similarly, breaking a capsule in half usually results in significant loss of medication. Some oral preparations should not be opened, broken, scored, or crushed because this would change the drug's action. If a dose smaller than one-half of a scored tablet or any portion of an unscored tablet or capsule is needed, try to substitute a commercially available solution or suspension or one that's prepared by the pharmacist.

Ratios and proportions

Calculating the number of tablets or capsules to administer lends itself to the use of ratios and proportions. To do this, follow this four-step process:

1. Set up the first ratio with the known tablet strength.

2. Set up second ratio with X, the unknown quantity.

3. Use these ratios in a proportion.

4. Solve for X by applying the principle that the product of the means equals the product of the extremes.

Practice in calculating number of tablets

A drug order calls for propranolol 100 mg P.O. q.i.d., but the only available form of propranolol is 40-mg tablets. How many tablets must you administer?

- Set up the first ratio with the known tablet (tab) strength:

$$40 \text{ mg:1 tab}$$

Set up the second ratio with the desired dose and the unknown number of tablets:

$$100 \text{ mg:X tab}$$

- Use these ratios in a proportion:

$$40 \text{ mg:1 tab} :: 100 \text{ mg:X tab}$$

- Solve for X by applying the principle that the product of the means equals the product of the extremes:

$$1 \text{ tab} \times 100 \text{ mg} = 40 \text{ mg} \times \text{X tab}$$

$$\text{X} = \frac{1 \text{ tab} \times 100 \cancel{\text{mg}}}{40 \cancel{\text{mg}}}$$

■

Determining the amount of liquid medication to give

You'll frequently need to administer medications in liquid form, either suspensions or elixirs. To calculate the amount of solution to administer, you can use either the ratio or the fraction method. To do so, use a four-step process similar to the one described for determining the number of capsules or tablets to administer:

1. Set up a ratio or fraction with the known solution strength.
2. Set up a ratio or fraction with X, the unknown quantity.
3. Use these ratios or fractions in a proportion.
4. Solve for X, either by applying the principle that the product of the means equals the product of the extremes (if the ratio approach is used) or by cross multiplying (if the fraction method is used).

Calculating the amount of liquid medication

A patient is to receive 750 mg of amoxicillin oral suspension. The label reads "Amoxicillin (Amoxicillin trihydrate) 250 mg/5 ml. Bottle contains 100 ml." How many milliliters of amoxicilin solution should the patient receive?

- Set up a fraction with the known solution strength:

$$\frac{5 \text{ ml}}{250 \text{ mg}}$$

- Set up a fraction with the unknown quantity:

$$\frac{X \text{ ml}}{750 \text{ mg}}$$

- Set up the proportion:

$$\frac{X \text{ ml}}{750 \text{ mg}} = \frac{5 \text{ ml}}{250 \text{ mg}}$$

- Solve for X by cross multiplying:

$$X \text{ ml} \times 250 \text{ mg} = 750 \text{ mg} \times 5 \text{ ml}$$

$$X = \frac{3{,}750 \text{ ml}}{250}$$

$$X = 15 \text{ ml}$$

■

Determining how many suppositories to give

You'll commonly need to adminster medications in suppository form, especially if your patient can't take drugs orally. You can calculate the number of suppositories to administer by using either the ratio or the fraction method already described for capsules, tablets, and solutions.

Although the doctor usually orders drugs in the dosage provided by one suppository, two suppositories occasionally are needed to provide the ordered amount of medication. If you calculate that more than one is needed, you should recheck the calculations and then have another nurse perform the calculations. You should also contact the pharmacy to find out whether the medicated suppository is available in other dosages. If more than two suppositories are needed to provide one dose, contact the doctor.

Patient teaching

Teaching the patient about the purpose of the medications he is receiving is especially important when the medication is in suppository form. Many patients, for instance, presume that suppositories are given solely to promote bowel evacuation; in trying to comply with the presumed treatment, they move their bowels, thus expelling thc suppository and receiving little if any medication.

Calculating the number of suppositories

The doctor's order calls for "Tylenol supp. gr $\overline{x}$ q 4h p.r.n. temp. 101° F." The package label states that each suppository contains 10 gr of Tylenol. How many suppositories (supp) must you administer?

- Set up the proportion:

$$X \text{ supp:}10 \text{ gr} :: 1 \text{ supp:}10 \text{ gr}$$

- Solve for X, the unknown factor:

$$X \text{ supp} \times 10 \text{ gr} = 10 \text{ gr} \times 1 \text{ supp}$$

$$10 \text{ gr} = \frac{10 \text{ gr} \times 1 \text{ supp}}{10 \text{ gr}}$$

$$X = 1 \text{ supp}$$

DOSAGE CALCULATIONS IN PARENTERAL DRUG THERAPY

Administering drugs in varied concentrations

When administering medications, you'll use the same ratio or fraction techniques you use for administering enteral drugs. To avoid dosage errors, remember to include the drug's concentration in your calculations.

Drugs such as epinephrine, heparin, and allergy serums are available in varied concentrations. So you must consider the drug's concentration when calculating dosages. Otherwise, you could make a serious — even lethal — medication error. To avoid a dosage error, make sure that drug concentrations are part of the calculation.

For example, a drug order calls for 0.2 mg epinephrine S.C. stat. The ampule is labeled "1 ml of 1:1,000 epinephrine." You need to calculate the correct volume of drug to inject:

1. Determine the strength of the solution based on its unlabeled ratio:

$$1{:}1{,}000 \text{ epinephrine} = 1\text{g}/1{,}000 \text{ ml}$$

2. Set up a proportion with this information and the desired dose:

$$1 \text{ g:}1{,}000 \text{ ml} :: 0.2 \text{ mg:X ml}$$

Before you can perform this calculation, however, you must convert grams to milligrams by using the conversion 1 g = 1,000 mg.

3. Restate the proportion with the converted units and solve for X:

$$1{,}000 \text{ mg:}1{,}000 \text{ ml} :: 0.2 \text{ mg:X ml}$$

$$1{,}000 \text{ ml} \times 0.2 \text{ mg} = 1{,}000 \text{ mg} \times X \text{ ml}$$

$$1{,}000 \text{ ml} \times 0.2 \text{ mg} = \frac{X}{1{,}000 \text{ mg}}$$

$$0.2 \text{ ml} = X$$

Calculating I.V. drip rates

To determine the I.V. drip rate, first set up a fraction showing the volume of infusion over the number of minutes in which that volume is to be infused. For example, if a patient is to receive 100 ml of solution within 1 hour, the fraction would be written as:

$$\frac{100 \text{ ml}}{60 \text{ min}}$$

Next, multiply the fraction by the drip factor (the number of drops contained in 1 ml) to determine the number of drops (gtt) per minute to be infused. The drip factor varies among I.V. administration sets; follow the manufacturer's guidelines (found on the administration set package) for the drip factor. Standard administration sets have drip factors of 10, 15, or 20 gtt/ml. A microdrip (minidrip) set has a drip factor of 60 gtt/ml. Which set you use depends on the rate and purpose of the infusion. (See *Determining I.V. tubing type*, page 126.)

Use the following equation to determine the drip rate per minute (min) of an I.V. solution:

$$\frac{\text{Total ml}}{\text{total min}} \times \begin{matrix}\text{drip}\\\text{factor}\end{matrix} = \begin{matrix}\text{drops/}\\\text{min}\end{matrix}$$

Note that the equation applies both to large-volume solutions that infuse over many hours and to small-volume solutions that infuse in less than 1 hour.

Flow rate

You can modify the equation by first determining the flow rate (the number of milliliters to be infused over 1 hour). For example, if the patient is to receive 1,000 ml over 8 hours, the fraction would be:

$$\text{flow rate} = \frac{1{,}000 \text{ ml}}{8 \text{ hours}}$$

In this example, the flow rate is 125 ml/hour. You will also use the flow rate when working with I.V. infusion pumps to set the number of milliliters to be delivered in 1 hour. You then divide the flow rate by 60 minutes. This fraction would be:

$$\text{rate per min} = \frac{125 \text{ ml /hour}}{60 \text{ min}}$$

In this example, the rate is 2.08 ml/minute, which can be rounded off to 2.1 ml/minute. The rate per minute is then multiplied by the drip factor (found on the administration tubing set package) to determine the number of drops per minute.

For example, if the drip factor of the administration set that you're using is 15 gtt/ml, the equation would be:

$$\begin{matrix}\text{drip}\\\text{rate}\end{matrix} = 2.1 \text{ ml/min} \times 15 \text{ gtt/ml}$$

In this example, the drip rate is 31.5 gtt/minute, which

Determining I.V. tubing type

Most health care facilities stock I.V. tubing in several sizes. Microdrip (minidrip) tubing delivers 60 gtt/ml, and standard or macrodrip tubing delivers 10, 15, or 20 gtt/ml, depending on the manufacturer.

Microdrip or macrodrip

The rate and purpose of the infusion determine whether the microdrip or macrodrip tubing should be used. For example, if a patient is to receive a solution at a rate of 125 ml/hour, macrodrip tubing is preferred. If microdrip tubing were used in this instance, the drip rate would be 125 gtt/minute, which is difficult to assess.

Conversely, if a patient is to receive a solution at a rate of 10 ml/hour, microdrip tubing is preferred. If macrodrip tubing with a drip factor of 15 gtt/ml were used, the drip rate would be 3 gtt/minute. Maintaining I.V. patency at this rate is nearly impossible.

Rule of thumb

A good rule of thumb for selecting I.V. tubing is to use a macrodrip tubing for any infusion with a rate of at least 80 ml/hour and microdrip tubing for any infusion with a rate of less than 80 ml/hour. Follow your facility's protocols.

Other factors

Usually only microdrip tubing is used with pediatric patients to prevent fluid overload.

When I.V. controllers and pumps are used, you must use the tubing specifically manufactured to work with that pump.

can be rounded off to 32 gtt/minute.

In practice, you may observe the drip rate for 15 seconds — sufficient time to determine whether the rate needs to be adjusted. To calculate the drip rate for 15 seconds (sec), divide the drip rate per minute by 4. In the example, the equation would be:

$$\text{drip rate for 15 sec} = \frac{32 \text{ gtt/min}}{4}$$

In this example, the drip rate is 8 gtt/15 seconds. You would then observe the drip chamber for 15 seconds to ensure that 8 drops are delivered.

Shortcuts
You also can use these quicker methods to compute I.V. infusion rates. For example, when using a microdrip set, determine the flow rate for 60 minutes. When you multiply by the drip factor (60 gtt/minute), the fractions cancel each other out: The flow rate equals the drip rate. For example, if the flow rate is 125 ml/60 minutes, the equation would be:

$$\begin{matrix}\text{125 gtt/min} \\ \text{(drip rate)}\end{matrix} = \frac{125 \text{ ml}}{60 \text{ min}} \times \frac{60 \text{ gtt}}{1 \text{ ml}}$$

In this example, the number of drops per minute (125) is the same as the number of milliliters of fluid per hour. Rather than spend time calculating the equation, you can simply use the number assigned to the flow rate as the drip rate.

For I.V. administration sets that deliver 10 gtt/ml, divide the flow rate by 6 to find the drip rate. For sets that deliver 15 gtt/ml, divide the flow rate by 4 to find the drip rate.

For sets that deliver 20 gtt/ml, divide the flow rate by 3 to find the drip rate. For example, if the ordered flow rate is 125 ml/hour and you're using an administration set with a drip factor of 10 gtt/ml), the equation would be:

$$\frac{125 \text{ ml}}{6} = 20.8 \text{ gtt/min}$$

In this example, the drip rate is 20.8 gtt/minute, which can be rounded off to 21 gtt/minute. The drip rate obtained is the same whether you use this quick method or one of the longer ones.

Practicing drip rate calculations

- A doctor's order calls for 500 ml of D_5W in 0.45% sodium chloride solution to infuse over 12 hours. You need to determine the drip rate for an administration set that delivers 15 gtt/ml.

  Use this equation:

$$X = \frac{500 \text{ ml}}{12 \text{ hours} \times 60 \text{ min}} \times 15 \text{ gtt/ml}$$

Multiply the number of hours by 60 minutes in the denominator of the fraction.

Divide the fraction and solve for X, the unknown factor:

$$X = 0.69 \text{ ml/min} \times 15 \text{ gtt/ml}$$
$$X = 10.35 \text{ gtt/min}$$

The drip rate is 10.35 gtt/minute, which can be rounded off to 10 gtt/minute.

- A doctor's order calls for 1,000 ml of D_5W given I.V. over 12 hours. You'll be using a Cutter administration tubing set (drip factor is 20 gtt/ml). What is the flow rate (the amount infused in 1 hour) and the drip rate?

To calculate the flow rate, set up this proportion, and solve for X:

$$\frac{1{,}000 \text{ ml}}{12 \text{ hours}} = \frac{X \text{ ml}}{1 \text{ hour}}$$

The flow rate is 83.3 ml/hour, which can be rounded off to 83 ml/hour.

To find the drip rate, set up this equation and solve for X:

$$X = \frac{83 \text{ ml}}{60 \text{ min}} \times \frac{20 \text{ gtt}}{1 \text{ ml}}$$

The drip rate is 27.6 gtt/minute, which can be rounded off to 28 gtt/minute. ■

Reconstituting a powder

Although the pharmacist may reconstitute powders for parenteral use, you may have to perform this task. If so, keep the following points in mind.

When reconstituting powders for injection, consult the drug label. It will give the total quantity of drug in the vial or ampule, the amount and type of diluent to add to the powder, and the strength and shelf life (expiration date) of the resulting solution.

When diluent is added to a powder, the powder increases the fluid volume. For this reason, the label calls for less diluent than the total volume of the prepared solution. For example, you may have to add 1.7 ml of diluent to a vial of powdered drug to obtain a 2-ml total volume of prepared solution. Follow the directions on the drug label.

Solution concentration

To determine how much solution to administer, use the manufacturer's information about the concentration of the solution.

For example, if you want to administer 500 mg of a drug and the concentration of the prepared solution is 1 g (1,000 mg) per 10 ml, you can set up a fraction proportion as follows:

$$\frac{X \text{ ml}}{500 \text{ mg}} = \frac{10 \text{ ml}}{1{,}000}$$

Solve for X, the unknown factor:

$$X \text{ ml} \times 1{,}000 \text{ mg} = 500 \text{ mg} \times 10 \text{ ml}$$

$$X = \frac{5{,}000 \text{ ml}}{1{,}000}$$

$$X = 5 \text{ ml}$$

If you prefer the ratio method, set up the proportion as follows:

$$X \text{ ml} : 500 \text{ mg} :: 10 \text{ ml} : 1{,}000 \text{ mg}$$

Solve for X, the unknown factor:

$$X \text{ ml} \times 1{,}000 \text{ mg} = 500 \text{ mg} \times 10 \text{ ml}$$

$$X = \frac{5{,}000 \text{ ml}}{1{,}000}$$

$$X = 5 \text{ ml}$$

By using either method (fraction or ratio), you would calculate that 5 ml of solution must be given so the patient receives 500 mg of the drug.

Practicing calculations

The doctor orders 500 mg of ampicillin for a patient. A 1-g vial of ampicillin as a powder is available. The label says, "Add 4.5 ml sterile water to yield 1 g/5 ml." How many milliliters of reconstituted ampicillin should you give the patient?

First, dilute the powder according to the instructions.

- The concentration listed on the label provides the first part of the proportion:

$$\frac{1 \text{ g}}{5 \text{ ml}}$$

- Next, make sure the same units of measure appear in both denominators of the proportion. In this case, the units must both be grams or milligrams. If you use milligrams and the fraction method, the proportion would be:

$$\frac{X \text{ ml}}{500 \text{ mg}} = \frac{5 \text{ ml}}{1{,}000 \text{ mg}}$$

- Solve for X:

$$X \text{ ml} \times 1{,}000 \text{ mg} = 500 \text{ mg} \times 5 \text{ ml}$$

$$X = \frac{2{,}500 \text{ ml}}{1{,}000}$$

$$X = 2.5 \text{ ml}$$

Give 2.5 ml of the solution, which will deliver 500 mg of ampicillin.

Some medications that require reconstitution are packaged in vials that have two chambers separated by a rubber stopper. The upper chamber contains the diluent and the lower chamber contains the powdered drug. When you depress the top of the vial, the rubber stopper between the two chambers dislodges, allowing the diluent to flow into the lower chamber, where it mixes with the powdered drug. Then you can remove the correct amount of solution with a syringe. ■

PART TWO

DRUG ALERTS

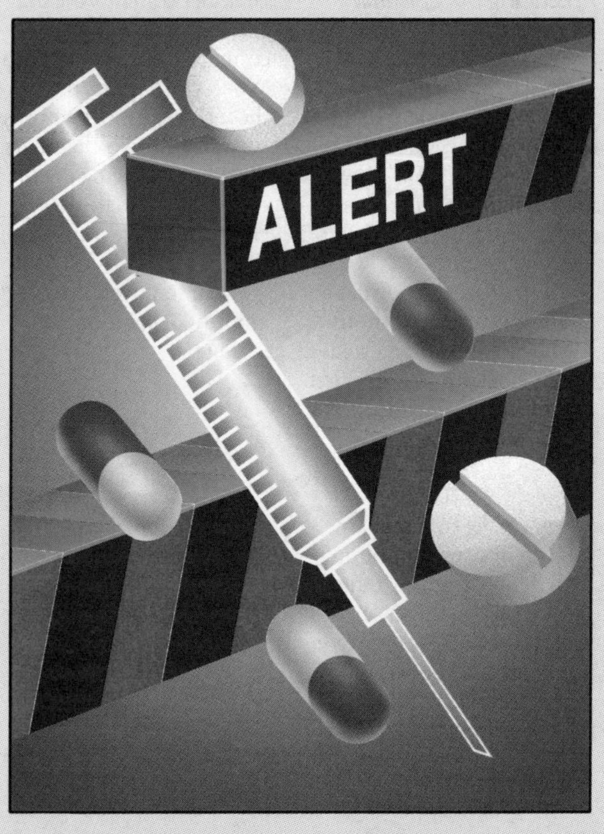

CHAPTER 5

GIVING LIFE-SUPPORT DRUGS

CHOOSING THE ROUTE

I.V. infusion

An I.V. line lets you administer drugs quickly during cardiopulmonary arrest. Typically, an infusion of D_5W maintains I.V. access. However, using normal saline or lactated Ringer's solution causes fewer complications.

If the patient is suffering from acute blood loss, fluids may also be administered to expand circulating blood volume. Whole blood; crystalloid solutions, such as lactated Ringer's or normal saline solution; or colloid solutions, such as human serum albumin, may all be used.

Using a peripheral vein
If the patient doesn't already have a patent I.V. line, start a peripheral I.V. line as soon as possible after beginning cardiopulmonary resuscitation (CPR), performing defibrillation (when indicated), and establishing a patent airway. A peripheral vein is usually chosen because resuscitation efforts would have to be interrupted to insert a central line.

The peripheral line is inserted through the antecubital or external jugular veins. Once the line is inserted, administer medications by rapid I.V. push, following each drug with a bolus of 20 ml of I.V. fluid. Keep in mind that drugs require 1 to 2 minutes to reach the central circulation through peripheral veins, so peak drug levels will be lower and circulation time will be increased when using a peripheral line instead of a central line.

To speed the drug's circulation time, elevate the patient's extremity.

Using a central line
A central line allows drugs to arrive more rapidly at their site of action. If spontaneous circulation doesn't return after initial drug administration through a peripheral vein, the doctor may insert a central line into the supraclavicular subclavian or internal jugular vein. Either one of these central-line routes causes less interruption of chest compressions than the infraclavicular route.

The doctor may also choose to pass a peripherally inserted central catheter, extending above the diaphragm, into the femoral vein. (A short femoral venous line should not be used for administering drugs during CPR because little cephalad flow occurs below the diaphragm.) ■

Endotracheal administration

If you can't immediately obtain venous access and if the patient has an endotracheal (ET) tube, you can administer drugs through it. Lidocaine, epinephrine, and atropine may all be administered through an ET tube.

Drugs administered via an ET tube require 2 to 2½ times the recommended I.V. dose.

To administer, dilute the drug with 10 ml of normal saline solution or distilled water. Then, during a pause in chest compressions, slide a catheter beyond the tip of the ET tube, attach the medication-filled syringe with the needle removed, and quickly spray in the drug. Give several quick insufflations to aerosolize the medication and hasten absorption; then resume chest compressions. ■

Intraosseous administration

Drugs may be given by the intraosseous route when I.V. access isn't readily available. This is especially desirable in pediatric patients. The intraosseous dose is the same as the I.V dose. However, some evidence suggests that a higher dose may be necessary, especially when giving intraosseous epinephrine. ■

GIVING DRUGS THAT CONTROL HEART RATE AND RHYTHM

Adenosine

Because this drug depresses activity of the AV node and sinus node, it's not useful in treating atrial flutter, atrial fibrillation, or atrial or ventricular tachycardia. However, by producing transient AV or ventriculoatrial block, adenosine can confirm the diagnosis of one of these conditions.

Special considerations

- Administration of adenosine is contraindicated in patients receiving dipyridamole and carbamazepine.
- Patients taking theophylline may require a higher dosage of adenosine.
- Common but transient side effects include flushing, dyspnea, and chest pain (which should resolve within 1 to 2 minutes).
- After adenosine therapy to treat supraventricular tachycardia, transient periods of sinus bradycardia may occur. ■

Atropine

This drug reverses hypotension and systemic vascular resistance. Useful in treating sinus bradycardia, it may also help treat AV block at the nodal level or ventricular asystole.

Special considerations

- Atropine increases oxygen demand and can also trigger tachyarrhythmias. Therefore, only patients in complete cardiac arrest should receive the total vagolytic dose.
- Also use caution when administering atropine to patients with acute myocardial ischemia or infarction. An excessive increase in heart rate may worsen the ischemia or increase the zone of infarction. ■

Bretylium

This drug treats resistant ventricular tachycardia and ventricular fibrillation that doesn't respond to defibrillation, epinephrine, or lidocaine.

Special considerations

- Initially after injection, bretylium triggers the release of catecholamines. This is followed by a postganglionic adrenergic action, which frequently induces hypotension.
- The patient may also receive a continuous infusion of bretylium. During such an infusion, continue cardiac and hemodynamic monitoring. ■

Diltiazem

This calcium channel blocker slows conduction and increases refraction in the AV node. Diltiazem may also control the ventricular response rate in patients with atrial fibrillation, atrial flutter, or multifocal atrial tachycardia.

As effective as verapamil, diltiazem also causes less myocardial depression. It may also be used as a maintenance I.V. infusion to control the ventricular rate in atrial fibrillation.

Special consideration

Because diltiazem also decreases contractility in the myocardium, it can exacerbate CHF in patients with severe left ventricular dysfunction. ■

Isoproterenol

This drug increases cardiac output and myocardial work, which can worsen ischemia and arrhythmias in patients with ischemic heart disease. Therefore, isoproterenol should only be given to patients with refractory torsades de pointes or to control symptomatic bradycardia in heart transplant patients until a pacemaker can be inserted. However, it is not the drug of choice for either of these conditions.

Special considerations

- At low doses, isoproterenol can raise blood pressure. However, at high doses, it is harmful.
- Isoproterenol shouldn't be used to treat hypotension or cardiac arrest. ■

Lidocaine

Lidocaine is the antiarrhythmic drug of choice for treating ventricular ectopy, ventricular tachycardia (VT), and ventricular fibrillation (VF). Prophylactic administration of lidocaine in uncomplicated acute MI is no longer recommended unless VT and VF persist after defibrillation and administration of epinephrine.

Special considerations

- Keep in mind that the half-life of lidocaine increases after 24 to 48 hours. Therefore, check with the patient's doctor about either reducing the patient's dose after 24 hours or monitoring the patient's blood level of the drug.
- Also monitor the patient for signs of drug efficacy and toxicity. Signs of toxicity include slurred speech, altered level of consciousness, muscle twitching, and seizures. If any of these occur, call the patient's doctor immediately. ■

Magnesium

Because a lack of magnesium can trigger arrhythmias, this drug is often used to treat ventricular fibrillation, ventricular tachycardia, and torsades de pointes. Magnesium may also be given to patients after MI to reduce the incidence of ventricular arrhythmias.

Special consideration

Administer cautiously to prevent severe hypotension or asystole. ■

Procainamide

This drug suppresses PVCs and recurrent ventricular tachycardia. Procainamide is typically given when lidocaine is either contraindicated or fails to suppress ventricular ectopy.

Special considerations

- Give the drug slowly while monitoring the patient's ECG and blood pressure. Hypotension may occur with rapid administration.

- Patients with renal failure should receive a reduced maintenance dose.
- Monitor blood levels in patients with renal failure and in patients receiving a constant infusion of more than 3 mg/minute for more than 24 hours.
- Procainamide should not be used in patients with preexisting QT prolongation and torsades de pointes. It should be used cautiously in patients with acute MI. ■

Verapamil

This calcium channel blocker slows conduction and increases refraction in the AV node. This makes verapamil effective for treating patients with atrial fibrillation, atrial flutter, or multifocal atrial tachycardia. Although not the drug of choice, verapamil can also help treat narrow-complex paroxysmal supraventricular tachycardia.

Special consideration
Because verapamil may decrease myocardial contractility, it can aggravate CHF in patients with severe left ventricular dysfunction. ■

GIVING DRUGS THAT IMPROVE CARDIAC OUTPUT AND BLOOD PRESSURE

Dobutamine

Used to treat heart failure, dobutamine increases myocardial contractility and reduces reflex peripheral vasodilation. In high doses, when the heart rate is increased more than 10%, dobutamine may exacerbate myocardial ischemia.

Special consideration
During administration, monitor the patient's hemodynamic status to optimize the effectiveness of the drug. ■

Dopamine

At low doses, dopamine dilates renal and mesenteric blood vessels and increases cardiac output without significantly increasing heart rate, blood pressure, or pulmonary occlusive pressure.

However, higher doses may cause vasoconstriction as well as increased pulmonary occlusive pressure. During resuscitation, dopamine is used to treat hypotension occurring with symptomatic bradycardia or after the return of spontaneous circulation.

Special considerations

- During administration, closely monitor the patient's hemodynamic status. If tachycardia results, notify the patient's doctor. The dosage may have to be reduced or drug administration stopped.
- Always taper the dose gradually. Never abruptly withdraw the drug.
- Because alkaline solutions inactivate dopamine, never mix it in the same I.V. line as sodium bicarbonate. ■

Epinephrine

This drug increases cardiac and cerebral blood flow. It's the first drug given when the patient fails to respond to initial cardiopulmonary resuscitation, intubation and ventilation, and initial defibrillations. And, although it's not the drug of choice, it can also help treat symptomatic bradycardia.

Special consideration

Don't administer epinephrine in the same line with alkaline solutions. ■

Nitroglycerin

This drug relaxes vascular smooth muscle. It's the treatment of choice for angina pectoris (given sublingually) and CHF and unstable angina (given I.V.). When used along with dobutamine, it improves the patient's hemodynamic status while reducing the risk of ischemic damage.

Special considerations

- Low doses produce vasodilation; higher doses may also cause arteriolar dilation. However, as a general rule, the effect of nitroglycerin depends more on the patient's intravascular volume status than on the drug dosage. For example, hypovolemia will dull the hemodynamic effects of nitroglycerin, resulting in an increased risk of hypotension.
- Hypotension, which may exacerbate myocardial ischemia, is the main toxic effect of nitroglycerin. (Drug-induced hypotension usually responds well to fluid replacement therapy, however.) Other toxic effects of nitroglycerin include tachycardia, paradoxical bradycardia, hyperemia, methemoglobinemia, and headache.
- When administering nitroglycerin to a patient with

CHF, closely monitor his hemodynamic status. ■

Sodium bicarbonate

This drug may help patients with preexisting metabolic acidosis, hyperkalemia, or TCA or phenobarbital overdose.

Give sodium bicarbonate only after defibrillation, cardiac compression, intubation, ventilation, and more than one trial of epinephrine have been used.

Special consideration
After administration, obtain an arterial blood gas (ABG) analysis. By providing information about the patient's base deficit or bicarbonate concentration, ABG analysis will help guide bicarbonate therapy. ■

Sodium nitroprusside

A fast-acting and powerful direct peripheral vasodilator, sodium nitroprusside is used to treat heart failure and hypertension. It works by reducing peripheral arterial resistance (afterload) while increasing cardiac output, which minimizes the drop in systemic blood pressure and heart rate. This results in the following effects:

- direct vasodilation
- decreased left ventricular filling
- relief of pulmonary congestion
- decreased left ventricular volume and pressure
- enhanced systolic emptying
- reduced left ventricular volume and wall stress
- reduced pulmonary pressure, leading to a relief of pulmonary congestion
- decreased myocardial oxygen consumption.

Special considerations

- Use an infusion pump to administer nitroprusside and, because the drug deteriorates when exposed to light, wrap the tubing in opaque material.
- During administration, closely monitor the patient's hemodynamic status.
- Hypotension is the major complication of nitroprusside administration. Other possible side effects include headache, nausea, vomiting, and abdominal cramping.
- Be alert for signs of cyanide or thiocyanate toxicity, particularly in patients with renal or hepatic insufficiency. Signs of cyanide toxicity include confusion, hyperreflexia, and seizures. If such signs occur, stop the infusion and notify the patient's doctor immediately.
- Sodium nitrite and sodium thiosulfate may be administered if the patient shows signs of toxicity. ■

ADMINISTERING LIFE-SUPPORT DRUGS

ALERT

Giving life-support drugs to adults

DRUG, ROUTE, AND DOSAGE	PRECAUTIONS
adenosine *I.V. push:* 6 mg I.V. initially by rapid bolus over 1 to 3 seconds. If no response in 1 to 2 min, give 12 mg I.V.	▪ Contraindicated in patients receiving dipyridamole and carbamazepine. ▪ Patients receiving theophylline may require larger doses.
atropine ***To treat bradycardia*** *I.V. push*: 0.5 to 1.0 mg I.V. q 3 to 5 min, up to 3 mg total. ***To treat asystole*** *I.V. push:* 1 mg I.V.; repeat in 3 to 5 min if asystole persists. *I.V. infusion:* Not recommended. *Endotracheal:* May be used 2 to 2½ times the I.V. dose diluted in 10 ml of normal saline solution or sterile water.	▪ Lower doses (<0.5 mg) may cause bradycardia. ▪ Higher doses (>3 mg) may cause full vagal blockage. ▪ Use cautiously in presence of acute MI or ischemia.
bretylium *I.V. push:* Rapidly administer 5 mg/kg; can be increased to 10 mg/kg and repeated q 5 min. Maximum dose is 30 to 35 mg/kg. *I.V. infusion:* 500 mg diluted with at least 50 ml D_5W or dextrose 5% in normal saline solution; infuse at 1 to 2 mg/min.	▪ Not typically used to treat ventricular fibrillation (VF) or ventricular tachycardia (VT) unless other drugs fail. ▪ May lower blood pressure.

(continued)

ALERT

Giving life-support drugs to adults *(continued)*

DRUG, ROUTE, AND DOSAGE	PRECAUTIONS
calcium chloride *I.V. push:* Administer 2 to 4 mg/kg of 10% solution; can be repeated q 10 min. *I.V. infusion:* Not generally recommended. (Calcium gluceptate in dose of 5 to 7 ml and calcium gluconate 5 to 8 ml.)	▪ Contraindicated in patients with hypercalcemia. ▪ Infiltration may cause severe tissue damage. ▪ Use cautiously in patients receiving digoxin; may cause arrhythmias. ▪ Don't give to patients with high serum phosphate levels; may produce fatal calcium deposits. ▪ Don't mix with other medications. ▪ Administration is probably helpful in calcium channel blocker toxicity or in presence of hyperkalemia or hypocalcemia; otherwise should not be used.
dobutamine hydrochloride *I.V. push:* Not recommended. *I.V. infusion:* Reconstitute with D5W or normal saline solution; then prepare standard dilution, and administer 2 to 20 mcg/kg/min.	▪ Don't use with beta blockers such as propranolol. ▪ Drug is incompatible with alkaline solutions. ▪ Patients with atrial fibrillation should receive digoxin first, or they may develop rapid ventricular response. ▪ Infiltration may cause severe tissue damage.

ALERT

Giving life-support drugs to adults *(continued)*

DRUG, ROUTE, AND DOSAGE	PRECAUTIONS
dopamine hydrochloride *I.V. push:* Not recommended. *I.V. infusion:* Standard dilution. May use with D_5W, dextrose 5% in normal saline solution, or combination of D_5W and normal saline solution; administer 2.5 to 5 mcg/kg/min; then titrate to desired effect with a final dosage of 5 to 20 mcg/kg/min.	▪ May precipitate vasoconstriction in high doses. ▪ May induce tachycardia. ▪ Drug is incompatable with alkaline solutions. ▪ Infiltration may cause severe tissue damage. ▪ Norepinephrine should be added if dopamine dosage exceeds 20 mcg/kg/min.
epinephrine *I.V. push:* Administer 10 ml of 1:10,000 solution (1 mg) q 3 to 5 min, then 20 ml of I.V. fluid to ensure delivery. *Intracardiac:* Administer 5 ml of 1:10,000 solution. *I.V. infusion:* 30 ml of 1:10,000 solution in 250 ml of normal saline solution or D_5W at 100 ml/hr. *Endotracheal:* 2 to 2½ times the I.V. dose.	▪ Increases intraocular pressure. ▪ May exacerbate CHF, arrhythmias, angina pectoris, hyperthyroidism, and emphysema. ▪ May cause headaches, tremors, or palpitations. ▪ Don't administer with alkaline solutions.

(continued)

ALERT

Giving life-support drugs to adults *(continued)*

DRUG, ROUTE, AND DOSAGE	PRECAUTIONS
lidocaine *I.V. push:* 1.0 to 1.5 mg/kg initially, then boluses of 0.5 to 1.5 mg/kg q 5 to 10 min to total of 3 mg/kg. Total dose should not exceed 300 mg/hr. *I.V. infusion:* Standard dilution. Administer 2 to 4 mg/min.	▪ Don't mix with sodium bicarbonate. ▪ Don't use if patient has high-grade SA or AV block. ▪ Discontinue if PR interval or QRS complex widens or if arrhythmias worsen. ▪ May lead to CNS toxicity.
procainamide *I.V. push:* Give 20 mg/min, up to total of 17 mg/kg (in emergency, may give up to 30 mg/min, up to total of 17 mg/kg). *I.V. infusion:* Administer 1 to 4 mg/min.	▪ Too-rapid injection can cause precipitous hypotension. ▪ Avoid use in patients with preexisting QT prolongation and torsades de pointes.
sodium bicarbonate *I.V. push:* 1 mEq/kg initially, then a half dose q 10 min.	▪ Don't mix with epinephrine, dopamine, or dobutamine. ▪ Forms an insoluble precipitate when mixed with calcium salts.
sodium nitroprusside *I.V. push:* 0.1 to 5 mcg/kg/min (up to total of 10 mcg/kg/min).	▪ May cause cyanide or thiocyanate toxicity in patients with hepatic or renal insufficiency. ▪ Wrap solution and tubing in opaque material to prevent deterioration when exposed to light. ▪ Use an infusion pump. ▪ May cause hypotension.

ALERT

Giving life-support drugs to children

DRUG, ROUTE, AND DOSAGE	PRECAUTIONS
adenosine ***To treat supraventricular tachycardia*** *I.V. push:* 0.1 to 0.2 mg/kg given as rapid bolus. Maximum single dose is 12 mg.	▪ Very effective. ▪ Minimal side effects.
atropine sulfate ***To treat bradycardia accompanied by poor perfusion or hypotension*** *I.V. push:* 0.02 mg/kg per dose. Minimum dose is 0.1. mg. Maximum single dose is 0.5 mg in a child and 1 mg in an adolescent.	▪ I.V. dose may be administered endotracheally but absorption is unreliable. ▪ Used to treat bradycardia only after ensuring adequate oxygenation and ventilation. ▪ Tachycardia may follow use of atropine in children but drug is usually well tolerated.
bretylium ***To correct ventricular fibrillation (VF) if defibrillation and lidocaine are ineffective*** *I.V. push:* 5 mg/kg rapidly; may be increased to 10 mg/kg if VF persists after second defibrillation attempt.	▪ Has been effective in adults with VF unresponsive to electrical defibrillation. No published data available on effectiveness in children.

(continued)

ALERT

Giving life-support drugs to children *(continued)*

DRUG, ROUTE, AND DOSAGE	PRECAUTIONS
calcium chloride 10% *I.V. push emergency dose:* 0.2 ml/kg to provide 20 mg/kg of the salt and 5.4 mg/kg of elemental calcium.	▪ Give slowly and repeat in 10 minutes if necessary. ▪ Calcium chloride is preparation of choice because it provides greater bioavailability than calcium gluconate. ▪ Recommended for treatment of electromechanical dissociation and systole, but this use has not been proved. ▪ Currently only indicated for documented hypocalcemia, hyperkalemia, and calcium channel blocker overdose.
dobutamine hydrochloride ***To treat low cardiac output and poor myocardial function*** *I.V. infusion:* 2 to 20 mcg/kg/min titrated to patient response.	▪ Response to drug varies widely. ▪ Higher-than-recommended infusion rates may produce tachycardia or ventricular ectopy.
dopamine hydrochloride ***To treat circulatory shock after resuscitation or when shock is unresponsive to fluid administration*** *I.V. infusion:* 2 to 20 mcg/kg/min.	▪ Infuse through a well-estabished I.V. line. ▪ Infiltration into tissues can produce local necrosis. ▪ If still ineffective when dose is 20 mcg/kg/min, administer epinephrine or dobutamine rather than increase dopamine dose above 20 mcg/kg/ min.

ALERT

Giving life-support drugs to children *(continued)*

DRUG, ROUTE, AND DOSAGE	PRECAUTIONS
epinephrine ***For bradycardia*** *I.V. push or intraosseous:* 0.01 mg/kg (1:10,000). *Endotracheal:* 0.1 mg/kg (1:1,000).	▪ When using different concentrations of epinephrine in the same patient, take care to avoid errors.
For asystolic or pulseless arrest First dose *I.V. push or intraosseous:* 0.01 mg/kg (1:10,000). *Endotracheal:* 0.1 mg/kg (1:1,000). Doses as high as 0.2 mg/kg may be effective. Subsequent doses *I.V. push, intraosseous, or endotracheal:* 0.1 mg/kg (1:1,000). Doses as high as 0.2 mg/kg may be effective.	▪ Be aware of effective dose of preservatives administered (if preservatives are present in the epinephrine preparation) when high doses are used. ▪ Administer second dose within 3 to 5 min after initial dose. Repeat doses q 3 to 5 min during resuscitation.
To maintain spontaneous circulation *I.V. infusion:* Begin at 0.1 mcg/kg/min; then titrate to desired effect (0.1 mcg/kg/min). In cases of asystole, may infuse a higher dose.	▪ Infuse only through a well-established I.V. line and preferably through a central line. ▪ Monitor infusion site closely for infiltration. ▪ Inactivated in alkaline solutions; never mix epinephrine with sodium bicarbonate. ▪ High doses may produce excessive vasoconstriction, resulting in compromised mesenteric, renal, and extremity blood flow.

(continued)

ALERT

Giving life-support drugs to children *(continued)*

DRUG, ROUTE, AND DOSAGE	PRECAUTIONS
lidocaine ***To treat ventricular ectopy and raise VF threshold*** *I.V. push:* 1 mg/kg per dose. *I.V. infusion:* 20 to 50 mcg/kg/min.	▪ If possible, administer before synchronized cardioversion of ventricular tachycardia that occurs with a pulse. ▪ Lidocaine infusion rate should not exceed 20 mcg/kg/min in patients with reduced drug clearance ability (shock, CHF, or cardiac arrest).
sodium bicarbonate ***To treat metabolic acidosis accompanying prolonged cardiac arrest*** *I.V. push or intraosseous:* 1 mEq/kg per dose or 0.3 × kg × base deficit.	▪ Infuse slowly and only if patient has adequate ventilation. ▪ In cardiac arrest, administer after effective ventilation is established and epinephrine plus chest compressions provide maximum circulation. ▪ Subsequent doses should be based on arterial blood gas (ABG) analysis but may be considered after every 10 minutes of cardiac arrest if ABG analysis is unavailable. ▪ A dilute solution (0.5 mEq/ml) may be used in neonates. ▪ Irrigate the I.V. tubing carefully between infusion of catecholamines or calcium and sodium bicarbonate.

CHAPTER 6

HEEDING CAUTIONS AND WARNINGS

Recognizing drug hazards

Observing cautions

RECOGNIZING DRUG HAZARDS

Drug expiration dates and storage recommendations

To ensure that a drug is as potent and therapeutically effective as intended, carefully observe expiration dates, and follow storage recommendations provided by the manufacturer or pharmacy.

Importance of heeding expiration dates

Federal regulations require that expiration dates appear on all drug containers. The regulations stipulate that at least 90% of the active ingredient must be available up to the expiration date, ensuring that a patient doesn't receive a drug that's no longer therapeutically active or that has degraded to toxic compounds. Hospital pharmacists relabel expiration dates on oral drugs that are repackaged for hospital use. Parenteral drugs are given new expiration dates after being reconstituted or mixed with I.V. fluids.

Importance of storing drugs properly

Drug storage can affect stability and, ultimately, therapeutic effectiveness. Drugs degrade more rapidly in warm, humid conditions. The USP uses these terms to describe drug storage conditions:

- *Freeze:* Store below 0° C (32° F).
- *Store in a cold place:* Temperature should not exceed 15° C (59° F).
- *Refrigerate:* Store at 2° to 15° C (36° to 59° F).
- *Avoid excessive heat:* Temperature should not exceed 40° C (104° F).

Tablets and capsules can be stored safely at room temperature unless otherwise specified. Room temperature is generally accepted as being between 15° and 30° C (59° and 86° F).

Liquid dose forms and injectable drugs sometimes require refrigeration. Use medication refrigerators only for drug storage, and keep a thermometer inside to monitor the temperature. Return expired drugs or drugs belonging to discharged patients to the pharmacy.

Some drugs also must be protected from light. For example, nitroglycerin should be stored in light-resistant bottles. Remind patients to store medications in a cabinet or other dark place. Tell them not to transfer medications to different containers to take to work or on vacation. Always check labels for storage requirements. ■

ALERT

Dialyzable drugs

The amount of a drug removed by dialysis differs among patients and depends on several factors, including the patient's condition, the drug's properties, the length of dialysis and the dialysate used, the rate of blood flow or the dwell time, and the purpose of dialysis. The chart below provides general guidelines: Don't assume a dosage adjustment should be made until you consult the patient's doctor or pharmacist.

DRUG	REDUCED BY HEMODIALYSIS
acetaminophen	Yes (may not influence toxicity)
acyclovir	Yes
allopurinol	Yes
alprazolam	No
amikacin	Yes
aminoglutethimide	Yes
amiodarone	No
amitriptyline	No
amoxicillin	Yes
amoxicillin/clavulanate potassium	Yes
amphotericin B	No
ampicillin	Yes
ampicillin/clavulanate potassium	Yes
aspirin	Yes

ALERT

Dialyzable drugs *(continued)*

DRUG	REDUCED BY HEMODIALYSIS
atenolol	Yes
azathioprine	Yes
azlocillin	Yes
aztreonam	Yes
bretylium	Yes
captopril	Yes
carbamazepine	No
carbenicillin	Yes
carmustine	No
carprofen	No
cefaclor	Yes
cefadroxil	Yes
cefamandole	Yes
cefazolin	Yes
cefonicid	Yes (only slightly [20%])
cefoperazone	Yes
cefotaxime	Yes
cefotetan	Yes (only slightly [20%])
cefoxitin	Yes
ceftazidime	Yes

(continued)

ALERT

Dialyzable drugs *(continued)*

DRUG	REDUCED BY HEMODIALYSIS
ceftizoxime	Yes
ceftriaxone	No
cefuroxime	Yes
cephalexin	Yes
cephalothin	Yes
cephapirin	Yes
cephradine	Yes
chloral hydrate	Yes
chlorambucil	No
chloramphenicol	Yes
chlordiazepoxide	No
chloroquine	No
chlorpheniramine	No
chlorpromazine	No
chlorprothixene	No
chlorthalidone	No
cimetidine	Yes
ciprofloxacin	Yes (only slightly [20%])
cisplatin	Maybe (within 3 hours after administration)
clindamycin	No

ALERT

Dialyzable drugs *(continued)*

DRUG	REDUCED BY HEMODIALYSIS
clofibrate	No
clonazepam	No
clonidine	No
clorazepate	No
cloxacillin	No
colchicine	No
cortisone	No
co-trimoxazole	Yes
cyclophosphamide	Yes
diazepam	No
diazoxide	No
diclofenac	No
dicloxacillin	No
digitoxin	No
digoxin	No
diphenhydramine	No
dipyridamole	Yes
disopyramide	Yes
doxepin	No
doxorubicin	No

(continued)

ALERT

Dialyzable drugs *(continued)*

DRUG	REDUCED BY HEMODIALYSIS
doxycycline	No
enalapril	Yes
erythromycin	No
ethacrynic acid	No
ethambutol	Yes (only slightly [20%])
ethchlorvynol	Yes
ethosuximide	Yes
famotidine	No
fenoprofen	No
flecainide	No
flucytosine	Yes
fluorouracil	Yes
flurazepam	No
furosemide	No
ganciclovir	Yes
gentamicin	Yes
glutethimide	Yes
glyburide	No
haloperidol	No
heparin	No
hydralazine	No

ALERT

Dialyzable drugs *(continued)*

DRUG	REDUCED BY HEMODIALYSIS
hydrochlorothiazide	No
hydroxyzine	No
ibuprofen	No
imipenem/cilastatin	Yes
imipramine	No
indomethacin	No
insulin	No
isoniazid	Yes
isosorbide	No
kanamycin	Yes
ketoconazole	No
ketoprofen	Maybe (substantial removal by dialysis is unlikely because the drug is highly [99%] protein bound)
labetalol	No
lidocaine	No
lithium	Yes
lomustine	No
lorazepam	No
mechlorethamine	No
mefenamic acid	No

(continued)

ALERT

Dialyzable drugs *(continued)*

DRUG	REDUCED BY HEMODIALYSIS
mercaptopurine	Yes
methadone	No
methicillin	No
methotrexate	Yes
methyldopa	Yes
methylprednisolone	Yes
metoclopramide	No
metolazone	No
metoprolol	No
metronidazole	Yes
mexiletine	No
mezlocillin	Yes
miconazole	No
minocycline	No
minoxidil	Yes
morphine	No
nadolol	Yes
nafcillin	No
naproxen	No
netilmicin	Yes
nifedipine	No

ALERT

Dialyzable drugs *(continued)*

DRUG	REDUCED BY HEMODIALYSIS
nitroglycerin	No
nitroprusside	Yes
nortriptyline	No
oxacillin	No
oxazepam	No
penicillin G	Yes
pentazocine	Yes
phenobarbital	Yes
phenylbutazone	No
phenytoin	No
piperacillin	Yes
prazepam	No
prazosin	No
prednisone	No
primidone	Yes
procainamide	Yes
propoxyphene	No
propranolol	No
protriptyline	No
quinidine	No

(continued)

ALERT

Dialyzable drugs *(continued)*

DRUG	REDUCED BY HEMODIALYSIS
ranitidine	Yes
reserpine	No
rifampin	No
streptomycin	Yes
sucralfate	No
sulbactam	Yes
sulfamethoxazole	Yes
temazepam	No
terfenadine	No
theophylline	Yes
ticarcillin	Yes
timolol	No
tobramycin	Yes
tocainide	Yes
tolbutamide	No
triazolam	No
trimethoprim	Yes
valproic acid	No
vancomycin	No
verapamil	No
vidarabine	Yes

Drugs whose forms can't be altered

Patients who have trouble ingesting tablets or capsules often prefer that their medication be crushed or altered in some way. But this isn't always possible. Because of their release rates, unusual dosages, or other peculiarities, certain drugs must be swallowed whole, and their forms shouldn't be altered.

Sustained-release tablets and capsules

Medications that come in these forms are designed to dissolve and release medication slowly. In reality, they release a drug at a constant rate or periodically over time and have two advantages: They are long-lasting and cause few side effects. Crushing them, however, releases too much of the drug too quickly, which may in turn cause side effects. Moreover, the positive effects of the drug may not last as long, and the patient's symptoms may recur before his next scheduled dose.

You can open sustained-release capsules and mix their contents carefully with a liquid or soft food. But don't mix the beads too vigorously or they'll break, causing the same undesirable effects as tablet crushing.

Some terms that indicate sustained-release drugs include Dura-Tab, Extentabs, Gradumets, Gyrocaps, Repetabs, Sequels, Spansules, and Tembids. Similarly, the following abbreviations indicate that drugs are sustained-release: Bid, CR, Dur, LA, Plateau Cap, SA, Span, and SR.

Some examples of sustained-release tablets and capsules include Artane Sequels, Compazine Spansules, Desoxyn Gradumets, and Dimetane Extentabs.

Enteric-coated tablets

This type of medication is specially treated to break down in the small intestine. Examples include bisacodyl and ferrous sulfate. If the outer coating of the tablet is destroyed, the drug is absorbed in the stomach and may be inactivated or cause side effects. Thus, besides preventing premature drug release, the tablet's coating protects the stomach from irritation; crushing the tablet destroys the coating.

Not all covered tablets are enteric. For example, sugar- and film-coated tablets can be crushed. Some examples of enteric-coated tablets are Azulfidine En-Tabs, Dulcolax, Ecotrin, and E-Mycin.

Sublingual and buccal tablets
These tablets, such as nitroglycerin and isosorbide, are intended to be absorbed by veins under the tongue or in the cheek. The sublingual and buccal routes allow the drug to bypass the liver (avoiding the first-pass effect) and protect the drug from contact with other drugs, food, and GI secretions that affect its potency or bioavailability. Crushing these tablets causes the drug to be inactivated because most of it is rapidly metabolized elsewhere — for example, in the liver. These routes produce higher blood levels than the oral route, so dosages are usually smaller.

Miscellaneous drugs
Some drugs can't be altered because of their active properties or peculiar dosages. Depakene, for example, comes in a liquid-filled capsule that, when opened, irritates the lining of the mouth. Some other drugs that can't be altered are Ery-Tab, Inderal LA, Nitrospan, and Ritalin-SR.

Administration guidelines
To determine whether a drug can be altered, read the package labeling or instructions inside. Then ask your pharmacist, who will know whether a drug can be crushed or if it's available in a liquid. He can also suggest transdermal patches or rectal suppositories, but if you substitute these, the dosage may need adjustment. If no alternatives are available, the patient's doctor may prescribe a different drug. ■

Chemotherapeutic drugs

Staff members who prepare and give chemotherapeutic drugs face a significant risk. Although the extent of the risk hasn't been fully determined, antineoplastics increase the handler's risk of reproductive abnormalities and may also cause hematologic problems. Long-term exposure to chemotherapeutic drugs may damage the liver and chromosomes, and direct exposure may burn and damage the skin. These drugs also pose certain environmental dangers. Therefore, take special care whenever handling chemotherapeutic drugs.

OSHA guidelines
The Occupational Safety and Health Administration (OSHA) has set guidelines to help ensure the safety of both the handler and the environment. These guidelines include two basic requirements:

- All health care workers who handle chemotherapeutic drugs should be specifically trained for this task, with an emphasis on reducing exposure while handling these drugs.
- The drugs must be prepared within a class II biological safety cabinet. This type of cabinet uses vertical air flow (instead of laminar or horizontal air flow) that creates an air barrier in the cabinet's work area. Any powder or liquid that escapes from the drug vials is trapped by the vertical air flow and drawn into filters.

Safety equipment

To protect yourself and the environment, wear a long-sleeved gown, latex surgical gloves, a mask, and a face shield or goggles. Make sure you have eyewash, a plastic absorbent pad, alcohol sponges, sterile gauze pads, shoe covers, and an impervious container with a biohazard label for the disposal of any unused drug or equipment.

Also keep a chemotherapeutic spill kit available. To create such a kit, you need a water-resistant, nonpermeable, long-sleeved gown with cuffs and back closure; shoe covers; two pairs of high-grade, extra-thick latex gloves (for double-gloving); a face shield or goggles; a mask; a disposable dustpan and a plastic scraper (for collecting broken glass); plastic-lined or absorbent towels; a container of desiccant powder or granules (to absorb wet contents); two disposable sponges; a puncture-proof, leakproof container with a biohazard-waste label; and a container of 70% isopropyl alcohol for cleaning the spill area.

Drug preparation

Prepare the prescribed chemotherapeutic drugs according to current product instructions and with attention to compatibility, stability, and reconstitution technique.

Wash your hands before and after drug preparation and administration. Prepare the drugs in a class II biological safety cabinet. Wear protective garments, including gloves, as required by the facility's policy. Don't wear these garments outside the preparation area. Never eat, drink, smoke, or apply cosmetics in the drug preparation area.

Before and after preparing the drug, clean the inside of the cabinet with 70% isopropyl alcohol and a disposable towel, which you should discard in a leakproof chemical-waste container. Then cover the work surface with a clean, plastic absorbent pad to minimize contamination by droplets or spills. Change the pad at the end of each shift and after any spill.

All drug preparation equipment and any unused drug are considered hazardous waste. Dispose of them according to the facility's policy. Place all chemotherapeutic waste products in leakproof, sealable plastic bags or another suitable container, and make sure the container is appropriately labeled.

Reduce your exposure to chemotherapeutic drugs by following the guidelines listed below.

Prevent systemic absorption

- Remember that systemic absorption can occur through ingestion of contaminated materials, contact with the skin, or inhalation. You can accidentally inhale a drug while opening a vial, expelling air from a syringe, or discarding leftover drug that splashes.
- Drug absorption can also result from handling contaminated feces or body fluids. Use a biological safety cabinet.
- Mix all chemotherapeutic drugs in an approved, class II biological safety cabinet required by OSHA. Prime all I.V. bags containing these drugs under such a cabinet, and leave the blower on 24 hours a day, 7 days a week.
- The biological safety cabinet should be examined every 6 months (and whenever it's moved) by a company that specializes in certifying such equipment.
- Vent vials with a hydrophobic filter, which is a vented access that allows the withdrawal of fluid in a vial without injecting air into the vial. (The hydrophobic filter repels the chemotherapy solution, which prevents a wicking action that would otherwise expose the solution to the air in the cabinet.)

Or use negative-pressure techniques, which involves withdrawing fluid from a vial without replacing the fluid with air. This prevents the accidental aerosolization of chemotherapy solution into the work area.

- Take care with needles, syringes, and I.V. sets. Use needles with hydrophobic filters to remove the solution from vials. Break ampules by wrapping a sterile gauze pad or alcohol sponge around the ampule's neck to decrease the chances of droplet contamination.
- Use only syringes and I.V. sets with luer-lock fittings. Mark all chemotherapeutic drugs with chemotherapy hazard labels.
- Don't clip needles, break syringes, or remove needles from syringes used in drug preparation. Use a gauze pad

when removing syringes and needles from I.V. bags of chemotherapeutic drugs.

- Place used syringes, needles, and other sharp or breakable items in a puncture-proof container.

Prevent skin and eye contact

- Change gloves every 30 minutes and whenever you spill a drug solution or puncture or tear a glove. Wash your hands before donning new gloves and anytime you remove your gloves.
- If the drug contacts your skin, wash the area thoroughly with soap (not a chemical germicidal agent) and water. Plain soap and water is least likely to cause a potential chemical skin reaction (possible between some chemotherapy agents and various germicidal agents).
- If eye contact occurs, hold the eyelid open, and flood the eye with water or isotonic eyewash for at least 5 minutes. Obtain a medical evaluation as soon as possible after accidental exposure.

Other critical precautions

- Use a chemotherapeutic spill kit to clean up after a major spill.
- Discard disposable gowns and gloves in an appropriately marked, leakproof receptacle whenever they become contaminated or you leave the work area.
- Never place food or drinks in a refrigerator that contains chemotherapeutic drugs.
- Understand drug excretion patterns and take precautions when handling a chemotherapy patient's body fluids.
- Wear disposable latex surgical gloves when handling body fluids or soiled linens. Provide male patients with a urinal with a tight-fitting lid. Before flushing the toilet, place a waterproof pad over the toilet bowl to prevent splashing. Place soiled linens in designated isolation bags.
- Remember that women who are pregnant, trying to conceive, or breast-feeding should exercise extreme caution when handling chemotherapeutic drugs.
- Document each exposure incident according to the facility's policy.

Home care considerations

- Advise the patient to obtain the chemotherapeutic drugs from a hospital pharmacy or a specialized retail pharmacy. Drugs should be sealed in a plastic bag.
- Before starting chemotherapy, check the patient's insurance, and make sure that home administration is a covered expense. Remember that if chemotherapy requires a 24-hour continuous infusion, it's typically administered through a portable in-

fusion pump; shorter infusions are commonly given through an implanted port.

- Instruct the patient or caregiver to put soiled linens in a washable pillowcase, separate from other household items, and to launder the pillowcase twice.
- Advise the patient or caregiver to arrange for pickup and proper disposal of contaminated waste.
- Tell the patient or caregiver to place all treatment equipment in a leakproof container before disposal.
- Advise the patient or caregiver to dispose of waste products in the toilet, emptying the container close to the water to minimize splashing. Advise them to close the lid and flush two or three times. ■

Most dangerous drugs

Almost any drug can cause side effects in some patients. But the following drugs cause roughly 90% of all reported reactions.

Anticoagulants
- heparin
- warfarin

Antimicrobials
- cephalosporins
- penicillins
- sulfonamides

Bronchodilators
- sympathomimetics
- theophylline

Cardiac drugs
- antihypertensives
- digoxin
- diuretics
- quinidine

CNS drugs
- analgesics
- anticonvulsants
- neuroleptics
- sedative-hypnotics

Diagnostic agents
- X-ray contrast media

Hormones
- corticosteroids
- estrogens
- insulin ■

OBSERVING CAUTIONS

Adrenergics: Direct and indirect-acting

Drugs in this class include albuterol, bitolterol, dobutamine, dopamine, ephedrine epinephrine, epinephryl, isoetharine, isoproterenol, metaproterenol, metaraminol, metaxalone, naphazoline, norepinephrine, phenylephrine, pirbuterol, pseudoephedrine, terbutaline, tetrahydrozoline, and xylometazoline.

When administering direct and indirect-acting adrenergics, heed the following cautions:

- If used as a vasopressor, correct fluid volume depletion before administration. Adrenergics are not a substitute for blood, plasma, fluid, or electrolytes.
- Monitor blood pressure, pulse, and respiratory and urinary output carefully during therapy.
- Tachyphylaxis or tolerance may develop after prolonged or excessive use.
- The preservative sodium bisulfite is present in many adrenergic formulations. Patients with a history of allergy to sulfites should avoid preparations that contain this preservative.
- For unknown reasons, paradoxical airway resistance (manifested by sudden increase in dyspnea) may result from repeated use of isoetharine. If this occurs, the patient should discontinue the drug and use alternative therapy (such as epinephrine).
- Adrenergic inhalation may be alternated with other drugs (steroids, other adrenergics), if necessary, but shouldn't be administered simultaneously because of the risk of excessive tachycardia.
- Don't use discolored or precipitated solutions.
- Protect solutions from light, freezing, and heat. Store them at controlled room temperature.
- Rarely, systemic absorption can follow application to nasal and conjunctival membranes. If symptoms of systemic absorption occur, the patient should stop the drug.
- Prolonged or too-frequent use may cause tolerance to bronchodilating and cardiac stimulant effect. Rebound bronchospasm may occur.
- Excessive increase in blood pressure is a major side effect of systemically administered alpha agonists.
- Alpha agonists also interfere with lactation and may cause nausea, vomiting, sweating, piloerection, rebound congestion, rebound miosis, difficult urination, and headache.
- Ophthalmic use may cause mydriasis and photophobia.
- Patients known to be more sensitive to the effects of these drugs include elderly people, infants, and patients with thyrotoxicosis or cardiovascular disease.
- Lower doses of adrenergics are recommended for use in children.
- Use of adrenergics during breast-feeding usually isn't recommended. ■

Adrenocorticoids: Nasal and oral

Nasal adrenocorticoids include beclomethasone, budesonide, dexamethasone, and flunisolide. Oral agents include triamcinolone acetonide.

When administering these drugs, heed the following cautions:

- Therapeutic effects of intranasal inhalants, unlike those of sympathomimetic decongestants, aren't immediate. Full therapeutic benefit requires regular use and is usually evident within a few days, although a few patients may require up to 3 weeks of therapy for maximum benefit.
- Use of nasal or oral inhalation therapy may occasionally allow a patient to discontinue systemic corticosteroid therapy. Therapy should be discontinued by gradually tapering the dosage while carefully observing the patient for signs of adrenal insufficiency (joint pain, lassitude, or depression).
- After the desired clinical effect is obtained, the maintenance dose should be reduced to the smallest amount necessary to control symptoms.
- Discontinue the drug if the patient develops signs of systemic absorption (including Cushing's syndrome, hyperglycemia, or glucosuria), mucosal irritation or ulceration, hypersensitivity, or infection. (If antifungals or antibiotics are being used with corticosteroids and the infection doesn't respond immediately, discontinue corticosteroids until the infection is controlled.)
- Localized infections with *Candida albicans* or *Aspergillus niger* commonly occur in the mouth and pharynx and occasionally in the larynx. Instruct the patient to gargle and rinse his mouth with water after using an oral steroid inhaler.
- Systemic absorption may occur, possibly leading to hypothalamic-pituitary-adrenal axis suppression with large doses or with combined nasal and oral corticosteroid therapy. ■

Adrenocorticoids: Ophthalmic

Drugs in this class include dexamethasone, fluorometholone, medrysone, and prednisolone.

When administering ophthalmic adrenocorticoids, heed the following cautions:

- Ophthalmic products may initially cause sensitivity to bright light. This may be minimized by wearing sunglasses.

- Monitor the patient's response by observing the area of inflammation and eliciting patient comments concerning pruritus and vision. Inspect the eye and surrounding tissues for infection and additional irritation.
- Discontinue the drug if the patient develops signs of systemic absorption (including Cushing's syndrome, hyperglycemia, or glucosuria), skin irritation or ulceration, hypersensitivity, or infection. (If antivirals or antibiotics are being used with corticosteroids and the infection doesn't respond immediately, stop the corticosteroids until the infection is controlled.)
- Topical ophthalmic corticosteroids may cause increased intraocular pressure.
- Patients with diabetes mellitus, preexisting glaucoma, or significant myopia are at much greater risk for increased intraocular pressure.
- Prolonged use (more than 2 years) may result in posterior subcapsular cataracts that don't regress when the drugs are discontinued. ■

Adrenocorticoids: Systemic

Drugs in this class include betamethasone, cortisone, dexamethasone, hydrocortisone, methylprednisolone, paramethasone, prednisolone, prednisone, and triamcinolone.

When administering systemic adrenocorticoids, heed the following cautions:

- Establish baseline blood pressure, fluid intake and output, weight, and electrolyte status. Watch for any sudden weight gain, edema, or change in blood pressure or electrolyte status.
- During times of physiologic stress (trauma, surgery, or infection), the patient may require additional steroids and may experience signs of steroid withdrawal; patients who were previously steroid-dependent may need systemic corticosteroids to prevent adrenal insufficiency.
- After long-term therapy, the drug should be reduced gradually. Rapid reduction may cause withdrawal symptoms.
- Be aware of the patient's psychological history and watch for any behavioral changes.
- Observe for signs of infection or delayed wound healing. ■

Adrenocorticoids: Topical

Drugs in this class include alclometasone, amcinonide, betamethasone, clobetasol, clocortolone, desonide, desoximetasone, dexamethasone, diflorasone, fluocinolone, fluocinonide, flurandrenolide, fluticasone, halcinonide, halobetasol, hydrocortisone, methylprednisolone, mometasone, and triamcinolone.

When administering topical adrenocorticoids, heed the following cautions:

- Wash your hands before and after applying the drug.
- Gently clean the area. Washing or soaking the area before application may increase drug penetration.
- Apply the drug sparingly in a light film; rub it in lightly. Avoid contact with the patient's eyes, unless using an ophthalmic product.
- Avoid prolonged application in areas near the eyes, genitals, rectum, on the face, and in skin folds. High-potency topical corticosteroids are more likely to cause striae and atrophy in these areas because of their higher rates of absorption.
- Monitor the patient's response. Observe the area of inflammation, and elicit the patient's comments concerning pruritus. Inspect his skin for infection, striae, and atrophy. Skin atrophy is common and may be clinically significant within 3 to 4 weeks of treatment with high-potency preparations; it also occurs more readily at sites where percutaneous absorption is high.
- Don't apply occlusive dressings over topical corticosteroids because this may lead to secondary infection, maceration, atrophy, striae, or miliaria caused by increasing steroid penetration and potency.
- To use with an occlusive dressing if necessary: Apply cream; then cover with a thin, pliable, noninflammable plastic film; seal to adjacent unaffected skin with hypoallergenic tape. Minimize side effects by using the occlusive dressing intermittently. Don't leave it in place longer than 16 hours each day.
- For patients with eczematous dermatitis who may develop irritation from adhesive material, hold dressings in place with gauze, elastic bandages, stockings, or stockinette.
- Stop the drug if the patient develops signs of systemic absorption (including Cushing's syndrome, hyperglycemia, or glucosuria), skin irritation or ulceration, hypersensitivity, or infection. (If antifungals or antibiotics are being used with corticosteroids and the infection doesn't respond immediately, corticosteroids should be stopped until the infection is controlled.)

- Prolonged application around the eyes may lead to cataracts or glaucoma. ■

Alkylating agents

Drugs in this class include altretamine, busulfan, carboplatin, carmustine, chlorambucil, cisplatin, cyclophosphamide, dacarbazine, ifosfamide, lomustine, mechlorethamine, melphalan, pipobroman, streptozocin, thiotepa, and uracil mustard.

When administering alkylating agents, heed the following cautions:

- Follow all established procedures for the safe and proper handling, administration, and disposal of chemotherapeutic agents.
- Monitor vital signs and patency of catheter or I.V. line throughout administration.
- Treat extravasation promptly.
- Attempt to alleviate or reduce anxiety in the patient and family before treatment.
- Monitor BUN, hematocrit, platelet count, ALT, AST, LD, serum bilirubin, serum creatinine, uric acid, WBC and differential counts, and other levels as required for the specific agent.
- Immunizations should be avoided if possible.
- Be alert for signs of bone marrow depression, leukopenia, thrombocytopenia, fever, chills, sore throat, nausea, vomiting, diarrhea, flank or joint pain, anxiety, swelling of feet or lower legs, loss of hair, and redness or pain at injection site. ■

Alpha-adrenergic blockers

Nonselective agents include dihydroergotamine, ergotamine tartrate, phenoxybenzamine, phentolamine, and tolazoline. Selective agents include doxazosin, prazosin, and terazosin.

When administering alpha-adrenergic blockers, heed the following cautions:

- Nonselective alpha-adrenergic blockers typically cause postural hypotension, tachycardia, palpitations, fluid retention (from excess renin secretion), nasal and ocular congestion, and aggravation of the signs and symptoms of respiratory infection.
- Use of these agents is contraindicated in patients with severe cerebral and coronary atherosclerosis and in those with renal insufficiency.
- Selective alpha-adrenergic blockers may cause severe postural hypotension and syncope, especially with the first dose; the most common side effects of $alpha_1$ blockade are dizziness, headache, and malaise.

- Monitor vital signs, especially blood pressure.
- Give doses at bedtime to reduce the likelihood of dizziness or light-headedness.
- To avoid first-dose syncope, begin with a small dose. ■

Aminoglycosides

Drugs in this class include amikacin, gentamicin, kanamycin, neomycin, netilmicin, streptomycin, and tobramycin.

When administering aminoglycosides, heed the following cautions:

- First, assess the patient's allergy history; don't give an aminoglycoside to a patient with a history of hypersensitivity reactions to any aminoglycoside; monitor the patient continuously for this and other side effects.
- Perform culture and sensitivity tests before the first dose; however, therapy may begin before results are available. Repeat tests periodically to assess drug efficacy.
- Monitor vital signs, electrolyte levels, and renal function studies before and during therapy. Make sure the patient is well hydrated to minimize chemical irritation of renal tubules; watch for signs of declining renal function.
- Keep peak serum levels and trough serum levels at recommended concentrations, especially in patients with decreased renal function. Draw blood for peak level 1 hour after I.M. injection (30 minutes to 1 hour after I.V. infusion); for trough level, draw blood just before the next dose. Note the time and date on all blood samples. Don't use heparinized tubes to collect blood samples; heparin interferes with results.
- Evaluate the patient's hearing before and during therapy; monitor for complaints of tinnitus, vertigo, or hearing loss.
- Avoid concomitant use of aminoglycosides with other ototoxic or nephrotoxic drugs.
- Usual duration of therapy is 7 to 10 days; if no response occurs in 3 to 5 days, drug should be discontinued and cultures repeated for reevaluation of therapy.
- Closely monitor patients on long-term therapy — especially elderly and debilitated patients and those receiving immunosuppressant or radiation therapy — for possible bacterial or fungal superinfection; monitor especially for fever.
- Don't add or mix other drugs with I.V. infusions — particularly penicillins, which will inactivate aminoglycosides; the two groups

are chemically and physically incompatible. If other drugs must be given I.V., temporarily stop the infusion of the primary drug.

- Oral aminoglycosides may be absorbed systemically in patients with ulcerative GI lesions; significant absorption may endanger patients with decreased renal function.
- To ensure the correct dosage, shake oral suspensions well before administering.
- Administer I.M. doses deep into large muscle mass (gluteal or midlateral thigh). Rotate injection sites to minimize tissue injury; don't inject more than 2 g of drug into each injection site. Apply an ice pack to the site to relieve pain.
- Too-rapid I.V. administration may cause neuromuscular blockade. Infuse an I.V. drug continuously or intermittently over 30 to 60 minutes for adults, 1 to 2 hours for infants; dilution volume for children is determined individually.
- Solutions should always be clear, colorless to pale yellow (in most cases, darkening indicates deterioration), and free of particles; don't give solutions containing precipitates or other foreign matter.
- Amikacin, gentamicin (without preservatives), kanamycin, and tobramycin have been administered intrathecally or intraventricularly. Some clinicians prefer intraventricular administration to ensure adequate CSF levels in the treatment of ventriculitis.
- Nephrotoxicity usually begins on the 4th to 7th day of therapy and appears to be dose-related.
- Parenterally administered forms of aminoglycosides may cause vein irritation, phlebitis, and sterile abscess. ■

Aminoquinolines

Drugs in this class include chloroquine, hydroxychloroquine, and primaquine.

When administering aminoquinolines, heed the following cautions:

- Give the drug immediately before or after meals to minimize GI side effects.
- Obtain a baseline ECG, blood counts, and an ophthalmologic examination, and check periodically for changes.
- Monitor the patient for signs of cumulative effects, such as blurred vision, increased sensitivity to light, muscle weakness, impaired hearing, tinnitus, fever, sore throat, unusual bleeding or bruising, unusual pigmentation of the oral mucous membranes, and jaundice.

Maximal effects may not occur for 6 months.

- Muscle weakness and altered deep tendon reflexes may require discontinuing the drug. ■

Amphetamines

Drugs in this class include amphetamine, benzphetamine, dextroamphetamine, diethylpropion, fenfluramine, methamphetamine, phendimetrazine, phenmetrazine, and phentermine.

When administering amphetamines, heed the following cautions:

- The patient should receive the lowest effective dose with the dosage adjusted individually according to response; after long-term use, the dosage should be lowered gradually to prevent acute rebound depression.
- Amphetamines may impair ability to perform tasks requiring mental alertness, such as driving a car.
- Check vital signs regularly for increased blood pressure or other signs of excessive stimulation; avoid late-day or evening dosing, especially of long-acting dosage forms, to minimize insomnia.
- Amphetamines are not recommended as first-line therapy for obesity; make sure patients taking amphetamines for weight reduction are on a low-calorie diet.
- Amphetamine therapy should be discontinued when tolerance to anorexigenic effects develops; dosage shouldn't be increased.
- Encourage the patient to get adequate rest; unusual compensatory fatigue may result as the drug's effects diminish.
- Follow the manufacturer's directions for reconstitution, storage, and administration of all preparations.
- If overdose occurs, protect the patient from excessive noise or stimulation.
- Amphetamines have a high potential for abuse. They are not recommended to combat fatigue caused by exhaustion or the need for sleep but are often abused for this purpose by students, athletes, and truck drivers.
- Amphetamines are contraindicated in patients with symptomatic cardiovascular disease, hyperthyroidism, nephritis, angina pectoris, any degree of hypertension, arteriosclerosis-induced parkinsonism, certain types of glaucoma, advanced arteriosclerosis, agitated states, or a history of substance abuse.
- Amphetamine use for analeptic effect is discouraged; CNS stimulation superimposed on CNS depression may cause neuronal instability and seizures.

- Amphetamines should be used cautiously in patients with diabetes mellitus; in elderly, debilitated, or hyperexcitable patients; and in children with Tourette syndrome. Avoid long-term therapy when possible because of the risk of psychological dependence or habituation.
- Prolonged administration of CNS stimulants to children with attention deficit disorders may be associated with temporary decreased growth. ■

Anabolic steroids

Drugs in this class include nandrolone, oxandrolone, oxymetholone, stanozolol, testolactone, and testosterone.

When administering anabolic steroids, heed the following cautions:

- Watch for signs of virilization in women. If possible, discontinue therapy when virilization first becomes apparent because some side effects (deepening of voice or clitoral enlargement) are irreversible.
- Edema usually is controllable with salt restriction, diuretics, or both. Monitor weight routinely.
- Watch for symptoms of jaundice. Dosage adjustment may reverse this condition. Periodic liver function tests are recommended.
- Observe the patient on concomitant anticoagulant therapy for ecchymotic areas, petechiae, or abnormal bleeding. Monitor PT.
- Watch for symptoms of hypoglycemia in patients with diabetes. Change of antidiabetic drug dosage may be required.
- Hypercalcemia symptoms may be difficult to distinguish from symptoms of the condition being treated unless anticipated. Hypercalcemia is most likely to occur in patients with metastatic breast cancer and may indicate bone metastasis.
- Patients with metastatic breast cancer should have regular determinations of serum calcium levels to identify the potential for serious hypercalcemia.
- Anabolic steroids may alter many laboratory test results during therapy and for 2 to 3 weeks after therapy is stopped.
- Offer the patient small, frequent meals — high in calories and protein — unless contraindicated.
- Anabolic steroids are contraindicated in premature infants and in patients with hypersensitivity to these drugs; prostatic hyperplasia with obstruction; prostatic or male breast cancer; cardiac,

hepatic, or renal decompensation; or nephrosis.

- Anabolic steroids should *not* be used to improve athletic performance. Risks associated with their use for this purpose far outweigh any possible benefits. Proof of anabolic steroid use is grounds for disqualification in many athletic events. Some states impose criminal penalties on doctors who prescribe anabolic steroids for this purpose. Anabolic steroids are now classified as schedule III controlled substances, and their distribution is regulated by the Drug Enforcement Agency.
- Use cautiously in prepubertal boys, in patients with diabetes or coronary disease, and in patients taking adrenocorticotropic hormone, corticosteroids, or anticoagulants. ■

Angiotensin-converting enzyme inhibitors

Drugs in this class include benazepril, captopril, enalapril, fosinopril, lisinopril, quinapril, and ramipril.

When administering ACE inhibitors, heed the following cautions:

- Discontinue diuretic therapy 2 to 3 days before beginning ACE inhibitor therapy to reduce the risk of hypotension; if the ACE inhibitor fails to adequately control blood pressure, resume diuretic therapy.
- Common side effects of therapeutic doses of ACE inhibitors are headache, fatigue, hypotension, tachycardia, dysgeusia, proteinuria, hyperkalemia, rash, cough, and angioedema of the face and extremities.
- Severe hypotension may occur at toxic drug levels.
- Use potassium supplements with caution because ACE inhibitors may cause potassium retention.
- ACE inhibitors should be used cautiously in patients with impaired renal function or serious autoimmune disease and in patients taking other drugs known to depress the WBC count or immune response. Periodically monitor WBC counts.
- Lower dosage is necessary in patients with impaired renal function.
- Discontinue ACE inhibitors if pregnancy is detected. These drugs may harm the fetus or cause fetal death during the second or third trimesters. ■

Antibiotic antineoplastics

Drugs in this class include bleomycin, dactinomycin, daunorubicin, doxorubicin, idarubicin, mitomycin, mitoxantrone, plicamycin, procarbazine, and streptozocin.

When administering antibiotic antineoplastics, heed the following cautions:

- Monitor vital signs and patency of catheter or I.V. line throughout administration.
- Carefully follow all established procedures for the safe and proper handling, administration, and disposal of chemotherapeutic agents.
- Treat extravasation promptly.
- Attempt to ease anxiety in the patient and family before treatment.
- Monitor BUN, hematocrit, platelet count, ALT, AST, LD, serum bilirubin, serum creatinine, uric acid, and total and differential WBC counts.
- Avoid immunizations if possible. Warn the patient to avoid close contact with people who have taken the oral poliovirus vaccine.
- The most common side effects include nausea, vomiting, diarrhea, fever, chills, sore throat, anxiety, confusion, flank or joint pain, swelling of feet or lower legs, loss of hair, redness or pain at injection site, bone marrow depression, and leukopenia. ■

Anticholinergics

Drugs in this class include atropine, benztropine, biperiden, clidinium, dicyclomine, glycopyrrolate, hyoscyamine, isopropamide, mepenzolate, methantheline, methscopolamine, oxyphenonium, procyclidine, propantheline, scopolamine, and trihexyphenidyl.

When administering anticholinergics, heed the following cautions:

- Give medication 30 minutes to 1 hour before meals and at bedtime to maximize therapeutic effects. In some instances, drugs should be administered with meals; always follow dosage recommendations.
- Monitor the patient's vital signs and urine output, and check for visual changes and signs of impending toxicity.
- Signs of drug toxicity include CNS signs resembling psychosis (disorientation, confusion, hallucinations, delusions, anxiety, agitation, and restlessness) and such peripheral effects as dilated, nonreactive pupils; blurred vision; hot, dry, flushed skin; dry mucous membranes; dysphagia; decreased or absent bowel sounds; urine re-

tention; hyperthermia; tachycardia; hypertension; and increased respiratory rate.

- The safety of anticholinergic therapy during pregnancy has not been determined. Use by pregnant women is indicated only when the drug's benefits outweigh potential risks to the fetus. ■

Antimetabolites

Drugs in this class include cytarabine, floxuridine, fludarabine, fluorouracil, hydroxyurea, mercaptopurine, methotrexate, thioguanine, and trimetrexate.

When administering antimetabolites, heed the following cautions:

- Follow all established procedures for the safe and proper handling, administration, and disposal of chemotherapeutic agents.
- Monitor vital signs and patency of catheter or I.V. line throughout administration.
- Treat extravasation promptly.
- Attempt to alleviate or reduce anxiety in the patient and family before treatment.
- Monitor BUN, hematocrit, platelet count, ALT, AST, LD, serum bilirubin, serum creatinine, uric acid, total and differential WBC counts, and other laboratory values as required.
- Avoid immunizations if possible. ■

Barbiturates

Drugs in this class include amobarbital, aprobarbital, butabarbital, mephobarbital, metharbital, methohexital, pentobarbital, phenobarbital, primidone, secobarbital, and thiopental.

When administering barbiturates, heed the following cautions:

- Dosage of barbiturates must be individualized for each patient because different rates of metabolism and enzyme induction occur.
- Parenteral solutions are highly alkaline; avoid extravasation, which may cause local tissue damage and tissue necrosis. Inject I.V. or deep I.M. only. Don't exceed 5 ml per I.M. injection site to avoid tissue damage.
- Too-rapid I.V. administration of barbiturates may cause respiratory depression, apnea, laryngospasm, or hypotension. Have resuscitation equipment available. Assess the I.V. site for signs of infiltration or phlebitis.
- Barbiturates may be given rectally if oral or parenteral route is inappropriate.
- Death is common with an overdose of 2 to 10 g; it may

occur at much smaller doses if alcohol is also ingested.

- Assess level of consciousness before and frequently during therapy to evaluate effectiveness of drug. Monitor neurologic status for possible alterations or deteriorations.
- Institute seizure precautions as necessary. Monitor for changes in seizure character, frequency, and duration.
- Check vital signs frequently, especially during I.V. administration.
- Assess the patient's sleeping patterns before and during therapy to ensure effectiveness of drug.
- Anticipate possible rebound confusion and excitatory reactions in patient.
- Assess bowel elimination patterns; monitor for complaints of constipation. Advise a high-fiber diet, if indicated.
- Monitor PT carefully in patients taking anticoagulants; dosage of anticoagulant may require adjustment to counteract possible interaction.
- Observe the patient to prevent hoarding or self-dosing, especially in depressed or suicidal patients, or those who are or have a history of being drug-dependent.
- Barbiturates can cause paradoxical excitement at low doses, confusion in elderly patients, and hyperactivity in children.
- Withdrawal symptoms may occur after as little as 2 weeks of uninterrupted therapy.
- Abrupt discontinuation may cause withdrawal symptoms; discontinue slowly.
- Avoid administering barbiturates to patients with status asthmaticus.
- Barbiturates should be used cautiously, if at all, in patients who are mentally depressed or who have suicidal tendencies or a history of drug abuse. ■

Benzodiazepines

Drugs in this class include alprazolam, chlordiazepoxide, clonazepam, diazepam, estazolam, flurazepam, halazepam, lorazepam, midazolam, oxazepam, prazepam, quazepam, temazepam, and triazolam.

When administering benzodiazepines, heed the following cautions:

- Assess level of consciousness and neurologic status before and frequently during therapy for changes. Monitor for paradoxical reactions, especially early in therapy.
- Institute seizure precautions if the drug is prescribed as an adjunct to treatment for seizure disorder.
- Assess vital signs frequently during therapy. Significant

changes in blood pressure and heart rate may indicate impending toxicity.

- Give the drug with milk or immediately after meals to prevent GI upset. Give an antacid, if needed, at least 1 hour before or after a dose to prevent an interaction and ensure maximum drug absorption and effectiveness.
- Monitor renal and hepatic function periodically to ensure adequate drug removal and prevent cumulative effects.
- As needed, institute safety measures (raised side rails and ambulatory assistance) to prevent injury. Anticipate possible rebound excitement.
- Observe the patient to prevent drug hoarding or self-dosing, especially by a depressed or suicidal patient or by one who has a history of being drug-dependent. Check the patient's mouth to make sure he has swallowed the tablet or capsule.
- After prolonged use, discontinue the drug gradually; abrupt discontinuation may cause withdrawal symptoms.
- Visual disturbances and cardiovascular irregularities are common.
- Continuing problems with short-term memory, confusion, severe depression, shakiness, vertigo, slurred speech, staggering, bradycardia, shortness of breath or difficulty breathing, and severe weakness usually indicate a toxic dose level. ■

Beta-adrenergic blockers

$Beta_1$ blockers include acebutolol, atenolol, betaxolol, bisoprolol, esmolol, metoprolol and tartrate. $Beta_1$ and $beta_2$ blockers include carteolol, labetalol, levobunolol, metipranolol, nadolol, penbutolol, pindolol, propranolol, and timolol. (See *Comparing beta-adrenergic blockers.*)

When administering beta-adrenergic blockers, heed the following cautions:

- Check apical pulse rate daily; discontinue drug, and reevaluate therapy if extremes occur (for example, a pulse rate below 60 beats/minute).
- Monitor blood pressure, ECG, and heart rate and rhythm frequently; be alert for progression of AV block or severe bradycardia.
- Weigh patients with CHF regularly; watch for gains of more than 5 lb (2.2 kg) per week.
- Because beta blockers mask signs of hypoglycemic shock, watch diabetic patients for sweating, fatigue, and hunger.
- Don't discontinue these drugs before surgery for pheochromocytoma; before any surgical procedure, notify the anesthesiologist that

Comparing beta-adrenergic blockers

DRUG	HALF-LIFE (hr)	LIPID SOLUBILITY	MEMBRANE-STABILIZING ACTIVITY	INTRINSIC SYMPATHOMIMETIC ACTIVITY
Nonselective				
carteolol	6	Low	0	++
labetalol	6 to 8	Moderate	0	0
metipranolol	4	Low to moderate	0	0
nadolol	20	Low	0	0
penbutolol	5	High	0	+
pindolol	3 to 4	Moderate	+	+++
propranolol	4	High	++	0
timolol	4	Low to moderate	0	0
Beta$_1$-selective				
acebutolol	3 to 4	Low	+	+
atenolol	6 to 7	Low	0	0
betaxolol	14 to 22	Low	+	0
esmolol	0.15	Low	0	0
metoprolol	3 to 7	Moderate	*	0

* Drug produces membrane-stabilizing effects only in higher-than-usual doses.

the patient is taking a beta-adrenergic blocker.

- Glucagon may be prescribed to reverse signs and symptoms of beta blocker overdose.
- Don't administer to patients with asthma. ■

Calcium channel blockers

Drugs in this class include amlodipine, bepridil, diltiazem, felodipine, isradipine, nicardipine, nifedipine, nimodipine, and verapamil. (See *Comparing oral calcium channel blockers.*)

When administering calcium channel blockers, heed the following cautions:

- Monitor heart rate and rhythm and blood pressure carefully when initiating therapy or increasing dose.
- Total serum calcium concentrations are not affected by calcium channel blockers.
- Concomitant use of calcium supplements may decrease the effectiveness of calcium channel blockers.
- Verapamil may cause cardiac conduction disturbances, including bradycardia and various degrees of heart block. It also may exacerbate heart failure and cause hypotension after rapid I.V. administration.
- Prolonged oral verapamil therapy may cause constipation.
- Most side effects of nifedipine, such as hypotension (commonly accompanied by reflex tachycardia), peripheral edema, flushing, lightheadedness, and headache, result from its potent vasodilatory properties. These effects are reduced when the sustained-release form is used.
- Diltiazem most commonly causes anorexia and nausea, and it may also induce various degrees of heart block, bradycardia, CHF, and peripheral edema.
- Use these drugs cautiously in patients with impaired left ventricular function. ■

Carbonic anhydrase inhibitors

Drugs in this class include acetazolamide, dichlorphenamide, and methazolamide.

When administering carbonic anhydrase inhibitors, heed the following cautions:

- In treating edema, intermittent dosage schedules may minimize tendency to cause metabolic acidosis and permit diuresis.
- Because they alkalinize urine, these drugs may cause false-positive results on tests for proteinuria.

Comparing oral calcium channel blockers

DRUG	ONSET	PEAK SERUM LEVEL (hr)	HALF-LIFE (hr)	THERAPEUTIC SERUM LEVEL (ng/ml)
bepridil	1 hr	2 to 3	24	1 to 2
diltiazem	15 min	0.5	3 to 4	50 to 200
felodipine	2 to 5 hr	2.5 to 5	11 to 16	unknown
nicardipine	20 min	1	8.6	28 to 50
nifedipine	5 to 30 min	0.5 to 2	2 to 5	25 to 100
nimodipine	unknown	<1	1 to 2	unknown
verapamil	30 min	1 to 2.2	6 to 12	80 to 300

- Establish baseline blood pressure and pulse rate before therapy, and monitor for changes. Impose safety measures until the patient's response to the drug is known.
- Establish baseline values for and periodically review the following laboratory tests: CBC, including WBC count; BUN and serum electrolyte, carbon dioxide, and creatinine levels; and especially liver function tests. Patients with liver disease are especially susceptible to diuretic-induced electrolyte imbalances; in severe cases, stupor, coma, and death can result.
- Administer diuretics in the morning so that most diuresis occurs before bedtime. To prevent nocturia, don't administer diuretics after 6 p.m.
- Consider reduced dosage for patients with hepatic dysfunction and those taking other antihypertensives; increased dosage for patients with renal impairment, oliguria, or decreased diuresis (inadequate urine output may result in circulatory overload, causing water intoxication, pulmonary edema, and CHF); and increased

dosage of insulin or oral antidiabetic drugs in diabetic patients.

- Monitor the patient for signs of toxicity: postural hypotension; muscle weakness and cardiac arrhythmias (signs of hypokalemia); leg cramps, nausea, muscle weakness, dry mouth, and dizziness (hyponatremia); lethargy, confusion, stupor, muscle twitching, increased reflexes, and seizures (water intoxication); severe weakness, headache, abdominal pain, malaise, nausea, and vomiting (metabolic acidosis); sore throat, rash, or jaundice (blood dyscrasia from hypersensitivity); and joint swelling, redness, and pain (hyperuricemia).
- Monitor the patient for edema. Observe lower extremities of ambulatory patients and the sacral area of patients on bed rest. Check abdominal girth with tape measure to detect ascites. Dosage adjustment may be indicated. Weigh the patient every morning immediately after voiding and before breakfast, in the same type of clothing and on the same scale. Weight provides an index for dosage adjustments.
- The patient may need a high-potassium diet or a potassium supplement.
- Many side effects associated with carbonic anhydrase inhibitors are dose-related and respond to lowered dosage; each drug has a slightly different side-effect profile, and patients who can't tolerate one of the drugs may be able to tolerate another.
- Drug use in glaucoma may be limited because of availability of other agents and its propensity for causing metabolic acidosis. Signs and symptoms of metabolic acidosis include weakness, malaise, headache, abdominal pain, nausea, vomiting, and poor skin turgor. ■

Cephalosporins

First-generation cephalosporins include cefadroxil, cefazolin, cephalexin, cephalothin, cephapirin, and cephradine. Second-generation cephalosporins include cefaclor, cefamandole, cefmetazole, cefonicid, cefotetan, cefoxitin, cefpodoxime, cefprozil, and cefuroxime. Third-generation cephalosporins include cefixime, cefoperazone, cefotaxime, ceftazidime, ceftizoxime, and ceftriaxone. (See *Comparing cephalosporins,* page 184.)

When administering cephalosporins, heed the following cautions:

- Give cephalosporins at least 1 hour before giving bacteriostatic antibiotics (tetracyclines, erythromycins, and chloramphenicol); these drugs inhibit bacterial cell growth, decreasing cephalosporin uptake by bacterial cell walls.

- Elderly patients commonly have renal impairment and may require lower dosages of cephalosporins.
- Cephalosporins are excreted in breast milk; use with caution in breast-feeding women.
- Hypersensitivity reactions range from mild rashes, fever, and eosinophilia to fatal anaphylaxis, and are more common in patients with penicillin allergy.
- Hematologic reactions include positive direct and indirect antiglobulin (Coombs' test), thrombocytopenia or thrombocythemia, transient neutropenia, and reversible leukopenia.
- Renal side effects may occur with any cephalosporin; they are most common in older patients, those with decreased renal function, and those taking other nephrotoxic drugs. GI reactions include nausea, vomiting, diarrhea, abdominal pain, glossitis, dyspepsia, and tenesmus. Liver function test results are occasionally elevated.
- Local venous pain and irritation are common after I.M. injection; such reactions occur more often with higher doses and long-term therapy.
- Disulfiram-type reactions occur when cefamandole, cefoperazone, cefonicid, or cefotetan are administered within 48 to 72 hours of alcohol ingestion.
- Obtain results of culture and sensitivity tests before administering the first dose, but don't delay therapy; check test results periodically to assess drug efficacy.
- Monitor renal function studies; dosages of certain cephalosporins must be lowered in patients with severe renal impairment.
- In decreased renal function, monitor BUN levels, serum creatinine levels, and urine output for significant changes.
- Monitor the patient's PT and platelet count, and assess him for signs of hypoprothrombinemia, which may occur — with or without bleeding — during therapy with cefamandole, cefoperazone, cefonicid, or cefotetan, usually in elderly, debilitated, or malnourished patients.
- Monitor patients on long-term therapy for possible bacterial and fungal superinfection, especially elderly and debilitated patients and those receiving immunosuppressants or radiation therapy.
- Monitor susceptible patients receiving sodium salts

(Text continues on page 186.)

Comparing cephalosporins

DRUG AND ROUTE	ELIMINATION HALF-LIFE (hr)	
	Normal renal function	End-stage renal disease
cefaclor oral	0.5 to 1	3 to 5.5
cefadroxil oral	1 to 2	20 to 25
cefamandole I.M., I.V.	0.5 to 2	12 to 18
cefazolin I.M., I.V.	1.2 to 2.2	12 to 50
cefixime oral	3 to 4	11.5
cefmetazole I.V.	1.2	Unknown
cefonicid I.M., I.V.	3.5 to 5.8	100
cefoperazone I.M., I.V.	1.5 to 2.5	3.4 to 7
ceforanide I.M., I.V.	2.5 to 3.5	5.5 to 25
cefotaxime I.M., I.V.	1 to 1.5	11.5 to 56
cefotetan I.M., I.V.	2.8 to 4.6	13 to 35
cefoxitin I.M., I.V.	0.5 to 1	6.5 to 21.5
cefpodoxime oral	2 to 3	9.8

SODIUM (mEq/g)	C.S.F. PENETRATION
No data available	No
No data available	No
3.3	No
2	No
No data available	Unknown
49	Unknown
3.7	No
1.5	Sometimes
No data available	No
2.2	Yes
3.5	No
2.3	No
No data available	Unknown

(continued)

Comparing cephalosporins *(continued)*

DRUG AND ROUTE	ELIMINATION HALF-LIFE (hr)	
	Normal renal function	End-stage renal disease
cefprozil oral	1 to 1.5	5.2 to 5.9
ceftazidime I.M., I.V.	1.5 to 2	35
ceftizoxime I.M., I.V.	1.5 to 2	30
ceftriaxone I.M., I.V.	5.5 to 11	15.7
cefuroxime I.M., I.V.	1 to 2	15 to 22
cephalexin oral	0.5 to 1	7.5 to 14
cephalothin I.M., I.V.	0.5 to 1	19
cephapirin I.M., I.V.	0.5 to 1	1 to 1.5
cephradine oral, I.M., I.V.	0.5 to 2	8 to 15

of cephalosporins for possible fluid retention.

- Cephalosporins cause false-positive results in urine glucose tests that use cupric sulfate solutions (Benedict's reagent or Clinitest); glucose oxidase tests (Clinistix or Tes-Tape) are not affected.
- Don't give a cephalosporin to any patient with a history of hypersensitivity reactions to cephalosporins.
- Administer cautiously to patients with penicillin allergy because they're more susceptible to such reactions. ■

SODIUM (mEq/g)	C.S.F. PENETRATION
No data available	Unknown
2.3	Yes
2.6	Yes
3.6	Yes
2.4	Yes
No data available	No
2.8	No
2.4	No
6	No

Cholinergics

Drugs in this class include acetylcholine, bethanechol, carbachol, and methacholine.

When administering cholinergics, heed the following cautions:

- These drugs may precipitate asthma attacks in susceptible patients.
- Clinical effects of overdose primarily involve muscarinic symptoms, such as nausea, vomiting, diarrhea, abdominal discomfort, involuntary defecation, urinary urgency, increased bronchial and salivary secretions, respiratory

depression, skin flushing or heat sensation, and bradycardia; cardiac arrest has also occurred.

- Regularly monitor the patient's vital signs, especially heart rate and respirations, and fluid intake and output.
- Evaluate the patient for changes in muscle strength, and observe closely for side effects or signs of acute toxicity.
- All cholinergics are contraindicated in pregnant women. They are also contraindicated in breast-feeding women because some cholinergics may be excreted in breast milk, possibly causing toxicity in infants.
- Use cautiously in elderly patients because they may be more sensitive to the drug's effects. A lower dosage may be indicated. ■

Cholinesterase inhibitors

Drugs in this class include ambenonium, echothiophate, edrophonium, neostigmine, physostigmine, pyridostigmine, and tacrine.

When administering cholinesterase inhibitors, heed the following cautions:

- Wide variations in response may occur, even in the same patient; give cautiously because the first sign of side effects may be subtle.
- Systemic side effects may occur even after topical application because of systemic absorption.
- Administer oral forms with food or milk to reduce muscarinic side effects by slowing down absorption and reducing peak serum levels.
- Observe patients closely for cholinergic reactions, especially with parenteral forms.
- Administer atropine before or concurrently with large doses of parenteral anticholinesterases to counteract muscarinic side effects.
- Dosage must be individualized according to severity of disease and patient response.
- Myasthenic patients may become refractory to these medications after prolonged use; however, responsiveness may be restored by reducing the dosage or discontinuing the drug for a few days. ■

Digitalis glycosides

Drugs in this class include digitoxin and digoxin.

When administering digitalis glycosides, heed the following cautions:

- Monitor heart rate daily because of the drug's effects on the cardiac conduction system. Slowing of the heart rate (60 beats/minute or less) may be an early sign of toxicity (except in patients with chronically slow heart rate).

- Observe for GI side effects, such as nausea, anorexia, and vomiting, which may be early signs of toxicity.
- Obtain serum drug levels before administering the morning dose, or at least 6 to 12 hours after a dose because of the drug's slow distribution.
- The drug should be discontinued at least 24 hours before elective cardioversion or as advised by the doctor.
- Higher-than-usual dosage and serum drug levels may be needed to adequately control atrial arrhythmias.
- Before prescribing additional drugs for patients currently receiving a digitalis glycoside, review drug interactions, which are numerous and may seriously affect therapy.
- These drugs have a narrow therapeutic index; also, signs and symptoms of the underlying disease may be difficult to distinguish from those indicating toxicity.
- Drug effects on the cardiac conduction system may lead to multiple arrhythmias, ranging from various degrees of AV block to complex ventricular ectopy.
- Long-term therapy may cause gynecomastia.
- Digitalis glycosides are a major cause of poisoning in children. ■

Diuretics, loop

Drugs in this class include bumetanide, ethacrynate, ethacrynic acid, furosemide, and torsemide. (See *Comparing loop diuretics,* page 190.)

When administering loop diuretics, heed the following cautions:

- Administer diuretics in the morning so that most diuresis occurs before bedtime.
- Notify the patient's doctor about possible dosage adjustment in certain conditions, such as reduced dosage for patients with hepatic dysfunction; increased dosage in patients with renal impairment, oliguria, or decreased diuresis (inadequate urine output may result in circulatory overload, causing water intoxication, pulmonary edema, and CHF); increased dosages of insulin or oral antidiabetic drugs in diabetic patients; and reduced dosages of other antihypertensives.
- Loop diuretics may cause metabolic and electrolyte disturbances, particularly potassium depletion.
- Loop diuretics may also cause hypochloremic alkalosis, hyperglycemia, hyperuricemia, and hypomagnesemia.

Comparing loop diuretics

DRUG AND ROUTE	ONSET (min)	PEAK (hr)	DURATION (hr)	USUAL DOSAGE
bumetanide				
I.V.	≤ 5	¼ to ¾	4 to 6	0.5 to 1 mg ≤ t.i.d
P.O.	30 to 60	1 to 2	4 to 6	0.5 to 2 mg/day
ethacrynic acid				
I.V.	≤ 5	¼ to ½	2	50 mg/day
P.O.	≤ 30	2	6 to 8	50 to 100 mg/day
furosemide				
I.V.	≤ 5	⅓ to 1	2	20 to 40 mg q 2 hr p.r.n.
P.O.	30 to 60	1 to 2	6 to 8	20 to 80 mg ≤ b.i.d.

- Rapid parenteral administration of loop diuretics may cause hearing loss (including deafness) and tinnitus.
- High dosages may produce profound diuresis, leading to hypovolemia and cardiovascular collapse.
- Establish baseline blood pressure and pulse rate before therapy, monitor regularly (especially during rapid diuresis), and watch for significant changes.
- Establish baseline values for, and periodically review the CBC, including the WBC count; serum electrolytes; carbon dioxide; magnesium; BUN and serum creatinine; and liver function tests.
- Patients taking a digitalis glycoside are at increased risk for digitalis toxicity from potassium depletion.
- Ototoxicity may follow prolonged use or administration of large doses.
- Patients with liver disease are especially susceptible to diuretic-induced electrolyte imbalances; in severe cases,

stupor, coma, and death can result.

- Elderly and debilitated patients require close observation because they are more susceptible to drug-induced diuresis.
- Use loop diuretics with caution in neonates; give the usual pediatric dose but extend the dose intervals.
- Loop diuretics should not be used by breast-feeding women. ■

Diuretics, osmotic

Drugs in this class include mannitol and urea.

When administering osmotic diuretics, heed the following cautions:

- Urea, unlike mannitol, penetrates the eyes and may cause a rebound increase in intraocular pressure (IOP) if plasma urea levels fall below that in the vitreous humor.
- Because urea penetrates the eyes, it shouldn't be used when irritation is present.
- When infusing mannitol, use a filter needle to capture any crystal fragments in the mannitol solution.
- The most severe side effects associated with mannitol are fluid and electrolyte imbalances.
- Circulatory overload may follow administration of mannitol to patients with inadequate urine output.
- The most common side effects associated with urea are headache, nausea, and vomiting; a rebound increase in IOP also may occur.
- Elderly or debilitated patients will need close observation and may require lower dosages. ■

Diuretics, potassium-sparing

Drugs in this class include amiloride, spironolactone, and triamterene.

When administering potassium-sparing diuretics, heed the following cautions:

- Potassium-sparing diuretics are less potent than many others; in particular, amiloride and triamterene have little clinical effect when used alone. However, because they protect against potassium loss, they're used with other more potent diuretics.
- Hyperkalemia may occur with all drugs in this class and can lead to cardiac arrhythmias.
- Other side effects include nausea, vomiting, headache, weakness, fatigue, bowel disturbances, cough, and dyspnea.
- Ask the doctor about appropriate dosage adjustments — for example, a reduced dosage for patients

with hepatic dysfunction and for those taking other antihypertensives, an increased dosage for patients with renal impairment, and changes in insulin requirements for diabetic patients.

- Patients with hepatic disease are especially susceptible to diuretic-induced electrolyte imbalances; in severe cases, coma and death can result.
- Elderly and debilitated patients need monitoring because they're more susceptible to drug-induced diuresis and hyperkalemia. Reduced dosages may be indicated.
- Watch for hyperkalemia and cardiac arrhythmias; monitor serum potassium and other electrolyte levels frequently, and check for significant changes.
- Establish baseline values for, and periodically monitor the following: CBC, including WBC count; carbon dioxide; BUN and creatinine levels; and especially liver function studies.
- Monitor patients with hepatic disease in whom mild drug-induced acidosis may be hazardous; watch for mental confusion, lethargy, or stupor.
- Use these drugs with caution in children because they're more susceptible to hyperkalemia.
- Drug may be excreted in breast milk.
- Potassium-sparing diuretics are contraindicated in patients with serum potassium levels above 5.5 mEq/L, in those receiving other potassium-sparing diuretics or potassium supplements, and in patients with anuria, acute or chronic renal insufficiency, diabetic nephropathy, or known hypersensitivity to the drug.
- Use these drugs cautiously in patients with severe hepatic insufficiency, because electrolyte imbalance may precipitate hepatic encephalopathy, and in patients with diabetes, who are at increased risk for hyperkalemia. ■

Diuretics, thiazide and thiazide-like

Thiazide diuretics include bendroflumethiazide, benzthiazide, chlorothiazide, hydrochlorothiazide, hydroflumethiazide, methyclothiazide, polythiazide, and trichlormethiazide.

Thiazide-like diuretics include chlorthalidone, indapamide, metolazone, and quinethazone. (See *Comparing thiazides.*)

When administering thiazide and thiazide-like diuretics, heed the following cautions:

Comparing thiazides

Under most conditions, thiazide diuretics differ mainly in their duration of action. The onset for each of the following is within 2 hours, except for cyclothiazide, whose onset is within 6 hours.

DRUG	EQUIVALENT DOSE (mg)	PEAK (hr)	DURATION (hr)
bendroflumethiazide	5	4	6 to 12
benzthiazide	50	4 to 6	6 to 12
chlorothiazide	500	4	6 to 12
cyclothiazide	2	7 to 12	18 to 24
hydrochlorothiazide	50	4 to 6	6 to 12
hydroflumethiazide	50	4	6 to 12
methyclothiazide	5	4 to 6	24
polythiazide	2	6	24 to 48
trichlormethiazide	2	6	24

- Efficacy and toxicity profiles of thiazide and thiazide-like diuretics are equivalent at comparable dosages; the single exception is metolazone, which may be more effective in patients with impaired renal function.
- Usually, thiazide and thiazide-like diuretics are less effective than loop diuretics in patients with renal insufficiency.
- Therapeutic doses of thiazide diuretics cause electrolyte and metabolic disturbances, the most common being potassium depletion; patients may require potassium supplements.

- Other side effects include hypochloremic alkalosis, hypomagnesemia, hyponatremia, hypercalcemia, hyperuricemia, elevated cholesterol levels, and hyperglycemia.
- Overdose of thiazides may produce lethargy, which can progress to coma within a few hours.
- Thiazide and thiazide-like diuretics (except metolazone) are ineffective in patients with a glomerular filtration rate below 25 ml/minute.
- Because thiazides may increase lipid levels, consider an alternative agent in patients with significant hyperlipidemia.
- Patients also taking a digitalis glycoside have an increased risk of digitalis toxicity from the potassium-depleting effect of these diuretics.
- Thiazides may be used with potassium-sparing diuretics to prevent potassium loss.
- Because thiazides may cause hyperglycemia, diabetic patients may need adjustments in insulin or oral antidiabetic drug dosage.
- These drugs are not as effective if the patient's serum creatinine and BUN levels are more than twice the normal levels.
- In patients with a history of gout, these agents may cause an increase in uric acid levels.
- Antihypertensive effects persist for approximately 1 week after discontinuation of the drug.
- Many nonprescription drugs contain sodium and potassium and can cause electrolyte imbalances, and many diet aids and cold preparations contain drugs that may raise blood pressure.
- Thiazide-related photosensitivity reaction occurs 10 days to 2 weeks after initial sun exposure.
- Elderly and debilitated patients require close observation and may require reduced dosages.
- Thiazides are distributed in breast milk; their safety and effectiveness in breast-feeding women have not been established. ■

Nitrates

Drugs in this class include amyl nitrite, erythrityl, isosorbide, nitroglycerin, and pentaerythritol.

When administering nitrates, heed the following cautions:

- Nitrates relax all smooth muscle, not just vascular smooth muscle, regardless of autonomic innervation, including bronchial, biliary, GI, ureteral, and uterine smooth muscle.

- Because individual nitrates have similar pharmacologic and therapeutic properties, the best nitrate to use in a specific situation depends mainly on the onset of action and duration of effect required.
- If combination therapy is required (sedatives and nitrates), each drug should be adjusted individually; fixed combinations of oral nitrates and sedatives should be avoided.
- Dosage should be titrated to patient response. Patients should avoid switching brands after they're stabilized on a particular formulation.
- The dissolution rate varies with the buccal route but usually ranges from 3 to 5 hours. Hot liquids will increase the dissolution rate and should be avoided.
- Only the sublingual and translingual forms should be used to relieve an acute angina attack.
- Although a burning sensation was formerly an indication of the drug's potency, many current preparations don't produce this sensation.
- The most common side effect is headache (possibly severe), which usually occurs early in therapy and improves rapidly.
- Postural hypotension may occur and result in dizziness or weakness. Patients who are especially sensitive to these drugs' antihypertensive effects may experience nausea, vomiting, weakness, restlessness, pallor, cold sweats, tachycardia, syncope, or cardiovascular collapse. Alcohol may intensify these effects.
- Transient flushing may occur.
- GI upset may be controlled by a temporary dosage reduction. Ask the patient's doctor.
- If blurred vision, dry mouth, or rash develops, notify the patient's doctor, who may wish to discontinue therapy (rash occurs more commonly with pentaerythritol).
- Repeated or prolonged use may result in both dependence and tolerance to these drugs.
- Tolerance to both the vascular and antianginal effects of these drugs can develop, and cross-tolerance between nitrates and nitrites has been demonstrated.
- Tolerance is associated with a high or sustained plasma drug concentration and occurs most frequently with oral, I.V., and topical therapy. It rarely occurs with intermittent S.L. use.
- Patients taking oral isosorbide dinitrate or topical nitroglycerin have not exhibited cross-tolerance to S.L. nitroglycerin.

- If serious side effects develop in patients using ointment or the transdermal system, wipe the ointment from the skin or remove the product at once, and notify the patient's doctor. Be sure to avoid touching the ointment.
- Be sure to remove the transdermal patch before performing defibrillation. Because of the patch's aluminum backing, electric current may cause the patch to explode. ■

Nonsteroidal anti-inflammatory drugs

Drugs in this class include diflunisal, etodolac, fenoprofen calcium, flurbiprofen, ibuprofen, indomethacin, ketoprofen, ketorolac tromethamine, meclofenamate, mefenamic acid, nabumetone, naproxen, oxaprozin, oxyphenbutazone, phenylbutazone, piroxicam, sulindac, and tolmetin.

When administering NSAIDs, heed the following cautions:

- NSAIDs offer only symptomatic relief of rheumatoid conditions by reducing pain, stiffness, swelling, and tenderness; they don't reverse or arrest the disease process.
- Administer oral NSAIDs with a full 8-oz (240-ml) glass of water to ensure adequate passage into stomach. Have the patient sit up for 15 to 30 minutes after taking the drug to prevent it from becoming lodged in the esophagus.
- Patients who don't respond to one NSAID may respond to another.
- Use of an NSAID with an opioid analgesic has an additive effect. A lower dosage of the opioid analgesic may be possible.
- Side effects of oral NSAIDs chiefly involve the GI tract, particularly erosion of the gastric mucosa, which commonly causes dyspepsia, heartburn, epigastric distress, nausea, and abdominal pain.
- GI symptoms usually occur in the first few days of therapy and often subside with continuous treatment.
- CNS side effects (headache, dizziness, or drowsiness) may also occur.
- Fluid retention may aggravate preexisting hypertension or CHF.
- NSAIDs may mask the signs and symptoms of acute infection (fever, myalgia, or erythema); carefully evaluate patients at high risk for infection (for example, those with diabetes).
- Monitor the patient for signs and symptoms of bleeding. Assess bleeding time if surgery is required.
- Monitor ophthalmic and auditory function before and

periodically during therapy to prevent toxicity.

- Monitor CBC, platelet count, PT, and liver and kidney function studies periodically to detect abnormalities.
- Use NSAIDs cautiously in patients with a history of GI disease, increased risk of GI bleeding, or decreased renal function.
- Patients with known "triad" symptoms (aspirin hypersensitivity, rhinitis or nasal polyps, and asthma) are at high risk for bronchospasm.
- Pregnant patients should avoid the use of all NSAIDs, especially during the third trimester, when prostaglandin inhibition may cause prolonged gestation, dystocia, and delayed parturition.
- Patients over age 60 may be more susceptible to the toxic effects of NSAIDs because of decreased renal function.
- NSAIDs may cause fluid retention and edema, especially in elderly patients with CHF.
- Don't use NSAIDs for prolonged periods in children under age 14; safety of such use hasn't been established.
- NSAID therapy isn't recommended during breast-feeding. ■

Opioid (narcotic) agonist-antagonists

Drugs in this class include buprenorphine, butorphanol, dezocine, nalbuphine, and pentazocine.

When administering opioid agonist-antagonists, heed the following cautions:

- The opioid agonist-antagonists, as well as the opioid antagonists, can reverse the desired effects of opioids; thus, drugs from these two groups (for example, meperidine and buprenorphine) should not be prescribed at the same time.
- Parenteral administration of opioid agonist-antagonists provides better analgesia than does oral dosing.
- I.V. forms should be given by very slow injections, preferably in diluted solution.
- Rapid I.V. injection increases the incidence of side effects.
- Give I.M. or S.C. injections cautiously to patients who are chilled, hypovolemic, or in shock because decreased perfusion may lead to accumulation.
- Major hazards of agonist-antagonists are respiratory depression, apnea, shock, and cardiopulmonary arrest, possibly leading to death.
- All opioid agonist-antagonists can cause respiratory depression, but the severity

of depression that each drug can cause has a "ceiling." For example, each drug depresses respiration to a certain point, but increased dosages won't depress it further.

- Respiratory depression may last longer than the drug's analgesic effect.
- All of the opioid agonist-antagonists have been reported to cause withdrawal symptoms after abrupt discontinuation of long-term use; they appear to have some addiction potential, but less than that of the pure opioid agonists.
- CNS effects, the most common side effects, may include drowsiness, sedation, light-headedness, dizziness, hallucinations, disorientation, agitation, euphoria, dysphoria, insomnia, confusion, headache, tremor, miosis, and seizures.
- Cardiovascular side effects may include tachycardia, bradycardia, palpitations, chest wall rigidity, hypertension, hypotension, syncope, and edema.
- GI side effects may include nausea, vomiting, and constipation (most common), dry mouth, anorexia, and biliary spasms (colic). Other effects include urinary retention or hesitancy, decreased libido, flushing, rash, pruritus, and pain at the injection site.
- Opioid agonist-antagonists may obscure the signs and symptoms of an acute abdominal condition or worsen gallbladder pain.
- These drugs may cause orthostatic hypotension in ambulatory patients.
- Opioid agonist-antagonists can produce morphinelike dependence and thus have abuse potential.
- Psychological and physical dependence with drug tolerance can develop with long-term use.
- Patients with dependence or tolerance to these drugs usually experience an acute abstinence syndrome or withdrawal signs and symptoms, the severity of which is related to the degree of dependence, the abruptness of withdrawal, and the specific drug used.
- Common signs and symptoms of withdrawal are yawning, lacrimation, and diaphoresis (early); mydriasis, piloerection, flushing of face, tachycardia, tremor, irritability, and anorexia (intermediate); and muscle spasms, fever, nausea, vomiting, and diarrhea (late).
- Tolerance to the opioid's agonist activity (but not to its antagonist activity) may develop.
- The first sign of tolerance to the therapeutic effect of agonist-antagonists is usually a reduced duration of effect.
- Opioid agonist-antagonists are contraindicated in pa-

tients with known hypersensitivity to any drug of the same chemical group.

- Use these drugs with extreme caution in patients with supraventricular arrhythmias.
- Avoid these drugs or administer them with extreme caution in patients with head injury or increased intracranial pressure because neurologic parameters are obscured; and during pregnancy and labor because these drugs cross the placenta readily (premature neonates are especially sensitive to respiratory and CNS depressant effects).
- Use opioid agonist-antagonists cautiously in patients with renal or hepatic dysfunction because accumulation or prolonged duration of action may occur; and in patients with pulmonary disease (asthma or COPD) because these drugs depress respiration and suppress the cough reflex.
- Use cautiously in patients undergoing biliary tract surgery because biliary spasm may occur; in patients with seizure disorders because drug may precipitate seizures; in elderly and debilitated patients, who are more sensitive to both the therapeutic and side effects of these drugs; and in patients prone to physical or psychological addiction because of the high risk of addiction.
- Administering an opioid agonist-antagonist to the mother shortly before delivery may cause respiratory depression in the neonate.
- Lower dosages are usually indicated for elderly patients, who may be more sensitive to these drugs' therapeutic and side effects.
- Opioid agonist-antagonists have a lower potential for abuse than do opioid agonists, but the risk still exists.
- Usually, these drugs are not recommended for use in breast-feeding women. ■

Opioid (narcotic) antagonists

Drugs in this class include naloxone and naltrexone.

When administering opioid antagonists, heed the following cautions:

- Nausea and vomiting may occur with high doses.
- Abrupt reversal of opioid agonists may result in nausea, vomiting, sweating, tachycardia, increased blood pressure, and tremulousness.
- In postoperative patients, an excessive dose may reverse analgesia and cause excitement, with arrhythmias and fluctuations in blood pressure.
- When given to a narcotic addict, opioid antagonists

may produce an acute abstinence syndrome. The drug should be discontinued if signs of this syndrome appear.

- Because naloxone's duration of activity is shorter than that of most narcotics, vigilance and repeated doses are usually necessary to manage an acute narcotic overdose in a nonaddicted patient.
- Use with extreme caution in patients with head injury, increased intracranial pressure, seizures, asthma, alcoholism, prostatic hyperplasia, severe hepatic or renal disease, acute abdominal conditions, cardiac arrhythmias, hypovolemia, or psychiatric disorders; and in elderly or debilitated patients. Reduced dosage may be necessary.
- Opioid antagonists should not be used in narcotic addicts, including mothers with narcotic dependence and their newborns; these patients may develop an acute abstinence syndrome. ■

Opioids (previously called narcotic agonists)

Drugs in this class include alfentanil, codeine, difenoxin, diphenoxylate, fentanyl, hydromorphone, levomethadyl, levorphanol, meperidine, methadone, morphine, oxycodone, oxymorphone, propoxyphene, and sufentanil.

When administering opioids, heed the following cautions:

- Some of the opioids are well absorbed after oral or rectal administration; others must be administered parenterally.
- I.V. administration is the most rapidly effective and reliable route; absorption after I.M. or S.C. administration may be erratic.
- Parenteral administration of opioids provides better analgesia than oral administration.
- Parenteral injections by I.M. or S.C. route should be given cautiously to patients who are chilled, hypovolemic, or in shock, because decreased perfusion may lead to accumulation of the drug and toxic effects.
- Opioids vary in onset and duration of action; they're removed rapidly from the bloodstream and distributed, in decreasing order of concentration, into the skeletal muscle, kidneys, liver, intestinal tract, lungs, spleen, and brain; they readily cross the placenta.
- Be alert for possible interactions with other drugs the patient is taking.
- Because opioids decrease gastric, biliary, and pancreatic secretions and delay diges-

tion, constipation is a common side effect.

▪ Respiratory depression and, to a lesser extent, circulatory depression (including orthostatic hypotension) are the major hazards of treatment with opioids.

▪ Rapid I.V. administration increases the incidence and severity of these serious side effects. Respiratory arrest, shock, and cardiac arrest have occurred. It's likely that equianalgesic doses of individual opioids produce a comparable degree of respiratory depression, but their duration may vary.

▪ Respiratory depression may last longer than the drug's analgesic effect.

▪ Other CNS side effects include dizziness, visual disturbances, mental clouding or depression, sedation, coma, euphoria, dysphoria, weakness, faintness, agitation, restlessness, nervousness, seizures and, rarely, delirium and insomnia. Side effects seem to be more prevalent in ambulatory patients and those not experiencing severe pain.

▪ GI side effects include nausea, vomiting, and constipation as well as increased biliary tract pressure that may result in biliary spasm or colic.

▪ Opioids may cause orthostatic hypotension in ambulatory patients. Have the patient sit or lie down to relieve dizziness or fainting.

▪ Opioids may obscure the signs and symptoms of an acute abdominal condition or worsen gallbladder pain.

▪ Psychological or physical dependence (addiction) or tolerance may follow prolonged, high-dose therapy (more than 100 mg of morphine daily for more than 1 month).

▪ The first sign of tolerance to the therapeutic effect of opioids is usually a shortened duration of effect.

▪ These drugs shouldn't be used to treat pulmonary edema resulting from a chemical respiratory stimulant. Opioids decrease peripheral resistance, causing pooling of blood in the extremities and decreased venous return, cardiac workload, and pulmonary venous pressure; blood is thus shifted from the central to the peripheral circulation.

▪ Routine use of opioids for preoperative sedation in patients without pain is not recommended because it may cause complications during and after surgery.

▪ Administer with extreme caution to patients with head injury, increased intracranial pressure, seizures, asthma, COPD, alcoholism, prostatic hyperplasia, severe hepatic or renal disease, acute abdominal conditions, cardiac ar-

rhythmias, hypovolemia, or psychiatric disorders, and to elderly or debilitated patients. Reduced dosage may be necessary.
- Administering an opioid to a woman shortly before delivery may cause respiratory depression in the neonate. Monitor closely and be prepared to resuscitate.
- Use opioids with extreme caution during pregnancy and labor because they readily cross the placenta.
- Premature neonates appear especially sensitive to respiratory and CNS depressant effects when opioids are used during delivery.
- Opioids have a high potential for addiction and should always be administered with caution in patients prone to physical or psychological dependence.
- Codeine, meperidine, methadone, morphine, and propoxyphene are excreted in breast milk and should be used with caution in breast-feeding women.
- Methadone has been shown to cause physical dependence in breast-feeding infants of women maintained on methadone. ■

Oxazolidinedione derivatives

Drugs in this class include paramethadione, pemoline, and trimethadione.

When administering oxazolidinedione derivatives, heed the following cautions:
- These drugs cause CNS sedation, which may lead to ataxia at high doses; paramethadione has the least sedative effect.
- Warn the patient to avoid drinking alcoholic beverages while taking any of these drugs. Alcohol may decrease the drug's effectiveness and increase CNS side effects.
- These drugs have no value in treating tonic-clonic seizures and may precipitate a first tonic-clonic seizure.
- The most common side effects of oxazolidinediones include blurred vision, drowsiness, and such GI disturbances as nausea and vomiting.
- Toxic effects include fatal hematologic and renal reactions, lupuslike syndrome, and lymphadenopathy resembling malignant lymphoma.
- Strict medical supervision is necessary during the 1st year of treatment.
- Because of their potential teratogenicity and toxic side effects, these drugs should be reserved for severely refractory seizure disorders.

- Drug should be discontinued if neutrophil count falls below 2,500/µl or if any of the following occur: hypersensitivity, scotomata, hepatitis, systemic lupus erythematosus, lymphadenopathy, rash, nephrosis, alopecia, or generalized tonic-clonic seizures.
- Anticonvulsants should not be discontinued abruptly.
- Oxazolidinediones are contraindicated during pregnancy because of their potential for causing fetal malformations, and in patients with a known hypersensitivity to these drugs.
- These drugs should be used with caution in patients with renal or hepatic dysfunction, severe blood dyscrasias, and retinal or optic nerve disease because they may cause severe toxic effects in these organs and systems.
- These drugs are not recommended for children under age 2. Be sure to give children only the dosage forms prepared for pediatric use.
- It's not known whether oxazolidinediones are excreted in breast milk; therefore, an alternative feeding method is recommended during therapy. ■

Pancreatic enzymes

Drugs in this class include pancreatin and pancrelipase.

When administering pancreatic enzymes, heed the following cautions:

- These drugs aren't effective in GI disorders unrelated to enzyme deficiency.
- For maximal effect, administer the patient's dose just before or during a meal.
- The preparations are coated to protect the enzymes from gastric juices; don't crush them, and advise the patient not to chew them.
- Antacids or histamine$_2$ blockers, such as cimetidine or ranitidine, may be administered concurrently to prevent inactivation of non-enteric-coated drug products.
- Enteric coating on some products may reduce availability of the enzyme in the upper portion of the jejunum.
- Because pancreatic enzymes are not absorbed, side effects are confined to the GI tract and usually consist of nausea, vomiting, diarrhea, and stomach cramps.
- These drugs are contraindicated in patients with a severe hypersensitivity to pork. ■

Penicillins

Aminopenicillins include amoxicillin, ampicillin, and bacampicillin. Extended-spectrum penicillins include carbenicillin, mezlocillin, piperacillin, and ticarcillin. Natural penicillins include penicillin G and penicillin V. Penicillinase-resistant penicillins include cloxacillin, dicloxacillin, methicillin, nafcillin, and oxacillin. (See *Comparing penicillins.*)

When administering penicillins, heed the following cautions:

- Hypersensitivity reactions occur with all penicillins; they range from mild rashes, fever, and eosinophilia to fatal anaphylaxis.
- Hematologic reactions include hemolytic anemia, transient neutropenia, leukopenia, and thrombocytopenia.
- Certain side effects are more common with specific classes of penicillin.
- Acute interstitial nephritis is reported most often with methicillin.
- GI side effects are most common with, but not limited to, ampicillin.
- High doses, especially of penicillin G, irritate the CNS in patients with renal disease, causing confusion, twitching, lethargy, dysphagia, seizures, and coma.
- Hepatotoxicity is most common with penicillinase-resistant penicillins; hyperkalemia and hypernatremia, with extended-spectrum penicillins.
- Jarisch-Herxheimer reaction can occur when penicillin G is used in secondary syphilis; signs and symptoms include chills, fever, headache, myalgia, tachycardia, malaise, diaphoresis, hypotension, and sore throat.
- Local irritation from parenteral therapy may be severe enough to require discontinuation of the drug or administration by subclavian catheter if drug therapy is to continue.
- Keep in mind that a negative history for penicillin hypersensitivity does not preclude future allergic reactions.
- Coagulation abnormalities, even frank bleeding, can follow high doses, especially of extended-spectrum penicillins; monitor PT and platelet counts, and assess the patient for signs of occult or frank bleeding.
- Patients on long-term therapy, especially elderly and debilitated patients and others receiving immunosuppressants or radiation therapy, may develop superinfection.

(Text continues on page 208.)

Comparing penicillins

DRUG, DOSAGE, AND ROUTE	FREQUENCY	PENICILLINASE RESISTANT
amoxicillin		
250 to 500 mg P.O.	q 8 hr	No
3 g P.O. with 1 g probenecid (for gonorrhea)	Single dose	
amoxicillin/clavulanate potassium		
250 to 500 mg P.O.	q 8 hr	Yes
ampicillin		
2 to 14 g daily I.M. or I.V.	Divided doses given q 4 to 6 hr	No
250 to 500 mg P.O.	q 6 hr	
2.5 g P.O. with 1 g probenecid (for gonorrhea)	Single dose	
ampicillin sodium/sulbactam sodium		
2.5 to 3 g I.M. or I.V.	q 6 to 8 hr	Yes
azlocillin		
200 to 350 mg/kg I.V. daily	Divided doses given q 4 to 6 hr	No
bacampicillin		
400 to 800 mg P.O.	q 12 hr	No

(continued)

Comparing penicillins *(continued)*

DRUG, DOSAGE, AND ROUTE	FREQUENCY	PENICILLINASE RESISTANT
carbenicillin		
200 mg/kg I.M. or I.V. daily (for urinary tract infections)	Divided doses given q 4 to 6 hr	No
30 to 40 g I.M. or I.V. daily (for systemic infections)	Divided doses given q 4 to 6 hr	
382 to 764 mg P.O.	q 6 hr	
cloxacillin		
250 mg to 1 g P.O.	q 6 hr	Yes
dicloxacillin		
125 to 500 mg P.O.	q 6 hr	Yes
methicillin		
1 to 2 g I.M. or I.V.	q 4 to 6 hr	Yes
mezlocillin		
3 to 4 g I.M. or I.V.	q 4 to 6 hr	No
nafcillin		
250 mg to 2 g I.M. or I.V.	q 4 to 6 hr	Yes
500 mg to 1 g P.O.	q 6 hr	
oxacillin		
250 mg to 2 g I.M., I.V.	q 4 to 6 hr	Yes
500 mg to 1 g P.O.	q 6 hr	

Comparing penicillins *(continued)*

DRUG, DOSAGE, AND ROUTE	FREQUENCY	PENICILLINASE RESISTANT
penicillin G benzathine 1.2 to 2.4 million units I.M.	Single dose	No
penicillin G potassium 200,000 to 4 million units I.M. or I.V.	q 4 hr	No
400,000 to 800,000 units P.O.	q 6 hr	
penicillin G procaine 600,000 to 1.2 million units I.M.	q 1 to 3 days	No
4.8 million units with 1 g probenecid (for syphilis)	Single dose for primary, secondary, and early latent syphilis; weekly for 3 weeks for late latent syphilis	
penicillin G sodium 200,000 to 4 million units I.M. or I.V.	q 4 hr	No
penicillin V potassium 250 to 500 mg P.O.	q 6 to 8 hr	No
piperacillin 100 to 300 mg/kg I.M. or I.V. daily	Divided doses given q 4 to 6 hr	No

(continued)

Comparing penicillins *(continued)*

DRUG, DOSAGE, AND ROUTE	FREQUENCY	PENICILLINASE RESISTANT
piperacillin sodium/ tazobactam sodium 3.375 g I.V.	q 6 hr	Yes
ticarcillin disodium 150 to 300 mg/kg I.M. or I.V. daily	Divided doses given q 3 to 6 hr	No
ticarcillin disodium/ clavulanate potassium 3 g I.V.	q 4 to 6 hr	Yes

- Don't add or mix other drugs — particularly aminoglycosides — with I.V. infusions of penicillin. These drugs will be inactivated if mixed with penicillins; they are chemically and physically incompatible.
- In patients with renal impairment, dosage should be reduced if creatinine clearance is less than 10 ml/ minute. ■

Phenothiazines

Phenothiazines are divided into five chemical groups: aliphatic derivatives, piperidine derivatives, piperazine derivatives, pyrrolidine derivatives, and thioxanthene derivatives.

Aliphatic derivatives include chlorpromazine, ethopropazine, promazine, promethazine, propiomazine, triflupromazine, and trimeprazine. Piperidine derivatives include mesoridazine and thioridazine. Piperazine derivatives include acetophenazine, fluphenazine, perphenazine, prochlorperazine, thiethylperazine, and trifluoperazine. Pyrrolidine derivatives include methdilazine. Thioxanthene derivatives include chlorprothixene and thiothixene.

When administering phenothiazines, heed the following cautions:

- These drugs are structurally similar to TCAs and share many of their side effects.
- A patient who doesn't respond to one phenothiazine may respond to another.
- Onset of full therapeutic effect requires 6 weeks to 6 months of therapy; therefore, dosage should not be adjusted more than once a week.
- Phenothiazines may cause pink to brown discoloration of urine.
- Phenothiazines may produce extrapyramidal symptoms (dystonic movements, torticollis, oculogyric crises, parkinsonian symptoms) ranging from akathisia during early treatment to tardive dyskinesia after long-term use.
- In some cases, extrapyramidal symptoms can be alleviated by dosage reduction or treatment with diphenhydramine, trihexyphenidyl, or benztropine mesylate.
- Dystonia usually occurs after initial therapy or after increased dosage in children and younger adults.
- Parkinsonian symptoms and tardive dyskinesia more often affect elderly patients, especially women.
- A neuroleptic malignant syndrome resembling severe parkinsonism may occur (most often in young men taking fluphenazine). It consists of rapid onset of hyperthermia, muscular hyperreflexia, marked extrapyramidal and autonomic dysfunction, arrhythmias, diaphoresis, and several other unpleasant reactions. Although rare, this condition has a 10% mortality rate and requires immediate treatment, including cooling blankets, neuromuscular blockers such as dantrolene, and supportive measures.
- Other side effects are similar to those seen with TCAs, including varying degrees of sedative and anticholinergic effects, orthostatic hypotension with reflex tachycardia, fainting and dizziness, and arrhythmias.
- Allergic manifestations are usually marked by elevation of liver enzyme levels that progresses to obstructive jaundice.
- The piperidine derivatives mesoridazine and thioridazine have the most pronounced cardiovascular effects, and the piperazine derivatives have the least.
- Parenteral administration is more often associated with cardiovascular effects because of more rapid absorption.
- Seizures are most common with aliphatic derivatives.
- Phenothiazines are contraindicated in patients with

known hypersensitivity to phenothiazines and related compounds, including allergic reactions involving hepatic function, and in patients with blood dyscrasias or bone marrow depression.

- These drugs are also contraindicated in patients with coma, brain damage, CNS depression, circulatory collapse, or cerebrovascular disease because additive CNS depression and accompanying blood pressure alteration may seriously worsen these states. Phenothiazines should not be given in conjunction with adrenergic blockers or spinal or epidural anesthesia because of the potential for postural hypotension.
- Phenothiazines should be used cautiously in patients with cardiac disease (arrhythmias, CHF, angina pectoris, valvular disease, or heart block) to avoid further compromise of cardiac function from alpha-adrenergic blockade. Such reactions are particularly likely in patients with preexisting cardiac compromise or a history of arrhythmias.
- Phenothiazines should be used cautiously in patients with encephalitis, Reye's syndrome, or head injury because their antiemetic and CNS depressant effects may mask signs and symptoms and obscure diagnosis.
- These drugs should be used cautiously in patients with respiratory disease to minimize the risk of respiratory depression and suppression of the cough reflex from additive CNS depression; and in patients with seizure disorders because these drugs lower seizure threshold and may require increased dosage of anticonvulsants.
- Phenothiazines should be used cautiously in patients with glaucoma, prostatic hyperplasia, paralytic ileus, or urine retention because they have significant antimuscarinic effects that may exacerbate these conditions.
- Phenothiazines should be used cautiously in patients with hepatic or renal dysfunction to prevent drug accumulation; in patients with Parkinson's disease because these drugs may aggravate tremors and other symptoms; in patients with pheochromocytoma because of possible adverse cardiovascular effects; and in patients with hypocalcemia because of increased risk of extrapyramidal symptoms.
- Don't withdraw the drug abruptly; although physical dependence does not occur with antipsychotic drugs, rebound exacerbation of psychotic symptoms may occur, and many drug effects persist.

▪ Unless otherwise specified, antipsychotics are not recommended for children under age 12. Use caution when using phenothiazines for nausea and vomiting because acutely ill children (those with chickenpox, measles, CNS infections, or dehydration) are at increased risk for dystonic reactions.
▪ If feasible, the patient should not breast-feed while taking a phenothiazine. Most phenothiazines are excreted in breast milk and have a direct effect on prolactin levels. The benefit to the mother must outweigh the hazard to the infant. ■

Salicylates

Drugs in this class include aspirin, choline magnesium trisalicylate, choline salicylate, magnesium salicylate, salicylamide, salsalate, sodium salicylate, and sodium thiosalicylate.

When administering salicylates, heed the following cautions:
▪ In rheumatoid conditions, salicylates offer only symptomatic relief by reducing pain, stiffness, swelling, and tenderness. They don't reverse or arrest the disease process.
▪ Side effects of salicylates involve primarily the GI tract, particularly the gastric mucosa.
▪ GI side effects occur more frequently with aspirin than with other salicylates. The most common symptoms are dyspepsia, heartburn, epigastric distress, nausea, and abdominal pain.
▪ GI reactions usually occur in the first few days of therapy, often subside with continuous treatment, and can be minimized by administering salicylates with meals or food, antacids, or an 8-oz (240-ml) glass of water or milk.
▪ The incidence and severity of GI bleeding are exposure-related.
▪ Chronic salicylate intoxication (salicylism) may occur with prolonged therapy at high doses. Signs and symptoms include tinnitus, hearing loss, hepatotoxicity, moderate to severe noncardiogenic edema, and adverse renal reactions.
▪ Salicylate-induced bronchospasm, with or without urticaria and angioedema, may occur in patients with hypersensitivity to these drugs, particularly those with the "triad" of aspirin sensitivity: rhinitis, nasal polyps, and asthma.
▪ A significant incidence of cross-sensitivity has been observed with tartrazine; 5% of allergic patients also exhibit cross-sensitivity with acet-

aminophen. (However, most clinicians consider acetaminophen an acceptable alternative in patients with documented aspirin or NSAID sensitivity.)
▪ Use salicylates with caution in patients with a history of GI disease (especially peptic ulcer disease), increased risk of GI bleeding, or decreased renal function.
▪ Salicylates may mask the signs and symptoms of acute infection (fever, myalgia, and erythema); carefully evaluate patients at risk for infections, such as those with diabetes.
▪ Warn patients who are or could become pregnant to avoid the use of all salicylates, especially during the third trimester, when prostaglandin inhibition can adversely affect fetal cardiovascular development.
▪ Patients over age 60 may be more susceptible to the toxic effects of salicylates because of possible impaired renal function.
▪ Children may be more susceptible to toxic effects of salicylates; therefore, use with caution.
▪ Because of epidemiologic association with Reye's syndrome, the CDC recommends that children with chickenpox or flulike symptoms not be given salicylates.
▪ Don't use long-term salicylate therapy in children under age 14; safety of this use hasn't been established.
▪ Salicylates are distributed into breast milk and should be avoided during breast-feeding. ■

Succinimide derivatives

Drugs in this class include ethosuximide, methsuximide, and phensuximide.

When administering succinimide derivatives, heed the following cautions:
▪ The most common side effects of succinimides involve the CNS and include drowsiness, headache, and blurred vision.
▪ Other side effects include acute dermatologic reactions (Stevens-Johnson syndrome), blood dyscrasias, renal dysfunction, and systemic lupus erythematosus.
▪ Obtain baseline liver, renal function, and blood studies and monitor frequently.
▪ Repeat CBCs every 3 months and urinalysis and liver function tests every 6 months.
▪ Succinimide anticonvulsants should not be discontinued abruptly.
▪ Succinimides add to CNS depressant effects of alcohol, narcotics, anxiolytics, antidepressants, and tranquilizers.
▪ Capsules should be protected from excessive heat, so

avoid storing them in a closed car or near a heat source.

- Succinimides are contraindicated in patients with known hypersensitivity to them.
- They should be used with caution in patients with acute intermittent porphyria.
- Also use with caution in patients with hepatic or renal dysfunction, in elderly patients (who metabolize and excrete all drugs slowly and may obtain therapeutic effect from a lower dosage), and in children.
- Women should discontinue breast-feeding while taking these drugs. ■

Sulfonamides

Drugs in this class include co-trimoxazole, sulfacetamide, sulfacytine, sulfadiazine, sulfamethizole, sulfamethoxazole, sulfasalazine, and sulfisoxazole.

When administering sulfonamides, heed the following cautions:

- Resistance to sulfonamides is common if therapy continues beyond 2 weeks.
- Resistance to one sulfonamide usually means cross-resistance to others.
- Sulfonamides may interact with other drugs (oral anticoagulants, cyclosporine, digoxin, folic acid, hydantoins, methotrexate, and sulfonylureas) and may alter test results.
- Sulfonamides alter results of tests using cupric sulfate.
- Sulfonamides cause side effects affecting many organs and systems; many of these are caused by hypersensitivity, including rash, fever, pruritus, erythema multiforme, erythema nodosum, Stevens-Johnson syndrome, Lyell's syndrome, exfoliative dermatitis, photosensitivity, joint pain, conjunctivitis, leukopenia, and bronchospasm.
- Hematologic reactions include granulocytopenia, thrombocytopenia, agranulocytosis, hypoprothrombinemia and, in G6PD deficiency, hemolytic anemia.
- Renal effects usually result from crystalluria (precipitation of the sulfonamide in the renal system).
- GI side effects include anorexia, stomatitis, pancreatitis, diarrhea, and folic acid malabsorption.
- Oral therapy commonly causes nausea and vomiting.
- Hepatotoxicity and CNS reactions (dizziness, confusion, headache, ataxia, drowsiness, and insomnia) are rare.
- Patients with AIDS have a much higher incidence of side effects.
- Patients on long-term therapy, especially elderly and debilitated patients, and those

receiving immunosuppressants or radiation therapy may develop superinfection.

- Photosensitization (photoallergy or phototoxicity) may occur.
- Elderly patients are susceptible to bacterial and fungal superinfection, are at greater risk for folate-deficiency anemia after sulfonamide therapy, and commonly are at greater risk for renal and hematologic effects because of diminished renal function.
- Don't administer a sulfonamide to any patient with a history of hypersensitivity to sulfonamides or to any other drug containing sulfur (such as thiazides, furosemide, and oral sulfonylureas).
- Sulfonamides are also contraindicated in patients with severe renal or hepatic dysfunction or porphyria, during pregnancy (at term, when they displace bilirubin at the binding site and may cause kernicterus in neonates), and during breast-feeding.
- Sulfonamides may cause kernicterus in infants because they displace bilirubin at the binding site, cross the placenta, and are excreted in breast milk.
- Because sulfonamides are excreted in breast milk, the doctor must decide whether to discontinue breast-feeding or discontinue the drug, taking into account the importance of the drug to the mother.
- Don't use in infants less than 2 months old (except as adjunctive therapy with pyrimethamine to treat congenital toxoplasmosis).
- Premature infants, infants with hyperbilirubinemia, and those with G6PD deficiency are at risk for kernicterus.
- Sulfacytine isn't recommended for use in children less than 14 years old.
- Administer sulfonamides with caution to patients with the following conditions: mild to moderate renal or hepatic impairment, urinary obstruction (because of the risk of drug accumulation), severe allergies, asthma, blood dyscrasias, or G6PD deficiency.
- Give sulfonamides with caution to children with the fragile X chromosome associated with mental retardation, because they are vulnerable to psychomotor depression from folate depletion. ■

Sulfonylureas

Drugs in this class include acetohexamide, chlorpropamide, glipizide, glyburide, tolazamide, and tolbutamide.

When administering sulfonylureas, heed the following cautions:

- These drugs can be used only in patients with functioning pancreatic beta cells.
- Administer sulfonylureas 30 minutes before the morning meal for once-daily dosing, or 30 minutes before the morning and evening meals for twice-daily dosing.
- These oral antidiabetic drugs are not effective in insulin-dependent (Type I, juvenile-onset) diabetes mellitus.
- Administration of oral antidiabetic drugs has been associated with increased cardiovascular mortality compared with treatment by diet alone or diet plus insulin, according to a long-term prospective clinical trial conducted by the University Group Diabetes Program.
- Patients transferring from one sulfonylurea (except chlorpropamide) to another usually need no transition period.
- Non-insulin-dependent diabetics may require insulin therapy during periods of increased stress, such as infection, fever, surgery, or trauma. Monitor patients closely for hyperglycemia in these situations.
- Dose-related side effects, which aren't usually serious and respond to decreased dosage, include headache, nausea, vomiting, anorexia, heartburn, weakness, and paresthesia.
- Hypoglycemia may follow excessive dosage, increased exercise, decreased food intake, or consumption of alcohol.
- Signs and symptoms of overdose include anxiety, chills, cold sweats, confusion, cool pale skin, difficulty in concentration, drowsiness, excessive hunger, headache, nausea, nervousness, rapid heartbeat, shakiness, unsteady gait, weakness, and unusual fatigue.
- These agents are contraindicated in treating insulin-dependent, brittle, or severe diabetes; diabetes mellitus adequately controlled by diet; and maturity-onset diabetes complicated by ketosis, acidosis, diabetic coma, Raynaud's gangrene, renal or hepatic impairment, or thyroid or other endocrine dysfunction.
- Use cautiously in patients with sulfonamide hypersensitivity.
- Sulfonylurea antidiabetic drugs shouldn't be used during pregnancy because of reportedly prolonged, severe hypoglycemia lasting from 4 to 10 days in neonates born to mothers taking these drugs.
- Use of insulin permits more rigid control of blood glucose levels, which should reduce the incidence of congenital abnormalities, mor-

tality, and morbidity caused by abnormal glucose levels.

- Elderly patients and those with renal insufficiency may be more sensitive to these agents because of decreased metabolism and excretion. They usually require lower dosages and should be closely monitored.
- Hypoglycemia may be more difficult to recognize in elderly patients, although it usually causes neurologic symptoms in such patients.
- Agents with prolonged duration of action should be avoided in elderly patients.
- Oral antidiabetic drugs are excreted in breast milk in minimal amounts and may cause hypoglycemia in the breast-feeding infant. ■

Tetracyclines

Drugs in this class include demeclocycline, doxycycline, minocycline, oxytetracycline, and tetracycline.

When administering tetracyclines, heed the following cautions:

- The most common side effects of tetracyclines involve the GI tract and are dose related. They include anorexia; flatulence; nausea; vomiting; bulky, loose stools; epigastric burning; and abdominal discomfort.
- Hypersensitivity reactions are infrequent and may include urticaria, rash, pruritus, eosinophilia, and exfoliative dermatitis.
- Photosensitivity reactions may be severe; they're most common with demeclocycline and rare with minocycline.
- Renal effects are minor and include occasional elevations in BUN levels (without rise in serum creatinine level)and a reversible diabetes insipidus syndrome (reported only with demeclocycline).
- Renal failure has been attributed to Fanconi's syndrome after use of outdated tetracycline.
- Rare side effects include hepatotoxicity, leukocytosis, thrombocytopenia, hemolytic anemia, leukopenia, neutropenia, and atypical lymphocytes.
- There have also been reports of vaginal candidiasis, microscopic thyroid discoloration (after chronic use), light-headedness, dizziness, and drowsiness.
- Tetracyclines may affect certain laboratory tests.
- Elderly patients are more susceptible to superinfection.
- Don't give any tetracycline antibiotic to a patient with a history of hypersensitivity to any other tetracycline.
- Children age 8 and under should not receive tetracyclines unless there's no alter-

native. Tetracyclines can cause permanent discoloration of teeth, enamel hypoplasia, and reversible decrease in bone calcification.
- When possible, tetracyclines should be avoided by breast-feeding women. ■

Thrombolytic enzymes

Drugs in this class include alteplase, anistreplase, streptokinase, and urokinase. (See *Comparing thrombolytic enzymes,* page 218.)

When administering thrombolytic enzymes, heed the following cautions:
- Thrombolytics act only on fibrin clots, not on those formed by a precipitated drug.
- Follow your facility's policy and instructions for reconstitution precisely. Pass the solution through a 0.45-micron (or smaller) filter to remove any filaments.
- Don't use dextran concomitantly because it can interfere with coagulation as well as with blood typing and crossmatching.
- Obtain pretherapy baseline determinations of thrombin time, PT, activated PTT, hematocrit, and platelet count for subsequent blood monitoring.
- During systemic thrombolytic therapy, as in pulmonary embolism or venous thrombosis, PT or thrombin time after 4 hours of therapy should be approximately twice the pretreatment value.
- Keep venipuncture sites to a minimum; apply pressure dressings for at least 15 minutes to prevent bleeding and hematoma.
- For arterial puncture (except intracoronary), use upper extremities, which are more accessible for pressure dressings. Apply pressure for at least 30 minutes after arterial puncture.
- Administer thrombolytics by infusion pump to ensure accuracy.
- I.M. injections are contraindicated during therapy because of increased risk of bleeding at the injection site.
- Stop therapy if bleeding is evident; pretreatment with heparin or drugs that affect platelets increases risk.
- Side effects of these agents are essentially an extension of their actions; hemorrhage is the most common side effect.
- These agents cause bleeding twice as often as does heparin.
- Streptokinase is more likely to cause an allergic reaction than urokinase.
- Patients age 75 or older are at greater risk for cerebral hemorrhage because they're more likely to have preexisting cerebrovascular disease. ■

Comparing thrombolytic enzymes

Thrombolytic enzymes dissolve clots by accelerating the formation of plasmin by activated plasminogen. Plasminogen activators, found in most tissues and body fluids, help plasminogen (an inactive enzyme) convert to plasmin (an active enzyme), which dissolves the clot.

Thrombolytic enzymes in current use include streptokinase, urokinase, tissue plasminogen activator (t-PA or alteplase), and anistreplase. Dosages of these enzymes may vary according to the patient's condition.

DRUG AND ACTION	INITIAL DOSE	MAINTENANCE THERAPY
alteplase Directly converts plasminogen to plasmin	*I.V. bolus:* 6 to 10 mg over 1 to 2 min	*I.V. infusion:* 50 to 54 mg/hr over 1st hour; 20 mg (20 ml)/hr over next 2 hr; then discontinue
anistreplase Directly converts plasminogen to plasmin	*I.V. push:* 30 units over 2 to 3 min	Not necessary
streptokinase Indirectly activates plasminogen, which converts to plasmin	*Intracoronary bolus:* 15,000 to 20,000 IU *I.V. bolus:* none needed	*Intracoronary infusion:* 2,000 to 4,000 IU/min over 60 min *I.V. infusion:* 1,500,000 units over 60 min
urokinase Directly converts plasminogen to plasmin	*Intracoronary bolus:* none needed	*Intracoronary infusion:* 2,000 units/lb/hr (4,400 units/kg/hr); rate of 15 ml of solution/hr for total of 12 hr (total volume should not exceed 200 ml)

Thyroid hormone antagonists

Drugs in this class include methimazole, propylthiouracil (PTU), and radioactive iodine 131).

When administering thyroid hormone antagonists, heed the following cautions:

- Therapeutic doses can cause fever, chills, sore throat, weakness, backache, swelling of feet, joint pain, and unusual bleeding or bruising.
- Toxic doses can cause constipation, cold intolerance, dry puffy skin, headache, sleepiness, muscle aches, and unusual weight gain.
- Signs and symptoms of overdose or hypothyroidism include mental depression; menstrual changes; cold intolerance; constipation; dry, puffy skin; headache; listlessness; muscle aches; nausea; vomiting; weakness; fatigue; hard, non-pitting edema; and weight gain.
- Signs of thyrotoxicosis or inadequate thyroid suppression include diarrhea, fever, irritability, listlessness, rapid heartbeat, vomiting, and weakness.
- Treatment with antithyroid drugs requires CBCs periodically to detect impending leukopenia, thrombocytopenia, or agranulocytosis.
- Thyroid hormone antagonists should be used cautiously with careful thyroid function monitoring in pregnant patients.
- Pregnant patients may require less drug as pregnancy progresses. Thyroid hormones may be added to the regimen. In some patients, thyroid hormone antagonists may be discontinued during the last few weeks of pregnancy.
- Drug should be discontinued if patient develops severe rash or enlarged cervical lymph nodes.
- Patients should avoid breast-feeding during treatment with thyroid hormone antagonists. ■

Thyroid hormones

Drugs in this class include levothyroxine sodium (T_4), liothyronine sodium (T_3), liotrix, thyroid USP (desiccated), and thyrotropin (TSH).

When administering thyroid hormones, heed the following cautions:

- Thyroid hormone dosage varies widely among patients; therefore, treatment should start at the lowest dose and be titrated to higher doses according to the patient's symptoms and laboratory data until a euthyroid state is reached.

- Patients taking anticoagulants usually require a lower dosage.
- Side effects of thyroid hormones are extensions of their pharmacologic properties. Signs of overdose include nervousness, insomnia, tremor, tachycardia, palpitations, nausea, headache, fever, and diaphoresis.
- Signs of thyrotoxicosis or inadequate dosage include diarrhea, fever, irritability, listlessness, rapid heartbeat, vomiting, and weakness.
- In patients over age 60, the initial dosage should be 25% less than the usual recommended starting dosage.
- During the first few months of therapy, children may suffer partial hair loss.
- Minimal amounts of exogenous thyroid hormones are excreted in breast milk. However, no problems have been reported in breast-feeding infants. ■

Tricyclic antidepressants

Drugs in this class include amitriptyline, amoxapine, clomipramine, desipramine, doxepin, imipramine, maprotiline, nortriptyline, protriptyline, and trimipramine.

When administering TCAs, heed the following cautions:

- Patients may respond to some TCAs and not to others; if a patient doesn't respond to one drug, another should be tried.
- Side effects of TCAs are similar to those seen with phenothiazines, including varying degrees of sedation, anticholinergic effects, and orthostatic hypotension.
- The tertiary amines have the strongest sedative effects; tolerance to these effects usually develops within a few weeks.
- Protriptyline has the least sedative effect (and may be stimulatory) but, along with the tertiary amines, has the most pronounced effect on blood pressure and cardiac tissue.
- Maprotiline and amoxapine are most likely to cause seizures, especially in an overdose.
- Desipramine has a greater margin of safety in patients with prostatic hyperplasia, paralytic ileus, glaucoma, or urine retention because of its relatively low level of anticholinergic activity.
- TCAs impair the patient's ability to perform tasks requiring mental alertness, such as driving a car.
- Check vital signs regularly for decreased blood pressure or tachycardia; observe the

patient carefully for other side effects and report changes. Check the ECG in patients over age 40 before initiating therapy. Ask the doctor about having the patient take the first dose in the office to allow close observation for side effects.

- Check for anticholinergic side effects (urine retention or constipation), which may require dosage reduction.
- Observe patients for mood changes to monitor progress; drug benefits may not be apparent for 3 to 6 weeks.
- Don't withdraw the drug abruptly; gradually reduce the dosage over a period of weeks to avoid rebound effect or other side effects.
- Because suicidal overdosage with TCAs is commonly fatal, prescribe only small amounts.
- Lower dosages are indicated in elderly patients because they're more sensitive to both the therapeutic and side effects of TCAs.
- TCAs are not recommended for children under age 12. ■

Vinca alkaloids

Drugs in this class include vinblastine, vincristine, and vindesine.

When administering vinca alkaloids, heed the following cautions:

- Vinblastine and vindesine may cause bone marrow depression, which is usually dose-related. Effects may include leukopenia, which occurs 4 to 10 days after a dose, with recovery within 10 to 21 days.
- Vincristine may cause neurotoxicity, which is usually dose-related. Effects may include peripheral neuropathy with loss of deep tendon reflexes, weakness, vocal cord paralysis, and paralytic ileus.
- The vinca alkaloids can cause life-threatening acute bronchospasm.
- These drugs are potent vesicants and can cause severe tissue necrosis if they extravasate. Take special care to avoid extravasation. If it occurs, treatment includes liberal injection of hyaluronidase into the site, followed by warm compresses to minimize the spread of the reaction.
- The agents in this class have similar names. Don't confuse one drug with another.
- Elderly patients may be more sensitive to the neurotoxic and myelosuppressant effects of vinca alkaloids.
- Because of the risk of serious side effects, mutagenicity, and carcinogenicity in infants, breast-feeding is not recommended. ■

Vitamins

Fat-soluble vitamins include vitamin A_1 (retinol), vitamin A_2 (dehydroretinol), vitamin A acid (retinoic acid), provitamin A (carotene), vitamin D, vitamin D_2 (ergocalciferol), vitamin D_3 (cholecalciferol), vitamin E, vitamin K (menadione or phytonadione), and tocopherol and tocotrienols (alpha, beta, gamma, and delta).

Water-soluble vitamins include vitamin B_1 (thiamine), vitamin B_2 (riboflavin), vitamin B_3 (niacin), vitamin B_5 (pantothenic acid), vitamin B_6 (pyridoxine), vitamin B_9 (folic acid or folacin), vitamin B_{12} (cyanocobalamin), vitamin C (ascorbic acid), and biotin. (See *Recommended daily allowances for adults ages 23 to 50.*)

When administering vitamins, heed the following cautions:

- Multiple vitamins may be indicated for patients taking oral contraceptives, estrogens, prolonged antibiotic therapy, isoniazid, or for patients receiving prolonged total parenteral nutrition.
- People with increased metabolic requirements (such as infants) and those suffering severe injury, trauma, major surgery, or severe infection also require vitamin supplements.
- Other indications for multiple vitamin therapy include prolonged diarrhea, severe GI disorders, malignant disease, surgical removal or resection of GI tract, obstructive jaundice, cystic fibrosis, and other conditions leading to reduced or poor absorption.
- The most common side effects seen with both types of vitamins include nausea, vomiting, diarrhea, fatigue, weakness, headache, loss of appetite, skin rash, and itching.
- Vitamins containing iron may cause constipation and black, tarry stools.
- Excessive fluoride supplements can result in hypocalcemia and tetany.
- Excessive amounts of vitamins, particularly in neonates, may be toxic. ■

Xanthine derivatives

Drugs in this class include aminophylline, caffeine, dyphylline, and theophylline. (See *Comparing xanthine derivatives,* page 224.)

When administering xanthine derivatives, heed the following cautions:

- The xanthines stimulate the CNS and heart while relaxing smooth muscle. This produces such reactions as hypotension, palpitations, arrhythmias, restlessness, irrita-

Recommended daily allowances for adults ages 23 to 50

VITAMIN	MALES	FEMALES	PREGNANT FEMALES	LACTATING FEMALES*
A	1,000 mcg	800 mcg	800 mcg	1,300 mcg
B_1	1.5 mg	1.1 mg	1.5 mg	1.6 mg
B_2	1.7 mg	1.3 mg	1.6 mg	1.8 mg
B_6	2 mg	1.6 mg	2.2 mg	2.1 mg
B_{12}	2 mcg	2 mcg	2.2 mcg	2.6 mcg
C	60 mg	60 mg	70 mg	95 mg
D	200 IU	200 IU	400 IU	400 IU
E	10 IU	8 IU	10 IU	12 IU
K	80 mcg	65 mcg	65 mcg	65 mcg
folic acid	200 mcg	180 mcg	400 mcg	280 mcg
niacin	19 mg	15 mg	17 mg	20 mg

*For the first 6 months

bility, nausea, vomiting, urine retention, and headache.

- Side effects are dose-related, except for hypersensitivity, and can be controlled by dosage adjustment and monitored via serum levels.
- Many dosage forms and agents are available; select the form that offers maximum potential for compliance and minimal toxicity.
- Timed-release preparations shouldn't be crushed or chewed.
- Dosage should be calculated from lean body weight because theophylline isn't distributed into fatty tissue.
- Individuals metabolize theophylline at different rates.
- Daily dosage may need to be adjusted in patients with CHF or hepatic disease and

Comparing xanthine derivatives

The table below compares the varying theophylline content of several common xanthine derivatives. (Dyphylline isn't included because although it has the same pharmacologic action as theophylline, it is a chemical derivative and not a true theophylline salt.)

DRUG	APPROXIMATE THEOPHYLLINE CONTENT	EQUIVALENT DOSE
theophylline anhydrous	100%	100 mg
theophylline monohydrate	90.7% (±1.1%)	110 mg
aminophylline anhydrous	85.7% (±1.7%)	116 mg
aminophylline dehydrate	78.9% (±1.6%)	127 mg
theophylline sodium glycinate	45.9% (±1.4%)	217 mg

in elderly patients. Monitor blood levels carefully.

- Aminophylline and theophylline release theophylline in the blood; theophylline blood levels are used to monitor therapy.
- Dyphylline is a theophylline analogue, and special blood tests are used to monitor dyphylline therapy. ■

■ CHAPTER 7

MANAGING SIDE EFFECTS

UNDERSTANDING PREDISPOSING FACTORS

Patient factors

A patient's therapeutic responses to a drug result from the interplay among patient characteristics, the drug's characteristics, and exogenous (external) factors. Patient, drug, and exogenous factors can alter that interplay to cause drug side effects.

Patient factors include extremes of age, extremes of body weight, genetic variations, the patient's temperament and attitudes, circadian rhythms, changes associated with disease, and changes associated with pregnancy.

Extremes of age

The absorption, distribution, metabolism, and excretion of drugs are different in infants and elderly patients than in young adults. Infants lack certain drug-metabolizing enzymes and have decreased renal blood flow. These physiologic factors increase drug and metabolite blood levels. The breast-feeding infant also may develop side effects to drugs that pass into the mother's breast milk.

Elderly patients have decreased blood flow to all organs, especially the liver and kidneys. These conditions result in increased drug levels as well as changes in drug distribution and a greater risk of toxicity.

Extremes of body weight

Recommended dosages typically are based on the average-sized adult. Therefore, an extremely thin or obese patient requires an individualized dosage calculation to prevent overdosing or underdosing. Abnormal thinness or obesity may alter drug distribution, resulting in higher- or lower-than-expected drug levels in tissues and at receptor sites.

Genetic variations

Genetic variations that alter enzyme activity or cause enzyme deficiency affect drug metabolism or drug action.

Acetylation

Isoniazid, hydralazine, and procainamide are metabolized in the liver by a pathway known as *acetylation,* a process that proceeds at a rate that's partially genetically determined.

In most patients, acetylation occurs either quickly or slowly. A slow acetylator will display a higher blood level of a given drug dose than a fast acetylator and may have a drug side effect as a result.

G6PD

G6PD (glucose-6-phosphate dehydrogenase) plays a vital role in RBC stability. A deficiency of this enzyme, which is common in individuals of African, Mediterranean, or Asian descent, is an inherited defect that alters the action of drugs. In a patient with G6PD deficiency, aspirin and other drugs can precipitate hemolysis. (For more information, see *How genetic variations affect drug response,* page 228.)

Cholinesterase

Various other genetic variations may produce side effects to specific drugs. An autosomal recessive disorder that causes pseudocholinesterase in the plasma can lead to apnea when the patient receives succinylcholine.

Glaucoma and malignant hyperthermia

An unknown mechanism may lead to glaucoma and increased intraocular pressure when corticosteroids are administered. A similar mechanism may result in malignant hyperthermia (severe hyperpyrexia and muscle rigidity, possibly resulting in death) when the patient receives an anesthetic such as halothane, methoxyflurane, cyclopropane ether, or succinylcholine.

Allergies

An inherited predisposition to allergies increases the patient's risk of an allergic response to a drug. Especially at risk is the patient with a history of eczema, angioedema, asthma, hay fever, or hives.

Rare variations

Some rare genetic variations include warfarin insensitivity, unstable hemoglobin Zurich, and unstable hemoglobin H, which cause hematologic side effects to certain drugs.

Temperament and attitudes

Psychological factors and personal values and beliefs can predispose a patient to drug side effects. For example, a patient who exhibits emotional, excitable, and hypochondriacal behavior may report drug side effects more frequently than someone without these psychological factors.

Attitudes can shape a patient's patterns of taking drugs and lead to erratic and unsafe self-medication. The patient also may feel community and cultural pressures when interpreting drug effects and reporting undesirable reactions. A patient's expectations of a drug's action

How genetic variations affect drug response

GENETIC VARIATION AND FREQUENCY	AFFECTED DRUGS	SIDE EFFECTS
Slow acetylation (50% of U.S. population)	dapsone, hydralazine, isoniazid, phenelzine	Polyneuritis
G6PD deficiency (common in Africans, Mediterraneans, and Asiatics)	analgesics, antimalarials, nitrofurantoin, sulfonamides, other drugs	Hemolysis
Glaucoma (common)	corticosteroids	Increased intraocular pressure
Reduced cholinesterase (approximately 1 in 2,500 patients)	succinylcholine	Apnea
Malignant hyperthermia (approximately 1 in 20,000 anesthetized patients)	anesthetics, such as ether, cyclopropane, halothane, methoxyflurane, and succinylcholine	Severe hyperpyrexia, muscle rigidity, death
Warfarin insensitivity (rare)	warfarin	Insufficient anticoagulation response to drug dose
Unstable hemoglobin Zurich (rare)	sulfonamides	Hemolysis
Unstable hemoglobin H (rare)	sulfisoxazole	Hemolysis

also can affect his response. These patient characteristics can affect the incidence of self-diagnosed side effects and the frequency and thoroughness of reporting patterns.

Circadian rhythms

Normal physiologic rhythms can influence drug action and lead to drug side effects. Research suggests that normal human biological rhythms can alter the absorption, metabolism, and excretion of certain drugs. Researchers are studying the contribution of sleep rhythms, hormone secretion, urinary excretion, and other regulatory processes to drug effectiveness and drug side effects.

Diseases

Pathophysiologic changes associated with various diseases may cause drug side effects. Diseases of organs responsible for drug absorption, metabolism, and excretion can alter a drug's actions and effects. For instance, cirrhosis of the liver may alter a drug's pharmacokinetic properties, especially its metabolism, thereby leading to abnormal drug concentration levels.

Diseases also can alter physiologic states unfavorably. For example, hypoalbuminemia can alter the availability of protein-binding drugs by decreasing the number of available plasma protein-binding sites. As a result, a drug's distribution, binding, and excretion are altered.

Pregnancy

Although many physiologic changes occur during pregnancy, the pregnant patient isn't necessarily at higher risk for side effects. However, changes in drug distribution and excretion rates may reduce blood levels of drugs (such as anticonvulsants) in pregnant women, necessitating dosage adjustments.

Although many drugs cross the placenta, the type of drug, its concentration, and fetal age determine the potential for side effects in the fetus. ■

Drug factors

Several drug factors, including bioavailability, additives, degradation, dosage, administration, and the number of drugs administered, influence side effects.

Bioavailability, additives, and degradation

Among different brands of the same drug, bioavailability may vary because of differences in manufacturing. Differences in onset of action, peak concentration, and duration of action among different products may lead to drug side effects. The doctor and pharmacist must exercise caution when substituting different forms of such drugs as anticonvulsants, anticoagulants, digitalis glycosides, and endocrine agents.

Dyes, buffering preparations, stabilizing agents, and other additives can cause drug side effects in certain patients. When an additive causes widespread side effects, the manufacturer may reformulate the product, removing the offending substance or substituting a less toxic compound.

Although uncommon, drug side effects can occur when a patient uses a drug after its expiration date or uses one that's been stored in an unfavorable environment.

Dosage

A patient who receives a higher drug dose for a prolonged period may be at increased risk for side effects. For example, a patient taking the antihypertensive hydralazine may be more likely to develop drug-induced systemic lupus erythematosus when the dosage exceeds 200 mg P.O. daily and the therapy lasts longer than 6 months.

Administration routes and techniques

Parenteral treatment causes more frequent side effects because a parenterally administered drug doesn't have to be absorbed through the GI tract before distribution into the blood. That makes the drug more quickly available at receptor sites. Toxicity (a condition caused by excessive amounts of a drug in the body) and hypersensitivity occur more commonly in these circumstances.

Drugs are manufactured for administration via designated routes. Administration via unrecommended routes may cause drug side effects. For example, instilling an otic solution into the eye may cause pain and irritation because the otic solution isn't formulated to the pH of the eye. Suspensions intended for I.M. or S.C. injection may be lethal if administered I.V.

Even when the appropriate route is used, improper technique can cause drug side effects. For example, administering some I.V. drugs too rapidly can alter distribution and produce a toxic response, and administering an excessive amount I.M. may cause tissue necrosis.

Number of drugs

The risk of drug side effects increases in direct relationship to the number of drugs administered to the patient. Complex interactions between drugs also may minimize some therapeutic effects and enhance others. ■

Exogenous factors

Dietary and environmental factors also influence a patient's predisposition to drug side effects.

Diet

Substances in foods may interfere with the activity of certain drugs. For example, tyramine, found in some cheeses, in beer, and in red wine, can precipitate a hypertensive crisis when ingested while a patient is taking an MAO inhibitor. Green, leafy vegetables may interfere with oral anticoagulants because of their high vitamin K content.

Dietary factors also can influence the pharmacokinetics of a drug. Certain foods, such as charcoal-broiled meats, vegetables from the *Brassica* family (cabbage and broccoli), and those containing caffeine, can stimulate the activity of liver enzymes, increasing a drug's metabolism rate.

The presence of food in the patient's stomach can alter drug absorption. Tetracycline absorption is decreased by food; carbamazepine absorption is increased. Foods can bind drugs and delay gastric emptying times.

Environment

A patient's environment may influence the relationship between physiologic function and a drug's effects and contribute to side effects. Pesticides, tobacco, and alcohol may alter the pharmacokinetics of certain drugs and increase the patient's risk of drug side effects. ■

RECOGNIZING TYPES OF SIDE EFFECTS

Type A effects

This type of effect results from an exaggerated but otherwise normal pharmacologic action of a drug in its usual therapeutic dose. Examples of this effect include orthostatic or exercise-induced hypotension from guanethidine and drowsiness from phenobarbital. The incidence of injury from a type A reaction is high, but the mortality is generally low.

Type A reactions are usually predictable. Consideration of a drug's properties along with its dose (most type A reactions are dose-dependent) strongly suggests the type of reaction that will result.

In some cases, a doctor prescribes a drug because it causes a type A effect. For example, although atropine is used to treat symptomatic bradycardia, doctors also prescribe it before surgery specifically to diminish secretions.

Another example is diphenhydramine. Initially, many patients who took this drug for its antihistamine properties complained of excessive drowsiness. Instead of abandoning the drug, manufacturers started using it as an ingredient in sleep aids. What's more, they found that diphenhydramine is safer than benzodiazepine sedative-hypnotics (such as flurazepam) prescribed for the same purpose. ■

Type B effects

Type B effects aren't as predictable as type A effects. They're unusual and unexpected, and they occur even when a drug is given in its normal therapeutic dose to a patient who should be able to tolerate it. For example, it's uncertain which patients will develop malignant hyperthermia from general anesthetics.

Many immune reactions (allergic and hypersensitivity reactions) fall into this category. Anaphylaxis is a classic type B hypersensitivity reaction. Because it's potentially life-threatening, anaphylaxis is one of the most serious drug side effects. It commonly occurs after a drug has been injected, but it may develop with any administration route. ■

IDENTIFYING DRUGS WITH ADDITIVES

Drugs with sulfite additives

Sulfites, used as a drug preservative, can cause allergic reactions in certain patients. The list below identifies sulfite-containing drugs:

- amikacin sulfate
- aminophylline
- amphotericin B
- amrinone lactate
- atropine sulfate with meperidine hydrochloride
- betamethasone sodium phosphate
- bupivacaine hydrochloride with epinephrine 1:200,000
- carisoprodol, aspirin, and codeine phosphate
- chlorpromazine, chlorpromazine hydrochloride
- dexamethasone acetate
- dexamethasone sodium phosphate

- dihydroxyacetone
- diphenhydramine hydrochloride
- dobutamine hydrochloride
- dopamine hydrochloride
- epinephrine, epinephrine bitartrate, epinephrine hydrochloride, racepinephrine hydrochloride
- epinephrine bitartrate 1% with pilocarpine hydrochloride 1%
- epinephrine bitartrate 1% with pilocarpine hydrochloride 2%
- epinephrine bitartrate 1% with pilocarpine hydrochloride 3%
- epinephrine bitartrate 1% with pilocarpine hydrochloride 4%
- epinephrine bitartrate 1% with pilocarpine hydrochloride 6%
- etidocaine hydrochloride with epinephrine bitartrate 1:200,000
- heparin calcium, heparin sodium
- hydralazine hydrochloride
- hydrocortisone sodium phosphate
- hyoscyamine sulfate
- imipramine hydrochloride
- influenza virus vaccine
- isoetharine hydrochloride, isoetharine mesylate
- isoproterenol hydrochloride, isoproterenol sulfate
- lidocaine hydrochloride with epinephrine hydrochloride
- mafenide acetate
- metaraminol bitartrate
- methotrimeprazine hydrochloride
- methyldopa, methyldopate hydrochloride
- metoclopramide hydrochloride
- orphenadrine citrate, orphenadrine hydrochloride
- oxycodone hydrochloride with acetaminophen
- pentazocine hydrochloride, pentazocine hydrochloride with acetaminophen
- perphenazine
- phenylephrine hydrochloride
- procainamide hydrochloride
- procaine hydrochloride
- prochlorperazine
- prochlorperazine edisylate, prochlorperazine maleate
- promazine hydrochloride
- propoxycaine hydrochloride with procaine hydrochloride 2% and levonordefrin 1:20,000
- propoxycaine hydrochloride with procaine hydrochloride 2% and norepinephrine bitartrate 1:30,000
- ritodrine hydrochloride
- scopolamine hydrobromide with phenylephrine hydrochloride 10%
- tetracycline hydrochloride 0.22% topical
- thiethylperazine maleate
- trifluoperazine hydrochloride
- tubocurarine chloride. ■

Drugs with benzyl alcohol additives

Used as a preservative in certain parenteral drugs, benzyl alcohol has reportedly caused neonatal kernicterus when given in large amounts. The list below identifies drugs containing benzyl alcohol:

- aminocaproic acid
- atracurium
- chlordiazepoxide
- chlorpheniramine injection
- chlorpromazine
- clindamycin
- co-trimoxazole
- cytarabine
- diazepam
- doxapram
- erythromycin
- etoposide
- fluphenazine decanoate injection
- fluphenazine enanthate
- glycopyrrolate
- heparin
- hydromorphone injection
- hyoscyamine injection
- leuprolide
- lincomycin
- lorazepam
- methotrexate
- netilmicin
- pancuronium
- penicillin G procaine
- phenobarbital sodium injection
- phenoxybenzamine
- physostigmine salicylate
- procainamide
- prochlorperazine edisylate injection
- promethazine
- pyridostigmine
- sodium tetradecyl sulfate
- sodium thiosalicylate injection
- spectinomycin
- succinylcholine
- trifluoperazine
- tubocurarine
- vecuronium
- vinblastine sulfate
- vincristine sulfate. ■

Drugs with tartrazine additives

Also known as FD&C Yellow No. 5, tartrazine is a common agent in some drugs. It's usually harmless but can provoke a severe allergic reaction in some people. The list below identifies drugs containing tartrazine:

- benzphetamine hydrochloride
- butabarbital sodium
- carisoprodol
- chlorphenesin
- chlorprothixene
- clindamycin
- desipramine hydrochloride
- dextroamphetamine sulfate
- dextrothyroxine
- fluphenazine hydrochloride
- haloperidol
- hexocyclium
- hydralazine
- hydromorphone hydrochloride
- imipramine

- mepenzolate
- methamphetamine hydrochloride
- methenamine hippurate
- methysergide maleate
- niacin
- paramethadione
- penicillin G benzathine
- penicillin G potassium
- penicillin V potassium
- pentobarbital sodium
- procainamide
- promazine hydrochloride
- rauwolfia serpentina
- uracil mustard. ■

Drugs with ethanol additives

Many liquid drug preparations for oral use contain ethanol, which produces a slight sedative effect but isn't harmful to most patients and can in fact be beneficial. But ingesting ethanol is undesirable and even dangerous in some circumstances. The list below identifies drugs containing ethanol:

- acetaminophen
- acetaminophen with codeine elixir
- belladonna tincture
- bitolterol
- brompheniramine elixir
- chlorpheniramine elixir
- clemastine fumarate
- co-trimoxazole
- cyproheptadine
- dexchlorpheniramine maleate
- dextroamphetamine
- diazepam
- diazoxide
- digoxin
- dihydroergotamine mesylate injection
- diphenhydramine
- epinephrine
- ergoloid mesylates
- esmolol
- ferrous sulfate elixirs
- fluphenazine hydrochloride
- hydromorphone cough syrup
- hyoscyamine
- indomethacin suspension
- isoetharine
- isoproterenol
- mesoridazine besylate
- methadone hydrochloride oral solution
- methdilazine
- methyldopa suspension
- minocycline
- molindone hydrochloride
- nitroglycerin infusion
- nystatin
- opium alkaloid hydrochlorides
- oxycodone hydrochloride
- paramethadione
- pentobarbital injection
- perphenazine
- phenobarbital injection
- phenytoin sodium injection
- promethazine
- pyridostigmine
- sodium butabarbital
- thioridazine
- thiothixene
- trimeprazine
- trimethoprim
- tripelennamine citrate. ■

DEALING WITH SIDE EFFECTS

Understanding your role

You have an essential role in preventing, detecting, and treating side effects. By working closely with the doctor, the pharmacist, the patient, and the patient's family, you can ensure more precise, individualized prescription; more knowledgeable and accurate administration practices; and the most comfortable and safest course of drug therapy possible.

Note predisposing factors

You may identify factors that predispose the patient to side effects during your assessment, such as a history of allergies. Use information obtained during the physical assessment and the health history to collaborate with the doctor in developing an appropriate drug regimen and later to modify the regimen, if necessary. Along with the doctor and pharmacist, you should analyze patient, drug, and situational factors to determine a therapeutic regimen with the least potential for triggering side effects.

Teach about drug therapy

You can also help by educating the patient and family about the effects of a prescribed drug, its administration, and any necessary precautions. The patient who understands the correct dosage, route, timing, and required precautions can minimize his risk of side effects.

Watch for side effects

Despite meticulous assessment and precautions, you can't prevent all side effects. Should the patient experience a side effect, you assume responsibility for detecting it early and managing symptoms. Because of frequent, close contact with the patient, you're usually the first to detect such common side effects as anorexia, nausea and vomiting, itching, constipation, and diarrhea.

Take quick action

By quickly and accurately reporting the evolving problem to the doctor, you ensure prompt attention to necessary changes in the drug regimen and efforts to control or treat the side effects.

At times, the patient must tolerate side effects as part of the drug therapy, as when a drug that can cure a disease or maintain life causes unavoidable reactions. In such circumstances, you can develop interventions to offset or minimize the patient's discomfort. ■

Responding to extravasation

Extravasation is the leakage of infused solution from a vein into surrounding tissue. It may result from a needle puncture in the vessel wall or leakage around a venipuncture site. Extravasation of I.V. solution may be referred to as *infiltration* because the fluid infiltrates the tissues.

Effects of extravasation

Extravasation causes local pain and itching, edema, blanching, and decreased skin temperature in the affected extremity.

Extravasation of a small amount of isotonic fluid or a nonirritating drug usually causes only minor discomfort. Treatment involves routine comfort measures, such as the application of warm compresses. However, extravasation of some drugs, such as vesicants, may lead to local tissue damage which in turn may lead to prolonged healing, infection, multiple debridements, cosmetic disfigurement, or loss of function. In these cases, emergency measures must be taken to minimize tissue damage and necrosis, prevent the need for skin grafts or, rarely, avoid amputation.

Prevention

- Use an existing I.V. line only when you're sure that it's patent. If indicated, perform a new venipuncture to ensure correct needle placement and vein patency.
- Select the site carefully. Use a distal vein first in case repeated needle sticks are necessary. Areas to avoid include the hand's dorsum, wrist, and fingers and previously damaged areas. Don't choose an area with poor circulation.
- Avoid probing for a vein. Instead, stop and begin again at another spot.
- After performing the venipuncture, apply a transparent dressing, which allows for inspection of the site.
- Then infuse D_5W or normal saline solution, checking for extravasation before beginning the prescribed infusion. To do so, apply a tourniquet above the needle to occlude the vein, and observe whether the flow continues. If not, the solution isn't infiltrating. You can also lower the I.V. container and check for blood backflow. Bear in mind that the needle may have punctured the opposite vein wall but may still rest in the vein. Flush the needle to ensure patency. If swelling occurs at the I.V. site, infiltration has occurred. ■

- During infusion, observe for signs of erythema or infiltration. Tell the patient to report burning, stinging, pain, or temperature changes.
- When administering potentially tissue-damaging drugs by I.V. bolus or push, infuse a small amount of normal saline solution to check for signs of infiltration before injecting the drug. When giving multiple drugs, administer vesicants last, preferably using an infusion pump.

Treatment

A health care facility's policy dictates extravasation treatment, which may include some or all of these steps:

- Stop the infusion, and remove the I.V. needle unless you need the route to infiltrate the antidote. Carefully estimate the amount of extravasated solution, and notify the doctor.
- Disconnect the tubing from the I.V. needle. Attach a 5-ml syringe to the needle and try to withdraw 3 to 5 ml of blood to remove any medication or blood in the tubing or needle and to provide a path to the infiltrated tissues.
- Clean the area around the I.V. site with an alcohol sponge or a 4″ × 4″ gauze pad soaked in an antiseptic agent. Then insert the needle of an empty tuberculin syringe into the subcutaneous tissue around the site, and gently aspirate as much solution as possible from the tissue.
- Instill the prescribed antidote into the subcutaneous tissue around the site. (See *Antidotes to vesicant extravasation.*) Then, if ordered, slowly instill an anti-inflammatory drug S.C. to help reduce inflammation and edema.
- If ordered, instill the prescribed antidote through the I.V. needle.
- Apply cold compresses to the affected area for 24 hours, or apply an ice pack for 20 minutes every 4 hours, to cause vasoconstriction, which may localize the drug and slow cell metabolism. After 24 hours, apply warm compresses, and elevate the affected extremity to reduce discomfort and promote fluid reabsorption. If the extravasated drug is a vasoconstrictor, such as norepinephrine or metaraminol bitartrate, apply warm compresses only.
- Continuously monitor the I.V. site for signs of abscess or necrosis. ■

ALERT

Antidotes to vesicant extravasation

The following chart lists common antidotes you may administer. Some will be used in combination with others.

ANTIDOTE	DOSE	EXTRAVASATED DRUG
ascorbic acid injection	50 mg	▪ dactinomycin
edetate calcium disodium (calcium EDTA)	150 mg	▪ cadmium ▪ copper ▪ manganese ▪ zinc
hyaluronidase 15 units/ml	Mix a 150-unit vial with 1 ml of normal saline solution for injection; withdraw 0.1 ml and dilute with normal saline solution to get 15 units/ml; give five 0.2-ml S.C. injections around site	▪ aminophylline ▪ calcium solutions ▪ contrast media ▪ dextrose solutions (concentrations of 10% or more) ▪ nafcillin ▪ potassium solutions ▪ total parenteral nutrition solutions ▪ vinblastine ▪ vincristine ▪ vindesine

(continued)

ALERT

Antidotes to vesicant extravasation *(continued)*

ANTIDOTE	DOSE	EXTRAVASATED DRUG
hydrocortisone sodium succinate 100 mg/ml, then topical 1% hydro-cortisone cream	50 to 200 mg (25 to 50 mg/ml of extravasate)	▪ doxorubicin ▪ vincristine
phentolamine mesylate	Dilute 5 to 10 mg with 10 ml of normal saline solution for injection	▪ dopamine ▪ epinephrine ▪ metaraminol ▪ norepinephrine
sodium bicarbon-ate 8.4%	5 ml	▪ carmustine ▪ daunorubicin ▪ doxorubicin ▪ vinblastine ▪ vincristine
sodium thiosul-fate 10%	Dilute 4 ml with 6 ml of sterile water for injec-tion; administer 10 ml	▪ dactinomycin ▪ mechloreth-amine ▪ mitomycin ▪ plicamycin

ALERT

Identifying and treating toxic drug reactions

Anemia, aplastic
Caused by altretamine, aspirin (long-term therapy), carbamazepine, chloramphenicol, co-trimoxazole, ganciclovir, gold salts, hydrochlorothiazide, mephenytoin, penicillamine, phenothiazines, phenylbutazone, triamterene, and zidovudine

Assessment findings
- Bleeding from mucous membranes, ecchymoses, and petechiae
- Fatigue, pallor, progressive weakness, shortness of breath, and tachycardia progressing to CHF
- Fever, oral and rectal ulcers, and sore throat without characteristic inflammation

Interventions
- Stop drug if possible, as ordered.
- Give vigorous supportive care, including transfusions, neutropenic isolation, antibiotics, and oxygen.
- Colony-stimulating factors may be given.
- In severe cases, bone marrow transplant may be needed.

Anemia, hemolytic
Caused by carbidopa-levodopa, levodopa, mefenamic acid, penicillins, phenazopyridine, primaquine, and sulfonamides

Assessment findings
- Chills, fever, back and abdominal pain (hemolytic crisis)
- Jaundice, malaise, and splenomegaly
- Signs of shock

Interventions
- Stop drug as ordered.
- Give supportive care, including transfusions and oxygen.
- Obtain a blood sample for Coombs' tests, as ordered.

Bone marrow toxicity (agranulocytosis)
Caused by ACE inhibitors, aminoglutethimide, carbamazepine, co-trimoxazole, flucytosine, gold salts, penicillamine, phenothiazines, phenylbutazone, phenyt-

(continued)

MANAGING SIDE EFFECTS

ALERT

Identifying and treating toxic drug reactions *(continued)*

oin, procainamide, propylthiouracil, and sulfonylureas

Assessment findings

- Enlarged lymph nodes, spleen, and tonsils
- Septicemia and shock
- Progressive fatigue and weakness, then sudden overwhelming infection with chills, fever, headache, and tachycardia
- Pneumonia
- Ulcers in the colon, mouth, and pharynx

Interventions

- Stop drug as ordered.
- Begin antibiotic therapy while awaiting culture and sensitivity test results.
- Give supportive care, including neutropenic isolation, warm saline gargles, and oral hygiene.

Bone marrow toxicity (thrombocytopenia)
Caused by anistreplase, ciprofloxacin, cisplatin, colfosceril, etretinate, floxuridine, flucytosine, ganciclovir, gold salts, heparin, interferon alfa-2a and alfa-2b, lymphocyte immune globulin, methotrexate, penicillamine, procarbazine, tetracyclines, and valproic acid

Assessment findings

- Fatigue, weakness, lethargy, and malaise
- Hemorrhage, loss of consciousness, shortness of breath, and tachycardia
- Sudden onset of ecchymoses or petechiae; large blood-filled bullae in the mouth

Interventions

- Stop drug or reduce dosage as ordered.
- Administer corticosteroids and platelet transfusions.

Cardiomyopathy
Caused by cytosine arabinoside, daunorubicin, doxorubicin, idarubicin, and mitoxantrone

Assessment findings

- Acute hypertension
- Arrhythmias
- Chest pain
- CHF
- Chronic cardiomyopathy
- Pericarditis-myocarditis syndrome

ALERT

Identifying and treating toxic drug reactions *(continued)*

Interventions
- Discontinue drug as ordered.
- Closely monitor patients receiving concurrent radiation therapy.
- Begin cardiac monitoring at earliest sign of problems.
- If patient is receiving doxorubicin, limit cumulative dose to less than 500 mg/m^2.

Dermatologic toxicity
Caused by androgens, barbiturates, corticosteroids, gold salts, hydralazine, interferons, iodides, pentamidine, phenolphthalein, phenothiazines, phenylbutazone, procainamide, psoralens, sulfonamides, sulfonylureas, tetracyclines, and thiazides

Assessment findings
- May range from phototoxicity to acneiform eruptions, alopecia, exfoliative dermatitis, lupuslike reactions, and toxic epidermal necrolysis

Interventions
- Stop drug as ordered.
- Administer topical antihistamines and analgesics as ordered.

Hepatotoxicity
Caused by amiodarone, asparaginase, carbamazepine, chlorpromazine, chlorpropamide, ciprofloxacin (parenteral), cytosine arabinoside, dantrolene, erythromycin estolate, ifosfamide, ketoconazole, leuprolide, methotrexate, methyldopa, mitoxantrone, niacin, plicamycin, and sulindac

Assessment findings
- Abdominal pain and hepatomegaly
- Abnormal levels of ALT, AST, LD, and serum bilirubin
- Bleeding, low-grade fever, mental changes, and weight loss
- Dry skin, pruritus, and rash
- Jaundice

Interventions
- Reduce dosage or stop drug as ordered.
- Monitor vital signs, blood levels, weight, intake and output, and fluids and electrolytes.

(continued)

ALERT

Identifying and treating toxic drug reactions *(continued)*

- Promote rest.
- Assist with hemodialysis if needed.
- Give symptomatic care: vitamins A, B complex, D, and K; potassium for alkalosis; salt-poor albumin for fluid and electrolyte balance; neomycin for GI flora; stomach aspiration for blood; reduced dietary protein and lactulose for blood ammonia.

Nephrotoxicity

Caused by aminoglycosides, cephalosporins, cisplatin, contrast media, corticosteroids, cyclosporine, gallium, gold salts (parenteral), nitrosoureas, NSAIDs, penicillin, pentamidine isethionate, plicamycin, and vasopressors or vasoconstrictors

Assessment findings

- Altered creatinine clearance
- Blurred vision, dehydration, edema, mild headache, and pallor
- Casts, albumin, or RBCs or WBCs in urine
- Dizziness, fatigue, irritability, and slowed mental processes
- Electrolyte imbalances
- Elevated BUN level
- Oliguria

Interventions

- Reduce dosage or stop drug as ordered.
- Assist with hemodialysis if needed.
- Monitor vital signs, weight changes, and urine volume.
- Give symptomatic care: fluid restriction and loop diuretics to reduce fluid retention and I.V. solutions to correct electrolyte imbalances.

Neurotoxicity

Caused by aminoglycosides, cisplatin, cytosine arabinoside, isoniazid, nitroprusside, polymyxin B injection, and vinca alkaloids

Assessment findings

- Akathisia
- Bilateral or unilateral palsies
- Muscle twitching and tremor
- Paresthesia
- Seizures
- Strokelike syndrome
- Unsteady gait
- Weakness

ALERT

Identifying and treating toxic drug reactions *(continued)*

Interventions
- Notify doctor as soon as changes appear.
- Reduce dosage or stop drug as ordered.
- Monitor carefully for any changes in patient's condition.
- Give symptomatic care: Remain with the patient, reassure him, and protect him during seizures. Provide a quiet environment, draw shades, and speak in soft tones. Maintain the airway, and ventilate the patient as needed.

Ocular toxicity
Caused by amiodarone, antibiotics such as chloramphenicol, anticholinergic agents, chloroquine, clomiphene, corticosteroids, cyclophosphamide, cytarabine, digitalis glycosides, ethambutol, lithium carbonate, methotrexate, phenothiazines, quinidine, quinine, rifampin, tamoxifen, and vinca alkaloids

Assessment findings
- Acute glaucoma
- Blurred, colored, or flickering vision
- Cataracts
- Corneal deposits
- Diplopia
- Miosis
- Mydriasis
- Optic neuritis
- Scotomata
- Vision loss

Interventions
- Notify doctor as soon as changes appear.
- Stop drug as ordered. (Some oculotoxic drugs used to treat serious conditions may be given again at a reduced dosage after the eyes are rested and have returned to near normal.)
- Monitor carefully for changes in symptoms.
- Treat effects symptomatically.

Ototoxicity
Caused by aminoglycosides; antibiotics, such as colistimethate sodium, gentamicin, kanamycin, streptomycin, and chloroquine; cisplatin; loop diuretics; minocycline; quinidine; quinine; salicylates; and vancomycin

(continued)

ALERT

Identifying and treating toxic drug reactions *(continued)*

Assessment findings
- Ataxia
- Hearing loss
- Tinnitus
- Vertigo

Interventions
- Notify doctor as soon as changes appear.
- Stop drug or reduce dosage as ordered.
- Monitor carefully for toxic effects.

Pseudomembranous colitis
Caused by antibiotics

Assessment findings
- Abdominal pain
- Colonic perforation
- Fever
- Hypotension
- Severe dehydration
- Shock
- Sudden and copious diarrhea (watery or bloody)

Interventions
- Notify doctor as soon as changes appear.
- Immediately discontinue drug as ordered.
- Give another antibiotic, such as vancomycin, metronidazole, or bacitracin.
- Maintain fluid and electrolyte balance. Check serum electrolyte levels daily. If pseudomembranous colitis is mild, give an ion exchange resin as ordered.
- Record intake and output.
- Monitor vital signs, skin color and turgor, urine output, and level of consciousness.
- Immediately report signs of shock.
- Observe for signs of hypokalemia, especially malaise and weak, rapid, and irregular pulse.

ALERT

Reversing anaphalaxis

DRUG AND ACTION	DOSAGE AND ADMINISTRATION GUIDELINES
aminophylline (Aminophyllin) ▪ Causes bronchodilation ▪ Stimulates respiratory drive ▪ Dilates constricted pulmonary arteries ▪ Causes diuresis ▪ Strengthens cardiac contractions ▪ Increases vital capacity ▪ Causes coronary vasodilation	*Severe anaphylaxis* *I.V.:* 5 to 6 mg/kg as a loading dose, followed by 0.4 to 0.9 mg/kg/min by infusion ▪ Monitor blood pressure, pulse, and respirations. ▪ Monitor intake and output, hydration status, and aminophylline and electrolyte levels. ▪ Monitor patient for arrhythmias. ▪ Use I.V. controller to reduce risk of overdose. ▪ Maintain serum levels at 10 to 20 mcg/ml.
cimetidine (Tagamet) ▪ Competes with histamine for H_2 receptor sites ▪ Prevents laryngeal edema	*Severe anaphylaxis* (experimental use) I.V.: 600 mg diluted in D_5W and administered over 20 min ▪ Be aware that cimetidine is incompatible with aminophylline. ▪ Reduce dosage for patients with impaired renal or hepatic function.
diphenhydramine (Benadryl) ▪ Competes with histamine for H_1 receptor sites ▪ Prevents laryngeal edema ▪ Controls localized itching	*Mild anaphylaxis* *P.O.:* 25 to 100 mg t.i.d. *I.V.:* 25 to 50 mg q.i.d. ▪ Administer I.V. doses slowly to avoid hypotension. ▪ Monitor patient for hypotension. ▪ Caution patient about driving; drug causes drowsiness and slows reflexes. ▪ Give fluids as needed. Drug causes dry mouth.

(continued)

MANAGING SIDE EFFECTS

ALERT

Reversing anaphalaxis *(continued)*

DRUG AND ACTION	DOSAGE AND ADMINISTRATION GUIDELINES
epinephrine (Adrenalin) *Alpha-adrenergic effects* ▪ Increases blood pressure ▪ Reverses peripheral vasodilation and systemic hypotension ▪ Decreases angioedema and urticaria ▪ Improves coronary blood flow by raising diastolic pressure ▪ Causes peripheral vasoconstriction *Beta-adrenergic effects* ▪ Causes bronchodilation ▪ Causes positive inotropic and chronotropic cardiac activity ▪ Decreases synthesis and release of chemical mediator	*Severe anaphylaxis* (drug of choice) *Initial infusion:* 0.2 to 0.5 mg of epinephrine (0.2 to 0.5 ml of 1:1,000 strength diluted in 10 ml normal saline solution) given I.V. slowly over 5 to 10 min, followed by continuous infusion *Continuous infusion:* 1 to 4 mcg/min (mix 1 ml of 1:1,000 epinephrine in 250 ml of D_5W to get concentration of 4 mcg/ml) ▪ Select large vein for infusion. ▪ Use infusion controller to regulate drip. ▪ Check blood pressure and heart rate. ▪ Monitor patient for arrhythmias. ▪ Check solution strength, dosage, and label before administering. ▪ Watch for signs of extravasation at infusion site. ▪ Monitor intake and output. ▪ Assess color and temperature of extremities.
hydrocortisone (Solu-Cortef) ▪ Prevents neutrophil and platelet aggregation ▪ Inhibits synthesis of mediators ▪ Decreases capillary permeability	*Severe anaphylaxis* *I.V.:* 100 to 200 mg q 4 to q 6 hr ▪ Monitor fluid and electrolyte balance, intake and output, and blood pressure closely. ▪ Maintain patient on ulcer and antacid regimen prophylactically.

CHAPTER 8

DEALING WITH INTERACTIONS

CLASSIFYING INTERACTIONS

Beneficial or harmful interactions

When one drug administered in combination with or shortly after another drug alters the effect of one or both drugs, this is known as a *drug interaction.* Usually, the effect of one drug is increased or decreased. For instance, one drug may inhibit or stimulate the metabolism or excretion of the other; or it may release another from plasma protein-binding sites, freeing it for further action.

Beneficial interactions

Combination drug therapy is based on drug interaction. One drug, for example, may be given to potentiate another. Probenecid, which blocks the excretion of penicillin, is sometimes given with penicillin to maintain adequate blood levels of penicillin for a longer period. Often, two drugs with similar actions are given together precisely because of the additive effect that results. For instance, aspirin and codeine, both analgesics, are often given in combination because together they provide greater pain relief than either alone.

Drug interactions are sometimes used to prevent or antagonize certain side effects. Hydrochlorothiazide and spironolactone, both diuretics, are often administered in combination because the former is potassium-depleting, whereas the latter is potassium-sparing.

Harmful interactions

But not all drug interactions are beneficial. Multiple drugs can interact to produce effects that are often undesirable and sometimes hazardous. Harmful drug interactions decrease efficacy or increase toxicity.

A hypersensitive patient who's well controlled with guanethidine may see his blood pressure rise again if he takes the antidepressant amitriptyline at the same time. Such a drug effect is known as *antagonism.* Drug combinations that produce these effects should be avoided if possible. Most harmful interactions can be prevented by checking and rechecking a medication and by understanding how reactions occur. ■

PREVENTING PHARMACOKINETIC INTERACTIONS

Interactions that alter absorption

Pharmacokinetic interactions are those in which the absorption, distribution, metabolism, or excretion of a drug is altered.

Decreased or delayed absorption of a drug from the GI tract can reduce a drug's effectiveness. Here are some specific pharmacokinetic interactions that result in altered drug absorption.

Tetracyclines and metals
When tetracyclines combine with metal ions (calcium, magnesium, aluminum, and iron, for example) in the GI tract, they form complexes that are poorly absorbed, causing them to lose some of their effectiveness. That's why tetracycline shouldn't be taken with milk, which contains calcium. Nor should it be taken concurrently with certain other drugs, such as antacids (most of which contain metals) and iron preparations. To avoid tetracycline-antacid interactions, always administer the two drugs at least 1 hour apart.

Fluoroquinolones and metals
Metals also form complexes with the fluoroquinolone derivatives — ciprofloxacin, enoxacin, lomefloxacin, norfloxacin, and ofloxacin — and may markedly reduce fluoroquinolone absorption. Patients taking fluoroquinolones should avoid metal-containing products (such as antacids) or, if both drugs are necessary, should take them at least 2 hours apart. Antacids and sucralfate shouldn't be taken within 4 hours of certain fluoroquinolones such as lomefloxacin.

Cholestyramine or colestipol and other drugs
Cholestyramine and colestipol are resinous antilipemics that bind with bile acids and prevent their reabsorption. They can also bind with other drugs in the GI tract and reduce absorption. Therefore, the interval between administration of cholestyramine or colestipol and another drug should be as long as possible.

Food and antibiotics
Because food in the GI tract can affect absorption, you should give penicillins, tetracyclines, and fluoroquinolones, as well as several other antibiotics, at least 1 hour before or 2 hours after meals. Exceptions include penicillin

V, amoxicillin, cephalosporins, doxycycline, lomefloxacin, minocycline, and certain formulations of erythromycin. Absorption of these drugs isn't appreciably affected by food.

Food may also greatly reduce the absorption of the antihistamine astemizole and the antiviral drug didanosine. Therefore, they must be administered on an empty stomach. ■

Interactions that alter distribution

Another type of pharmacokinetic interaction can occur when the patient receives two drugs that bind to the same plasma protein. The drug with the greater affinity for the binding sites will displace the other, altering distribution of the second drug. Because only the unbound, or free, portion of a drug is pharmacologically active, the displacement of even a small fraction of a highly protein-bound drug may substantially alter the effects of the drug. Take for instance the following drugs.

Warfarin and phenylbutazone

If administered concurrently, phenylbutazone displaces much of the warfarin from protein-binding sites. This action significantly increases the amount of active warfarin that's distributed throughout the body and puts the patient at risk for hemorrhage.

Valproic acid and salicylates

Salicylates, such as aspirin, may displace valproic acid from plasma protein–binding sites and alter valproic acid's metabolism. The increased serum concentration of unbound valproic acid may be toxic, and its dosage may have to be reduced. ■

Interactions that alter metabolism

A number of drugs are metabolized in the liver. Many drug interactions result from one drug's altering (either increasing or inhibiting) the metabolism of another.

For example, a drug may cause enzyme induction — that is, it may increase the activity of liver enzymes. This causes a second drug that is metabolized by these enzymes to be metabolized and excreted faster than it normally would be, thereby reducing its effects. Some examples follow.

Warfarin and phenobarbital

By causing enzyme induction, phenobarbital can accelerate warfarin's metabolism. This reduces warfarin's effects, risking thrombus formation. To compensate for this risk, the warfarin dosage may be increased. Keep in mind that an equally hazardous situation could develop if the patient suddenly stopped taking phenobarbital and the warfarin dosage wasn't reduced.

Cyclosporine and enzyme inducers

Enzyme inducers such as the barbiturates, phenytoin, and rifampin may increase the metabolism rate and reduce the effects of cyclosporine. The cyclosporine dosage may have to be significantly increased if the two are given concurrently.

Mercaptopurine and allopurinol or azathioprine and allopurinol

Allopurinol reduces uric acid production by inhibiting the enzyme xanthine oxidase. This enzyme helps metabolize such potentially toxic drugs as mercaptopurine and azathioprine. If xanthine oxidase is inhibited because of allopurinol therapy, the effects of mercaptopurine or azathioprine may be dangerously increased. When allopurinol is given in dosages of 300 to 600 mg per day concurrently with either drug, the mercaptopurine or azathioprine dosage should be one-fourth to one-third the usual dosage.

Benzodiazepines and cimetidine

Cimetidine inhibits the hepatic oxidative metabolic pathways through which most benzodiazepines (diazepam, for example) are normally metabolized. If cimetidine is administered with a benzodiazepine, the sedative effect of the benzodiazepine may be increased. However, cimetidine is not likely to affect the activity of lorazepam, oxazepam, and temazepam, which makes them good alternative drugs for a patient receiving cimetidine.

Nonsedating antihistamines and macrolide antibiotics or ketaconazole

Certain anti-infectives, such as the macrolide antibiotics (erythromycin, for example) and the antifungal drug ketaconazole, block the metabolism of the nonsedating antihistamines (terfenadine and astemizole). Toxic serum levels result, and lethal arrhythmias can occur. ■

Interactions that alter excretion

A change in urine pH will influence the activity of certain drugs, causing them to be reabsorbed or excreted to a greater extent than normal. For example, salicylates such as aspirin will be excreted faster — and therefore be less effective — when they're taken with an antacid that can increase urine pH. Conversely, a more acidic urine will cause salicylates to diffuse more readily back into the blood, thereby enhancing their effects. Patients taking large doses of salicylates — for example, for arthritis — are most prone to drug interactions.

A drug's effects may also be increased or prolonged because another drug inhibits its excretion by the kidneys. Two examples follow.

Penicillins and probenecid
By blocking renal tubular secretion of penicillins, probenecid can increase the serum concentrations of these drugs and prolong their activity.

Digoxin and quinidine
Serum digoxin levels rise significantly when digoxin is administered with quinidine, mainly because quinidine reduces renal clearance of digoxin. Quinidine also may reduce clearance of digoxin from tissue-binding sites. ■

PREVENTING PHARMACODYNAMIC INTERACTIONS

Interactions that cause opposite or similar effects

Pharmacodynamic interactions can result from concurrent administration of drugs having opposite or similar effects. They also occur when one drug alters the tissue sensitivity or responsiveness of another.

Interactions caused by drugs having opposite effects should be easy to detect, but sometimes they can be overlooked.

Thiazides and insulin
The thiazides and other diuretics are known to elevate blood glucose concentrations. If one of these diuretics is prescribed for a diabetic patient being treated with insulin or a sulfonylurea, such as glyburide, it may partially counteract the hypoglycemic action of the antidiabetic drug. As a result, the insulin or sulfonylurea dosage may need to be increased.

Beta-adrenergic agonists and beta-adrenergic blockers
Management of pulmonary disorders may be complicat-

ed by beta blockers (such as propranolol); therefore, these drugs shouldn't be given to patients with conditions such as asthma. Concurrent use of a beta blocker and a beta-adrenergic agonist (for example, albuterol and metaproterenol sulfate) may reduce the effects of both drugs. The cardioselective beta blockers (for example, acebutolol, atenolol, and metoprolol tartrate) are less likely to cause complications of pulmonary disorders or to reduce the bronchodilating effect of the beta-adrenergic agonists.

CNS depressants

One of the most common drug interactions results when the patient receives two or more drugs that depress the CNS. Keep in mind that many drugs can depress the CNS — for example, sedative-hypnotics, antipsychotics, TCAs , certain analgesics, most antihistamines, and some antihypertensives.

Alcohol and sedatives

The increased depressant effect caused by drinking alcoholic beverages while taking a sedative is a long-standing drug-related problem. The response of a patient will depend on many factors, including his tolerance for alcohol.

Antipsychotics, antiparkinsonian drugs, and antidepressants

Watch for an additive effect when two or more drugs that cause similar side effects are administered to the same patient. For example, a patient being treated with an antipsychotic such as chlorpromazine may also receive an antiparkinsonian drug such as trihexyphenidyl to control extrapyramidal reactions. And because he is also depressed, a TCA such as amitriptyline may be added to the therapy.

Each of these three drugs produces anticholinergic effects, which only increase when they're given together. Excessive anticholinergic effects can cause an atropine-like delirium, especially in elderly patients. In the case of the patient described above, this could be mistaken for an exacerbation of his psychiatric disorder, which might be treated by increasing the dosages of the drugs that are actually causing the problem.

Drugs with hypotensive effects

Certain antihypertensives, such as prazosin, as well as other drug classes (TCAs and calcium channel blockers, for example) can cause orthostatic hypotension resulting in dizziness, light-headedness, and even fainting. Elderly patients are more susceptible to this type of response and its associated risks, such as falls and injuries. Institute appropriate precautions with these drugs, whether giving them alone or in combination. ■

Drugs that alter electrolyte levels

Several important pharmacodynamic interactions may occur when a drug alters the concentrations of electrolytes, such as potassium and sodium.

Digitalis glycosides and diuretics

Most diuretics can cause excessive potassium loss within the first 2 weeks of therapy. This effect is common among the thiazide derivatives as well as with bumetanide, chlorthalidone, ethacrynic acid, furosemide, indapamide, metolazone, and quinethazone.

Hypokalemia can cause cardiovascular problems, so check serum potassium concentrations during diuretic therapy. Be especially alert if a digitalis glycoside, such as digoxin, is also ordered. If the patient loses too much potassium, his heart will become overly sensitive to the effects of the digitalis glycoside, and he may develop arrhythmias.

To avoid potassium depletion, a potassium-sparing diuretic, such as amiloride, spironolactone, or triamterene, can be given in combination with a potassium-depleting diuretic.

ACE inhibitors and potassium-sparing diuretics

The ACE inhibitors (for example, captopril, enalapril, fosinopril, and lisinopril) may elevate a patient's serum potassium level. A potassium-sparing diuretic or a potassium supplement should be used concurrently only if hypokalemia is documented.

Lithium and diuretics

Sodium depletion, another effect of diuretics, reduces renal clearance of lithium. Even protracted diaphoresis or diarrhea can cause enough sodium loss to reduce the patient's tolerance for lithium, thereby risking toxicity. ■

Drugs that cause interactions at receptor sites

Pharmacodynamic interactions can occur at receptor sites. These include interactions involving the use of MAO inhibitors, such as isocarboxazid, phenelzine, and tranylcypromine, and drugs with significant MAO-inhibiting effects, such as procarbazine and furazolidone.

MAO inhibitors and sympathomimetics

A primary function of the enzyme MAO (monoamine oxidase) is to break down catecholamines such as norepinephrine. If MAO is inhibited, the body will produce and store more norepinephrine than usual at receptor sites in adrenergic neurons. So a patient receiving an MAO inhibitor shouldn't be taking an indirect-acting sympathomimetic (such as amphetamines) that might release this norepinephrine. If he does, he may experience severe headache, hypertension, and cardiac arrhythmias from the release of excessive norepinephrine.

MAO inhibitors and tyramine

Serious reactions, including hypertensive crisis, have occurred in patients receiving MAO inhibitors after they've eaten foods high in tyramine. These foods include certain cheeses (such as cheddar, Camembert, and Stilton), certain alcoholic beverages (such as Chianti), pickled herring, and yeast extracts.

Why do these reactions occur? Because tyramine is metabolized by MAO in the intestinal wall and liver. The enzyme provides a built-in protection against the pressor actions of amines in foods. When MAO is inhibited, large amounts of unmetabolized tyramine can accumulate, resulting in the release of norepinephrine from adrenergic neurons.

MAO inhibitors and other antidepressants

Severe atropine-like reactions, tremor, and hyperthermia may occur when an MAO inhibitor and a TCA (amitriptyline and imipramine, for example) are used concurrently. Concomitant therapy with these drugs is contraindicated. In fact, an MAO inhibitor shouldn't be given until 7 to 14 days after therapy with the other antidepressant has been discontinued (and vice versa). However, combination therapy is effective in some patients who haven't responded to either drug alone or to other antidepressants. Concomitant therapy should be prescribed only if the patient can be closely monitored and if the doctor is familiar with the risks involved.

Serious reactions and deaths have occurred in patients taking fluoxetine and an MAO inhibitor concurrently or in close proximity to each other, so the two should never be taken together except under strict medical supervision. ■

PINPOINTING INTERACTIONS AND THEIR EFFECTS

ALERT

Dangerous drug interactions

Two or more drugs can interact to produce effects that are often undesirable and sometimes hazardous. Such interactions can decrease therapeutic efficacy or cause toxicity. If possible, avoid administering the combinations shown here.

DRUG	INTERACTING DRUG	POSSIBLE EFFECT
Aminoglycosides amikacin gentamicin kanamycin neomycin netilmicin streptomycin tobramycin	*Cephalosporins* (parenteral) ▪ ceftazidime ▪ ceftizoxime ▪ cephalothin	Possible enhanced nephrotoxicity
	Loop diuretics ▪ bumetadine ▪ ethacrynic acid ▪ furosemide	Possible enhanced ototoxicity
Amphetamines amphetamine benzphetamine dextroamphetamine methamphetamine	*Urine alkalinizers* ▪ potassium citrate ▪ sodium acetate ▪ sodium bicarbonate ▪ sodium citrate ▪ sodium lactate ▪ tromethamine	Decreased urinary excretion of amphetamine
ACE inhibitors captopril enalapril lisinopril	indomethacin	Decreased antihypertensive effect of ACE inhibitors

ALERT

Dangerous drug interactions *(continued)*

DRUG	INTERACTING DRUG	POSSIBLE EFFECT
Barbiturate anesthetics methohexital thiamylal thiopental	Opiate analgesics	Enhanced CNS and respiratory depression
Barbiturates amobarbital aprobarbital butabarbital mephobarbital pentobarbital phenobarbital primidone secobarbital	valproic acid	Increased serum barbiturate levels
Beta-adrenergic blockers acebutolol atenolol betaxolol carteolol esmolol levobunolol metoprolol nadolol penbutolol pindolol propranolol timolol	verapamil	Enhanced pharmacologic effects of both beta-adrenergic blockers and verapamil
captopril	Food	Possible diminished GI absorption

(continued)

ALERT

Dangerous drug interactions *(continued)*

DRUG	INTERACTING DRUG	POSSIBLE EFFECT
carbamazepine	erythromycin	Increased risk of carbamazepine toxicity
carmustine	cimetidine	Enhanced risk of bone marrow toxicity
ciprofloxacin	Antacids containing magnesium or aluminum hydroxide	Decreased plasma levels and effectiveness of ciprofloxacin
clonidine	Beta-adrenergic blockers	Enhanced rebound hypertension following rapid clonidine withdrawal
cyclosporine	Hydantoin derivatives	Reduced plasma levels of cyclosporine
Digitalis glycosides	*Loop and thiazide diuretics* ▪ bendroflumethiazide ▪ benzthiazide ▪ chlorothiazide ▪ cyclothiazide ▪ hydrochlorothiazide ▪ hydroflumethiazide ▪ methyclothiazide ▪ polythiazide ▪ trichlormethiazide	Increased risk of cardiac arrhythmias due to hypokalemia

ALERT

Dangerous drug interactions *(continued)*

DRUG	INTERACTING DRUG	POSSIBLE EFFECT
Digitalis glycosides *(continued)*	*Thiazide-like diuretics* ▪ indapamide ▪ metolazone ▪ quinethazone	Increased therapeutic or toxic effects
	Antithyroid agents ▪ methimazole ▪ propylthiouracil	Increased therapeutic or toxic effects
digitoxin	quinidine	Decreased digitoxin clearance
digoxin	amiodarone verapamil	Elevated serum digoxin levels
	quinidine	Enhanced clearance of digoxin
dopamine	phenytoin	Hypertension and bradycardia
epinephrine	Beta-adrenergic blockers	Increased systolic and diastolic pressures; marked decrease in heart rate
erythromycin	astemizole terfenadine	Increased risk of arrhythmias
ethanol	disulfiram furazolidone metronidazole	Acute alcohol intolerance reaction

(continued)

ALERT

Dangerous drug interactions *(continued)*

DRUG	INTERACTING DRUG	POSSIBLE EFFECT
furazolidone	Amine-containing foods *Anorexiants* ▪ amphetamine ▪ benzphetamine ▪ dextroamphetamine ▪ diethylpropion ▪ fenfluramine ▪ mazindol ▪ methamphetamine ▪ phendimetrazine ▪ phenteramine	Inhibits MAO, possibly leading to hypertensive crisis
heparin	Salicylates	Enhanced risk of bleeding
insulin	ethanol	Enhanced antidiabetic effect
levodopa	furazolidone	Enhanced toxic effects of levodopa
lithium	Thiazide diuretics	Decreased lithium excretion
MAO inhibitors isocarboxazid pargylene phenelzine tranylcypromine	Amine-containing foods Anorexiants meperidine	Inhibit MAO, possibly leading to hypertensive crisis

ALERT

Dangerous drug interactions *(continued)*

DRUG	INTERACTING DRUG	POSSIBLE EFFECT
meperidine	MAO inhibitors	Cardiovascular instability and increased toxicity
methotrexate	probenecid	Decreased methotrexate elimination
	Salicylates	Increased risk of methotrexate toxicity
Nondepolarizing muscle relaxants	*Aminoglycosides* Inhalation anesthetics	Enhanced neuromuscular blockade
Oral anticoagulants warfarin	amiodarone	Increased risk of bleeding
	Androgens testosterone	Possible enhanced bleeding caused by increased hypoprothrombinemia
	Barbiturates carbamazepine	Reduced effectiveness of warfarin

(continued)

ALERT

Dangerous drug interactions *(continued)*

DRUG	INTERACTING DRUG	POSSIBLE EFFECT
Oral anticoagulants warfarin *(continued)*	*Cephalosporins (parenteral, with methyltetrazolthiol chain)* ▪ amitriptyline ▪ amoxapine ▪ cefamandole ▪ cefoperazone ▪ cefotetan ▪ chloral hydrate ▪ cholestyramine ▪ cimetidine ▪ clofibrate ▪ co-trimoxazole ▪ desipramine ▪ dextrothyroxine ▪ disulfiram ▪ doxepin ▪ erythromycin ▪ glucagon ▪ imipramine ▪ metronidazole ▪ nortriptyline ▪ phenylbutazone ▪ protriptyline ▪ quinidine ▪ quinine ▪ salicylates ▪ sulfinpyrazone ▪ thyroid drugs ▪ TCAs ▪ trimipramine	Increased risk of bleeding

ALERT

Dangerous drug interactions *(continued)*

DRUG	INTERACTING DRUG	POSSIBLE EFFECT
Oral anticoagulants warfarin *(continued)*	ethchlorvynol glutethimide griseofulvin	Decreased pharmacologic effect
	rifampin trazodone	Decreased risk of bleeding
	methimazole propylthiouracil	Increased or decreased risk of bleeding
Penicillins	Tetracyclines	Reduced effectiveness of penicillins
Potassium supplements	Potassium-sparing diuretics	Increased risk of hyperkalemia
quinidine	amiodarone	Increased risk of quinidine toxicity
Sympatho-mimetics	MAO inhibitors	Increased risk of hypertensive crisis
Tetracyclines	Antacids containing magnesium, aluminum, or bismuth salts	Decreased plasma levels and effectiveness of tetracyclines

ALERT

Drug and alcohol interactions

DRUG	EFFECTS
▪ Analgesics ▪ Antianxiety drugs ▪ Antidepressants ▪ Antihistamines ▪ Antipsychotics ▪ Hypnotics	Deepened CNS depression
▪ MAO inhibitors	Deepened CNS depression; possible hypertensive crisis with certain types of beer and wine containing tyramine (for example, Chianti)
▪ Oral antidiabetic drugs ▪ sulfonylurea	Disulfiram-like effects (facial flushing, headache), especially with chlorpropamide; inadequate food intake may trigger increased antidiabetic activity
▪ Cephalosporins ▪ metronidazole ▪ Some antibacterial agents	Disulfiram-like effects

Drug and smoking interactions

The polycyclic hydrocarbons in cigarette smoke may increase the activity of hepatic enzymes that metabolize certain drugs. Therefore, the effects of these drugs may be diminished if the patient smokes cigarettes or even lives or works in a smoke-filled environment. Conversely, if the patient suddenly stops smoking, the effects of the drug could be dangerously increased.

If a smoker is taking one of the following drugs, monitor plasma drug levels and watch for possible side effects.

Ascorbic acid
Smoking can result in low serum vitamin C levels as well as decreased oral absorption of vitamin C. Tell the patient to increase his vitamin C intake.

Chlordiazepoxide or chlorpromazine and diazepam
Possible effects of smoking include increased drug metabolism, resulting in reduced plasma levels, and decreased sedative effects. Watch for a decrease in the drug's effectiveness, and adjust the patient's drug dosage, if ordered.

Propoxyphene hydrochloride
Smoking increases the metabolism of this drug, resulting in diminished analgesic effects. Also, smokers seem to experience fewer side effects than do nonsmokers. In patients who smoke, watch for a decrease in the drug's effectiveness. Increase the dosage, if ordered.

Propranolol
Possible effects of smoking include increased metabolism, decreasing the drug's effectiveness. Furthermore, propranolol's effectiveness is hampered by the effects of smoking, which increases heart rate, stimulates catecholamine release from the adrenal medulla, raises arterial blood pressure, and increases myocardial oxygen consumption.

Monitor the patient's blood pressure and heart rate. Propranolol's and smoking's effects may diminish as the patient ages. To reduce drug and smoking interaction, the doctor may order a selective beta blocker such as atenolol.

Oral contraceptives containing estrogen and progestin
Side effects, such as headache, dizziness, depression, libido changes, migraine, hypertension, edema, worsen-

ing of astigmatism or myopia, nausea, vomiting, and gallbladder disease, are possible. Inform the patient of the increased risk of MI and cerebrovascular accident. Advise the patient to either stop smoking or use a different birth control method.

Theophylline
Smoking increases theophylline metabolism (from induction of liver microsomal enzymes), resulting in lower plasma theophylline levels. Monitor plasma theophylline levels, and watch for decreased therapeutic effect.

Increase theophylline dosage, if ordered. ■

ALERT

Drug and food interactions

The chart below describes how interactions with food may alter the absorption, excretion, or plasma level of specific drugs. Keep in mind that you may still need to give certain drugs, such as salicylates and NSAIDs, with food to prevent troublesome GI effects.

DRUG	FOOD CAUSING INTERACTION	EFFECT
acebutolol (Sectral)	Food in general	Slightly decreases drug absorption and peak levels
amiloride hydrochloride (Midamor)	Potassium-rich diet	May rapidly increase serum potassium levels
Antihypertensive drugs	Licorice	Decreases antihypertensive effect
astemizole (Hismanal)	Food in general	Reduces drug absorption by 60%

ALERT

Drug and food interactions *(continued)*

DRUG	FOOD CAUSING INTERACTION	EFFECT
bacampicillin (Spectrobid Powder for Oral Suspension)	Food in general	Decreases drug absorption
buspirone (BuSpar)	Food in general	May decrease presystemic drug clearance
caffeine (Caffedrine, NoDoz, Quick Pep, Tirend, Vivarin)	Caffeine-containing beverages and food	May cause sleeplessness, irritability, nervousness, and rapid heartbeat
calcium glubionate (Neo-Calglucon Syrup)	Bran, cereals (whole grain), dairy products, and spinach	Large quantities interfere with calcium absorption
captopril (Capoten)	Food in general	Reduces drug absorption by 30% to 40%
cefuroxime axetil (Ceftin Tablets)	Food in general	Increases drug absorption
choline and magnesium salicylate (Trilisate)	Food that lowers urine pH	Decreases urinary salicylate excretion and increases plasma levels
	Food that raises urine pH	Enhances renal salicylate clearance and decreases plasma salicylate concentration

(continued)

ALERT

Drug and food interactions *(continued)*

DRUG	FOOD CAUSING INTERACTION	EFFECT
demeclocycline hydrochloride (Declomycin)	Dairy products, food in general	Interferes with absorption of oral forms of demeclocycline
dextroamphetamine sulfate (Dexedrine Elixir)	Fruit juice	Decreases blood drug levels and efficacy
dicumarol	Diet high in vitamin K	Decreases PT
digoxin (Lanoxin Tablets, Lanoxicaps)	Food high in bran fiber	May reduce bioavailability of oral digoxin
	Food in general	Slows drug absorption rate
dyclonine hydrochloride (Dyclone 0.5% and 1% Topical Solutions, USP)	Food in general	Topical anesthesia may impair swallowing and thus enhance danger of aspiration; food shouldn't be ingested for 60 minutes.
erythromycin base (ERYC, PCE Dispertabs)	Food in general	Optimum blood levels are obtained on a fasting stomach; administration is preferable 30 minutes before or 2 hours after meals.

ALERT

Drug and food interactions *(continued)*

DRUG	FOOD CAUSING INTERACTION	EFFECT
estramustine phosphate sodium (Emcyt)	Dairy products, calcium-rich foods	Impair drug absorption
etodolac (Lodine)	Food in general	Reduces peak concentration by about 50% and delays peak concentration by 1.4 to 3.8 hours
etretinate (Tegison Capsules)	Dairy products, high-lipid diet	Increase drug absorption
famotidine (Pepcid Oral Suspension)	Food in general	Slightly increases bioavailability
felodipine (Plendil)	Grape juice (doubly concentrated)	Increases bioavailability more than twofold
fenoprofen calcium (Nalfon Pulvules and Tablets)	Dairy products, food in general	Delay and diminish peak blood levels
ferrous sulfate (Feosol, SlowFe)	Dairy products, eggs	Inhibit iron absorption

(continued)

ALERT

Drug and food interactions *(continued)*

DRUG	FOOD CAUSING INTERACTION	EFFECT
fluoroquinolone antibiotics, such as ciprofloxacin (Cipro), norfloxacin (Noroxin), ofloxacin (Floxin)	Food in general	May decrease absorption of oral fluoroquinolones
flurbiprofen (Ansaid)	Food in general	Alters rate of absorption but not extent of drug availability
fosinopril sodium (Monopril)	Food in general	May slow rate but not extent of drug absorption
glipizide (Glucotrol)	Food in general	Delays absorption by about 40 minutes
hydralazine (Apresoline Tablets)	Food in general	Increases plasma levels of drug
hydrochlorothiazide (Esidrix, HydroDIURIL)	Food in general	Enhances GI drug absorption
ibuprofen (Advil, Motrin, Nuprin)	Food in general	Reduces rate but not extent of drug absorption
isotretinoin (Accutane)	Dairy products, food in general	Increase absorption of oral isotretinoin

ALERT

Drug and food interactions *(continued)*

DRUG	FOOD CAUSING INTERACTION	EFFECT
isradipine (DynaCirc)	Food in general	Delays peak concentration by about 1 hour with no effect on bioavailabilty
ketoprofen (Orudis Capsules)	Food in general	Slows absorption rate, delays and reduces peak concentrations
levodopa-carbidopa (Sinemet Tablets)	High-protein diet	May impair levodopa absorption
	Food in general	Increases the extent of availability and peak concentrations of sustained-release levodopa-carbidopa
levothyroxine sodium (Synthroid Injection)	Soybean formula (infant's)	May cause excessive stools
lidocaine hydrochloride (Xylocaine)	Food in general	Topical anesthesia may impair swallowing and thus enhance danger of aspiration; avoid food ingestion for 60 minutes.

(continued)

ALERT

Drug and food interactions *(continued)*

DRUG	FOOD CAUSING INTERACTION	EFFECT
liotrix (Euthroid, Thyrolar)	Soybean formula (infant's)	May cause excessive stools
meclofenamate (Meclomen)	Food in general	Decreases rate and extent of drug absorption
methenamine mandelate (Mandelamine Granules)	Food that raises urine pH	Reduces essential antibacterial activity
methotrexate sodium (Rheumatrex)	Food in general	Delays absorption and reduces peak concentration of oral methotrexate sodium
minocycline hydrochloride (Minocin)	Dairy products	Slightly decrease peak plasma levels and delay them by 1 hour
misoprostol (Cytotec)	Food in general	Diminishes maximum plasma concentrations

ALERT

Drug and food interactions *(continued)*

DRUG	FOOD CAUSING INTERACTION	EFFECT
MAO inhibitors, such as isocarboxazid (Marplan Tablets), phenelzine (Nardil), or tranylcypromine (Parnate Tablets); drugs that also inhibit MAO, such as amphetamines, furazolidone (Furoxone), isoniazid (Laniazid), or procarbazine (Matulane Capsules)	Anchovies, avocados, bananas, beans (broad, fava), beer (including alcohol-free and reduced-alcohol), caviar, cheese (especially aged, strong, and unpasteurized), chocolate, cream (sour), figs (canned), herring (pickled), liqueurs, liver, meat extracts, meat prepared with tenderizers, raisins, sauerkraut, sherry, soy sauce, red wine, yeast extract, yogurt	Can cause hypertensive crisis
moricizine hydrochloride (Ethmozine)	Food in general	Administration 30 minutes after a meal delays rate but not extent of drug absorption.
nifedipine (Procardia XL Tablets)	Food in general	Slightly alters early rate of drug absorption

(continued)

ALERT

Drug and food interactions *(continued)*

DRUG	FOOD CAUSING INTERACTION	EFFECT
nitrofurantoin (Macrodantin Capsules)	Food in general	Increases drug bioavailability
pancrelipase (Creon Capsules)	Food with a pH > 5.5	Dissolves protective enteric coating
pentoxifylline (Trental)	Food in general	Delays drug absorption but doesn't affect total absorption
phenytoin (Dilantin)	Charcoal-broiled meats	May decrease blood drug levels
polyethylene glycol electrolyte solution (GoLYTELY, NuLYTELY)	Food in general	For best results, no solid food should be consumed for 3 to 4 hours before drinking solution.
propafenone hydrochloride (Rythmol)	Food in general	Increases peak blood levels and bioavailability in a single-dose study
propranolol hydrochloride (Inderal)	Food in general	Increases bioavailability of oral propranolol
ramipril (Altace)	Food in general	Reduces rate but not extent of drug absorption

ALERT

Drug and food interactions *(continued)*

DRUG	FOOD CAUSING INTERACTION	EFFECT
salsalate (Disalcid, Mono-Gesic, Salflex)	Food that lowers urine pH	Decreases urinary excretion and increases plasma levels
	Food that raises urine pH	Increases renal clearance and urinary excretion of salicylic acid
selegiline hydrochloride (Eldepryl)	Food with high concentration of tyramine	May precipitate hypertensive crisis if daily dose exceeds recommended maximum
sodium fluoride (Luride)	Dairy products	Form calcium fluoride, which is poorly absorbed
sulindac (Clinoril Tablets)	Food in general	Slightly delays peak plasma concentrations of biologically active sulfide metabolite
tetracycline hydrochloride (Achromycin V)	Dairy products, food in general	Interfere with absorption of tetracycline

(continued)

ALERT

Drug and food interactions *(continued)*

DRUG	FOOD CAUSING INTERACTION	EFFECT
theophylline (Constant-T, Quibron-T, Quibron SR, Respbid, Slo-Bid, Theo-Dur, Theo-24, Theolair-SR, TheoX, Uniphyl)	caffeine-containing beverages, chocolate	Large quantities increase side effects of theophylline.
	High-lipid diet	Reduces plasma levels and delays peak plasma levels
	Charcoal-broiled foods, especially meats; cruciferous vegetables (cabbage family); high-protein and low-carbohydrate diets	Large quantities may increase hepatic metabolism of theophylline.
tolmetin sodium (Tolectin)	Dairy products	Decrease total bioavailability by 16%
	Food in general	Decreases total bioavailability by 16% and reduces peak plasma concentrations by 50%

ALERT

Drug and food interactions *(continued)*

DRUG	FOOD CAUSING INTERACTION	EFFECT
trazodone hydrochloride (Desyrel)	Food in general	May affect bioavailability, including amount of drug absorbed and peak plasma levels
verapamil hydrochloride (Calan SR, Isoptin SR)	Food in general	Decreases bioavailability but narrows peak-to-trough ratio
warfarin sodium (Coumadin, Panwarfin)	Diet high in vitamin K	Decreases PT
	Charcoal-broiled meats	May decrease blood levels of drug

ALERT

Drug interference with test results

A drug in a blood or urine specimen may interact with laboratory test chemicals. Or a drug may cause a physiologic change altering the blood or urine level of the substance being tested. This chart identifies both types of interference.

DRUGS CAUSING CHEMICAL INTERFERENCE	DRUGS CAUSING PHYSIOLOGIC INTERFERENCE	
Alkaline phosphatase		
▪ albumin ▪ fluorides	*Increased test values* ▪ anticonvulsants ▪ hepatotoxic drugs	*Decreased test values* ▪ clofibrate
Ammonia, blood		
	Increased test values ▪ acetazolamide ▪ ammonium chloride ▪ asparaginase ▪ barbiturates ▪ diuretics, loop and thiazide ▪ ethanol	*Decreased test values* ▪ kanamycin, oral ▪ lactulose ▪ neomycin, oral ▪ potassium salts
Amylase, serum		
▪ chloride salts ▪ fluorides	*Increased test values* ▪ asparaginase ▪ azathioprine ▪ cholinergic agents ▪ contraceptives, oral ▪ contrast media with iodine ▪ corticosteroids ▪ loop and thiazide diuretics ▪ methyldopa ▪ narcotics	

ALERT

Drug interference with test results *(continued)*

DRUGS CAUSING CHEMICAL INTERFERENCE	DRUGS CAUSING PHYSIOLOGIC INTERFERENCE	
Aspartate aminotransferase		
▪ erythromycin ▪ methyldopa	*Increased test values* ▪ cholinergic agents ▪ hepatotoxic drugs ▪ opium alkaloids	
Bilirubin, serum		
▪ ascorbic acid ▪ dextran ▪ epinephrine ▪ pindolol	*Increased test values* ▪ hemolytic agents ▪ hepatotoxic drugs ▪ methyldopa ▪ rifampin	*Decreased test values* ▪ barbiturates
Blood urea nitrogen		
▪ chloral hydrate ▪ chloramphenicol ▪ streptomycin	*Increased test values* ▪ anabolic steroids ▪ nephrotoxic drugs	*Decreased test values* ▪ tetracyclines
Calcium, serum		
▪ aspirin ▪ heparin ▪ hydralazine ▪ sulfisoxazole	*Increased test values* ▪ asparaginase ▪ calcium salts ▪ diuretics, loop and thiazide ▪ lithium ▪ thyroid hormones ▪ vitamin D	*Decreased test values* ▪ acetazolamide ▪ anticonvulsants ▪ calcitonin ▪ cisplatin ▪ contraceptives ▪ corticosteroids ▪ laxatives ▪ magnesium salts ▪ plicamycin

(continued)

ALERT

Drug interference with test results *(continued)*

DRUGS CAUSING CHEMICAL INTERFERENCE	DRUGS CAUSING PHYSIOLOGIC INTERFERENCE	
Chloride, serum		
	Increased test values ▪ acetazolamide ▪ androgens ▪ estrogens ▪ NSAIDs	*Decreased test values* ▪ corticosteroids ▪ diuretics, loop and thiazide
Cholesterol, serum		
▪ androgens ▪ aspirin ▪ corticosteroids ▪ nitrates ▪ phenothiazines ▪ vitamin D	*Increased test values* ▪ beta-adrenergic blockers ▪ contraceptives, oral ▪ corticosteroids ▪ diuretics, thiazide ▪ phenothiazines ▪ sulfonamides	*Decreased test values* ▪ androgens ▪ captopril ▪ chlorpropamide ▪ cholestyramine ▪ clofibrate ▪ colestipol ▪ haloperidol ▪ neomycin, oral
Creatine kinase		
	Increased test values ▪ aminocaproic acid ▪ amphotericin B ▪ chlorthalidone ▪ clofibrate ▪ ethanol (long-term use)	
Creatinine, serum		
▪ cefoxitin ▪ cephalothin ▪ flucytosine	*Increased test values* ▪ cimetidine ▪ nephrotoxic drugs	

ALERT

Drug interference with test results *(continued)*

DRUGS CAUSING CHEMICAL INTERFERENCE	DRUGS CAUSING PHYSIOLOGIC INTERFERENCE	
Glucose, serum		
▪ acetaminophen ▪ ascorbic acid (urine) ▪ cephalosporins (urine)	*Increased test values* ▪ TCAs ▪ beta-blockers ▪ corticosteroids ▪ dextrothyroxine ▪ diazoxide ▪ diuretics, loop and thiazide ▪ epinephrine ▪ estrogens ▪ isoniazid ▪ lithium ▪ phenothiazines ▪ phenytoin ▪ salicylates	*Decreased test values* ▪ acetaminophen ▪ anabolic steroids ▪ clofibrate ▪ disopyramide ▪ ethanol ▪ gemfibrozil ▪ MAO inhibitors ▪ pentamidine
Magnesium, serum		
	Increased test values ▪ lithium ▪ magnesium salts	*Decreased test values* ▪ aminoglycosides ▪ amphotericin B ▪ calcium salts ▪ cisplatin ▪ digitalis glycosides ▪ diuretics, loop and thiazide ▪ ethanol

(continued)

ALERT

Drug interference with test results *(continued)*

DRUGS CAUSING CHEMICAL INTERFERENCE	DRUGS CAUSING PHYSIOLOGIC INTERFERENCE	
Phosphates, serum		
	Increased test values ▪ vitamin D (excessive amounts)	*Decreased test values* ▪ antacids, phosphate-binding ▪ mannitol
Potassium, serum		
	Increased test values ▪ aminocaproic acid ▪ ACE inhibitors ▪ antineoplastics ▪ diuretics, potassium-sparing ▪ isoniazid ▪ lithium ▪ mannitol ▪ succinylcholine	*Decreased test values* ▪ ammonium chloride ▪ amphotericin B ▪ corticosteroids ▪ diuretics, potassium-wasting ▪ glucose ▪ insulin ▪ laxatives ▪ penicillins, extended-spectrum ▪ salicylates
Protein, serum		
	Increased test values ▪ anabolic steroids ▪ corticosteroids ▪ phenazopyridine	*Decreased test values* ▪ contraceptives, oral ▪ estrogens ▪ hepatotoxic drugs

ALERT

Drug interference with test results *(continued)*

DRUGS CAUSING CHEMICAL INTERFERENCE	DRUGS CAUSING PHYSIOLOGIC INTERFERENCE	
Protein, urine		
▪ aminoglycosides ▪ cephalosporins ▪ contrast media ▪ magnesium sulfate ▪ miconazole ▪ nafcillin ▪ phenazopyridine ▪ sulfonamides ▪ tolbutamide ▪ tolmetin	*Increased test values* ▪ cephalosporins ▪ contrast media with iodine ▪ corticosteroids ▪ nafcillin ▪ nephrotoxic drugs ▪ sulfonamides	
Prothrombin time		
	Increased test values ▪ anticoagulants ▪ asparaginase ▪ aspirin ▪ azathioprine ▪ certain cephalosporins ▪ chloramphenicol ▪ cholestyramine ▪ colestipol ▪ cyclophosphamide ▪ hepatotoxic drugs ▪ propylthiouracil ▪ quinidine ▪ quinine ▪ sulfonamides	*Decreased test values* ▪ anabolic steroids ▪ contraceptives, oral ▪ estrogens ▪ vitamin K

(continued)

ALERT

Drug interference with test results *(continued)*

DRUGS CAUSING CHEMICAL INTERFERENCE	DRUGS CAUSING PHYSIOLOGIC INTERFERENCE	
Sodium, serum		
	Increased test values ▪ clonidine ▪ diazoxide ▪ guanabenz ▪ guanadrel ▪ guanethidine ▪ methyldopa ▪ NSAIDs ▪ steroids	*Decreased test values* ▪ ammonium chloride ▪ carbamazepine ▪ desmopressin ▪ diuretics ▪ lypressin ▪ vasopressin
Uric acid, serum		
▪ ascorbic acid ▪ caffeine ▪ levodopa ▪ theophylline	*Increased test values* ▪ acetazolamide ▪ cisplatin ▪ diazoxide ▪ diuretics ▪ epinephrine ▪ ethambutol ▪ ethanol ▪ levodopa ▪ niacin	*Decreased test values* ▪ acetohexamide ▪ allopurinol ▪ clofibrate ▪ contrast media with iodine ▪ diflunisal ▪ glucose infusions ▪ guaifenesin ▪ phenothiazines ▪ phenylbutazone ▪ salicylates (small doses) ▪ uricosuric agents

REVIEWING THE NURSE'S ROLE

Your role in preventing interactions

Besides being familiar with types of interactions, a key step to preventing interactions is communication — with the patient, his other nurses, his doctor, and above all, the pharmacist. Encourage the patient to express how he feels and whether he thinks the drug is helping him, making him worse, or causing other symptoms. Likewise, his other nurses, his doctor, and the pharmacist must contribute to an ongoing exchange of vital information.

Ask pertinent questions

The exchange of information begins with the data you collect when you take the patient's history. The first step in assessment, history taking provides an excellent opportunity to collect information that will help identify patients at risk for drug interactions.

Drug history

Begin by compiling a list of every drug that the patient is currently taking and every drug he has taken during the previous 2 weeks. This should include nonprescription as well as prescription medications. Consider asking the patient or his caregiver to bring in all his medications so that you can review them with him.

Ask specifically about vitamins and minerals, antacids, antidiarrheals, and laxatives. Is the patient taking medications for allergies, a cold or cough, or pain relief? Also note if he's using something to help him fall asleep at night or to stay awake.

Food, caffeine, alcohol, and smoking

Remember that food, caffeine, alcohol, and nicotine can affect drug therapy. So gather as much information as possible about the patient's eating, drinking, and smoking habits. Keep in mind that people often minimize what they consider to be bad habits. By winning your patient's trust, you should be able to get him to open up and possibly reveal something significant about these habits.

Other risk factors

Note any other factors that may increase the risk of a drug interaction — age, for example, and body build. Very young and very old patients are at increased risk. Also at risk are very thin or obese patients or patients whose weight fluctuates dramatically.

Ask the patient if he's being treated by more than one doctor. Does he have any other health problems — whether short- or long-term, medical, dental, or psychological? For example, hepatic or renal dysfunction, which will delay a drug's metabolism and excretion, must be documented.

Previous drug reactions

An obvious but sometimes overlooked question is whether the patient has ever had a problem in the past with a particular drug or drug combination. Has he had any reactions to certain dosages of a drug?

Patients often know instinctively when they need more or less than the prescribed amount of a drug. If the patient feels uncomfortable with the drug's effects or doesn't believe it's working for him, he's more likely not to cooperate with the drug regimen. Also, if a patient feels a drug is interfering with his lifestyle, he'll usually stop taking it as soon as he starts to feel a little better, no matter what he's told to the contrary.

Share information

Pass on all relevant information to the pharmacist and doctor — for example, the patient's weight, his diet, and any reactions he's had previously with medications. If possible, try to hold medication rounds with the pharmacist or, better yet, with both the doctor and the pharmacist. Try to arrange a time when they can come to the nursing unit and discuss each patient with you.

You have the right to ask the pharmacist for whatever information you need to monitor and evaluate drug therapy. Pharmacists keep detailed drug profiles of each patient. Some hospitals use computerized drug-interaction screening programs. At the very least, easy-to-use reference charts and handbooks should always be available to you.

Note on the plan of care any concerns you have about the drugs your patient is taking. That way, all the nurses caring for him will be warned to watch for possible interactions. If a drug needs to be given with or without food, or at a certain time before or after administration of another drug, note this on the plan of care as well.

Note troublesome drugs

Mentally flag those drugs that are most likely to be involved in interactions. Be especially alert when administering antacids, warfarin, aspirin, steroids, digoxin, phenytoin, aminophylline, quinidine, and MAO inhibitors. If your patient is receiving any of these drugs, evaluate his regimen carefully. Suggest therapeutic alternatives to the doctor if you note a possible interaction. Remember, the doctor may not be aware that the patient is receiving a potentially interactive drug prescribed by another doctor.

Monitor drug therapy

Throughout the course of drug therapy, assess your patient closely for both desired effects and side effects. If his condition should worsen, review his drug regimen with the pharmacist and doctor. The problem may be related to the medications he's receiving rather than to a deterioration of his condition. And, of course, report any unexpected or unusual side effects to the doctor.

Listen to your patient's concerns. How well will his sublingual drug be absorbed if his mouth is very dry? Can a systemic drug that's given as a suppository be expected to work effectively if his rectum is full of feces? What chance does his parenteral medication have of producing the desired therapeutic effect if the same site has been used repeatedly?

In many cases, a dosage adjustment will eliminate side effects. Or the doctor may want to prescribe smaller dosages of two drugs that produce the same desired effects as the drug the patient has been taking but with fewer side effects.

Manage common problems

Use traditional nursing measures to help the patient cope with common drug-related problems, such as nausea, constipation or diarrhea, itching, and postural hypotension. And look for ways to simplify the routine whenever possible — for example, use combination or long-acting products when appropriate.

Keeping down the cost of a patient's medication can also help foster patient cooperation. So, if a less-expensive generic form of a drug is available, alert both the patient and his doctor. Remember that many prescriptions are never filled because of the cost.

Include the family

Make sure both the patient and his family are aware of possible interactions related to his drug regimen. Write down all signs and symptoms that should be reported immediately. Inform the patient and his caregiver that any change in his condition might be related to his medications and should be communicated to his doctor. Home health care or office nurses should also review these concerns with the patient periodically.

Finally, if you feel uneasy about giving a drug because of a potential interaction — or for any other reason — discuss the problem with the pharmacist and doctor. Don't let anyone talk you into giving a drug that you think may harm your patient. ■

■ CHAPTER 9

PREVENTING INCOMPATIBILITIES

CLASSIFYING INCOMPATIBILITIES

Compatibility of I.V. drugs

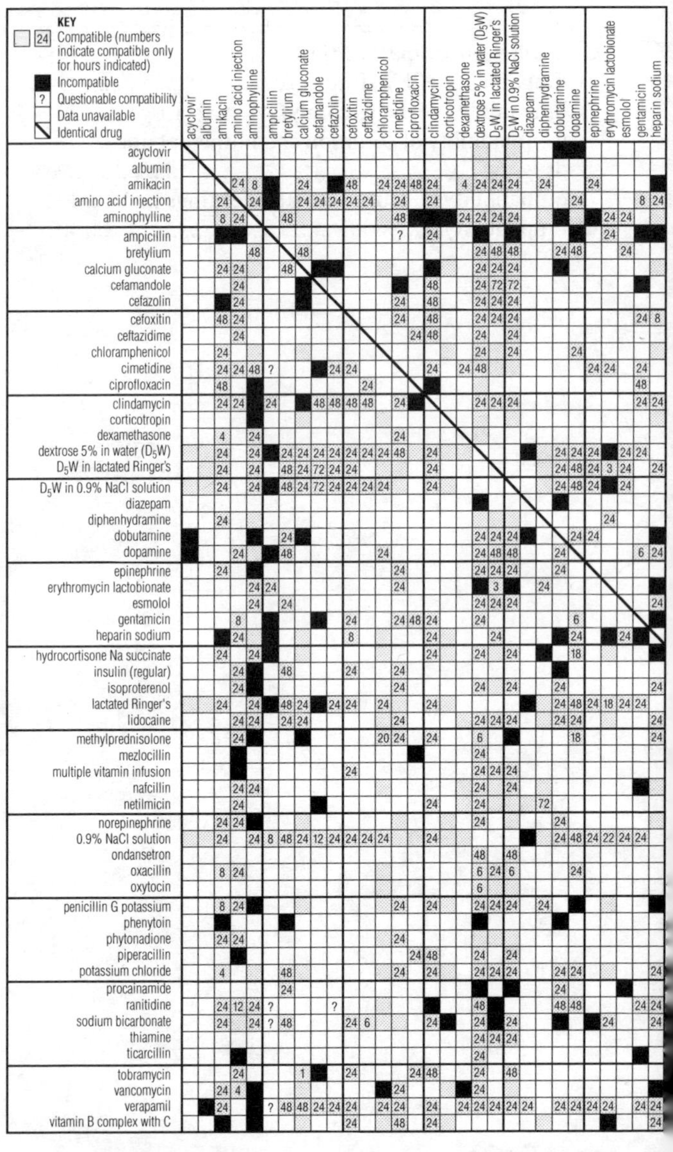

KEY
- ✓ / 24 Compatible (numbers indicate compatible only for hours indicated)
- ■ Incompatible
- ? Questionable compatibility
- (blank) Data unavailable
- ╲ Identical drug

	acyclovir	albumin	amikacin	amino acid injection	aminophylline	ampicillin	bretylium	calcium gluconate	cefamandole	cefazolin	cefoxitin	ceftazidime	chloramphenicol	cimetidine	ciprofloxacin	clindamycin	corticotropin	dexamethasone	dextrose 5% in water (D_5W)	D_5W in lactated Ringer's	D_5W in 0.9% NaCl solution	diazepam	diphenhydramine	dobutamine	dopamine	epinephrine	erythromycin lactobionate	esmolol	gentamicin	heparin sodium
acyclovir	╲																		✓		✓			■	■					
albumin		╲																	✓	✓	✓									
amikacin			╲	24	8	■		24		■	48		24	24	48	24		4	24	24	24		24			24				■
amino acid injection			24	╲	24	■		24	24	24	24	24		24		24									24				8	24
aminophylline			8	24	╲		48	✓					✓	48	■	■	■	24	24	24	24		✓	■	✓	■	24	24		✓
ampicillin			■	■		╲								?		24			■		■				■		24		■	■
bretylium					48		╲	48											24	48	48			24	48			24		
calcium gluconate			24	24	✓		48	╲	■	■			✓			■	✓		24	24	24			■						✓
cefamandole				24				■	╲					■		48			24	72	72								■	
cefazolin			■	24				■		╲				24		48			24	24	24									
cefoxitin			48	24							╲			24		48			24	24	24								24	8
ceftazidime				24								╲			24	48			24		24									
chloramphenicol			24		✓			✓					╲				✓		24	✓	24				24					✓
cimetidine			24	24	48	?			■	24	24			╲		24		24	48	✓	✓					24	24		24	
ciprofloxacin			48		■							24			╲	■			✓										48	
clindamycin			24	24	■	24		■	48	48	48	48		24	■	╲			24	24	24								24	24
corticotropin					■			✓					✓				╲		✓		✓									✓
dexamethasone			4		24									24				╲	✓											
dextrose 5% in water (D_5W)	✓	✓	24		24	■	24	24	24	24	24	24	24	48	✓	24	✓	✓	╲			■	✓	24	24	24	■	24	24	
D_5W in lactated Ringer's		✓	24		24		48	24	72	24	24		✓	✓		24				╲			✓	24	48	24	3	24		24
D_5W in 0.9% NaCl solution	✓	✓	24		24	■	48	24	72	24	24	24	24	✓		24	✓				╲		✓	24	48	24	■	24		
diazepam																			■			╲		■						
diphenhydramine			24		✓														✓	✓	✓		╲				24			
dobutamine	■				■		24	■											24	24	24	■		╲	24	24				■
dopamine	■			24	✓	■	48						24						24	48	48			24	╲				6	24
epinephrine			24		■									24					24	24	24			24		╲				
erythromycin lactobionate					24	24								24					■	3	■		24				╲			■
esmolol					24		24												24	24	24							╲		24
gentamicin				8		■			■		24			24	48	24			24						6				╲	■
heparin sodium			■	24	✓	■		✓			8		✓			24	✓			24				■	24		■	24	■	╲
hydrocortisone Na succinate			24		24	■		✓					✓			24	✓		24	✓	24		■		18		✓			■
insulin (regular)				24	■		48				24			24										■						
isoproterenol				24	■									24					24	✓	24			24						24
lactated Ringer's	✓	✓	24		24	■	48	24	■	24	24		24	✓		24	✓					■	✓	24	48	24	18	24	24	
lidocaine				24	24		24	24					✓	24				✓	24	24	24		✓	24	24		✓			24
methylprednisolone				24	■			■					20	24		24			6		■				18					24
mezlocillin				■											■				24											
multiple vitamin infusion				■							24								24	24	24									
nafcillin				24	24								✓					✓	24	✓	24		✓						■	✓
netilmicin				24					■							24		✓	24	✓	✓	✓	72							
norepinephrine			24	24	■			✓						✓			✓		24		✓			24						✓
0.9% NaCl solution	✓	✓	24		24	8	48	24	12	24	24	24	24	✓	✓	24	✓	✓				■	✓	24	48	24	22	24	24	
ondansetron																			48		48									
oxacillin			8	24									✓						6	24	6				24					
oxytocin													✓						6	✓	✓									
penicillin G potassium			8	24	■			✓					✓	24		24	✓		24	24	24		24		■		✓			■
phenytoin			■				■												■					■						
phytonadione			24	24									✓	24					✓	✓	✓									
piperacillin				■											24	48			24		24									
potassium chloride			4		✓		48	✓					✓	24		24	✓		24	24	24			24	24		✓			24
procainamide							24												■		■			24				■		
ranitidine			24	12	24	?				?			✓			■			48	■				48	48				24	24
sodium bicarbonate			24	✓	24	?	48				24	6	✓	✓		24	■		24	■	24			■		■	24			24
thiamine																			24	24	24									
ticarcillin				■															24										■	
tobramycin				24				1	■		24				24	48			24		48									
vancomycin			24	4	■			✓					■	24			✓	■	24		✓									■
verapamil		■	24		■	?	48	48	24	24	24		24	24		24		24	24	24	24	24		24	24	24	24		24	24
vitamin B complex with C			■		■			✓			24		✓	48		24	✓						✓				■			24

PREVENTING INCOMPATIBILITIES

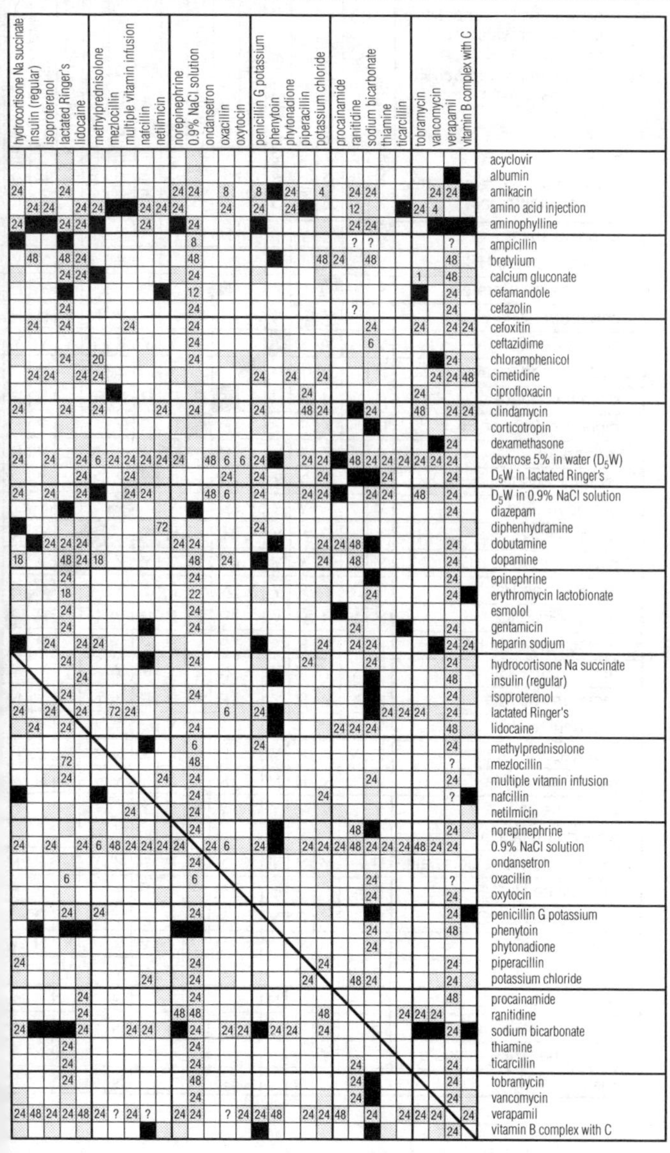

	hydrocortisone Na succinate	insulin (regular)	isoproterenol	lactated Ringer's	lidocaine	methylprednisolone	mezlocillin	multiple vitamin infusion	nafcillin	netilmicin	norepinephrine	0.9% NaCl solution	ondansetron	oxacillin	oxytocin	penicillin G potassium	phenytoin	phytonadione	piperacillin	potassium chloride	procainamide	ranitidine	sodium bicarbonate	thiamine	ticarcillin	tobramycin	vancomycin	verapamil	vitamin B complex with C
acyclovir																													
albumin																												■	
amikacin	24			24							24	24		8		8	■	24		4		24	24				24	24	■
amino acid injection		24	24		24	24	■	■	24	24	24			24		24		24	■			12			■	24	4		
aminophylline	24	■	■	24	24	■			24		■	24				■						24	24				■	■	■
ampicillin	■			■								8										?	?					?	
bretylium		48		48	24							48					■			48	24		48					48	
calcium gluconate				24	24	■						24														1		48	
cefamandole				■						■		12														■		24	
cefazolin				24								24										?						24	
cefoxitin		24		24				24				24											24			24		24	24
ceftazidime												24											6						
chloramphenicol				24		20						24															■	24	
cimetidine		24	24		24	24										24		24		24							24	24	48
ciprofloxacin							■												24							24			
clindamycin	24			24		24				24		24				24			48	24		■	24			48		24	24
corticotropin																							■						
dexamethasone																											■	24	
dextrose 5% in water (D_5W)	24		24		24	6	24	24	24	24	24		48	6	6	24	■		24	24	■	48	24	24	24	24	24	24	
D_5W in lactated Ringer's					24			24						24		24				24		■	■	24				24	
D_5W in 0.9% NaCl solution	24		24		24	■		24	24				48	6		24			24	24	■		24	24		48		24	
diazepam				■								■																24	
diphenhydramine	■									72						24													
dobutamine		■	24	24	24						24	24					■			24	24	48	■					24	
dopamine	18			48	24	18						48		24		■				24		48						24	
epinephrine				24								24											■					24	
erythromycin lactobionate				18								22											24					24	■
esmolol				24								24									■								
gentamicin				24					■			24										24			■			24	
heparin sodium	■		24		24	24										■				24		24	24				■	24	24
hydrocortisone Na succinate				24					■			24							24				24					24	
insulin (regular)					24												■						■					48	
isoproterenol				24								24											■					24	
lactated Ringer's	24		24		24		72	24						6		24	■						■	24	24	24		24	
lidocaine		24		24								24					■				24	24	24					48	
methylprednisolone									■			6				24												24	
mezlocillin				72								48																?	
multiple vitamin infusion				24						24		24											24					24	
nafcillin	■					■						24								24								?	■
netilmicin								24				24																	
norepinephrine												24					■					48	■					24	
0.9% NaCl solution	24		24		24	6	48	24	24	24	24		24	6		24	■		24	24	24	48	24	24	24	48	24	24	
ondansetron												24																	
oxacillin				6								6											24					?	
oxytocin																							24					24	
penicillin G potassium				24		24						24											■					24	■
phenytoin		■		■	■						■	■											24					48	
phytonadione																							24						
piperacillin	24											24								24								24	
potassium chloride									24			24							24			48	24					24	
procainamide					24							24																48	
ranitidine					24						48	48								48					24	24	24		
sodium bicarbonate	24	■	■	■	24			24	24		■	24		24	24	■	24	24		24						■	■	24	■
thiamine				24								24																	
ticarcillin				24								24										24						24	
tobramycin				24								48										24	■					24	
vancomycin												24										24	■					24	
verapamil	24	48	24	24	48	24	?	24	?		24	24		?	24	24	48		24	24	48		24		24	24	24		24
vitamin B complex with C									■							■							■					24	

PREVENTING INCOMPATIBILITIES

Compatibility of drugs combined in a syringe

KEY

Y = compatible for at least 30 minutes
P = provisionally compatible; administer within 15 minutes
$P_{(5)}$ = provisionally compatible; administer within 5 minutes
N = not compatible
* = conflicting data
(A blank space indicates no available data.)

	atropine sulfate	benzquinamide HCl	butorphanol tartrate	chlorpromazine HCl	cimetidine HCl	codeine phosphate	dimenhydrinate	diphenhydramine HCl	droperidol	fentanyl citrate	glycopyrrolate	heparin Na	hydromorphone HCl	hydroxyzine HCl	meperidine HCl
atropine sulfate		Y	Y	Y	Y		P	P	P	P	Y	$P_{(5)}$	Y	Y	Y
benzquinamide HCl	Y										Y			Y	Y
butorphanol tartrate	Y			Y	Y		N	Y	Y	Y				Y	P
chlorpromazine HCl	Y		Y		N		N	P	P	P	Y	N	Y	P	P
cimetidine HCl	Y		Y	N				Y	Y	Y	Y	Y	Y	Y	Y
codeine phosphate											Y			Y	
dimenhydrinate	P		N	N				P	P	P	N	$P_{(5)}$		N	P
diphenhydramine HCl	P		Y	P	Y		P		P	P	Y		Y	P	P
droperidol	P		Y	P	Y		P	P		P	Y	N		P	P
fentanyl citrate	P		Y	P	Y		P	P	P			$P_{(5)}$	Y	Y	P
glycopyrrolate	Y	Y		Y	Y	Y	N	Y	Y				Y	Y	Y
heparin Na	$P_{(5)}$			N	Y		$P_{(5)}$		N	$P_{(5)}$					N
hydromorphone HCl	Y			Y	Y			Y		Y	Y			Y	
hydroxyzine HCl	Y	Y	Y	P	Y	Y	N	P	P	Y	Y		Y		P
meperidine HCl	Y	Y	P	P	Y		P	P	P	P	Y	N		P	
metoclopramide HCl	P			P			P	Y	P	P		$P_{(5)}$		P	P
midazolam HCl	Y	Y	Y	Y	Y		N	Y	Y	Y	Y		Y	Y	Y
morphine sulfate	P	Y	Y	P	Y		P	P	P	P	Y	N*		Y	N
nalbuphine HCl	Y				Y				Y					Y	
pentazocine lactate	P	Y	Y	P	Y		P	P	P	P	N	N	Y	Y	P
pentobarbital Na	P	N	N	N	N		N	N	N	N	N		Y	N	N
perphenazine	Y		Y	Y	Y		Y	Y	Y	Y					P
phenobarbital Na		N										$P_{(5)}$			
prochlorperazine edisylate	P		Y	Y	Y		N	P	P	P	Y		N*	P	P
promazine HCl	P			P	Y		N	P	P	P	Y			P	P
promethazine HCl	P		Y	P	Y		N	P	P	P	Y	N	Y	P	Y
ranitidine HCl	Y			Y			Y	Y		Y	Y		Y	N	Y
scopolamine HBr	P	Y	Y	P	Y		P	P	P	P	Y		Y	Y	P
secobarbital Na		N			N						N				
sodium bicarbonate											N				
thiethylperazine maleate			Y										Y		
thiopental Na		N		N			N	N			N				N

midazolam HCl	morphine sulfate	nalbuphine HCl	pentazocine lactate	pentobarbital Na	perphenazine	phenobarbital Na	prochlorperazine edisylate	promazine HCl	promethazine HCl	ranitidine HCl	scopolamine HBr	secobarbital Na	sodium bicarbonate	thiethylperazine maleate	thiopental Na	
Y	P	Y	P	P	Y		P	P	P	Y	P					atropine sulfate
Y	Y		Y	N		N					Y	N			N	benzquinamide HCl
Y	Y		Y	N	Y		Y		Y		Y			Y		butorphanol tartrate
Y	P		P	N	Y		Y	P	P	Y	P				N	chlorpromazine HCl
Y	Y	Y	Y	N	Y		Y	Y	Y		Y	N				cimetidine HCl
																codeine phosphate
N	P		P	N	Y		N	N	N	Y	P				N	dimenhydrinate
Y	P		P	N	Y		P	P	P	Y	P				N	diphenhydramine HCl
Y	P	Y	P	N	Y		P	P	P		P					droperidol
Y	P		P	N	Y		P	P	P	Y	P					fentanyl citrate
Y	Y		N	N			Y	Y	Y	Y	Y	N	N		N	glycopyrrolate
	N*		N			P(5)			N							heparin Na
Y			Y	Y			N*		Y	Y	Y			Y		hydromorphone HCl
[illegible]	Y	Y	Y	N			P	P	P	N	Y					hydroxyzine HCl
Y	N		P	N	P		P	P	Y	Y	P				N	meperidine HCl
Y	P		P		P		P	P	P	Y	P		N			metoclopramide HCl
	Y	Y		N	N		N	Y	Y	N	Y			Y		midazolam HCl
			P	N*	Y		P*	P	P*	Y	P				N	morphine sulfate
				N			Y		Y	Y	Y			Y		nalbuphine HCl
	P			N	Y		P	Y	Y	Y	P					pentazocine lactate
[illegible]	N*	N	N		N		N	N	N		Y		Y		Y	pentobarbital Na
[illegible]	Y		Y	N			Y			Y						perphenazine
										N						phenobarbital Na
[illegible]	P*	Y	P	N	Y			P	P	Y	P				N	prochlorperazine edisylate
	P		Y	N			P		P	P						promazine HCl
	P*	Y	Y	N			P	P		Y	P				N	promethazine HCl
	Y	Y	Y		Y	N	Y	P	Y		Y			Y		ranitidine HCl
	P	Y	P	Y			P		P	Y					Y	scopolamine HBr
																secobarbital Na
				Y											N	sodium bicarbonate
		Y								Y						thiethylperazine maleate
	N			Y			N		N		Y		N			thiopental Na

ALERT

Incompatibility of common chemotherapeutic drugs

CHEMOTHERAPEUTIC DRUG	INCOMPATIBLE DRUGS
bleomycin	▪ aminophylline ▪ ascorbic acid ▪ cefazolin sodium ▪ diazepam ▪ hydrocortisone sodium succinate ▪ methotrexate ▪ mitomycin ▪ nafcillin sodium ▪ penicillin G sodium ▪ riboflavin ▪ terbutaline sulfate *Special consideration* ▪ Use caution when combining any divalent or trivalent cation with bleomycin sulfate.
carboplatin	aluminum *Special considerations* ▪ Combination causes precipitate formation and loss of potency. ▪ Use only aluminum-free administration equipment.
carmustine	sodium bicarbonate

ALERT

Incompatibility of common chemotherapeutic drugs *(continued)*

CHEMOTHERAPEUTIC DRUG	INCOMPATIBLE DRUGS
cisplatin	▪ aluminum ▪ bicarbonate solutions ▪ Drugs containing sodium thiosulfate, sodium metabisulfite, or sodium bisulfite ▪ Combinations of cisplatin 200 mg/L with fluorouracil 1 g/L or cisplatin 500 mg/L wtih fluorouracil 10 g/L in normal saline solution ▪ mesna *Special considerations* ▪ Aluminum causes precipitate formation. Use only aluminum-free administration equipment (needles, syringes, catheters), such as stainless steel. ▪ Bicarbonate enhances decomposition of cisplatin. ▪ Sodium thiosulfate, sodium metabisulfite, and sodium bisulfite may inactivate cisplatin. ▪ Fluorouracil may result in loss of potency in cisplatin.

(continued)

ALERT

Incompatibility of common chemotherapeutic drugs *(continued)*

CHEMOTHERAPEUTIC DRUG	INCOMPATIBLE DRUGS
cytarabine	▪ cephalothin sodium (2 g/L with cytarabine 100 mg/L in D_5W) ▪ fluorouracil ▪ gentamicin sulfate (240 mg/L with cytarabine 300 mg/L in D_5W) ▪ heparin sodium (10,000 units/L with cytarabine 500 mg/L in normal saline solution) ▪ heparin sodium (20,000 units/L with cytarabine 500 mg/L in D_5W) ▪ hydrocortisone sodium succinate (500 mg/L with cytarabine 360 mg/L in lactated Ringer's injection) ▪ insulin, regular (40 units/L with cytarabine 100 mg/L or cytarabine 500 mg/L in D_5W ▪ methylprednisolone sodium succinate (250 mg/L with cytarabine 360 mg/L in Ringer's injection and sodium lactate 1/6M) ▪ nafcillin sodium (4 g/L with cytarabine 100 mg/L in D_5W ▪ oxacillin sodium (2 g/L with cytarabine 100 mg/L in D_5W) ▪ penicillin G sodium (2 million units/L with cytarabine 200 mg/L in D_5W)
dacarbazine	▪ hydrocortisone sodium succinate ▪ sodium bicarbonate
dactinomycin	No information available.
daunorubicin	▪ dexamethasone sodium phosphate ▪ heparin sodium

ALERT

Incompatibility of common chemotherapeutic drugs *(continued)*

CHEMOTHERAPEUTIC DRUG	INCOMPATIBLE DRUGS
doxorubicin	▪ aminophylline ▪ cephalothin sodium ▪ dexamethasone sodium phosphate ▪ diazepam ▪ fluorouracil ▪ furosemide 10 mg/L ▪ heparin sodium 1,000 units/ml ▪ hydrocortisone sodium phosphate and sodium succinate *Special considerations* ▪ Combinations with fluorouracil and doxorubicin 10 mg/L in D_5W produce purple color. ▪ Combinations with furosemide and heparin sodium produce precipitate. ▪ Doxorubicin reacts with aluminum slowly and doesn't cause substantial loss of potency. Therefore, don't store reconstituted doxorubicin in syringes capped with aluminum-hubbed needles; however, the drug may be administered safely through an aluminum-hubbed needle.

(continued)

ALERT

Incompatibility of common chemotherapeutic drugs *(continued)*

CHEMOTHERAPEUTIC DRUG	INCOMPATIBLE DRUGS
fluorouracil	▪ cisplatin ▪ cytarabine ▪ diazepam ▪ doxorubicin ▪ droperidol (when mixed in a syringe with room-temperature fluorouracil [25 mg/0.5ml] or when injected sequentially into a Y-site with fluorouracil [50mg/ml], without flush in between) *Special consideration* ▪ There are conflicting compatibility reports for injecting fluorouracil with ondansetron via Y-site injection. Consult the primary literature for guidelines.
ifosfamide	No information available.
leucovorin	▪ droperidol (when combined in a syringe or injected sequentially into a Y-site without flush in between) causes precipitate formation. ▪ foscarnet (when injected via a Y-site)
mesna	cisplatin

ALERT

Incompatibility of common chemotherapeutic drugs *(continued)*

CHEMOTHERAPEUTIC DRUG	INCOMPATIBLE DRUGS
methotrexate sodium	▪ droperidol 2.5 mg/ml ▪ prednisolone sodium phosphate 200 mg/L ▪ ranitidine 25 mg/ml *Special consideration* ▪ There are conflicting compatibility reports for combining methotrexate sodium with heparin sodium or metoclopramide in a syringe. Consult the primary literature for instructions.
mitoxantrone	heparin sodium
plicamycin (mithramycin)	iron (plicamycin has a strong ability to chelate metal ions)
vinblastine	▪ furosemide 5 mg/0.5 ml (when combined in a syringe) ▪ furosemide 10 mg/ml (when injected sequentially into a Y-site without flush in between)
vincristine	furosemide

Compatibility of drugs with tube feedings

Some feeding formulas, such as Ensure, may chemically break down when combined with a drug such as Dimetapp Elixir. Increased formula viscosity and a clogged tube can occur from giving drugs such as Klorvess, Neo-Calglucon Syrup, Dimetane Elixir, Phenergan Syrup, or Sudafed Syrup with a feeding formula.

Drug preparations such as ferrous sulfate or potassium chloride liquids are incompatible with some formulas, causing clumping when mixed in a tube. Still other combinations may alter the bioavailability of some drugs, such as phenytoin.

Follow these guidelines:

- Never add a drug to a feeding formula container.
- Check the compatibility of a drug and the feeding formula before administering.
- Infuse 30 ml of water before and after giving a drug dose through a feeding tube.
- Flush the feeding tube with 5 ml of water between drug doses if you're giving more than one drug.
- Dilute highly concentrated liquids with 60 ml of water.
- Instill drugs in liquid form when possible. If you must crush a tablet, crush it into fine dust and dissolve it in warm water. (Never crush and liquefy enteric-coated tablets or timed-release capsules.) ■

Compatibility of insulins

Some insulins can be mixed together to fine-tune their onset, peak, and duration of action, helping to achieve glucose control. Most regular insulin can be combined in a syringe with all other types. Insulin zinc suspension (lente), prompt insulin zinc suspension (semilente), and extended insulin zinc suspension (ultralente) are compatible in any proportion.

Precautions

- Before drawing up insulin suspension, roll and invert the bottle to ensure even drug particle distribution.
- Don't shake bottle; foam or bubbles may develop in the syringe.

Incompatibilities

- Don't mix human zinc suspension insulin with insulin zinc suspension (lente) because their buffering systems aren't compatible.
- Don't mix insulins of different purities or origins. Prompt insulin zinc suspension (semilente insulin) cannot be mixed with neutral protamine (NPH) insulin. ■

CHAPTER 10

TREATING OVERDOSE AND SUBSTANCE ABUSE

REVIEWING OVERDOSE EFFECTS AND TREATMENTS

Acetaminophen overdose

In an acute acetaminophen overdose, plasma levels of 300 mcg/ml occurring 4 hours after ingestion or 50 mcg/ml occurring 12 hours after ingestion are associated with hepatotoxicity.

Clinical findings include cyanosis, anemia, jaundice, skin eruptions, fever, vomiting, CNS stimulation, delirium, and methemoglobinemia, progressing to CNS depression, coma, vascular collapse, seizures, and death. Acetaminophen poisoning develops in stages:

- *Stage 1* (12 to 24 hours after ingestion): nausea, vomiting, diaphoresis, anorexia
- *Stage 2* (24 to 48 hours after ingestion): clinically improved but elevated liver function tests
- *Stage 3* (72 to 96 hours after ingestion): peak hepatotoxicity
- *Stage 4* (7 to 8 days after ingestion): recovery.

Treatment

- To treat acetaminophen toxicity, immediately induce emesis with ipecac syrup (if the patient is conscious) or with gastric lavage.
- Administer activated charcoal via a nasogastric tube.
- Oral acetylcysteine, a specific antidote for acetaminophen poisoning, is most effective if started within 12 hours after ingestion but can still help if started as late as 24 hours after ingestion. Administer an acetylcysteine loading dose of 140 mg/kg P.O., followed by maintenance doses of 70 mg/kg P.O. every 4 hours for an additional 17 doses. Repeat doses vomited within 1 hour of administration.
- Remove charcoal by lavage before administering acetylcysteine because it may interfere with this antidote's absorption. Acetylcysteine minimizes hepatic injury by supplying sulfhydryl groups that bind with acetaminophen metabolites.
- Hemodialysis may be helpful in removing acetaminophen from the body.
- Monitor laboratory parameters and vital signs closely.
- Cimetidine has been used investigationally to block acetaminophen's metabolism to toxic intermediates.
- Provide symptomatic and supportive measures (respiratory support and correction of fluid and electrolyte imbalances).
- Determine plasma acetaminophen levels at least 4

hours after overdose. If they indicate hepatotoxicity, perform liver function tests every 24 hours for at least 96 hours. ■

Analeptic drug overdose

Individual responses to an analeptic drug overdose vary widely. Toxic doses also vary, depending on the specific drug and the route of ingestion.

Signs and symptoms of overdose include restlessness, tremor, hyperreflexia, tachypnea, confusion, aggressiveness, hallucinations, and panic; fatigue and depression usually follow the excitement stage. Other effects may include arrhythmias, shock, altered blood pressure, nausea, vomiting, diarrhea, and abdominal cramps; death is usually preceded by seizures and coma.

Treatment

- Treat an overdose symptomatically and supportively.
- If oral ingestion is recent (within 4 hours), use gastric lavage or ipecac syrup to empty the stomach and reduce further absorption. Follow with activated charcoal.
- Monitor vital signs and fluid and electrolyte balance.
- If the drug was smoked or injected, focus interventions on enhanced drug elimination and supportive care.
- Administer sedatives as needed.
- Urine acidification may enhance excretion.
- A saline cathartic (magnesium citrate) may hasten GI evacuation of an unabsorbed sustained-release drug. ■

Anticholinergic overdose

Clinical effects of an anticholinergic overdose include such peripheral effects as dilated, nonreactive pupils; blurred vision; flushed, hot, dry skin; dry mucous membranes; dysphagia; decreased or absent bowel sounds; urine retention; hyperthermia; tachycardia; hypertension; and increased respiratory rate.

Treatment

- Treat an overdose symptomatically and supportively, as needed.
- If the patient is alert, induce emesis (or use gastric lavage), and follow with a saline cathartic and activated charcoal to prevent further drug absorption.
- In severe cases, physostigmine may be administered to block central antimuscarinic effects.
- Give fluids as needed to treat shock.

▪ If urine retention occurs, catheterization may be necessary. ■

Anticoagulant overdose

Clinical effects of an oral anticoagulant overdose vary with severity. They may include internal or external bleeding or skin necrosis, but the most common sign is hematuria. Excessively prolonged PT or minor bleeding requires withdrawal of therapy; withholding one or two doses may be adequate in some cases.

Treatment

▪ To control bleeding, treatment may include oral or I.V. phytonadione (vitamin K_1) and, in severe hemorrhage, fresh frozen plasma or whole blood. Menadione (vitamin K_3) isn't as effective. Use of phytonadione may interfere with subsequent oral anticoagulant therapy. ■

Antihistamine overdose

Drowsiness is the usual clinical sign of an antihistamine overdose. Seizures, coma, and respiratory depression may occur with a severe overdose. Certain $histamine_1$ antagonists, such as diphenhydramine, also block cholinergic receptors and produce modest anticholinergic reactions, such as dry mouth, flushed skin, fixed and dilated pupils, and GI reactions, especially in children. Phenothiazine-type antihistamines, such as promethazine, also block dopamine receptors. Movement disorders mimicking Parkinson's disease may also be seen.

Treatment

▪ Treat overdose with gastric lavage followed by activated charcoal. Ipecac syrup is not generally recommended because acute dystonic reactions may increase the risk of aspiration. In addition, phenothiazine-type antihistamines may have antiemetic effects.

▪ Treat hypotension with fluids or vasopressors, and treat seizures with phenytoin or diazepam.

▪ Watch for arrhythmias and treat them appropriately. ■

Barbiturate overdose

A barbiturate overdose may cause an unsteady gait, slurred speech, sustained nystagmus, somnolence, confusion, respiratory depression, pulmonary edema, areflexia, and coma. Typical shock syndrome — with tachycardia, hypotension, jaundice, oliguria, and hypothermia followed by fever — may occur.

Treatment
- Maintain and support ventilation and pulmonary function as necessary.
- Support cardiac function and circulation with vasopressors and I.V. fluids as needed.
- If the patient is conscious and his gag reflex is present, induce emesis (if ingestion was recent) by administering ipecac syrup.
- If emesis is contraindicated, perform gastric lavage while a cuffed endotracheal tube is in place to prevent aspiration. Follow with administration of activated charcoal and saline cathartic.
- Measure intake and output, vital signs, and laboratory parameters.
- Maintain body temperature.
- Roll patient from side to side every 30 minutes to avoid pulmonary congestion.
- Alkalinization of urine may be helpful in removing drug from the body.
- Dialysis may be useful in severe overdose.

Benzodiazepine overdose

An overdose of benzodiazepines produces somnolence, confusion, coma, hypoactive reflexes, dyspnea, labored breathing, hypotension, bradycardia, slurred speech, and unsteady gait or impaired coordination.

Treatment
- Support blood pressure and respiration until drug effects subside.
- Monitor vital signs.
- Mechanical ventilation via an endotracheal (ET) tube may be required to maintain a patent airway and support adequate oxygenation.
- Flumazenil, a specific benzodiazepine antagonist, may be useful.
- Use I.V. fluids or vasopressors, such as dopamine and phenylephrine, to treat hypotension as needed.
- If the patient is conscious and his gag reflex is present, induce emesis (if ingestion was recent) by administering ipecac syrup. If emesis is contraindicated, perform gastric lavage while a cuffed ET tube is in place to prevent aspiration. After emesis or lavage, administer activated charcoal with a cathartic as a single dose.
- Dialysis is of limited value.

CNS depressant overdose

Signs of a CNS depressant overdose include prolonged

coma, hypotension, hypothermia followed by fever, and inadequate ventilation, sometimes without significant respiratory depression. Absence of pupillary reflexes, dilated pupils, loss of deep tendon reflexes, tonic muscle spasms, and apnea also may occur.

Treatment

- Overdose treatment involves support of respiration and cardiovascular function; mechanical ventilation may be necessary.
- Maintain adequate urine output with adequate hydration while avoiding pulmonary edema.
- Empty gastric contents by inducing emesis.
- For lipid-soluble drugs such as glutethimide, charcoal and resin hemoperfusion are effective in removing the drug; hemodialysis and peritoneal dialysis are of minimal value. Because of the significant storage of glutethimide in fatty tissue, blood levels commonly show large fluctuations with worsening of symptoms. ■

Digitalis glycoside overdose

Clinical effects of a digitalis glycoside overdose primarily affect the GI, cardiac, and central nervous systems.

Severe overdose may cause hyperkalemia, which may develop rapidly and result in life-threatening cardiac effects. Cardiac signs of digoxin toxicity may occur — with or without other toxicity signs — and commonly precede other toxic effects. Because cardiotoxic effects also can occur in heart disease, determining whether these effects result from an underlying heart disease or digoxin toxicity may be difficult.

Digoxin has caused almost every kind of arrhythmia; various combinations of arrhythmias may occur in the same patient. Patients with chronic digoxin toxicity commonly have ventricular arrhythmias, AV conduction disturbances, or both. Patients with digoxin-induced ventricular tachycardia have a high mortality because ventricular fibrillation or asystole may result.

Treatment

- If toxicity is suspected, the drug should be discontinued and serum drug level measurements obtained. Usually, the drug takes at least 6 hours to be distributed between plasma and tissue and to reach equilibrium. Plasma levels drawn earlier may show higher digoxin levels than those present after the drug is distributed into the tissues.

- Other treatment measures include immediate emesis induction, gastric lavage, and administration of activated charcoal to reduce absorption of the remaining drug. Multiple doses of activated charcoal (such as 50 g q 6 hours) may help reduce further absorption, especially of any drug undergoing enterohepatic recirculation.
- Some clinicians advocate cholestyramine administration if digoxin was recently ingested; however, this may not be useful if the ingestion is life-threatening.
- Any interacting drugs probably should be discontinued.
- Ventricular arrhythmias may be treated with I.V. potassium (in replacement doses, but not to patients with significant AV block) or I.V. phenytoin, lidocaine, or propranolol.
- Refractory ventricular tachyarrhythmias may be controlled with overdrive pacing.
- Procainamide may be used for ventricular arrhythmias that don't respond to the above treatments.
- In severe AV block, asystole, and hemodynamically significant sinus bradycardia, atropine restores a normal heart rate.
- Administration of digoxin-specific antibody fragments (digoxin immune Fab) is a promising new treatment for life-threatening digoxin toxicity. Each 40 mg of digoxin immune Fab binds about 0.6 mg of digoxin in the bloodstream. The complex is then excreted in the urine, rapidly decreasing serum levels and therefore cardiac drug concentrations. ■

Diphenhydramine overdose

Signs and symptoms of diphenhydramine overdose include tachycardia, hallucinations, seizures, coma, dry mucous membranes, and diplopia. Diphenhydramine is an active ingredient in sleeping pills, as well as an antipruritic and antihistamine.

Treatment

- Treatment includes administration of oxygen via a nasal cannula at a rate of 4 liters/minute and cardiac monitoring.
- Establish I.V. access with an 18G catheter and begin infusing normal saline solution.
- Draw blood for a CBC, serum chemistry, and blood alcohol level.
- Obtain a blood sample for arterial blood gas analysis and a urine specimen for toxicology studies.
- If the patient is conscious and his gag reflex is present,

induce emesis (if ingestion was recent) by administering ipecac syrup.

- If emesis is contraindicated, perform gastric lavage while a cuffed endotracheal tube is in place to prevent aspiration. Follow with administration of activated charcoal and magnesium sulfate cathartic to promote excretion of remaining diphenhydramine through the GI tract.
- If the patient's temperature exceeds 102° F (38.9° C), use a hypothermia blanket. ■

Iron supplement overdose

Iron supplements are a major cause of poisoning, especially in small children. In fact, as little as 1 g of ferrous sulfate can kill an infant.

Symptoms of iron poisoning result from its acute corrosive effects on the GI mucosa, as well as the adverse metabolic effects caused by iron overload. Four stages of acute iron poisoning have been identified, and signs and symptoms may occur within the first 10 to 60 minutes of ingestion or may be delayed several hours.

Stage 1

The first findings reflect acute GI irritation and include epigastric pain, nausea, and vomiting. Diarrhea may occur as green stools, followed by tarry stools and then melena. Hematemesis may be accompanied by drowsiness, lassitude, shock, and coma. Local erosion of the stomach and small intestine may further enhance the absorption of iron.

Stage 2

If death doesn't occur in the first phase, a second phase of apparent recovery may last 24 hours.

Stage 3

A third phase, which can occur 4 to 48 hours after ingestion, is marked by CNS abnormalities, metabolic acidosis, hepatic dysfunction, renal failure, and bleeding diathesis. This stage may progress to circulatory failure, coma, and death.

Stage 4

If the patient survives, the fourth phase consists of late complications of acute iron intoxication and may occur 2 to 6 weeks after the overdose. Severe gastric scarring, pyloric stenosis, or intestinal obstruction may be present.

Treatment

- Patients who develop vomiting, diarrhea, leukocytosis, or hyperglycemia and have an abdominal X-ray that's positive for iron within 6 hours of ingestion are likely to be at risk for serious toxicity. Empty the stomach by inducing emesis with ipecac syrup, and perform gastric lavage. If patients have had multiple episodes of vomiting or the vomitus contains blood, avoid ipecac and perform lavage.

- Some doctors add sodium bicarbonate to the lavage solution to convert ferrous iron to ferrous carbonate, which is poorly absorbed. Disodium phosphate has also been used; however, some children may develop life-threatening hyperphosphatemia or hypercalcemia.
- Other possible treatments include lavage with normal saline solution, administration of a saline cathartic, surgical removal of tablets, and chelation therapy with deferoxamine mesylate.
- Dialysis is of little value.
- Supportive treatment includes monitoring acid-base balance, maintaining a patent airway, and controlling shock and dehydration with appropriate I.V. therapy. ■

NSAID overdose

Clinical signs of an NSAID overdose include dizziness, drowsiness, paresthesia, vomiting, nausea, abdominal pain, headache, sweating, nystagmus, apnea, and cyanosis.

Treatment

- To treat an NSAID overdose, empty the stomach immediately by inducing emesis with ipecac syrup or by gastric lavage.
- Administer activated charcoal via a nasogastric tube.
- Provide symptomatic and supportive care (respiratory support and correction of fluid and electrolyte imbalances).
- Monitor laboratory parameters and vital signs closely.
- Alkaline diuresis may enhance renal excretion.
- Dialysis is of minimal value because ibuprofen is strongly protein-bound. ■

Opioid overdose

Rapid I.V. administration may result in an opioid overdose because of the delay in maximum CNS effect (30 minutes). The most common signs of morphine overdose are respiratory depression with or without CNS depression and pinpoint pupils.

Other acute toxic effects include hypotension, bradycardia, hypothermia, shock, apnea, cardiopulmonary arrest, circulatory collapse, pulmonary edema, and seizures.

Treatment

- Establish respiratory exchange via a patent airway and ventilation, as needed.
- Administer a narcotic antagonist (such as naloxone) to reverse respiratory depression. Because the duration of action of morphine is longer than that of naloxone, repeated doses of naloxone are necessary. Do not give naloxone except in clinically significant respiratory or cardiovascular depression.
- Monitor vital signs closely.
- If the patient seeks treatment within 2 hours of an oral overdose, induce emesis (with ipecac syrup) or use gastric lavage. Avoid aspiration.
- Give activated charcoal via a nasogastric tube for further removal of the drug.
- Provide symptomatic and continued respiratory support and correction of fluid or electrolyte imbalance.
- Monitor laboratory values, vital signs, and neurologic status. ■

Phenothiazine overdose

CNS depression is characterized by deep, unarousable sleep and possibly a coma, hypotension or hypertension, extrapyramidal symptoms, abnormal involuntary muscle movements, agitation, seizures, arrhythmias, ECG changes, hypothermia or hyperthermia, and autonomic nervous system dysfunction.

Treatment

- Maintain vital signs, a patent airway, stable body temperature, and fluid and electrolyte balance.
- Do not induce vomiting. Because phenothiazines inhibit the cough reflex, aspiration may occur. Use gastric lavage, then activated charcoal and saline cathartics.
- Regulate body temperature.
- Treat hypotension with I.V. fluids: Don't give epinephrine.
- Treat seizures with parenteral diazepam or barbiturates; arrhythmias with parenteral phenytoin; and extrapyramidal reactions with benztropine or parenteral diphenhydramine. ■

Salicylate overdose

Clinical effects of a salicylate overdose include metabolic acidosis with respiratory alkalosis, hyperpnea, and tachypnea, caused by increased carbon dioxide production and direct stimulation of the respiratory center.

Treatment

- To treat aspirin overdose, induce emesis with ipecac syrup (if the patient is conscious) or use gastric lavage.
- Administer activated charcoal via a nasogastric tube.
- Provide symptomatic and respiratory support and correction of fluid and electrolyte imbalances.
- Closely monitor laboratory values and vital signs.
- Enhance renal excretion by administering sodium bicarbonate to alkalinize urine. Apply a hypothermia blanket or cool soaks if the patient's rectal temperature is above 104° F (40° C).
- Hemodialysis is used only in severe poisoning or in a patient at risk for pulmonary edema. ■

TCA overdose

This overdose is commonly life-threatening, particularly when combined with alcohol. The first 12 hours after ingestion are characterized by agitation, irritation, confusion, hallucinations, hyperthermia, parkinsonian symptoms, seizures, urine retention, dry mucous membranes , pupillary dilation, constipation, and ileus.

This phase precedes CNS depressant effects, including hypothermia, decreased or absent reflexes, sedation, hypotension, cyanosis, and cardiac irregularities.

Severe toxicity is best indicated by a widened QRS complex. Metabolic acidosis may follow hypotension, hypoventilation, and seizures.

Treatment

- Maintain a patent airway, stable body temperature, and fluid and electrolyte balance.
- Induce emesis if the patient is conscious; follow with gastric lavage and activated charcoal.
- Treat seizures with parenteral diazepam or phenytoin, arrhythmias with parenteral phenytoin or lidocaine, and acidosis with sodium bicarbonate.
- Don't give barbiturates; they may enhance CNS and respiratory depressant effects.
- Treat arrhythmias with parenteral phenytoin or lidocaine.
- Treat acidosis with sodium bicarbonate. ■

ALERT

Administering antidotes in poisoning or overdose

ANTIDOTE AND INDICATIONS	DOSAGE
acetylcysteine Treatment of acetaminophen toxicity	▪ *Adults and children:* 140 mg/kg P.O. initially, followed by 70 mg/kg q 4 hr for 17 doses (total of 1,330 mg/kg).
activated charcoal Treatment of poisoning or overdose with most orally administered drugs, except caustic agents and hydrocarbons	▪ *Adults:* initially, 1 g/kg (30 to 100 g) P.O., or 5 to 10 times the amount of poison ingested as a suspension in 180 to 240 ml of water. ▪ *Children ages 1 to 12:* 20 to 50 g P.O. as single dose. ▪ *Children under age 1:* 1 g/kg P.O. as single dose.
aminocaproic acid Antidote for alteplase, anistreplase, streptokinase, or urokinase toxicity	▪ *Adults:* initially, 5 g P.O. or as slow I.V. infusion, followed by 1 to 1.25 g/hr until bleeding is controlled. Don't exceed 30 g daily.
amyl nitrite Antidote for cyanide poisoning	▪ *Adults:* 0.2 or 0.3 ml by inhalation for 30 to 60 seconds q 5 min until the patient regains consciousness.

NURSING CONSIDERATIONS

- Use cautiously in elderly or debilitated patients and in patients with asthma or severe respiratory insufficiency.
- Don't use with activated charcoal.
- Don't combine with amphotericin B, ampicillin, chymotrypsin, erythromycin lactobionate, hydrogen peroxide, iodized oil, oxytetracycline, tetracycline, or trypsin. Administer separately.

- Don't give to semiconscious or unconscious patients.
- If possible, administer within 30 minutes of poisoning. Administer larger dose if patient has food in his stomach.
- Don't give with syrup of ipecac because charcoal inactivates ipecac. If a patient needs syrup of ipecac, give charcoal after he has finished vomiting.
- Don't give in ice cream, milk, or sherbet because they reduce adsorption capacities of charcoal.
- Powder form is most effective. Mix with tap water to form thick syrup. You may add small amount of fruit juice or flavoring to make syrup more palatable.
- You may need to repeat dose if the patient vomits shortly after administration.

- Use cautiously with oral contraceptives and estrogens because they may increase risk of hypercoagulability.
- For infusion, dilute solution with sterile water for injection, normal saline injection, D_5W, or Ringer's solution.
- Monitor coagulation studies, heart rhythm, and blood pressure.

- Amyl nitrite is effective within 30 seconds, but its effects last only 3 to 5 minutes.
- To administer, wrap ampule in cloth and crush. Hold near the patient's nose and mouth so that he can inhale vapor.
- Monitor the patient for orthostatic hypotension.
- The patient may experience headache after administration.

(continued)

ALERT

Administering antidotes in poisoning or overdose *(continued)*

ANTIDOTE AND INDICATIONS	DOSAGE
atropine sulfate Antidote for anticholinesterase toxicity	▪ *Adults:* initially, 1 to 2 mg by direct I.V. injection, then 2 mg q 5 to 60 min until symptoms subside. In severe cases, initial dose may be as much as 6 mg q 4 to 60 min, as needed. Administer over 1 to 2 min.
botulism antitoxin, trivalent equine Treatment of botulism	▪ *Adults and children:* 2 vials I.V. Dilute antitoxin 1:10 in D_5W, $D_{10}W$, or normal saline solution before administration. Give first 10 ml of diluted solution over 5 min; after 15 min, you may increase rate.
deferoxamine mesylate Adjunctive treatment of acute iron intoxication	▪ *Adults and children:* initially, 1 g I.M. or I.V., followed by 500 mg I.M. or I.V. q 4 hr for two doses; then 500 mg I.M. or I.V. q 4 to 12 hr. Don't infuse more than 15 mg/kg/hr. Don't administer more than 6 g in 24 hr.

NURSING CONSIDERATIONS
• Atropine sulfate is contraindicated for patients with glaucoma, myasthenia gravis, obstructive uropathy, or unstable cardiovascular status. • Monitor intake and output to assess for urine retention.
• Obtain an accurate patient history of allergies, especially to horses, and of reactions to immunizations. • Test the patient for sensitivity (against a control of normal saline solution in opposing extremity) before administration. Read results after 5 to 30 minutes. A wheal indicates a positive reaction, requiring patient desensitization. • Keep epinephrine 1:1,000 available in case of allergic reaction.
• Don't administer the drug to patients with severe renal disease or anuria. Use cautiously in patients with impaired renal function. • Keep epinephrine 1:1,000 available in case of allergic reaction. • Use I.M. route if possible. Use I.V. route only when the patient is in shock. • To reconstitute for I.M. administration, add 2 ml of sterile water for injection to each ampule. Make sure the drug dissolves completely. To reconstitute for I.V. administration, dissolve as for I.M. use but in normal saline solution, D_5W, or lactated Ringer's solution. • Monitor intake and output carefully. Warn patient that his urine may turn red. • Reconstituted solution can be stored for up to 1 week at room temperature. Protect from light.

(continued)

ALERT

Administering antidotes in poisoning or overdose *(continued)*

ANTIDOTE AND INDICATIONS	DOSAGE
digoxin immune Fab (ovine) Treatment of potentially life-threatening digoxin or digitoxin intoxication	▪ *Adults and children:* give I.V. over 30 min or as a bolus if cardiac arrest is imminent. Dosage varies according to amount of drug ingested; average dose is 10 vials (400 mg), but if toxicity resulted from acute digoxin ingestion and neither serum digoxin level nor estimated ingestion amount is known, increase dose to 20 vials (800 mg).
edetate calcium disodium Treatment of lead poisoning in patients with blood levels over 50 mcg/dl	*For blood levels of 51 to 100 mcg/dl* ▪ *Adults and children:* 1 g/m^2 I.M. or I.V. daily for 3 to 5 days. For I.V. infusion, dilute in D_5W or normal saline solution. Give over 1 to 2 hr. *For blood levels over 100 mcg/dl* ▪ *Adults and children:* 1.5 g/m^2 I.M. or I.V. daily for 3 to 5 days, usually with dimercaprol. For I.V. infusion, dilute in D_5W or normal saline solution. Give over 1 to 2 hr. If needed, repeat course 2 to 3 weeks later.

NURSING CONSIDERATIONS

- Use cautiously in patients allergic to ovine proteins because the drug is derived from digoxin-specific antibody fragments obtained from immunized sheep. Perform skin test before administering.
- Use only in patients in shock or cardiac arrest with ventricular arrhythmias, such as ventricular tachycardia or fibrillation; with progressive bradycardia, such as severe sinus bradycardia; or with second- or third-degree AV block unresponsive to atropine.
- Infuse through a 0.22-micron membrane filter, if possible.
- Refrigerate powder for reconstitution. If possible, use reconstituted drug immediately, although you may refrigerate it for up to 4 hours.
- Drug interferes with digitalis immunoassay measurements, resulting in misleading standard serum digoxin levels until the drug is cleared from the body (about 2 days).
- Total serum digoxin levels may rise after administration of this drug, reflecting Fab-bound (inactive) digoxin.
- Monitor potassium levels closely.

- Don't give to patients with severe renal disease or anuria.
- Avoid using I.V. route in patients with lead encephalopathy because intracranial pressure may increase; use I.M. route.
- Avoid rapid infusion; I.M. route is preferred, especially for children.
- If giving a high dose, give with dimercaprol to avoid toxicity.
- Force fluids to facilitate lead excretion except in patients with lead encephalopathy.
- Before giving, obtain baseline intake and output, urinalysis, BUN, and serum alkaline phosphatase, calcium, creatinine, and phosphorus levels. Then monitor these values on first, third, and fifth days of treatment. Monitor ECG periodically.
- If procaine hydrochloride has been added to I.M. solution to minimize pain, watch for local reaction.

(continued)

ALERT

Administering antidotes in poisoning or overdose *(continued)*

ANTIDOTE AND INDICATIONS	DOSAGE
methylene blue Treatment of cyanide poisoning	▪ *Adults and children:* 1 to 2 mg/kg of 1% solution by direct I.V. injection over several minutes. May repeat dose in 1 hr.
naloxone hydrochloride ▪ Treatment of respiratory depression caused by opioid drugs ▪ Treatment of postoperative narcotic depression ▪ Treatment of asphyxia neonatorum	*For respiratory depression caused by opioid drugs* ▪ *Adults:* 0.4 to 2 mg I.V., S.C., or I.M. May repeat q 2 to 3 min p.r.n. *For postoperative narcotic depression* ▪ *Adults:* 0.1 to 0.2 mg I.V. q 2 to 3 min p.r.n. ▪ *Children:* 0.01 mg/kg I.V., I.M., or S.C. Repeat as necessary q 2 to 3 min. If patient doesn't improve with initial dose of 0.01 mg/kg, he may need up to 10 times this dose (0.1 mg/kg). *For asphyxia neonatorum* ▪ *Neonates:* 0.01 mg/kg I.V. into umbilical vein. Repeat q 2 to 3 min for three doses, if necessary.

NURSING CONSIDERATIONS

- Don't give to patients with severe renal impairment or hypersensitivity to drug.
- Use with caution in G6PD deficiency; may cause hemolysis.
- Avoid extravasation; S.C. injection may cause necrotic abscesses.
- Warn the patient that methylene blue will discolor his urine and stools and stain his skin. Hypochlorite solution rubbed on his skin will remove stains.

- Use cautiously in patients with cardiac irritability or narcotic addiction.
- Monitor respiratory depth and rate. Be prepared to provide oxygen, ventilation, and other resuscitation measures.
- If neonatal concentration (0.02 mg/ml) isn't available, dilute adult concentration (0.4 mg) by mixing 0.5 ml with 9.5 ml of sterile water or normal saline injection.
- Respiratory rate increases within 2 minutes. Effects last 1 to 4 hours.
- Duration of narcotic may exceed that of naloxone, causing the patient to relapse into respiratory depression.
- You may administer drug by continuous I.V. infusion to control side effects of epidurally administered morphine.
- You may see "overshoot" effect—the patient's respiratory rate after receiving drug exceeds his rate before respiratory depression occurred.
- Naloxone is the safest drug to use when the cause of respiratory depression is uncertain.
- This drug doesn't reverse respiratory depression caused by diazepam.
- Although generally believed ineffective in treating respiratory depression caused by nonopioid drugs, naloxone may reverse coma induced by alcohol intoxication, according to recent reports.

(continued)

ALERT

Administering antidotes in poisoning or overdose *(continued)*

ANTIDOTE AND INDICATIONS	DOSAGE
pralidoxime chloride Antidote for organophosphate poisoning and cholinergic drug overdose	▪ *Adults:* I.V. infusion of 1 to 2 g in 100 ml of normal saline solution over 15 to 30 min. If the patient has pulmonary edema, administer by slow I.V. push over 5 min. Repeat in 1 hr if weakness persists. If the patient needs additional doses, administer them cautiously. If I.V. administration isn't possible, give I.M. or S.C., or 1 to 3 g P.O. q 5 hr. ▪ *Children:* 20 to 40 mg/kg I.V.

NURSING CONSIDERATIONS

- Don't give to patients poisoned with carbaryl, a carbamate insecticide, because it increases carbaryl's toxicity.
- Use with caution in patients with renal insufficiency, myasthenia gravis, asthma, or peptic ulcer.
- Use in hospitalized patients only; have respiratory and other supportive equipment available.
- Administer antidote as soon as possible after poisoning. Treatment is most effective if started within 24 hours of exposure.
- Before administering, suction secretions and make sure airway is patent.
- Dilute drug with sterile water without preservatives. Give atropine along with pralidoxime.
- If the patient's skin was exposed, remove his clothing and wash his skin and hair with sodium bicarbonate, soap, water, and alcohol as soon as possible. A second washing may be needed. When washing the patient, wear protective gloves and clothes to avoid exposure.
- Observe the patient for 48 to 72 hours if he ingested poison. Delayed absorption may occur.
- Watch for signs of rapid weakening in the patient with myasthenia gravis being treated for overdose of cholinergic drugs. He may pass quickly from cholinergic crisis to myasthenic crisis and require more cholinergic drugs to treat the myasthenia. Keep edrophonium available.

(continued)

ALERT

Administering antidotes in poisoning or overdose *(continued)*

ANTIDOTE AND INDICATIONS	DOSAGE
protamine sulfate Treatment of heparin overdose	▪ *Adults:* usually 1 mg for each 78 to 95 units of heparin, based on coagulation studies. Dilute to 1% (10 mg/ml) and give by slow I.V. injection over 1 to 3 min. Don't exceed 50 mg in 10 min.
syrup of ipecac (ipecac syrup) Induction of vomiting in poisoning	▪ *Adults:* 15 ml P.O., followed by 200 to 300 ml of water. ▪ *Children over age 1:* 15 ml P.O., followed by about 200 ml of water or milk. ▪ *Children under age 1:* 5 to 10 ml P.O., followed by 100 to 200 ml of water or milk. Repeat dose once after 20 min, if necessary.

NURSING CONSIDERATIONS

- Use cautiously after cardiac surgery.
- Administer slowly to reduce side effects. Have equipment available to treat shock.
- Monitor the patient continuously, and check vital signs frequently.
- Watch for spontaneous bleeding (heparin "rebound"), especially in patients undergoing dialysis and in those who have had cardiac surgery.
- Protamine sulfate may act as an anticoagulant in extremely high doses.

- Ipecac syrup is contraindicated for semicomatose, unconscious, and severely inebriated patients and for those with seizures, shock, or absent gag reflex.
- Don't give after ingestion of petroleum distillates or volatile oils because of the risk of aspiration pneumonitis. Don't give after ingestion of caustic substances such as lye because further injury can result.
- Before giving, make sure you have ipecac syrup, not ipecac fluid extract (14 times more concentrated and deadly).
- If two doses don't induce vomiting, notify the doctor, who will probably order gastric lavage.
- If the patient also needs activated charcoal, give charcoal after he has vomited or charcoal will neutralize emetic effect.
- Tell parents of children over age 1 to keep 1 oz (30 ml) of syrup on hand.

ALERT

REVIEWING SUBSTANCE ABUSE EFFECTS AND TREATMENTS

Recognizing and treating acute substance abuse

SUBSTANCE	SIGNS AND SYMPTOMS
Alcohol (ethanol) ▪ Beer and wine ▪ Distilled spirits ▪ Other preparations, such as cough syrup, aftershave, or mouthwash	▪ Ataxia ▪ Seizures ▪ Coma ▪ Hypothermia ▪ Alcohol breath odor ▪ Respiratory depression ▪ Bradycardia ▪ Hypotension ▪ Nausea and vomiting

INTERVENTIONS

- Expect to induce vomiting or perform gastric lavage if ingestion occurred in the previous 4 hours. Give activated charcoal and a saline cathartic, as ordered.
- Start I.V. fluid replacement and administer D_5W, thiamine, B-complex vitamins, and vitamin C, as ordered, to prevent dehydration and hypoglycemia and to correct nutritional deficiencies.
- Pad bed rails, and apply cloth restraints to protect the patient.
- Give an anticonvulsant such as diazepam, as ordered, to control seizures.
- Watch for signs of withdrawal, such as hallucinations and alcohol withdrawal delirium. If these occur, give chlordiazepoxide, chloral hydrate, or paraldehyde, as ordered.
- Auscultate the patient's lungs frequently to detect crackles or rhonchi, possibly indicating aspiration pneumonia. If you note these breath sounds, expect to give antibiotics.
- Monitor the patient's neurologic status and vital signs every 15 minutes until he is stable. Assist with dialysis if his vital functions are severely depressed.

(continued)

ALERT

Recognizing and treating acute substance abuse *(continued)*

SUBSTANCE	SIGNS AND SYMPTOMS
Amphetamines ▪ amphetamine sulfate (Benzedrine), also known as bennies, greenies, and cartwheels ▪ dextroamphetamine sulfate (Dexedrine), also known as dexies, hearts, or oranges ▪ methamphetamine (Methadrin), also known as speed, meth, or crystal	▪ Dilated, reactive pupils ▪ Altered mental status (from confusion to paranoia) ▪ Hallucinations ▪ Tremor and seizure activity ▪ Hyperactive deep tendon reflexes ▪ Exhaustion ▪ ComaR▪ Dry mouth ▪ Shallow respirations ▪ Tachycardia ▪ Hypertension ▪ Hyperthermia ▪ Diaphoresis
Antipsychotics ▪ chlorpromazine (Thorazine) ▪ phenothiazines ▪ thioridazine (Mellaril)	▪ Constricted pupils ▪ Photosensitivity ▪ Extrapyramidal effects (dyskinesia, opisthotonos, muscle rigidity, and ocular deviatio ▪ Dry mouth ▪ Decreased level of consciousness (LOC) ▪ Decreased deep tendon reflexes ▪ Seizures ▪ Hypothermia or hyperthermia ▪ Dysphagia ▪ Respiratory depression ▪ Hypotension ▪ Tachycardia

INTERVENTIONS

- If the drug was taken orally, induce vomiting or perform gastric lavage; give activated charcoal and a sodium or magnesium sulfate cathartic, as ordered.
- Lower the patient's urine pH to 5 by adding ammonium chloride or ascorbic acid to his I.V. solution, as ordered.
- Force diuresis by giving the patient mannitol, as ordered.
- Expect to give a short-acting barbiturate, such as pentobarbital, to control stimulant-induced seizures.
- Restrain the patient if he's paranoid or hallucinating.
- Give haloperidol I.M., as ordered, to treat agitation or combative behavior.
- Give an alpha-adrenergic blocker such as phentolamine for hypertension, as ordered.
- Watch for cardiac arrhythmias. Notify the doctor if these develop, and expect to give propranolol or lidocaine to treat tachyarrhythmias or ventricular arrhythmias, respectively.
- Treat hyperthermia with tepid sponge baths or a hypothermia blanket, as ordered.
- Provide a quiet environment to avoid overstimulation.
- Be alert for signs of withdrawal, such as abdominal tenderness, muscle aches, and long periods of sleep.
- Observe suicide precautions, especially if the patient shows signs of withdrawal.

- Expect to perform gastric lavage if the patient ingested the drug within the past 6 hours. (Don't induce vomiting.) Give activated charcoal and a cathartic as ordered.
- Give diphenhydramine or benztropine, as ordered, to treat extrapyramidal effects.
- Give physostigmine salicylate, as ordered, to reverse anticholinergic effects in severe cases.
- Replace fluids I.V., as ordered, to correct hypotension; monitor the patient's vital signs often.
- Give supplemental oxygen to treat respiratory depression.
- Give an anticonvulsant, such as diazepam, or a short-acting barbiturate, such as pentobarbital sodium.

(continued)

ALERT

Recognizing and treating acute substance abuse *(continued)*

SUBSTANCE	SIGNS AND SYMPTOMS
Anxiolytic sedative-hypnotics ▪ benzodiazepines (Valium or Librium)	▪ Confusion ▪ Drowsiness ▪ Stupor ▪ Decreased reflexes ▪ Seizures ▪ Coma ▪ Shallow respirations ▪ Hypotension
Barbiturate sedative-hypnotics ▪ amobarbital sodium (Amytal), also known as blue angels, blue devils, or blue birds ▪ phenobarbital (Luminal), also known as phennies, purple hearts, or goofballs ▪ secobarbital sodium (Seconal), also known as reds, red devils, or seccy	▪ Poor pupil reaction to light ▪ Nystagmus ▪ Depressed LOC (from confusion to coma) ▪ Flaccid muscles and absent reflexes ▪ Hyperthermia or hypothermia ▪ Cyanosis ▪ Respiratory depression ▪ Hypotension ▪ Blisters or bullous lesions

INTERVENTIONS

- Induce vomiting or perform gastric lavage; give activated charcoal and a cathartic, as ordered.
- Give supplemental oxygen to correct hypoxia-induced seizures.
- Replace fluids I.V., as ordered, to correct hypotension; monitor the patient's vital signs often.
- If the patient has severe toxicity, give physostigmine salicylate, as ordered, to reverse respiratory and CNS depression.

- Induce vomiting or perform gastric lavage if the patient ingested the drug within 4 hours; give activated charcoal and a saline cathartic, as ordered.
- Maintain his blood pressure with I.V. fluid challenges and vasopressors, as ordered.
- If the patient has taken a phenobarbital overdose, give sodium bicarbonate I.V., as ordered, to alkalinize his urine and to speed the drug's elimination.
- Apply a hyperthermia or hypothermia blanket, as ordered, to help return the patient's temperature to normal.
- Prepare the patient for hemodialysis or hemoperfusion if toxicity is severe.
- Perform frequent neurologic assessments, and check your patient's pulse rate, temperature, skin color, and reflexes often.
- Notify the doctor if you see signs of respiratory distress or pulmonary edema.
- Watch for signs and symptoms of withdrawal, such as hyperreflexia, tonic-clonic seizures, and hallucinations. Provide symptomatic relief of withdrawal symptoms, as ordered.
- Protect the patient from injuring himself.

(continued)

ALERT

Recognizing and treating acute substance abuse *(continued)*

SUBSTANCE	SIGNS AND SYMPTOMS
Cocaine ▪ cocaine hydro-chloride ▪ crack ▪ freebase	▪ Dilated pupils ▪ Confusion ▪ Alternating euphoria and apprehension ▪ Hyperexcitability ▪ Visual, auditory, and olfactory hallucinations ▪ Spasms and seizures ▪ Coma ▪ Tachypnea ▪ Hyperpnea ▪ Pallor or cyanosis ▪ Respiratory arrest ▪ Tachycardia ▪ Hypertension or hypotension ▪ Fever ▪ Nausea and vomiting ▪ Abdominal pain ▪ Perforated nasal septum or mouth sores
Glutethimide (Doriglute) Also known as cibas, CD, or blues	▪ Small, reactive pupils ▪ Nystagmus ▪ Drowsiness ▪ Irritability ▪ Impaired thought processes (memory, judgment, and attention span) ▪ Slurred speech ▪ Twitching, spasms, and seizures ▪ Hypothermia ▪ Apnea ▪ Respiratory depression ▪ Hypotension ▪ Paralytic ileus ▪ Poor bladder control

INTERVENTIONS

- Calm the patient down by talking to him in a quiet room.
- If cocaine was ingested, induce vomiting or perform gastric lavage; give activated charcoal followed by a saline cathartic, as ordered.
- Give the patient a tepid sponge bath, and administer an antipyretic, as ordered, to reduce fever.
- Monitor his blood pressure and heart rate. Expect to give propranolol for symptomatic tachycardia.
- Administer an anticonvulsant such as diazepam, as ordered, to control seizures.
- Scrape the inside of the patient's nose to remove residual amounts of the drug.
- Monitor his heart rate and rhythm; ventricular fibrillation and cardiac standstill can occur as a direct cardiotoxic result of cocaine ingestion. Defibrillate the patient, and initiate cardiopulmonary resuscitation, if indicated.

- If the drug was taken orally, induce vomiting or perform gastric lavage; give activated charcoal and a cathartic, as ordered.
- Maintain the patient's blood pressure with I.V. fluid challenges and vasopressors, as ordered.
- Assist with hemodialysis or hemoperfusion if the patient has hepatic or renal failure or is in a prolonged coma.
- Administer an anticonvulsant such as diazepam for seizures, as ordered.
- Perform hourly neurologic assessments: Coma may recur because of the drug's slow release from fat deposits.
- Be alert for signs of increased intracranial pressure, such as decreasing LOC and widening pulse pressure. Give mannitol I.V., as ordered.
- Watch for signs and symptoms of withdrawal, such as hyperreflexia, tonic-clonic seizures, and hallucinations, and provide symptomatic relief of withdrawal symptoms.
- Protect the patient from injuring himself.

(continued)

ALERT

Recognizing and treating acute substance abuse *(continued)*

SUBSTANCE	SIGNS AND SYMPTOMS
Hallucinogens ▪ Lysergic acid diethylamide (LSD), also known as hawk, acid, or sunshine ▪ mescaline (peyote), also known as mese, cactus, or big chief	▪ Dilated pupils ▪ Intensified perceptions ▪ Agitation and anxiety ▪ Synesthesia ▪ Impaired judgment ▪ Hyperactive movement ▪ Flashbacks ▪ Hallucinations ▪ Depersonalization ▪ Moderately increased blood pressure ▪ Increased heart rate ▪ Fever
Narcotics ▪ codeine ▪ heroin, also known as junk, smack, H, or snow ▪ hydromorphone hydrochloride (Dilaudid), also known as D or lords ▪ morphine, also known as mort, monkey, M, or Miss Emma	▪ Constricted pupils ▪ Depressed LOC (but patient is usually responsive to persistent verbal or tactile stimuli) ▪ Seizures ▪ Hypothermia ▪ Slow, deep respirations ▪ Hypotension ▪ Bradycardia ▪ Skin changes (pruritus, urticaria, and flushed skin)

INTERVENTIONS

- Reorient the patient repeatedly to time, place, and person.
- Restrain the patient to protect him from injuring himself and others.
- Calm the patient down by talking to him in a quiet room.
- If the drug was taken orally, induce vomiting or perform gastric lavage; give activated charcoal and a cathartic, as ordered.
- Give diazepam I.V., as ordered, to control seizures.

- Give naloxone as ordered until the drug's CNS depressant effects are reversed.
- Replace fluids I.V., as ordered, to increase circulatory volume.
- Correct hypothermia by applying extra blankets; if the patient's body temperature doesn't increase, use a hyperthermia blanket, as ordered.
- Reorient the patient often.
- Auscultate the lungs often for crackles, possibly indicating pulmonary edema. (Onset may be delayed.)
- Administer oxygen via nasal cannula, mask, or mechanical ventilation to correct hypoxemia from hypoventilation.
- Monitor cardiac rate and rhythm, being alert for atrial fibrillation. (This should resolve when hypoxemia is corrected.)
- Be alert for signs of withdrawal, such as piloerection (goose flesh), diaphoresis, and hyperactive bowel sounds.

(continued)

ALERT

Recognizing and treating acute substance abuse *(continued)*

SUBSTANCE	SIGNS AND SYMPTOMS
Phencyclidine (PCP) Also known as angel dust, peace pill, or hog	▪ Blank stare ▪ Nystagmus ▪ Amnesia ▪ Decreased awareness of surroundings ▪ Recurrent coma ▪ Violent behavior ▪ Hyperactivity ▪ Seizures ▪ Gait ataxia ▪ Muscle rigidity ▪ Drooling ▪ Hyperthermia ▪ Hypertensive crisis ▪ Cardiac arrest

INTERVENTIONS

- If the drug was taken orally, induce vomiting or perform gastric lavage; instill and remove activated charcoal repeatedly, as ordered.
- Acidify the patient's urine with ascorbic acid, as ordered, to increase drug excretion. Do so for 2 weeks because signs and symptoms may recur when fat cells release PCP stores.
- Give diazepam and haloperidol, as ordered, to control agitation or psychotic behavior.
- Administer diazepam, as ordered, to control seizures.
- Provide a quiet environment and dimmed light.
- As ordered, give propranolol for hypertension and tachycardia, nitroprusside for severe hypertension.
- Closely monitor urine output and serial renal function tests; rhabdomyolysis, myoglobinuria, and renal failure may occur in severe intoxication.
- If renal failure develops, prepare the patient for hemodialysis.

PART THREE

DRUG ADMINISTRATION TIPS AND TECHNIQUES

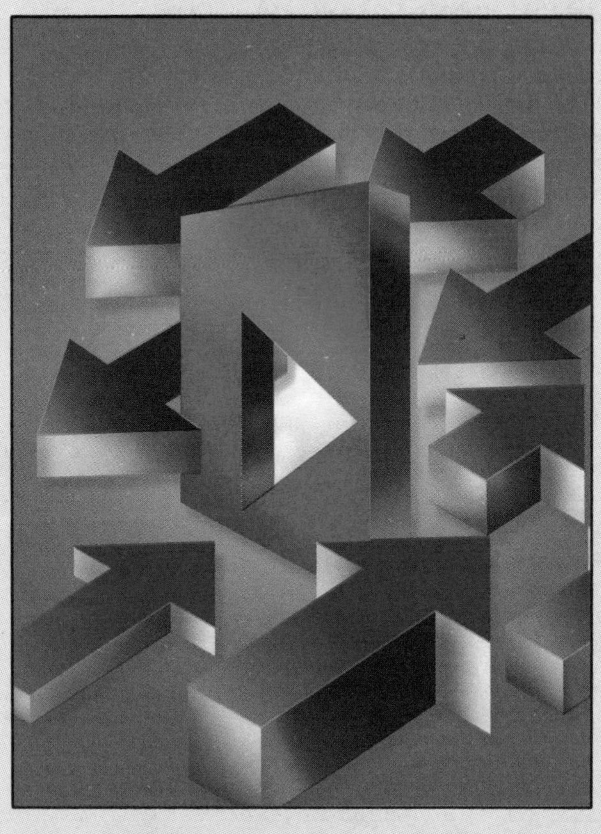

CHAPTER 11

GIVING ORAL DRUGS

TABLETS, CAPSULES, AND LIQUID MEDICATIONS

Giving tablets and capsules

To administer a drug orally, you'll need the patient's medication administration record; the ordered medication; a souffle cup or a plastic, graduated medicine cup; and gloves, if needed. Also obtain a glass of water or other liquid to help the patient swallow the medication. If you plan to crush a tablet, you'll need a mortar and pestle or pill-crushing device. To divide a scored tablet, you'll need a knife or scoring device and a paper towel.

- First, wash your hands. Then remove the unit-dose tablet or capsule from the patient's medication drawer, or select the prescribed bottle of tablets or capsules from the shelf. Open the container, and pour the required number of tablets or capsules into the container lid. If you pour too many, return the excess tablets and capsules to the container — without touching them.
- Next, place the correct number of tablets or capsules in the medicine cup.
- If you're using a unit-dose package, open the wrapper, and place the medication in the cup.
- If you're giving a chewable tablet, make sure that the patient chews it thoroughly before swallowing. Also, caution him not to chew other tablets, particularly coated ones.
- Next, check the patient's identification bracelet, and administer the medication.

Crushing tablets

- If you're using a mortar and pestle to crush a tablet, make sure that they're clean and that no remnants from a previously crushed tablet remain. Then place the tablet in the mortar, and crush it completely with the pestle. Place the crushed tablet into a medicine cup or directly into the fluid or food in which it will be mixed. Remove all drug particles from the mortar.

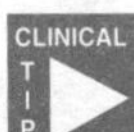

To save time, use the pestle to crush the tablet in its unopened wrapper. Be sure to remove all the medication before discarding the wrapper.

- If you're using a pill-crushing device, first place a souffle cup in the device, add the tablet, and place another souffle cup over the tablet. Then press the handle of the device to crush the tablet between the cups. Remove the top cup, and administer the medication.

Splitting tablets

- To split a scored tablet, use a paper towel to grasp both sides of the tablet. Then push down on the edges to break it. If the tablet is difficult to break or if it isn't scored, use the knife or scoring device to make a small slit in the center of the tablet.
- To use the scoring device, place the tablet in the device, and close the lid. Then place the correct dose in the medicine cup, and properly discard the unused portion. ■

Dispensing liquid medications

To give liquid medications, do the following:

- Take the bottle from the patient's medication drawer or shelf. If the medication is a suspension, shake it well. Then uncap the bottle, and place the cap upside down on a clean surface. Holding the graduated medicine cup at eye level, pour the medication into the cup up to the correct dose mark. Wipe the bottle lip with a damp paper towel, and replace the cap.
- Next, check the patient's identification bracelet, and administer the medication with whichever liquid or food you're using to help him swallow.

Giving liquid medication to an infant

- If you're giving a liquid medication to an infant, first put a bib under his chin. Then, hold him securely.
- With your free hand, withdraw the correct amount of medication from the bottle into the dropper by squeezing the bulb. Hold the dropper at eye level to check the amount. Squeeze any excess medication into a sink or waste receptacle; don't return it to the bottle.
- Hold the infant in the crook of your arm so that his head is elevated at a 45-degree angle. Gently instill the drops into his mouth. If the dropper isn't calibrated, hold it vertically over the infant's open mouth, and instill the prescribed number of drops.

  If you're using a calibrated dropper, instill the medication into the pocket between the infant's cheek and tongue. If the dropper touches the infant's mouth, wash the dropper thoroughly. Then return the dropper to the bottle and secure it. ■

Giving sublingual, buccal, and translingual drugs

When the doctor prescribes a drug in sublingual, buccal, or translingual form, he does so to prevent the drug's destruction or transformation in the stomach or small intestine. Sublingual, buccal, and translingual drugs act quickly because the oral mucosa's thin epithelium and abundant vasculature promote the drug's direct absorption into the bloodstream.

Drugs given sublingually include ergotamine tartrate, erythrityl tetranitrate, isoproterenol hydrochloride, isosorbide dinitrate, and nitroglycerin. A drug given buccally is erythrityl tetranitrate. Translingual drugs, which are sprayed onto the tongue, include nitrate preparations for patients with chronic angina. They may be administered prophylactically before stressful activities or at the onset of an attack.

Giving the medication
You'll need the patient's medication record, the ordered medication, and a medication cup. You'll also need gloves. To begin, match the drug order with the patient's medication administration record, and confirm the patient's identity. Do this by asking his name and checking his identification bracelet.

Before you give a sublingual or buccal drug, wash your hands, and put on gloves. Remove the tablet from the patient's medication drawer, and place it in the medication cup.

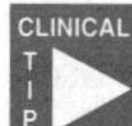

When you give a sublingual or buccal drug, observe your patient to ensure that he doesn't swallow the medication. Also, inspect his oral mucosa for irritation caused by continuous buccal administration. Remember to alternate placement sites and to administer sublingual or buccal tablets after you give all other oral drugs.

Sublingual administration
- To give a tablet sublingually, place it under the patient's tongue. Instruct the patient to leave it there until it dissolves completely and not to chew the tablet, drink water, or smoke for 1 hour (because nicotine's vasoconstrictive effects slow absorption).
- Sublingual drugs — erythrityl tetranitrate, for example — may cause a tingling sensation under the tongue. If the patient finds this bothersome, tell him that placing the drug in the buccal pouch instead may help.
- Tell the patient who's taking nitroglycerin tablets to wet the tablet with saliva before putting it in his mouth. This speeds absorption.

Buccal administration
- To administer a buccal medication, place the tablet between the patient's cheek and teeth. Instruct him to

close his mouth and hold the tablet against his cheek until it's absorbed.

- If your patient is taking buccal tablets that are absorbed slowly (some may take up to 1 hour), advise him not to eat or ingest liquids while the tablet is in the mouth. Otherwise, he might swallow the tablet.

Translingual administration

- Advise the patient who's using a translingual spray to familiarize himself with the position of the opening on the container. This opening can be identified by the finger rest on top of the container. Learning to handle the container is especially helpful when using the medication at night.
- To administer a translingual spray, tell the patient to hold the medication canister vertically, with the valve head uppermost and the spray opening as close to his mouth as possible. Instruct him to spray the dose onto the tongue by pressing the button firmly. ■

Are sugar-free cough preparations useful?

For some patients, such as those with diabetes, sugar-free cough preparations are desirable. Here's a list of brand names of sugar-free cough preparations. An asterisk indicates that the drug is available without a prescription.

- *Anamine HD syrup
- *Anatuss syrup (alcohol-free)
- Anatuss with Codeine syrup (alcohol-free)
- *Cerose-DM liquid
- Codiclear DH syrup (alcohol- and dye-free)
- *Codimal DM syrup
- *Dexafed Cough syrup (alcohol-free)
- Entus Tablets
- Entuss Expectorant liquid (alcohol-free)
- Entuss-D liquid (alcohol- and dye-free)
- Entuss-D tablets (dye-free)
- Kwelcof Liquid (alcohol- and dye-free)
- *Lanatuss Expectorant
- *Naldecon-DX Adult Liquid (alcohol-free)
- Naldecon-DX Pediatric Drops
- *Naldecon-EX Syrup
- *Naldecon Senior DX Liquid (alcohol-free)
- *Noratuss II Liquid (alcohol- and sodium-free)
- *Phanatuss syrup
- Ryna-C Liquid (alcohol- and dye-free)
- Ryna-CX Liquid (alcohol- and dye-free)
- *Scot-Tussin DM Liquid (alcohol-free)
- *Silexin Cough syrup (alcohol-free)
- Tolu-Sed Cough syrup
- *Tolu-Sed DM liquid

- *Tricodene liquid
- Trind liquid
- Tussar SF cough syrup
- Tussi-Organidin liquid
- Tussirex sugar-free (alcohol- and dye-free)
- Tussi-R-Gen DM liquid (alcohol-free)
- Tussi-R-Gen expectorant (alcohol-free) ■

How can I make tablets or capsules easier to swallow?

If a patient can't swallow a whole tablet or capsule, ask the pharmacist if the drug is available in liquid form or if it can be administered by another route. If not, ask him if you can crush the tablet or open the capsule and mix it with food. Keep in mind, however, that many enteric-coated or timed-release drugs and gelatin capsules should *not* be crushed. Remember to contact the doctor for an order to change the route of administration when necessary. ■

How can I make drugs more palatable?

Some drugs, especially those in liquid or powder form, have an unpleasant taste. To promote patient compliance, consider these tips:

- Mix the drug with fruit juice or cola syrup, if allowed. Have the patient sip the mixture through a straw.
- Use a syringe to instill the drug into the pocket between the patient's cheek and teeth.
- Suggest that the patient suck on ice chips just before taking the drug.
- Unless the patient is receiving a small amount of the drug, pour it over ice.
- Tell the patient to hold his nose while swallowing.
- Chill oily medications.
- Offer a piece of hard candy or chewing gum, or let the patient gargle or rinse his mouth after he swallows the drug, if allowed. ■

Which drugs shouldn't be crushed or dissolved?

When you're preparing solid drugs for administration, be careful not to crush or dissolve a drug if doing so can impair its effectiveness or absorption. Many drug forms (such as timed-release, enteric-coated, encapsulated beads, wax matrix, sublingual, buccal, and effervescent tablet preparations) are formulated to release their active ingredients for a specified duration or at a predetermined time after administration. Disrupting these formulations by crushing can dramatically affect the drug's absorption rate and increase the risk of side effects.

Other reasons not to crush a drug involve such considerations as taste, tissue irritation, and unusual formulation — for example, a capsule within a capsule, a liquid within a capsule, or a multiple, compressed tablet. Avoid crushing the drugs that are listed here by brand name, for the reasons noted beside them.

- Accutane (mucous membrane irritant)
- Acutrim 16 Hour (precision release)
- Aerolate Jr. (timed-release)
- Aerolate Sr. (timed-release)
- Aerolate III (timed-release)
- Allerest 12 Hour (extended-release)
- Artane Sequels (sustained-release)
- Atrohist Plus (sustained-release)
- Atrohist Sprinkle
- Azulfidine EN-Tabs (enteric-coated)
- Bayer Timed-Release Arthritic Pain Formula
- Betapen-VK (taste)
- Bisco-Lax (enteric-coated)
- Bontril Slow-Release
- Breonesin (liquid-filled)
- Brexin-L.A. (extended-release)
- Bromfed (extended-release)
- Bromfed-PD (slow-release)
- Calan SR (sustained-release)
- Cama Arthritis Pain Reliever (multiple compressed tablet)
- Carbiset-TR (timed-release)
- Cardizem
- Cardizem CD (sustained-release)
- Cardizem-SR (sustained-release)
- Carter's Little Pills (enteric-coated)
- Charcoal Plus (enteric-coated)
- chloral hydrate capsules (liquid within a capsule)
- Chlor-Trimeton Repetabs (timed-release)
- Choledyl SA (sustained-action)
- Cipro (taste)
- Codimal-L.A. (sustained-release)
- Colace (taste)
- Comhist LA (sustained-release)
- Compazine spansule (sustained-release)
- Congess JR (sustained-release)
- Congess SR (sustained-release)
- Contac (sustained-release)
- Cotazym-S (enteric-coated)
- Creon (enteric-coated)
- Dallergy (timed-release)
- Dallergy-Jr. (sustained-release)
- Deconamine SR (sustained-release)
- Deconsal Sprinkle (sustained-release)

- Deconsal II (sustained-release)
- Demazin Repetabs (timed-release)
- Depakene (mucous membrane irritant)
- Depakote (enteric-coated)
- Desoxyn Gradumet (long-acting)
- Desyrel (taste)
- Dexedrine Spansule (sustained-release)
- Diamox Sequels (sustained-release)
- Dilatrate-SR (sustained-release)
- Dimetane Extentabs (timed-release)
- Disobrom (sustained-release)
- Disophrol Chronotabs (sustained-release)
- Donnatal Extentabs (sustained-release)
- Donnazyme (enteric-coated)
- Drisdol (liquid-filled)
- Drixoral Allergy Sinus (sustained-release)
- Dulcolax (enteric-coated)
- Easprin (enteric-coated)
- Ecotrin (enteric-coated)
- E.E.S. (enteric-coated)
- Elixophyllin SR (sustained-release)
- E-Mycin (enteric-coated)
- Endafed (sustained-release)
- Entex LA (long-acting)
- Entozyme (enteric-coated)
- Equanil (taste)
- Ergostat (sublingual)
- ERYC (enteric-coated)
- Ery-Tab (enteric-coated)
- Erythrocin Stearate (enteric-coated)
- Erythromycin Base (enteric-coated)
- Eskalith CR (controlled-release)
- Feldene (mucous membrane irritant)
- Feocyte (prolonged-action)
- Feosol (enteric-coated)
- Feosol Spansule (sustained-release)
- Feratab (enteric-coated)
- Fero-Grad-500 Filmtabs (timed-release)
- Fero-Gradumet Filmtabs (timed-release)
- Ferralet S.R. (sustained-release)
- Feverall Sprinkle Caps (taste)
- Fumatinic (sustained-release)
- Geocillin (taste)
- Gris-PEG (crushing may cause precipitation as larger particles)
- Guaifed (timed-release)
- Guaifed-PD (timed-release)
- Humibid DM (sustained-release)
- Humibid DM Sprinkle (sustained-release)
- Humibid L.A. (sustained-release)
- Humibid Sprinkle (sustained-release)
- Hydergine (sublingual)
- Hydergine LC (liquid within a capsule)
- Hytakerol (liquid-filled)
- Iberet-500 Filmtabs (timed-release)

- Ilotycin (enteric-coated)
- Inderal LA (sustained-release)
- Indocin SR (sustained-release)
- Isoclor Timesules (sustained-release)
- Isoptin SR (sustained-release)
- Isordil (sublingual)
- Isordil Tembids (sustained-release)
- Isuprel Glossets (sublingual)
- Kaon-Cl (controlled-release)
- Klor-Con-10 (timed-release)
- Klotrix (controlled-release)
- K-Tab (controlled-release)
- K+10 (controlled-release)
- Levsinex Timecaps (timed-release)
- Meprospan (sustained-release)
- Mestinon Timespans (timed-release)
- Micro-K Extencaps (controlled-release)
- Motrin (taste)
- M S Contin (controlled-release)
- Naldecon (timed-release)
- Nico-400 (timed-release)
- Nicobid Tempules (timed-release)
- Nitro-Bid Plateau Caps (sustained-release)
- Nitrocine Timecaps (sustained-release)
- Nitroglyn (sustained-release)
- Nitrong (sublingual)
- Nitrostat (sublingual)
- Nolamine (sustained-release)
- Nolex LA (long-acting)
- Norflex (sustained-release)
- Norpace CR (controlled-release)
- Novafed (timed-release)
- Novafed A (sustained-release)
- Optilets-500 Filmtab (enteric-coated)
- Optilets-M-500 Filmtab (enteric-coated)
- Oramorph SR (sustained-release)
- Ornade Spansules (sustained-release)
- Pabalate (enteric-coated)
- Pancrease (enteric-coated)
- Pancrease MT (enteric-coated)
- Papaverine (timed-release)
- Pathilon (sustained-release)
- Pavabid Plateau Caps (sustained-release)
- PBZ-SR (sustained-release)
- Perdiem (wax-coated)
- Phenergan (taste)
- Phyllocontin (controlled-release)
- Plendil (extended-release)
- Polaramine (timed-release)
- Prelu-2 (sustained-release)
- Pro-Banthine (taste)
- Procan SR (sustained-release)
- Procardia (crushing delays absorption)
- Procardia XL (sustained-release)
- Pronestyl-SR (sustained-release)
- Proventil Repetabs (extended-release)

- Quadra Hist (sustained-release)
- Quibron-T/SR (sustained-release)
- Quinaglute Dura-tabs (sustained-release)
- Quinidex Extentabs (sustained-release)
- Respaire-60 SR (sustained-release)
- Respaire-120 SR (sustained-release)
- Respbid (timed-release)
- Ritalin-SR (sustained-release)
- Robimycin Robitab (enteric-coated)
- Rondec-TR (sustained-release)
- Roxanol SR (sustained-release)
- Ru-Tuss (timed-release)
- Ru-Tuss DE (timed-release)
- Sinemet CR (controlled-release)
- Slo-Bid Gyrocaps (timed-release)
- Slo-Niacin (timed-release)
- Slo-Phyllin Gyrocaps (timed-release)
- Slow Fe (slow-release)
- Slow K (controlled-release)
- Slow-Mag (sustained-release)
- Sorbitrate SA (extended-release)
- Sparine (taste)
- S-P-T (liquid gelatin suspension)
- Sudafed 12 Hour (extended-release)
- Sustaire (sustained-release)
- Tavist-D (multiple compressed tablet)
- Teldrin (timed-release)
- Tepanil Ten-Tab (sustained-release)
- Theobid Duracaps (timed-release)
- Theobid Jr. Duracaps (timed-release)
- Theochron (timed-release)
- Theoclear L.A. (timed-release)
- Theo-Dur (timed-release)
- Theo-Dur Sprinkle (timed-release)
- Theolair-SR (timed-release)
- Theo-Sav (timed-release)
- Theo-24 (timed-release)
- Theovent Long-Acting (timed-release)
- Theo-X (controlled-release)
- Therapy Bayer (enteric-coated)
- Thorazine Spansule (extended-release)
- Toprol-XL (extended-release)
- T-Phyl (timed-release)
- Trental (controlled-release)
- Triaminic TR (multiple compressed tablet)
- Triaminic-12 (extended-release)
- Triptone Caplets (long-acting)
- Tuss-LA (sustained-release)
- Tuss-Ornade Spansules (timed-release)
- Uniphyl (timed-release)
- ULR-LA (long-acting)
- Valrelease (extended-release)
- Verelan (extended-release)

- Wellbutrin (anesthetizes mucous membranes)
- Wygesic (taste)
- ZORprin (extended-release)
- Zymase (enteric-coated) ■

What should I teach about analgesics?

Three frequently prescribed analgesics include acetaminophen with codeine, propoxyphene napsylate and acetaminophen, and ibuprofen. Although they all relieve mild-to-moderate pain, they differ in mechanism of action, duration of action, and side effects. The choice depends on the cause of the pain and the patient's ability to tolerate side effects.

Acetaminophen with codeine and propoxyphene napsylate and acetaminophen

These two narcotic and nonnarcotic combination drugs are similar in action, analgesic potency, and side effects. Codeine and propoxyphene napsylate are narcotic analgesics that act through the CNS. Acetaminophen (an ingredient common to both combination drugs) is a nonnarcotic analgesic that relieves mild pain and reduces fever. Unlike aspirin or ibuprofen, acetaminophen doesn't have anti-inflammatory activity, so it's not as effective for relieving arthritic pain.

Side effects

Dizziness and sedation are the most common side effects of both these combination drugs.

Patient instructions

- Warn the patient to use caution when driving or performing other tasks that require alertness.
- Tell the patient not to take a higher dosage than the doctor prescribes; doing so could cause severe side effects, including respiratory depression.
- Instruct the patient to avoid drinking alcohol while taking any narcotic analgesic: This combination may cause severe sedation and respiratory depression.

Ibuprofen

Besides relieving pain, this NSAID reduces fever and inflammation. Because of its anti-inflammatory action, it's often prescribed for arthritic pain. It's available by prescription in 300-, 400-, 600-, and 800-mg tablets and in liquid form (100 mg/5 ml); or in nonprescription 200-mg tablets. The schedule for ibuprofen is 4 to 6 hours unlike most oral analgesics, which typically have a schedule of 3 to 4 hours.

Side effects
Possible effects include nausea, epigastric pain, heartburn, rash, and dizziness. Serious GI bleeding can occur with long-term use.

Patient instructions
▪ Tell the patient to take ibuprofen with food or milk to minimize GI upset.
▪ Teach the patient signs and symptoms of GI bleeding; if any occur, he should report them to his doctor immediately. He should also report weight gain, rash, and unusual bleeding or bruising.
▪ Warn the patient to avoid drinking alcohol while taking ibuprofen; alcohol may increase the risk of GI toxicity. ■

What should I teach about antibiotics?

Seven of the 25 most commonly prescribed drugs are antibiotics and, while no two are exactly alike, they're all used to prevent or treat infections caused by susceptible bacteria. When any antibiotic is prescribed for a patient, be sure to tell him to take it exactly as prescribed, or it may not be effective. For example, he shouldn't skip doses or discontinue the drug until it's all gone. If he thinks the drug isn't working or if he feels worse, he should contact his doctor.

Amoxicillin and amoxicillin/clavulanate
Amoxicillin is prescribed for systemic infections or for acute or chronic urinary tract infections (UTIs). A member of the penicillin family, amoxicillin is effective against many gram-positive and gram-negative bacteria. Amoxicillin has the same bactericidal activity as ampicillin, an antibiotic often administered I.V. for systemic infections. Patients who were receiving I.V. ampicillin in the hospital may go home with oral amoxicillin.

Amoxicillin/clavulanate is a combination drug that contains the bactericidal antibiotic amoxicillin and an enzyme inhibitor, clavulanate potassium. The addition of clavulanate makes the drug effective against beta-lactamase producing bacteria, which can resist amoxicillin alone. It's used to treat lower respiratory infections, otitis media, sinusitis, skin infections, systemic infections, and UTIs.

Side effects
Common to amoxicillin and amoxicillin/clavulanate, side effects include nausea, diarrhea, vomiting, and hypersensitivity reactions, such as rash, and urticaria. Avoid ad-

ministration of amoxicillin to the patient who's allergic to penicillin because anaphylaxis can occur.

Patient instructions

- Advise the patient to take the drug with food to prevent GI distress.
- Tell the patient to stop taking the drug and to notify his doctor immediately if he develops a rash or has difficulty breathing.
- Instruct the patient to report the signs and symptoms of superinfection, such as coated tongue, vaginal or rectal itching, and diarrhea.

Cephalexin and cefaclor

These two cephalosporins are used to treat otitis media and infections of the respiratory tract, urinary tract, skin, and soft tissues. Cephalexin also treats bone and joint infections.

Cephalexin is similar to cephalothin and cefazolin, which are administered by injection or infusion. Patients receiving those drugs in the hospital may be prescribed oral cephalexin at discharge. Likewise, oral cefaclor may replace cefoxitin and cefotetan, which are administered by injection. Cephalexin and cefaclor are usually well tolerated.

Side effects

The most common complaint is diarrhea. Other side effects include nausea, dizziness, headache, and anorexia. Because these drugs are chemically related to penicillin, sensitivity reactions can occur in patients who are sensitive to penicillin. If your patient wasn't being treated with a cephalosporin in the hospital, be sure to ask him if he's ever had a reaction to penicillin. If so, notify the doctor, who may prescribe another antibiotic.

Patient instructions

- Tell the patient to take the drug with food or milk to prevent GI upset.
- Warn the patient to discontinue the drug and to notify his doctor immediately if he develops a rash or has difficulty breathing.
- Instruct the patient to report signs and symptoms of superinfection (coated tongue, vaginal or rectal itching, or diarrhea).

Ciprofloxacin

This oral, broad-spectrum fluoroquinolone antibiotic may be prescribed to treat infections that usually require I.V. therapy in the hospital, such as infectious diarrhea and infections of the lower respiratory tract, urinary tract, skin, and bone.

Side effects

Ciprofloxacin is generally well tolerated, but side effects may include nausea, diarrhea, vomiting, abdominal pain, headache, rash, lightheadedness, crystalluria, and photosensitivity reactions.

Patient instructions

- Warn the patient to use caution when driving or performing other tasks that require alertness.
- Inform the patient that he may take the drug with or without food but to drink a glass of water with each dose (to reduce the risk of crystalluria).
- Advise the patient to use a sunscreen if he plans to be in the sun for extended periods.
- Instruct the patient not to take antacids containing magnesium or aluminum within 2 hours of taking ciprofloxacin — these antacids could inhibit ciprofloxacin's absorption.

Erythromycin

A macrolide antibiotic, erythromycin may be used to treat mild to moderately severe respiratory tract infections, acute pelvic inflammatory disease, Legionnaires' disease, intestinal dysenteric amebiasis, and skin infections. It's often prescribed for patients who are hypersensitive to penicillin or tetracycline.

Side effects

Such effects may include abdominal pain, cramping, rash, nausea, vomiting, and diarrhea.

Patient instructions

- Tell the patient to take each dose with food or milk to minimize GI upset.
- Instruct the patient to stop taking the drug and to notify his doctor immediately if he develops signs of a hypersensitivity reaction, such as a rash.

Trimethoprim and sulfamethoxazole

This antibiotic is prescribed for UTIs, shigellosis, *Pneumocystis carinii* pneumonia, chronic bronchitis, and otitis media. A combination drug, it contains sulfamethoxazole (a sulfonamide antibiotic) and trimethoprim (a urinary anti-infective).

Side effects

Possible reactions include nausea, vomiting, anorexia, diarrhea, rash, urticaria, and crystalluria. Severe reactions, which rarely occur, may include Stevens-Johnson syndrome, generalized skin eruption, epidermal necrosis, anaphylaxis, agranulocytosis, and aplastic anemia.

Patient instructions

- Instruct the patient to stop taking the drug and to notify his doctor immediately if he develops a rash, sore throat, fever, or mouth sores.

- Advise the patient to use a sunscreen when he's outdoors; some patients have photosensitivity reactions.
- Instruct the patient to drink a glass of water with each dose to minimize the risk of crystalluria. ■

What should I teach about anticonvulsants?

Phenytoin

This hydantoin anticonvulsant may be prescribed to control generalized motor and complex partial (psychomotor or temporal lobe) seizures. It's also used to prevent and treat seizures that occur after neurosurgery. Phenytoin is available in extended-release and immediate-release forms.

Side effects

Particularly in patients who take phenytoin for a long period, side effects frequently occur. Possible effects include ataxia, slurred speech, confusion, nystagmus, dizziness, insomnia, changes in vision, transient nervousness, motor twitching, headaches, nausea, and gingival hyperplasia. Many side effects are dose-related and may be relieved by reducing the dosage.

Patient instructions

- Instruct the patient to report any side effects; his doctor may want to adjust the drug dosage.
- Warn the patient not to stop taking the drug unless instructed to do so; abrupt withdrawal may cause seizures.
- Teach the patient to take the drug with food to reduce GI upset and to enhance absorption.
- Encourage the patient to brush and floss his teeth often. Good oral hygiene and gum massage can help to prevent gingival changes. Tell him to schedule regular appointments with his dentist and to tell his dentist he's taking phenytoin.
- Warn the patient not to drink alcohol with this drug. Heavy drinking may increase phenytoin's toxic effects.
- Tell the patient to consult his doctor or pharmacist before taking nonprescription drugs because many of them interact with phenytoin.
- Instruct the patient to make sure his pharmacist refills his prescription with the same brand each time. Different brands may exert slightly different therapeutic effects; a change could precipitate a seizure or increase the risk of side effects.
- Warn the patient not to drive or perform other tasks that require alertness and co-

ordination until he adjusts to this drug. ■

What should I teach about benzodiazepines?

Alprazolam and triazolam

These two short-acting benzodiazepines, which are chemically similar, act on the CNS. However, alprazolam is classified as an antianxiety drug and triazolam as a hypnotic.

Alprazolam relieves symptoms of anxiety caused by depression or anxiety disorders. It's usually prescribed for short-term use because, over time (more than 4 months), it may cause physical or psychological dependence.

Triazolam, which is prescribed for insomnia, induces sleep and prevents nocturnal and early morning awakenings. It's also usually prescribed for short-term use.

Side effects

For both drugs, side effects include daytime sleepiness, drowsiness, dizziness, lightheadedness, headache, and anterograde amnesia.

Patient instructions

- Warn the patient to use caution when driving or performing other tasks that require alertness.
- Advise the patient not to increase his dosage without consulting his doctor, even if he thinks the drug isn't working. Drug ineffectiveness after weeks of therapy may indicate drug tolerance.
- Tell the patient not to stop the drug abruptly, particularly if he takes it routinely, because withdrawal symptoms, such as rebound insomnia, may occur.
- Warn the patient not to drink alcohol while taking a benzodiazepine. The interaction may cause serious side effects, such as excessive CNS depression and rebound anxiety.
- Instruct the patient to check with his doctor or pharmacist before taking nonprescription drugs because some of them, such as antihistamines, may interact with benzodiazepines and cause increased sedation.
- Advise elderly patients to change body positions slowly to avoid ataxia.
- Tell a woman to notify her doctor immediately if she suspects she's pregnant. ■

What should I teach about bronchodilators?

Theophylline

This drug, a xanthine bronchodilator, relaxes bronchial smooth muscle. It's indicated to relieve or prevent asthma symptoms and reversible bronchospasm associated with chronic bronchitis and emphysema. Many dosage forms are available: immediate-release capsules, tablets, and liquids; extended-release capsules and tablets; and extended-release sprinkles.

Side effects
Common side effects include nausea, vomiting, diarrhea, dizziness, insomnia, and headache. However, these are usually dose-related and subside when the dosage is reduced. High doses may produce more serious problems, such as seizures and cardiac arrhythmias.

Patient instructions
- Teach the patient to take theophylline with food to minimize GI upset.
- Advise the patient to consume foods or beverages containing caffeine, such as coffee, tea, chocolate, and some soft drinks, in moderation; large amounts of caffeine may increase theophylline's side effects.
- Tell the patient who takes an extended-release tablet not to chew, crush, or dissolve it. He should swallow it whole to ensure its sustained action.
- Instruct a patient who takes the sprinkle form to open the capsule and spread the beads on a spoonful of soft food, such as applesauce or pudding. He should swallow the food without chewing the beads, then drink a glass of water or juice to make sure he's consumed all of the drug.
- Remind the patient to notify his doctor if he changes his smoking habits; smoking speeds the metabolism of theophylline, and his dosage may need to be changed. ■

What should I teach about cardiovascular drugs?

Atenolol and metoprolol
$Beta_1$-adrenergic blockers, atenolol and metoprolol are used to manage angina pectoris or hypertension. They may be prescribed alone or with other antihypertensives, such as a loop diuretic.

Side effects
These drugs are generally well tolerated, although some patients experience bradycardia, hypotension, vertigo, fatigue, nausea, and diarrhea.

Patient instructions
- Warn the patient against stopping the drug or skipping doses; abrupt withdrawal may precipitate or exacerbate angina.
- Advise the patient to consult his doctor or pharmacist

before taking nonprescription drugs. Some products, such as decongestants and diet aids, contain alpha-adrenergic stimulants, which may increase blood pressure.

Captopril and enalapril

These ACE inhibitors are often combined with thiazide and loop diuretics to treat hypertension. They may also be prescribed as adjunct therapy with digoxin and a diuretic for treating CHF.

Side effects

For both drugs, side effects include angioedema, agranulocytosis, hypotension, proteinuria, renal failure, tachycardia, palpitations, rash, cough, and dizziness. Side effects specific to enalapril include headache and fatigue; loss of taste is specific to captopril.

Patient instructions

- Warn the patient to stop taking the drug and to notify his doctor immediately if he experiences symptoms of angioedema, including breathing difficulty and swelling of the face, eyes, lips, or tongue.
- Emphasize the importance of taking the drug as prescribed because hypertension is often asymptomatic.
- Instruct the patient to consult his doctor or pharmacist before taking nonprescription drugs. Many of them, such as diet aids and allergy and cold products, contain sympathomimetics that may increase blood pressure.
- Tell the patient who takes captopril to consult his doctor before taking aspirin or ibuprofen, which may decrease captopril's antihypertensive effect.

Digoxin

This digitalis glycoside is prescribed for CHF, atrial fibrillation and flutter, and paroxysmal atrial tachycardia. It has a narrow therapeutic range, so the therapeutic serum level is close to the toxic serum level.

Side effects

These may be severe and include visual disturbances (such as yellow halos around images), headache, anorexia, nausea, vomiting, muscle weakness, fatigue, hallucinations, and agitation.

Patient instructions

- Tell your patient to notify his doctor immediately if he experiences any of the side effects mentioned above. They may accompany other serious symptoms that the patient may not notice.
- Warn him that digoxin may interact with other drugs, so he shouldn't take nonprescription medications without notifying his doctor or pharmacist.
- Tell your patient to make sure his pharmacist refills his

prescription with the same brand of digoxin. Absorption can vary from brand to brand, so a change could alter the therapeutic effect.

Diltiazem, nifedipine, and verapamil

The immediate-release dosage forms of these three calcium channel blockers are used to treat vasospastic (Prinzmetal's or variant) angina or chronic stable angina pectoris and to control the ventricular rate in supraventricular tachycardia. Extended-release forms are prescribed for hypertension.

Side effects

All three drugs may cause headache, dizziness, peripheral edema, CHF, pulmonary edema, dyspnea, rash, nausea, and constipation.

Patient instructions

- Tell the patient to take his drug with food to minimize GI upset.
- Instruct the patient not to chew an extended-release tablet or capsule. Chewing may destroy its sustained action.
- Warn the patient to rise from a lying or sitting position slowly to prevent orthostatic hypotension.
- Inform the patient that headaches are common during the first week or two of therapy, but they usually subside. If they continue or are severe, instruct him to notify his doctor.

Furosemide

A loop diuretic, furosemide is used to treat hypertension and edema associated with CHF, hepatic cirrhosis, or renal disease.

Side effects

Possible side effects include fluid and electrolyte imbalances (hypokalemia and dehydration), orthostatic hypotension, GI irritation, and glycosuria.

Patient instructions

- Teach the patient to take furosemide in the morning to reduce nocturnal urination and to take it with food to decrease GI upset.
- Recommend that the patient drink a glass of orange juice or eat a banana every day if he's not taking a potassium supplement.
- Tell the patient to rise slowly from a lying or sitting position to prevent orthostatic hypotension.
- Warn diabetic patients that furosemide may increase serum glucose levels. Tell them to report elevated blood or urine glucose test results to their doctors. ■

What should I teach about antiulcer drugs?

Cimetidine and ranitidine

These two H_2-receptor antagonists may be used to treat a benign gastric ulcer or an active duodenal ulcer. They're also prescribed for hypersecretion associated with Zollinger-Ellison syndrome and other pathologic hypersecretory conditions. Ranitidine is the only H_2-receptor antagonist approved to treat gastroesophageal reflux disease.

Side effects

Both drugs can cause similar side effects: headache, fatigue, dizziness, confusion, diarrhea, and mild gynecomastia (when used longer than 1 month).

Patient instructions

- Tell the patient to report severe headaches to his doctor, who may want to change the dosing schedule or medication.
- Warn the patient not to skip doses, even if he feels better; doing so may worsen his condition.
- If the patient is also taking an antacid (such as Maalox), tell him to take it 1 hour before or after ranitidine or cimetidine; antacids may reduce absorption of both drugs.
- If the patient smokes, explain that cigarette smoke hinders ulcer healing, and encourage him to quit.

Sucralfate

This cytoprotective drug, which forms a protective barrier over ulcerated tissue, is prescribed to treat duodenal ulcers. Therapy usually lasts 4 to 8 weeks.

Side effects

Most patients tolerate sucralfate well. Constipation is the most common side effect; other possible problems include GI discomfort, nausea, diarrhea, dizziness, and sleepiness.

Patient instructions

- Teach the patient to take sucralfate on an empty stomach.
- If the patient is taking an antacid concurrently, tell him to allow at least 1 hour between doses. The antacid could hinder sucralfate's absorption.
- If the patient is taking other drugs concurrently, instruct him to take them at least 2 hours before or after taking sucralfate. Sucralfate interferes with the absorption of some drugs.
- Warn the patient to take sucralfate exactly as ordered. Stopping it early or skipping doses may prevent the ulcer from healing completely. ■

CHAPTER 12

APPLYING TOPICAL DRUGS

EYE, EAR, AND NASAL ADMINISTRATION

Administering eyedrops or ointments

Ophthalmic drops or ointments are for diagnostic or therapeutic use. An eye patch enhances an ophthalmic drug's effects and protects ocular tissues. You'll give eyedrops to anesthetize the eye, dilate the pupil, or stain the cornea (to detect abrasions or scars) during an eye examination. You'll also give eyedrops to lubricate the eye or its socket, protect the vision of a newborn, and treat certain eye disorders — by giving pilocarpine for glaucoma, for example.

Getting ready

- Gather the equipment you'll need, including the patient's medication administration record (MAR) and chart, the prescribed eye medication, sterile cotton balls, gloves, warm water or normal saline solution, sterile gauze pads, facial tissue and, if necessary, an eye dressing.
- Then read the drug label to make sure that the medication is for ophthalmic use.
- If you're instilling an eyedrop solution, check the expiration date and inspect for cloudiness, discoloration, and precipitates. If the solution appears abnormal in any way, don't use it.
- If you're administering an ointment and the tip of the tube is crusty, wipe it with a sterile gauze pad to remove the crust. Also be sure to check the expiration date.

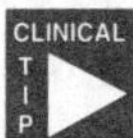

Keep in mind that some ophthalmic drugs are in suspension form and normally appear cloudy.

- Verify the order on the patient's MAR by checking it against the doctor's order on the patient's chart. Also check the medication label against the MAR. Make sure that you know which eye to treat because different medications or dosages may be ordered for each eye. Confirm the patient's identity by asking his name and checking the name, room number, and bed number on his identification bracelet.
- Explain the procedure to the patient, and provide privacy.
- Wash your hands, and put on gloves.
- If the patient has an eye dressing, remove it by gently pulling it down and away from his forehead.
- Remove any discharge by cleaning around the eye with sterile cotton balls or sterile gauze pads moistened with warm water or normal saline

solution. Clean from the inner canthus to the outer canthus, using a fresh sterile cotton ball or sterile gauze pad for each stroke.

- To remove crusted secretions around the eye, moisten a gauze pad with warm water or normal saline solution. Have the patient close his eye. Then place the moist pad over it for 1 or 2 minutes. Remove the pad, and reapply new, moist sterile gauze pads, as needed, until the secretions soften enough to be removed without injuring the mucosa.
- Have the patient tilt his head back and toward the side of the affected eye. This lets excess medication flow away from the tear duct, thus minimizing systemic absorption.
- Unless the bottle cap and eyedropper are a closed unit, remove the cap from the medication bottle, and draw the medication into the dropper, taking care not to contaminate it.

Instilling eyedrops

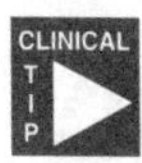

Before instilling eyedrops, ask the patient to look up and away. This moves the cornea away from the lower eyelid and minimizes the risk of touching the cornea with the dropper if the patient blinks.

- Steady the hand holding the medication bottle against the patient's forehead. Use your other hand to gently pull down the lower eyelid, and instill the drops in the conjunctival sac (as shown),

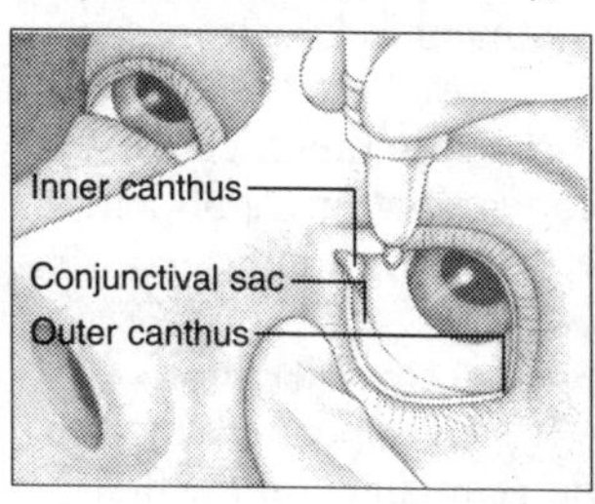

not directly onto the eyeball. Release the patient's eyelid, and have him blink to distribute the medication.

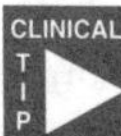

Because elderly patients may have difficulty sensing drops in the eye, suggest chilling the medication when instilling drops at home. The cold drops should enhance placement sensation.

Instilling eye ointment

- Squeeze a small ribbon of ointment on the edge of the conjunctival sac from the inner to the outer canthus (as shown). Avoid touching the

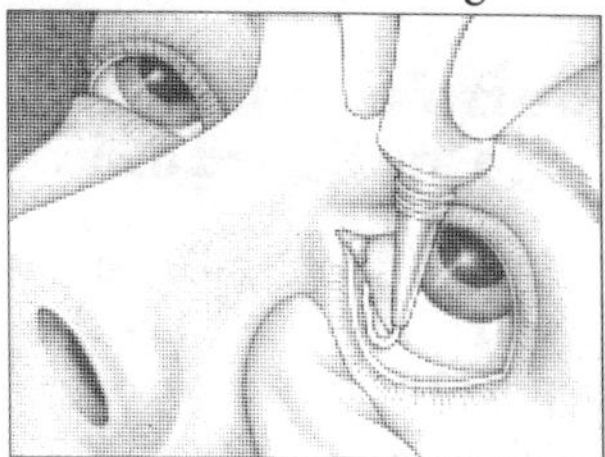

tube to the patient's eye. Cut off the ribbon by turning the tube. Then release the eyelid,

APPLYING TOPICAL DRUGS

and have the patient roll her eyes behind closed lids to distribute the medication.

- Use a clean tissue to remove any excess solution or ointment leaking from the eye. Use a fresh tissue for each eye to prevent cross-contamination. Apply a new eye dressing if indicated.

Special considerations

- If you're opening a medication container for the first time, write the date on the label because an opened container should be used within 2 weeks to avoid contamination.
- To prevent contamination, never use the same medication container for more than one patient.
- Keep in mind that certain drugs may cause eye disorders or other serious reactions. For example, anticholinergics, which are commonly used during eye examinations, may precipitate acute glaucoma in a predisposed patient. ■

Inserting and removing a medicated disk

Small and flexible, an oval, medicated eye disk consists of three layers: two soft outer layers and a middle layer that contains the medication. Floating between the eyelid and the sclera, the disk stays in the eye while the patient sleeps and even swims or plays sports. Once the disk is in place, eye fluid moistens it, releasing the medication for up to 1 week. Keep in mind that this device shouldn't be used if the patient has conjunctivitis, keratitis, a detached retina, or any condition in which pupillary constriction should be avoided.

Getting ready

- Explain to the patient possible side effects, such as a foreign-body sensation in the eye, mild tearing or redness, increased mucus discharge, eyelid redness and itching and, possibly, blurred vision, headaches, stinging, and swelling. Reassure him that mild side effects should subside within the first 6 weeks of therapy.
- Plan to insert the disk before the patient goes to bed. This minimizes the blurring that usually occurs immediately after disk insertion.

Inserting the disk

- Begin by gathering the medicated disk, a cotton-tipped applicator, and gloves.
- Wash your hands, and put on gloves.
- Press your fingertip against the oval disk so that it lies across your fingertip. It should stick to your finger. Lift the disk out of its packet.

▪ Gently pull the patient's lower eyelid away from the eye, and place the disk in the conjunctival sac, as shown. It should lie horizontally, not vertically.

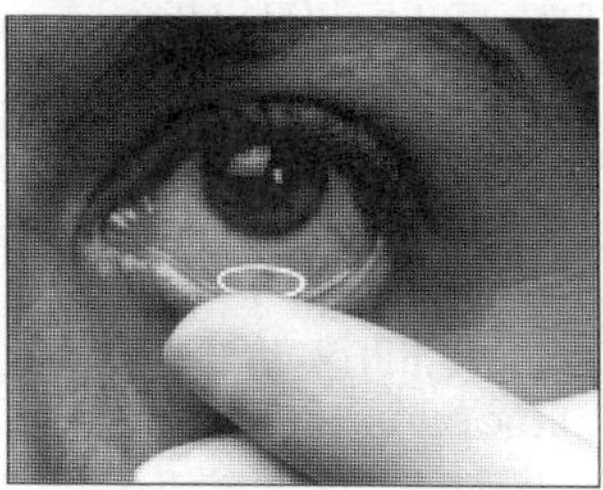

▪ Pull the lower eyelid out, up, and over the disk. Tell the patient to blink several times. If the disk is still visible, pull the lower eyelid out and over the disk again.

▪ Tell the patient that once the disk is in place, he can adjust its position by gently pressing his finger against his closed eyelid.

▪ If the disk falls out, wash your hands, put on gloves, rinse the disk in cool water, and reinsert it. If the disk appears bent, replace it. If it repeatedly slips out of position, reinsert it in the upper eyelid, using a cotton-tipped applicator to gently lift and evert the eyelid (as shown).

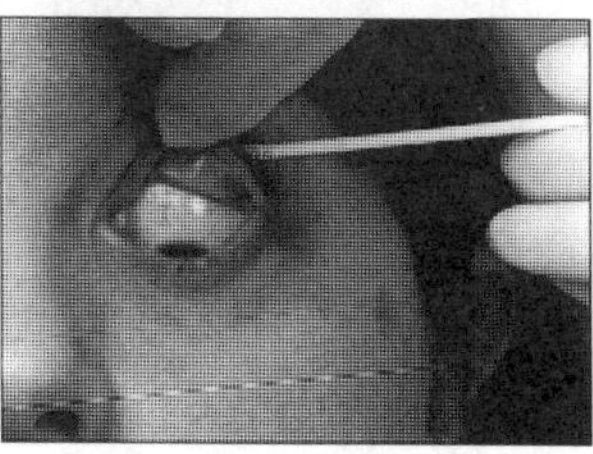

▪ If both of the patient's eyes are being treated with medication disks, replace both disks at the same time so that both eyes receive medication at the same rate.

Removing the disk

▪ To remove a disk using one finger, put on gloves, and evert the lower eyelid to expose the disk. Then use the forefinger of your other hand to slide the disk onto the eyelid and out of the patient's eye.

▪ To remove a disk using two fingers, evert the lower lid with one hand to expose the disk. Then pinch the disk with the thumb and forefinger of your other hand, and remove it from the eye.

Special considerations

▪ If the patient will continue therapy with an eye medication disk after discharge, teach him how to insert and remove it himself. To check his mastery of these skills, have him demonstrate insertion and removal techniques for you.

▪ Explain that mild reactions are common but should subside within the first 6 weeks of use. Foreign-body sensation in the eye, mild tearing or redness, increased mucus discharge, eyelid redness, and itching can occur. Blurred vision, stinging, swelling, and headaches can occur with pilocarpine specifically. Tell the patient to report persistent or severe symptoms.

Administering otic drugs

Otic drugs may be instilled to treat infections and inflammation, to soften cerumen for later removal, to produce local anesthesia, or to ease removal of a foreign object trapped in the ear.

Getting ready

- Gather the prescribed eardrops, the patient's medication administration record (MAR), a penlight, facial tissues (or cotton-tipped applicators), cotton balls, and an emesis basin for warm water.
- Verify the order on the patient's MAR by checking it against the doctor's order. Then check the medication label against the patient's MAR.
- To avoid side effects (such as vertigo, nausea, and pain) from instilling eardrops that are too cold, warm the medication to body temperature by submerging it in a basin of warm water. To avoid burning the patient's eardrum, don't overwarm the medication. If necessary, test its temperature by placing a drop on your wrist.

Instilling eardrops

- First wash your hands. Confirm the patient's identity by asking his name and checking the name, room number, and bed number on his identification bracelet.
- Explain the procedure. Then have the patient lie on his side so that his affected ear faces upward.
- Straighten the ear canal. For an adult, pull the auricle of the ear up and back.

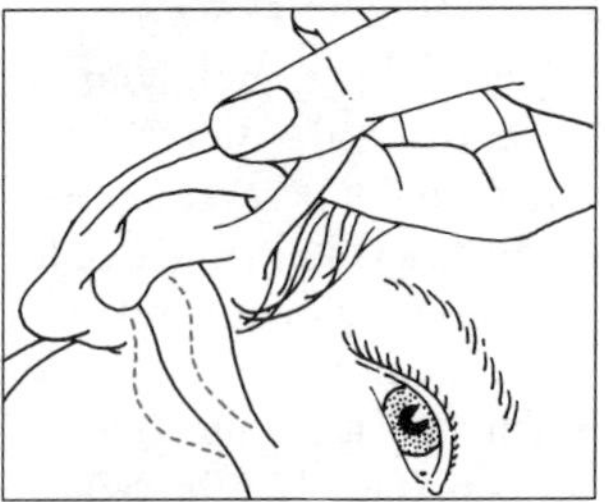

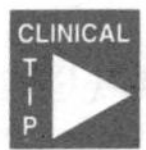

For an infant or a child under age 3, gently pull the auricle down and back because the ear canal in infants and toddlers is positioned differently.

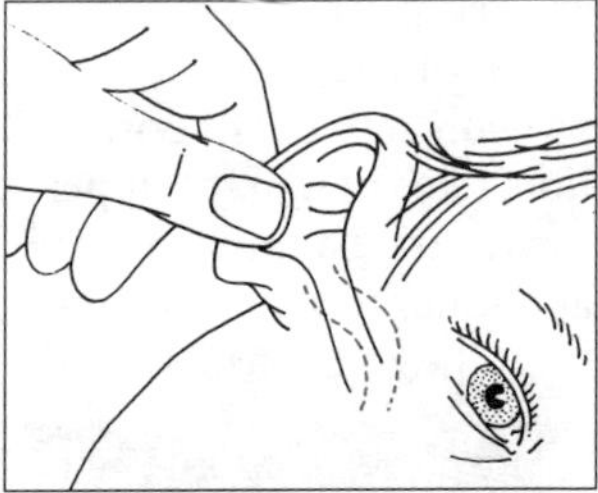

- Using the penlight, examine the ear canal for drainage, which can reduce the drug's effectiveness. If you find any, clean the canal with a cotton-tipped applicator.

- Straighten the patient's ear canal again, and instill the ordered number of drops. To avoid patient discomfort, aim the dropper so that the drops fall against the sides of the ear canal, not onto the eardrum. Hold the ear canal in position until you see the drug disappear. Then release the ear.
- Instruct the patient to remain on his side for 5 to 10 minutes to allow the drug to travel down the ear canal. If ordered, tuck a cotton ball loosely into the opening of the ear canal to contain the drug. Avoid inserting it too deeply because this would prevent secretions from draining and increase pressure on the eardrum.
- Then clean and dry the outer ear. Assist the patient into a comfortable position, and wash your hands.

Special considerations

- You probably wouldn't instill otic drugs in a patient with a perforated eardrum (although it may be permitted for some drugs and if sterile technique is used).
- Certain otic drugs may also be prohibited in other conditions because they may enhance the infectious organism's growth. For instance, medications that contain hydrocortisone shouldn't be prescribed for patients with herpes, another viral infection, or a fungal infection.
- Some conditions make the normally sensitive ear canal quite tender, so be especially gentle when instilling otic drugs.
- Also take special care not to injure the eardrum. Never insert an object, such as a cotton-tipped applicator, into the ear canal past the point where you can see the tip.
- If the patient has vertigo, keep the bed rails up, and assist him as necessary. Also, advise him to move about slowly to avoid increasing his vertigo.
- If necessary, teach the patient to instill the eardrops correctly so that he can continue treatment at home. Review the procedure, and let the patient try it himself while you observe. ■

Giving nasal drugs to an adult

Generally, nasal drugs produce local effects. Use drops to medicate a specific nasal area and sprays and aerosols to diffuse medication in the nasal passages.

The most commonly administered nasal drugs are vasoconstrictors, which coat and shrink swollen mucous membranes. Other nasal drugs include local anesthetics, which promote patient

Positioning the patient for nose drops

To ensure the maximum benefit of nasal medication, be sure to position the patient so that the drops don't flow into the pharynx.

Treating nasal congestion

- To relieve an ordinary stuffy nose, apply drops to the nasal mucosa.
- Help the patient into a reclining or supine position with his head slightly tilted toward the affected side.
- Aim the dropper upward toward the patient's eye, rather than downward toward his ear.

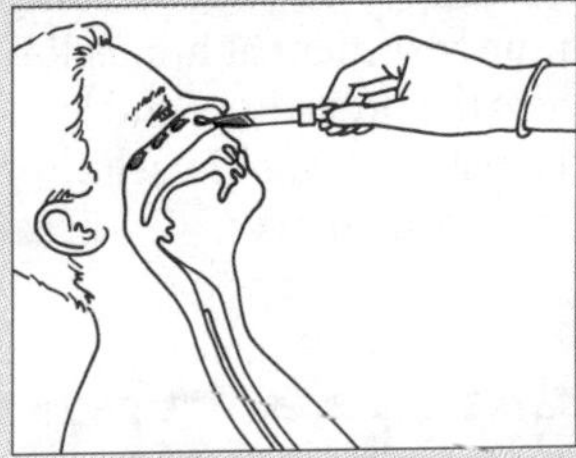

Treating the sinuses

- To treat the ethmoid and sphenoid sinuses, position the patient on his back with his neck hyperextended and his head tilted back over the edge of the bed. Support his head with one hand to prevent neck strain, as shown.

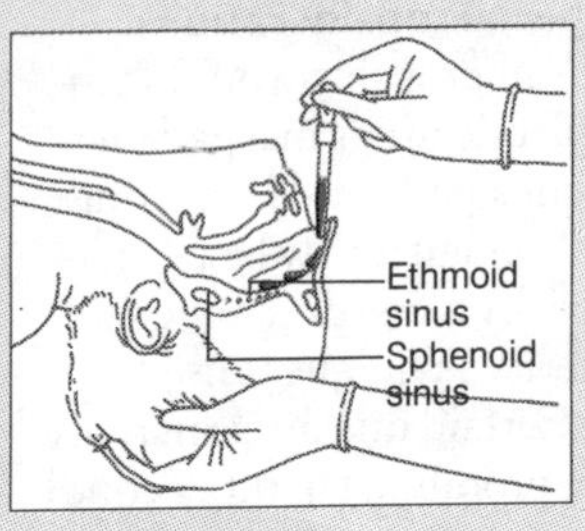

- To treat the maxillary and frontal sinuses, have the patient lie on his back with his head tilted toward the affected side and hanging over the edge of the bed. Ask him to turn his head sideways after he hyperextends his neck. Support his head with your hand to prevent neck strain.

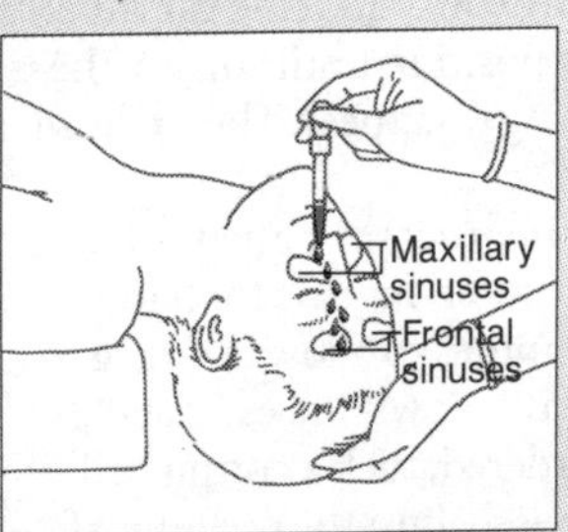

comfort during procedures such as bronchoscopy, and corticosteroids, which reduce inflammation from allergies, infections, and nasal polyps. For best effect, deliver nose drops directly onto the mucous membranes. (See *Positioning the patient for nose drops.*)

Getting ready

- After verifying the medication order, gather the equipment you'll need, including the prescribed medication, the patient's medication administration record, an emesis basin, facial tissues, and gloves.
- Verify the patient's identity, and explain the procedure to him. Position him as needed to ensure that the drops reach the intended site.

Instilling the medication

- Wash your hands, and put on gloves. Uncap the nose drop bottle, and squeeze the bulb on the nose dropper to withdraw the prescribed dose.
- Push up gently on the tip of the patient's nose to open his nostril completely.
- Place the dropper about ⅓″ (0.8 cm) inside the nostril. Slightly angle the tip of the dropper toward the inner corner of the patient's eye. Squeeze the dropper bulb to dispense the correct number of drops into each nostril. To minimize the risk of contamination, don't let the dropper touch the patient's nose.

Aftercare

- Stay with the patient. Encourage him to breathe through his mouth. If he coughs, help him to sit upright, and gently pat his back. For several minutes, observe him closely for possible respiratory problems.
- After you instill the prescribed number of drops, instruct the patient to keep his head tilted back for about 5 minutes. Encourage him to expectorate any medication that runs into his throat. Then document drug administration. ■

Giving nasal drugs to an infant or a child

When you administer nasal medication to an infant or child, you'll use different positioning techniques, depending on the patient's age and size.

Getting ready

Gather the necessary equipment, including the prescribed medication, the patient's medication administration record, an emesis basin, facial tissues, gloves and, if the patient is a child, a pillow. Warm the medication by holding the closed container under warm water. Then wash your hands, and put on gloves.

Instilling the medication

- If the patient is an infant, position him on your arm so that his head tilts back.
- Draw up the medication by squeezing the dropper's bulb until the correct dose fills the

dropper. Open the infant's nostril, taking care also to support his head.

- Instill the medication, and keep the infant's head tilted back for 5 minutes. Observe

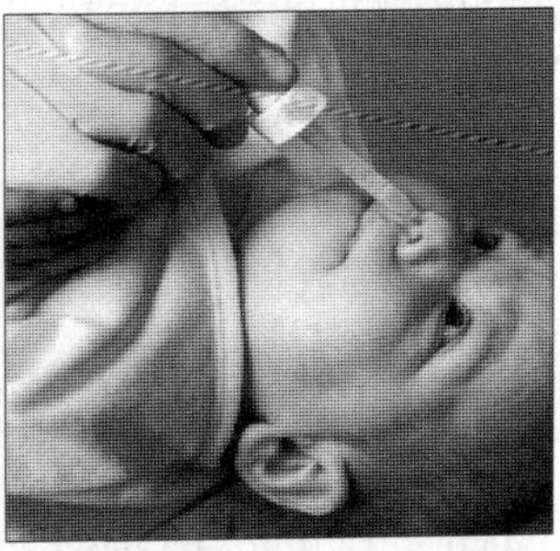

for signs of aspiration. If the infant begins to cough, hold him in an upright sitting position, and gently pat him on the back until he clears his lungs.

- If the child is too large to hold in your arms, have him lie on his back, and place a pillow under his shoulders. Gently tilt his head back, supporting it between your forearm and body. Use your other arm to steady his position and, if necessary, to restrain his arms and hands.

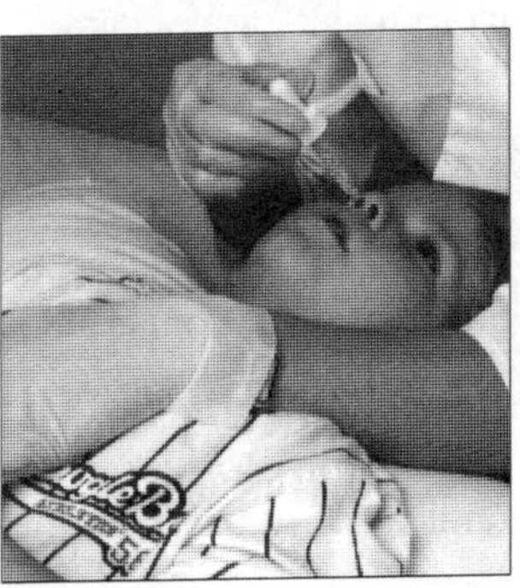

- Instill the medication, and keep the child's head tilted back for about 5 minutes.
- Document the procedure. ■

Delivering a nasal spray

A nasal sprays breaks down medication into small particles and distributes it evenly over the mucous membranes.

Getting ready

- Gather the needed equipment, including the prescribed medication in an atomizer, the patient's medication administration record, an emesis basin, facial tissues, and gloves.
- Wash your hands, and put on gloves. Have the patient sit up straight with his head upright.

CLINICAL TIP With many patients, you'll find administration to be more effective when you explain the procedure and have the patient perform it while you supervise.

Instilling the medication

- Occlude one nostril with your index finger. Place the tip of the atomizer about ½" (1 cm) inside the patient's open nostril, and position the tip straight up toward the inner corner of the eye.

- Depending on the drug, have the patient hold his breath or inhale. Then squeeze the atomizer once quickly and firmly — just enough for the medication to coat the inside of the nose. Excessive force may propel the medication into the patient's sinuses and cause a headache. Repeat the procedure in the other nostril, as ordered.
- Tell the patient to keep his head tilted back for several minutes so that the medication has time to work. Instruct him not to blow his nose during that time. ■

Administering an aerosol drug

Because nasal aerosol devices break down drug particles into even smaller particles than do atomizer sprays, they're especially suited for treating nasal polyps. Aerosol delivery effectively allows drug particles to reach inflamed areas. One of the most commonly used devices for delivering a metered dose of medication is the Turbinaire.

Getting ready

- Gather the equipment you'll need, including the prescribed medication, the plastic nasal adapter, the patient's medication administration record, facial tissues, and gloves. Wash your hands, and put on gloves.
- Explain the procedure to the patient. Demonstrate how to assemble the spray device by placing the stem of the medication cartridge into the plastic nasal adapter.

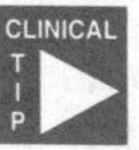

If you're inserting a refill cartridge, first remove the plastic cap from the stem.

- Have the patient blow her nose gently to remove excess mucus. At the same time, shake the cartridge well, and remove the protective cap from the adapter tip.

Instilling the medication

- Place the aerosol applicator tip inside the patient's nostril. Depending on the drug, tell her to hold her breath or inhale. Firmly press once on the cartridge and release it. Have the patient continue to hold her breath or inhale for several seconds afterward.

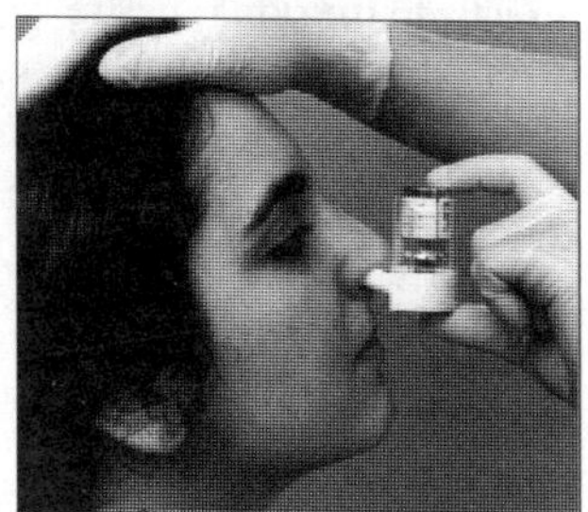

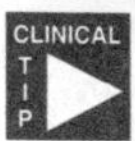

Remember to wear gloves, especially if the patient has heavy nasal discharge.

▪ Remove the adapter tip from the nostril, and have the patient exhale. If ordered, have her repeat the procedure. Direct the patient not to blow her nose for at least 2 minutes after the procedure.

Aftercare

▪ Rinse the equipment, replace the protective cap, and store the device in a plastic bag to keep it clean.
▪ Tell the patient to report any increased nasal irritation, bleeding, nasal congestion, headaches, or dizziness.
▪ Document the procedure. ■

ADMINISTRATION VIA THE SKIN

Applying a drug to the skin

Topical drugs, such as lotions and ointments, are applied directly to the skin. They're commonly used for local, rather than systemic, effects.

Getting ready

▪ Verify the order on the patient's medication administration record, explain the procedure, and provide privacy.
▪ Wash your hands to prevent cross-contamination, and put on gloves.
▪ Help the patient into a comfortable position that provides access to the affected area.
▪ Expose the affected area and place a linen-saver pad or towel under it.
▪ Make sure that the skin or mucous membrane is intact (unless the medication is for a skin lesion, such as an ulcer). If necessary, clean the area by removing crusts, epidermal scales, and old medication.
▪ Change your gloves if they become soiled or if you have cleaned debris from the area.

Applying a cream, paste, or lotion

▪ Open the medication container. Place the lid or cap upside down to protect the inside surface from contamination.
▪ Remove a tongue blade from its sterile wrapper, and cover one end with medication from the tube or jar. Transfer the medication from the tongue blade to your gloved hand. To prevent contamination, use a new tongue blade each time you take medication from the container.
▪ Apply the medication to the affected area, using long, smooth strokes in the direction of hair growth. This prevents you from forcing medication into the hair follicles, which may irritate them and

cause folliculitis. Avoid excessive pressure, which could abrade the skin.

- When applying medication to the face, use cotton-tipped applicators for small areas such as under the eyes. For larger areas, use a sterile gauze pad. Clean the patient's face with mild soap and water to remove any medication residue or exudate. Then apply the medication, as directed.

Removing ointment

- Like oil and water, ointment and water don't mix. To remove ointment from your patient's skin, you'll need a solvent, such as cottonseed oil, and sterile 4″ × 4″ gauze pads. Saturate one gauze pad with the cottonseed oil.
- Use this pad to swab the ointment gently from the patient's skin. Remove any remaining cottonseed oil by gently wiping the area with a clean sterile gauze pad. Don't wipe too hard, though, or you could irritate the skin.

Applying a spray or a powder

- Before applying a spray, shake the medication container. Hold the container 6″ to 12″ (15 to 30 cm) from the skin, or as directed by the product label, and begin spraying.
- To apply a powder, first dry the skin surface, making sure that you spread and dry any skin folds where moisture collects. Apply a thin layer of powder over the affected area.

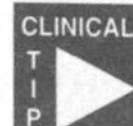

To protect the patient from inhaling any airborne powder unnecessarily, shake the powder onto your hand, and then apply it gently to his skin. ■

Applying a drug to the scalp

To apply a medicated lotion, cream, or shampoo to the patient's scalp, you proceed similarly; however, you should work a medicated shampoo into a lather, which you don't do with other scalp medications.

Getting ready

- Wash the patient's hair. After drying his hair and scalp with a towel, comb out any tangles.
- Using your fingertips, apply medication to the scalp, starting at the point where the hair parts naturally. Spread the medication evenly.
- Continue applying the medication every ½″ (1 cm), following instructions on the product label. If directed, massage the medication into the scalp, taking care not to

use your fingernails. Repeat as instructed.

Using medicated shampoo

- Read the label carefully to make sure that you apply the shampoo as directed and understand what corrective actions to take in an accident. (For instance, some shampoos contain selenium sulfide, which is toxic if ingested. Other products can harm the eyes and need to be flushed from the eyes promptly with water.)
- Shake the bottle of shampoo well. Wet the patient's hair thoroughly, and wring out excess water.
- Part the hair and apply the shampoo, working it into a lather and adding water as needed. Lather the scalp and hair for as long as instructed. Then rinse the hair.
- Remove excess moisture with a towel. Then comb or brush the hair. ■

Administering a transdermal drug

Given through an adhesive disk or measured dose of ointment applied to the skin, transdermal drugs deliver constant, controlled medication directly into the bloodstream for a prolonged systemic effect. (See *Understanding transdermal drugs.*)

Getting ready

- Verify the order on the patient's medication administration record (MAR). Then explain the procedure and provide privacy.
- Gather the patient's MAR and chart, medication disk or ointment, application strip or measuring tape (for nitroglycerin), gloves, plastic wrap, adhesive tape, and a transparent semipermeable dressing.
- Wash your hands, and put on gloves so that your hands don't absorb the drug.

Applying transdermal ointment

- Choose the application site — usually a dry, hairless spot on the patient's chest or arm. To promote absorption, wash the site with soap and warm water. If the patient has a previously applied medication strip, remove it, and wash the area to remove any drug residue. Dry the application site thoroughly.
- Squeeze the prescribed amount of ointment onto the application strip or measuring paper. Don't let any of the drug touch your skin.

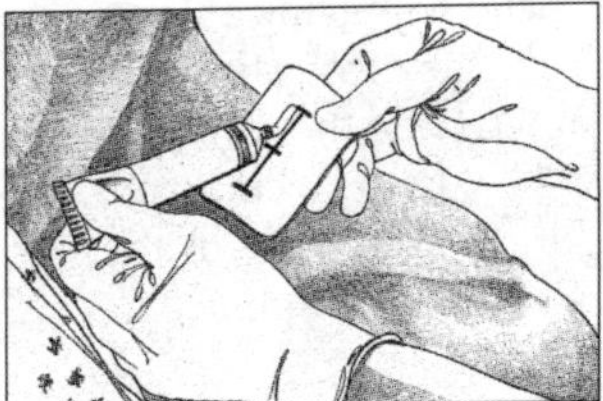

Understanding transdermal drugs

Through a measured dose of ointment or an adhesive patch applied to the skin, transdermal drugs deliver a constant, controlled medication directly into the bloodstream for prolonged systemic effect.

Medications currently available in transdermal form include nitroglycerin, used to control angina; nicotine, used to wean a person from smoking; scopolamine, used to treat motion sickness; estradiol, used for postmenopausal hormone replacement; clonidine, used to treat hypertension; and fentanyl, a narcotic analgesic used to control chronic pain.

Delivery times

Differences in transdermal forms usually reflect drug delivery times.

Transdermal nitroglycerin ointment dilates the coronary vessels for up to 4 hours, whereas a nitroglycerin patch (or disk) produces the same effect for as long as 24 hours. In patch form, scopolamine can relieve motion sickness for as long as 72 hours. Estradiol in a patch lasts for up to 1 week; clonidine, for 24 hours; and fentanyl, up to 72 hours.

Proper absorption

Ensuring proper absorption of these drugs depends on proper application along with appropriate patient teaching.

- To ensure effectiveness, instruct the patient to avoid applying a transdermal drug to broken or irritated skin, which would increase irritation, or to skin folds or scarred or calloused skin, which may impair absorption. Also avoid applying a disk below the elbow or knee.
- Advise the patient to alternate the application sites to avoid skin irritation.
- Instruct the patient to reapply daily transdermal medications at the same time every day to ensure a continuous effect. Bedtime application is ideal because body movement is reduced during the night. Tell him to apply a new disk about 30 minutes before removing the old one.
- Warn the patient not to get the disk wet. Tell him to discard the disk if it leaks or falls off, and then to clean the site and apply a new disk at a different site.

(continued)

Understanding transdermal drugs *(continued)*

- Advise the patient not to touch the ointment or gel because it may rub off onto his fingers. Remind him to wash his hands after application to remove medication that may have rubbed off inadvertently.
- Teach the patient what to do before reapplying nitroglycerin ointment. He should remove the plastic wrap, application strip, and any drug residue from the previous application site.

Side effects

- Inform the patient about possible side effects from transdermal delivery, such as skin irritation (pruritus or a rash).
- Instruct the patient who uses scopolamine patches not to drive or operate machinery until he's accustomed to his own response to the drug. Also mention that common side effects from scopolamine are dry mouth and drowsiness.
- Warn a patient who uses clonidine patches to check with the doctor before using any nonprescription cough preparations because they may counteract clonidine's effects. Mention that clonidine may cause severe rebound hypertension, especially if it's withdrawn suddenly.
- Explain that transdermal nitroglycerin medications may cause headaches and, in elderly patients, postural hypotension.
- Inform the patient that transdermal estradiol increases the risk of endometrial cancer, thromboembolic disease, and birth defects.

- Apply the strip, drug side down, directly to the skin. Maneuver the strip slightly to spread a thin layer of the ointment over a 3″ (8-cm) area, but don't rub the ointment into the skin.
- Secure the application strip by covering it with a semipermeable dressing or, if applying nitroglycerin ointment, the plastic wrap. Tape the plastic wrap in place.

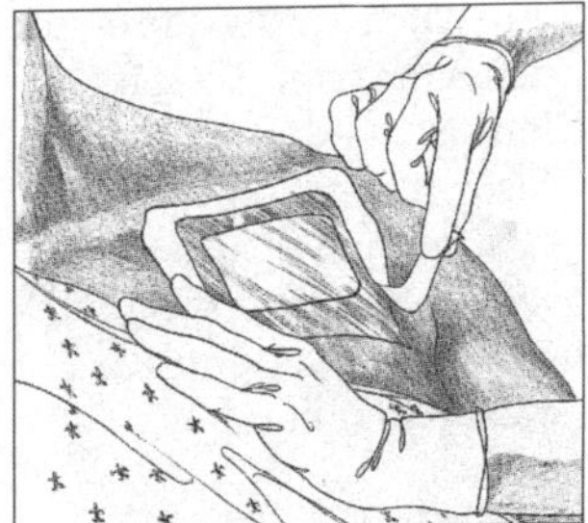

- If required by your facility's policy, label the strip with the date, time, and your initials. If you didn't wear gloves, wash your hands immediately to avoid absorbing the drug. Instruct the patient to keep the area around the patch as dry as possible.

Applying a transdermal patch

- Choose a dry, hairless application site. If necessary, clip any hair from the site, but don't shave the area. The most commonly used sites include the upper arm, chest, back, and behind the ears. Clean the application site with soap and warm water. Dry thoroughly. Open the drug package, and remove the patch.
- Without touching the adhesive surface, remove the clear plastic backing.
- Without touching the patch's adhesive layer, apply the patch to the site. If required by your facility's policy, label the site with the date, time, and your initials. ■

Which topical drug form should I use?

Different topical drug forms have distinct properties, making some more suitable than others for certain disorders or for particular skin areas, such as the scalp and face. Ointments, for instance, have a fatty base, making them an ideal form for antimicrobial and antiseptic drugs. Common topical drug forms, their effects, and appropriate nursing considerations include those that follow.

Cream

An oil-in-water semisolid emulsion, a cream acts as a barrier. To apply a cream, thoroughly massage it into clean, dry skin. After application, observe the patient's skin for irritation.

Paste

A stiff mixture of powder and ointment, paste provides a uniform coating of medication, thereby reducing and repelling moisture. Apply paste to clean, dry skin. Cover the medicated area to increase absorption and to protect the patient's clothing and bed linen.

Ointment

A semisolid suspension of oil and water, an ointment retains body heat and provides prolonged contact with a drug. To increase absorption, warm the patient's skin with hot packs or a warm bath before applying. As directed, apply a thin layer of ointment to clean, dry skin, and rub it in well. Use care when applying ointment to draining wounds.

Lotion
A suspension of insoluble powder in water or an emulsion without powder, lotion creates a sensation of dryness when applied to clean, dry skin. It leaves a uniform, powdery film that soothes, cools, and protects the skin. Before using, shake the container well. To increase absorption, warm the patient's skin with hot packs or a bath before application. Thoroughly massage lotion into the skin. After application, observe the skin for irritation.

Powder
An inert chemical that may contain medication, powder promotes skin drying and reduces moisture, maceration, and friction. Apply powder to clean, dry skin. To keep the patient from inhaling powder, instruct him to turn his head to the side during application. If you're applying powder to the patient's face or neck, give him a cloth or a piece of gauze to mask his mouth. Direct him to exhale as you apply the powder. ■

Which medicated dressing should I use?

You may need to apply a permeable, a semipermeable, or an occlusive medicated dressing to treat skin problems — especially when the patient can't tolerate a bath, when a skin problem affects an area that can't be soaked, or when the skin needs long-term treatment and protection.

A permeable dressing allows air to reach the wound, whereas a semipermeable dressing allows oxygen to reach the wound. An occlusive dressing, which is impermeable to oxygen, reduces wound pain, speeds reepithelialization, and stimulates debridement and healing. No matter which dressing you use, be sure to apply it correctly. Incorrect application can macerate the skin and stain clothing and bed linen.

Open, wet dressing
This permeable dressing is used for acute inflammatory skin conditions, erosions, ulcers, and skin lesions with oozing exudate. For example, you may use an open, wet dressing to apply a solution of water and aluminum sulfate. This type of dressing:
- delivers medication and softens and heals the skin
- absorbs pus and exudate

- decreases blood flow to inflamed areas
- helps promote drainage
- protects the site from contamination.

Leave this dressing uncovered after application; remoisten when the water in the medication evaporates.

Wet-to-dry dressing
This permeable dressing is used for wound debridement. For example, you may use a wet-to-dry dressing to apply sodium hypochlorite. This type of dressing:

- delivers medication and softens the skin
- absorbs pus, exudate, debris, and eschar.

Apply this dressing as you would apply any open, wet dressing; remove the dressing when the water evaporates (don't remoisten it).

Dry dressing
This semipermeable dressing is used for neurodermatitis and stasis dermatitis. For example, you may use a dry dressing with a debriding agent such as collagenase. This type of dressing protects the affected area from abrasion and contamination. Simply apply this ordinary gauze pad to the skin.

Closed, wet dressing
This occlusive dressing is used for such skin conditions as cellulitis, erysipelas, psoriasis, lichen simplex chronicus, and eczema. For example, you may use an occlusive dressing to apply desoximetasone and an insulated dressing to apply boric acid solution. This type of dressing:

- delivers medication, softens and heals the skin, and increases the effectiveness of medication
- absorbs pus and exudate
- increases blood flow to inflamed areas
- protects the site from contamination.

Apply this medication-soaked dressing to the skin, and cover it with an occlusive or insulated bandage to prevent water evaporation and heat loss. ■

RECTAL AND VAGINAL ADMINISTRATION

Inserting a rectal suppository

Medication may be administered rectally to a patient who's unconscious, vomiting, or otherwise unable to swallow. (See *Guide to rectal drug forms,* page 378.)

Advantages

- Rectal administration bypasses the upper GI tract so that medications aren't destroyed in the stomach or

Guide to rectal drug forms

DRUG FORM	LOCAL USES	SYSTEMIC USES
Suppository Supplying a solid drug in a firm base, such as cocoa butter, suppositories melt at body temperature. These drugs are molded in cylindrical shapes usually about 1½″ (4 cm) long (smaller for infants and children). Before using, keep suppositories refrigerated to prevent softening and possible decreased drug effectiveness.	▪ Relieves local pain and irritation ▪ Promotes astringent action ▪ Controls local itching ▪ Reduces inflammation ▪ Stimulates defecation ▪ Lubricates and cleans ▪ Relieves colic and flatus	▪ Reduces pain and discomfort ▪ Relieves nausea and vomiting ▪ Reduces fever ▪ Provides bronchodilation ▪ Produces sedation ▪ Promotes serenity and relaxation
Ointment This semisolid drug formulation may be applied externally to the anus or internally to the rectum.	▪ Reduces fever ▪ Promotes astringent action ▪ Relieves pain ▪ Reduces inflammation ▪ Kills bacteria	None
Enema This is a liquid given rectally for retention (for at least 30 minutes or until absorbed, or for at least 10 minutes and then expelled). Note: Enemas given to clean the lower bowel are not medicated.	▪ Destroys parasites ▪ Promotes astringent action ▪ Stimulates defecation ▪ Lubricates and cleans ▪ Kills bacteria ▪ Reduces inflammation	Reduces fever

small intestine by digestive enzymes.

- It doesn't irritate the upper GI tract, as some oral medications can.
- Rectal administration bypasses the portal system, thereby avoiding biotransformation in the liver.

Disadvantages

- The patient may experience discomfort or embarrassment.
- A rectal medication may be incompletely absorbed, especially if the patient can't retain it or if the rectum contains fecal matter.
- Because of incomplete absorption, the patient may require a higher dose than if he were taking the same drug in oral form.

Getting ready

- Gather the prescribed suppository, the patient's medication administration record (MAR) and chart, several 4″ × 4″ gauze pads, gloves, a linen-saver pad, water-soluble lubricant and, if indicated, a bedpan.

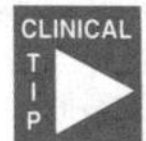

If the suppository softens too much for easy insertion, hold it (in its wrapper) under cold running water to harden it again.

- Match the patient's MAR with the doctor's order, and confirm the patient's identity.
- Explain the procedure, and provide privacy.
- Place the patient in Sims' position. Cover him with the bedcovers, exposing only the buttocks. Then place a linen-saver pad under the buttocks.

Inserting the suppository

- Put on gloves, and remove the suppository from its wrapper. Squeeze some water-soluble lubricant onto the suppository.
- Using your nondominant hand, lift the patient's upper buttock to expose the anus.
- Then, instruct the patient to take several deep breaths through his mouth to relax the anal sphincter and reduce anxiety or discomfort.
- Using your dominant hand, insert the suppository, tapered end first, into the rectum. Use your index finger to direct the suppository along the rectal wall toward the umbilicus. Continue to advance it about 3″ (8 cm), or about the length of your finger, until it passes the patient's internal anal sphincter.

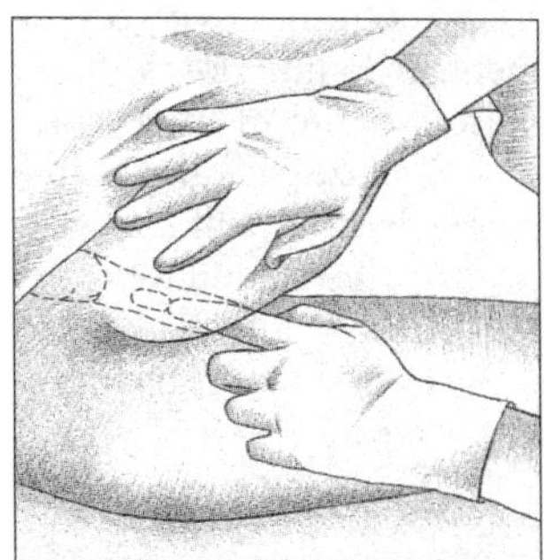

APPLYING TOPICAL DRUGS

Aftercare

- Ensure the patient's comfort. Encourage him to lie quietly and, if applicable, to retain the suppository for an appropriate time. A suppository given to relieve constipation should be retained as long as possible (at least 20 minutes) to be effective. If necessary, press on the anus with a gauze pad until the patient's urge to defecate passes. If the patient can't retain the

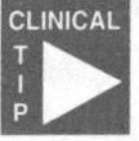

suppository, and, if pressing on the anus with a gauze pad fails to relieve the urge to defecate, place the patient on a bedpan. Inform him that the suppository may discolor his next bowel movement. ■

Applying a rectal ointment

Depending on your patient's needs, you may apply rectal ointment externally or internally.

Getting ready

- Gather the necessary equipment, including gloves, the prescribed ointment, several 4″ × 4″ gauze pads and, if applying the ointment internally, an applicator and water-soluble lubricant.
- Wash your hands, and put on gloves.

Applying the ointment

- For external application, squeeze a small amount of ointment on your finger.
- Spread the ointment over the anal area, using your gloved finger or a gauze pad.
- For internal application, remove the ointment tube's cap, and attach the applicator to the tube.
- Coat the applicator with water-soluble lubricant. Expect to use about 1″ (2.5 cm) of ointment. To judge the pressure needed to extract this amount, squeeze a small amount from the tube before you attach the applicator.
- With your nondominant hand, lift the patient's upper buttock to expose the anus. Gently insert the applicator, directing it toward the umbilicus. Then slowly squeeze the tube to eject the medication.

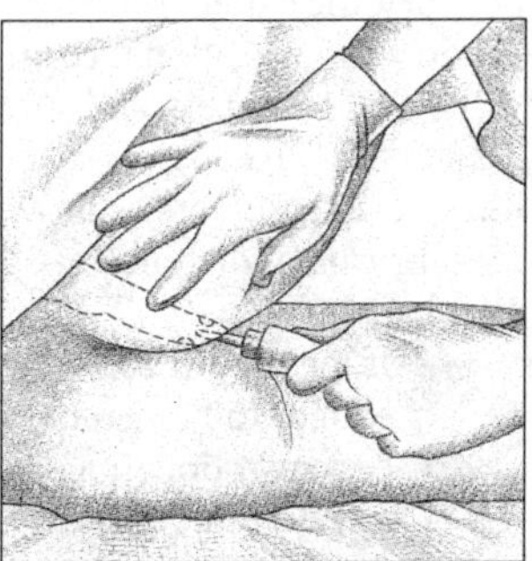

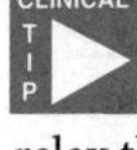

Direct the patient to breathe deeply through his mouth to relax the anal sphincter and to reduce anxiety or discomfort during insertion.

Aftercare

- Withdraw the applicator, and place a folded 4″ × 4″ gauze pad between the patient's buttocks to absorb excess ointment.
- Remove the applicator from the tube, and recap the tube. Clean the applicator with soap and water.
- Document the procedure. ■

Instilling a retention enema

Administering drugs by enema involves having the patient retain a solution in the rectum or colon for 30 to 60 minutes. An adult requires 150 to 300 ml (about 5 to 10 oz) of fluid; a child over age 6, about 75 to 150 ml (2½ to 5 oz). (These amounts are smaller than those used for irrigating enemas.)

Getting ready

- Gather the following equipment, including the prescribed solution (usually available in a premixed commercially prepared container), a disposable enema kit or an enema bag assembly, gloves, 4″ × 4″ gauze pads, a bedpan, toilet paper, an emesis basin, a linen-saver pad, and water-soluble lubricant.
- Explain the procedure to the patient. Stress the importance of retaining the solution until the medication is absorbed.
- To avoid stimulating peristalsis, have the patient empty his bladder and rectum before you begin.
- Place a linen-saver pad under him, and assist him into Sims' position. If he's uncomfortable in this position, reposition him on his right side or his back.

Administering a commercially prepared enema

- Put on gloves, and remove the cap from the rectal tube.
- Check the amount of lubricant already on the rectal tube. If needed, squeeze additional water-soluble lubricant onto a 4″ × 4″ gauze pad, and dip the rectal tube's tip in the lubricant.
- Gently squeeze the enema container to expel air.
- With your nondominant hand, lift the patient's upper buttocks to expose the anus. Instruct the patient to take a deep breath. As the patient inhales, insert the rectal tube into the rectum, pointing the tube toward the umbilicus. For an adult, advance the tube 3″ to 4″ (8 to 10 cm); for a child over age 6, advance the tube 2″ to 3″ (5 to 8 cm).
- Squeeze the enema container until the solution fills

the patient's rectum. Remove the rectal tube, and discard the used enema and original packaging properly. Tell the patient to retain the solution for the prescribed time.

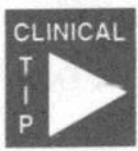
If the patient is apprehensive, position him on a bedpan, and let him hold toilet tissue or a rolled washcloth against his anus. If he needs to use the bathroom or commode later, instruct him to call for help before getting out of bed, especially if he feels weak or faint.

Using an enema bag

- Prepare the prescribed solution and warm it to 105° F (40.6° C). Test the temperature of the solution with a bath thermometer, or pour a small amount of solution over your wrist.
- Put on gloves. Close the clamp on the enema tubing, and fill the enema bag with the solution.
- Hang the enema bag on an I.V. pole so that it's slightly above the bed.
- Remove the protective cap from the end of the tubing. The tip of the tubing should be prelubricated. If it isn't, apply a small amount of water-soluble lubricant.
- Unclamp the tubing, flush the solution through the tubing, and then reclamp it.
- With your nondominant hand, lift the patient's upper buttock. With your other hand, insert the enema tubing into the patient's anus.

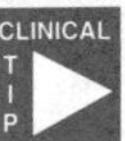
Before inserting the tubing, touch the patient's anal sphincter with the tip of the tube to stimulate contraction. Then, tell the patient to breathe deeply through the mouth while you gently advance the tube.

- Release the clamp on the tubing. Be sure to hold the tube in place throughout the entire procedure because bowel contractions and the pressure of the tube against the anal sphincter can displace the tube.
- Next, start the flow, and adjust the flow rate by lowering or raising the bag according to the patient's retention ability and comfort. However, don't raise it higher than 18″ (46 cm) for an adult, 12″ (30 cm) for a child, and 6″ to 8″ (15 to 20 cm) for an infant.

CLINICAL TIP If the flow stops, the tubing may be blocked with feces or compressed against the rectal wall. Gently turn the tubing to free it without stimulating defecation. If the tubing becomes clogged, withdraw it, flush with solution, and then reinsert.

- After administering most of the solution, clamp the tubing. Stop the flow before the container empties to avoid introducing air into the bowel. Remove the tubing and dispose of the setup.

- Instruct the patient to hold the solution for the prescribed time. If necessary, hold a 4″ × 4″ gauze pad against the anus until the patient's urge to defecate passes. Place him on a bedpan if doing so will make him more comfortable. ■

What should I remember when giving rectal drugs?

Remember these guidelines when giving rectal drugs:

- Before giving a retention enema, check the patient's elimination pattern. For example, a constipated patient may need a cleansing enema to prevent feces from interfering with drug absorption. A patient with a fecal impaction may need to have the drug delivered by another route. Also, a patient with diarrhea may be unable to retain the enema solution for the prescribed time.
- Because inserting a rectal suppository or an enema tube usually stimulates the vagus nerve, rectal drug administration is contraindicated in patients with cardiac arrhythmias or an MI. You also may need to avoid this route in patients who've had recent rectal, colon, or prostate surgery to minimize the risk of local trauma.
- Don't administer a rectal medication (or laxative) to a patient with undiagnosed abdominal pain. If the pain is caused by appendicitis, drug-induced peristaltic action could rupture the appendix.
- Before administering rectal medication, inspect the patient's rectum. If the tissue is inflamed, the drug could aggravate the condition. ■

Inserting a vaginal suppository

Among the forms of vaginal drugs are suppositories, creams, gels, ointments, and solutions. These medicated preparations can be inserted to treat infection (particularly *Trichomonas vaginalis* and monilial vaginitis) or inflammation. Or they may be used to prevent conception. Once in contact with the vaginal mucosa, suppositories melt, diffusing medication as effectively as creams, gels, and ointments.

Vaginal medications usually come with a disposable applicator to place the medication in the anterior and posterior fornices. Vaginal administration is most effective when the patient can lie down afterward to retain the medication.

Vaginal medications may be administered by you or by the patient herself.

Getting ready

- Gather the following equipment, including the patient's medication administration record, gloves, the prescribed drug and an applicator (if necessary), water-soluble lubricant, a small sanitary pad, an absorbent towel, a linen-saver pad, a small drape, cotton balls, a 4″ × 4″ gauze pad, and a paper towel. Soap and water may also be necessary.
- After verifying the medication order, confirm the patient's identity by asking her name and by checking the name, room number, and bed number on her identification bracelet.
- Explain the procedure to the patient, and provide privacy. Ask the patient to empty her bladder.
- Help the patient into the lithotomy position. Place a linen-saver pad under her buttocks and a small drape over her legs. Expose only her perineum.
- Wash your hands, and put on gloves. Then squeeze a small portion of water-soluble lubricant onto the 4″ × 4″ gauze pad. Unwrap the suppository, and coat it with lubricant.

Inserting the suppository

- Separate the labia. Examine the patient's perineum. If the perineum is excoriated, withhold the medication and notify the doctor. If you see any discharge, wash the area. To do this, soak several cotton balls in warm, soapy water. Then, while holding the labia open with one hand, clean the left side of the perineum, the right side and, finally, the center. Use a fresh cotton ball for each stroke.
- While the labia are still separated, insert the rounded tip of the suppository into the vagina, advancing it about 3″ to 4″ (8 to 10 cm) along the posterior wall of the vagina, or as far as it will go. ■

Using a vaginal applicator

Vaginal medications in the form of a cream, gel, foam, or a small suppository may require use of an applicator.

Getting ready

- Gather the following equipment, including the patient's medical administration record, gloves, the prescribed medication and an applicator (if necessary), water-soluble lubricant, a small sanitary pad, an absorbent towel, a linen-saver pad, a small drape, cotton balls, a 4″ × 4″ gauze pad, and a paper towel.

Soap and water may also be necessary.

- If your patient's medication doesn't come in a prepackaged applicator, fill the applicator with the prescribed drug. If the drug is in suppository form, place the suppository in the tip of the applicator.
- Wash your hands, and put on gloves. Clean the patient's perineum, and lubricate the applicator tip with water-soluble lubricant as you would when inserting a vaginal suppository.

Inserting the applicator

- Use your nondominant hand to separate the patient's labia. Use your dominant hand to insert the applicator about 2″ (5 cm) into the patient's vagina.
- Slowly press the plunger until you empty the applicator. Then, remove the applicator and place it on a paper towel to prevent the spread of microorganisms.
- Instruct the patient to remain lying down, with knees flexed, for 5 to 10 minutes so the medication can flow into the posterior fornix. Wash the applicator with soap and warm water, and store or discard it as appropriate. ■

Performing a vaginal irrigation

Vaginal medications can also be given by irrigation in the form of a douche. The procedure involves instilling a liquid into the vagina at low pressure. The liquid washes the vagina and immediately flows out without being retained by the patient. Vaginal irrigations help remove discharge, reduce inflammation, or prevent infection.

If a commercially prepared product isn't available, the solution can be instilled through a vaginal irrigation setup. As with other vaginal medications, the best time for administration is bedtime, when the patient can remain lying down.

Getting ready

- Gather the following equipment, including the patient's medication administration record, the prescribed medication, gloves, an irrigation bottle with a nozzle or a vaginal irrigation setup, a bedpan, a pillow or rolled blanket, and an I.V. pole (if necessary).
- Prepare the patient as you would to insert a suppository. Then place her on a bedpan, using a pillow or rolled blanket to support her lower back.

- Wash your hands, and put on gloves.
- If necessary, attach the nozzle tip to the irrigation bottle. Remove the protective cap, if applicable, and gently squeeze the bottle to ensure patency of the nozzle tip.

Using an irrigation bottle with a nozzle

- Use your nondominant hand to separate the labia. Use your dominant hand to insert the nozzle tip about 2″ (5 cm) into the vagina.
- Squeeze the bottle to instill the solution into the vagina. After the solution is infused, it should return freely into the bedpan.

Using an irrigation setup

- To administer the solution with an irrigation setup, clamp the irrigation tubing, and hang the container of irrigation fluid on the I.V. pole. Adjust the height of the I.V. pole so the bottom of the solution container is about 12″ (30 cm) above the vagina. This allows the solution to flow freely without injuring the vaginal lining.
- Hold the nozzle over the bedpan, and then unclamp the tubing. Allow solution to flow through the tubing to remove air and moisten the nozzle's tip. Then hold the nozzle over the patient's perineum to allow the solution to moisten and clean the perineal area. Clamp the tubing.
- Use your nondominant hand to separate the labia. Use your dominant hand to insert the nozzle into the vagina. Once the nozzle is inserted, direct it toward the patient's sacrum, and carefully advance it 3″ to 4″ (8 to 10 cm) into the vagina.
- Unclamp the tubing, and allow the solution to flow freely into the patient's vagina. Rotate the nozzle several times to irrigate all parts of the vagina.
- After administering all of the solution, remove the nozzle from the patient's vagina. Remove the bedpan, and pat the perineum and buttocks dry with a towel.
- To prevent the medication from soiling the patient's clothing and bed, provide a sanitary pad. Assist the patient with application, if necessary.
- Dispose of the irrigation equipment properly. Then remove your gloves, turning them inside out and placing them on the paper towel. Help the patient resume a comfortable position. ■

CHAPTER 13

GIVING INJECTIONS

INTRADERMAL ADMINISTRATION

Giving an intradermal injection

An intradermal (ID) injection delivers small amounts of a drug or an antigen (usually 0.5 ml or less) into the outer, superficial layers of the skin. Commonly performed to determine antigenic sensitivity by stimulating an immune response, an ID injection is used to produce a local effect, known as a *wheal.* Little systemic absorption occurs.

An ID injection allows identification of antibodies to such pathogens as the tubercle bacillus. For some patients, the doctor may order a local anesthetic injected intradermally before venipuncture, although this practice isn't endorsed by the Intravenous Nurses Society.

If you're giving an ID injection of lidocaine as the anesthetic, you'll administer only a small amount, and it will work in 2 to 3 seconds. Lidocaine injected intradermally numbs pain but allows the patient to feel touch and pressure.

The most common site for an ID injection is the ventral forearm because it's easily accessed and relatively hairless. For extensive allergy testing, the shoulder blades and the outer aspects of the upper arms may also be used. (See *Reading skin-test results.*)

Getting ready

- Gather a tuberculin syringe with a 26G or 27G ½″ or ⅝″ needle, the prescribed test antigen (or drug), gloves, a marking pen, alcohol sponges, and the patient's medication administration record (MAR).
- Verify the order on the patient's medication record by comparing it with the doctor's order.
- Prepare the medication, comparing the label with the patient's MAR to make sure you're giving the right drug.
- Verify the patient's identity by checking the name, room number, and bed number on his identification bracelet.
- Tell the patient where you'll give the injection. If it will be in the ventral forearm, instruct him to sit up. Then ask him to extend his arm and support it with the ventral surface exposed. He'll need to stay nearby for about 30 minutes after the injection (in case of anaphylaxis).
- Put on gloves. With an alcohol sponge, clean the surface of the ventral forearm about two or three fingerbreadths distal to the antecubital space. Make sure the test site

Reading skin-test results

Follow these general guidelines for reading skin test results easily and confidently:

- Feel the area around the injection site. It should be round and hard (induration). Observe the skin for flare (erythema), and assess its extent. Keep in mind that erythema without induration isn't significant.
- Measure the extent of the induration in millimeters.
- Record your findings.

Tuberculin test results

When testing for tuberculosis (TB), use a scale to measure your findings.

- If the induration is smaller than 5 mm in diameter, consider the test result *negative.*
- If the induration is 5 mm or more in diameter, consider the test result *positive* in any of the following circumstances:
  — The patient had recent close contact with a person with active, infectious TB.
  — The patient's chest X-ray shows pulmonary fibrotic lesions, suggesting old, healed TB lesions.
  — The patient has HIV or is at high risk for it.
- If the induration is 10 mm or more in diameter, consider the test result *positive* if the patient fails to meet the above criteria but has one or more of the following risk factors for TB:
  — He has a medical condition that increases his risk of active TB after infection has occurred (for example, COPD or AIDS).
  — He was born in Asia, Africa, Central America, or South America.
  — He is Black, Native American, or Hispanic *and* a member of a low socioeconomic or medically underserved group.
  — He uses I.V. drugs.
  — He is a resident or staff member of a congregate living arrangement, such as a prison, nursing home, or other long-term care facility.
  — He is a health care worker exposed to TB.
  — He is extremely young or old.
- If the induration is 15 mm or more in diameter, consider the test result *positive* even if the patient has no risk factors.

Note: A positive skin test result indicates infection with *Mycobacterium tuberculosis.* It doesn't necessarily indicate active disease.

(continued)

Reading skin-test results *(continued)*

Allergy test results
When testing for allergies, score the findings from 0 to 4+, as follows:
- Induration with a diameter of 2 mm or less — 0 (negative).
- Induration with a diameter of 3 to 5 mm (with erythema) — 1+.
- Induration with a diameter of 6 to 10 mm (with erythema) — 2+.
- Round induration with a diameter of 11 to 15 mm or more (with erythema) — 3+.
- Induration with a diameter of more than 15 mm, with erythema and pseudopods (asymmetrical branches) —4+.

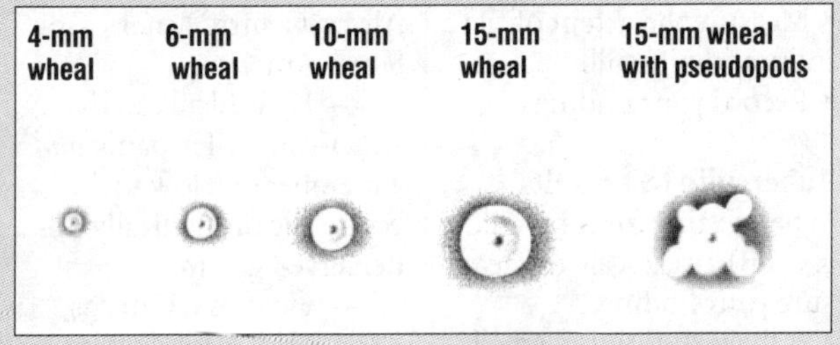

is free of hair and blemishes. Allow the skin to dry before giving the injection.

Injecting the drug
- Holding the patient's forearm in your nondominant hand, stretch the skin taut.
- With your dominant hand, hold the needle at a 15-degree angle to the patient's arm with the bevel facing up.
- Insert the needle about ⅛″ below the epidermis. Stop when the needle's bevel tip is under the skin, as shown in column two.
- Then gently inject the antigen. You should feel some resistance as you do this, and a wheal should form. If no wheal forms, you've probably injected the antigen too deeply. Withdraw the needle, and administer another test dose at least 2″ (5 cm) from the first site. If you're giving additional injections, be sure to space them about 2″ apart.

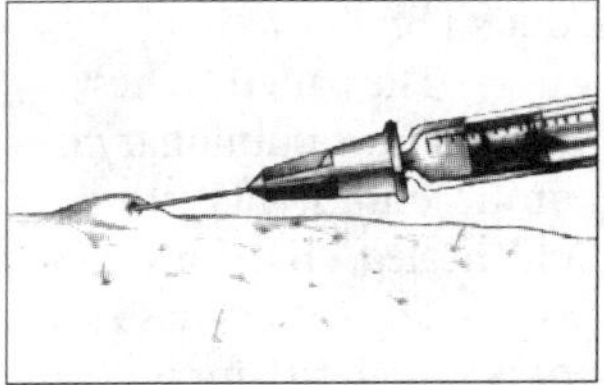

- Withdraw the needle at the same angle at which you inserted it. Don't rub the site.

This could irritate the underlying tissue, which could affect the test results.

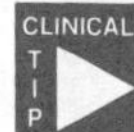

A patient who's hypersensitive to a test antigen may have a severe anaphylactic reaction. Be prepared to inject epinephrine immediately and to perform other emergency resuscitation procedures.

Aftercare

- Circle each test site with a marking pen, and label each site to recall the antigen given. Instruct the patient not to wash off the markings until the test period ends.
- Dispose of needles and syringes according to your facility's policy. Remove and discard your gloves.
- Document the name of the medication or antigen and the amount administered.
- Have the patient stay nearby for 30 minutes to allow you to observe for anaphylaxis. Notify the doctor immediately if an allergic reaction occurs. In most cases, a reaction occurs within 72 hours. ■

SUBCUTANEOUS ADMINISTRATION

Giving an S.C. injection

A drug injected subcutaneously into the adipose (fatty) tissue beneath the skin reaches the bloodstream more quickly than a drug taken by mouth. An S.C. injection also allows slower, more sustained drug absorption than an I.M. injection. What's more, this method causes minimal tissue trauma and poses little risk of injuring large blood vessels and nerves.

Absorbed mainly through the capillaries, drugs recommended for S.C. injection include nonirritating aqueous solutions and suspensions contained in 0.5 to 2 ml of fluid. Give drugs and solutions for S.C. injection through a short needle, using sterile technique. You can give S.C. injections in any part of the body that has relatively few sensory nerve endings and no bones or large blood vessels near the surface. (See *Locating S.C. injection sites*, page 392.)

Getting ready

Assemble the equipment you'll need, including the prescribed medication; the patient's medication administration record (MAR); a needle of appropriate gauge and length (usually a 25G ⅝″ needle for an average adult and a 25G to 27G ½″ needle for an infant, a child, or an elderly or thin patient); gloves; a 1- to 3-ml syringe; and alcohol sponges. Optional sup-

Locating S.C. injection sites

Indicated by dotted areas in the photographs, S.C. injection sites include the fat pads on the abdomen, upper hips, upper back, and lateral upper arms and thighs. To perform effective S.C. injections, follow these guidelines:

- For drugs that must be administered repeatedly, such as insulin, rotate sites. Choose one injection site in one area, move to a corresponding injection site in the next area, and so on. When returning to an area, choose a new site in that area. Use a site rotation chart, and don't use the same site more than once every 2 months.

  Preferred injection sites for insulin are the arms, abdomen, thighs, and upper hips.
- Heparin administration sites differ from other S.C injection sites because heparin should be injected only in the lower abdominal fat pad, about 2″ (5 cm) beneath the iliac crests. Giving heparin at this site reduces local capillary bleeding.

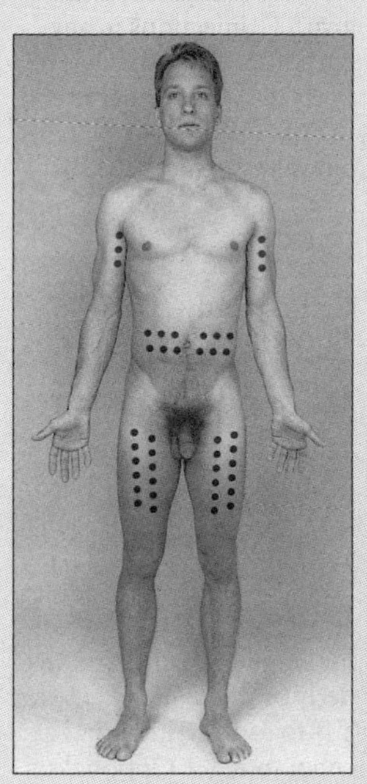

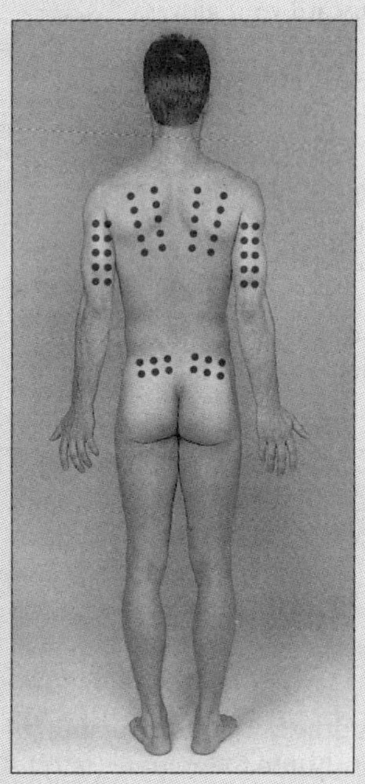

plies include an antiseptic cleaning agent, a filter needle, and an insulin syringe.

- Obtain the prescribed medication, and check it against the patient's MAR and the doctor's order.
- Prepare the medication, comparing the label with the MAR to make sure that you're giving the right drug.
- Verify the patient's identity by checking his identification bracelet.
- Then inspect the medication to make sure that it's not abnormally discolored or cloudy and that it doesn't contain precipitates.
- Select an appropriate injection site, remembering to rotate sites when the patient's regimen requires repeated injections. Use different body areas unless contraindicated by the drug.
- Also select a needle of proper gauge and length. To determine the needle size exactly, use your thumb and forefinger to form a skin fold at the site. Measure the fold from base to crest. If it measures more or less than ⅝″ (1.6 cm), remove the ⅝″ needle from the syringe, and replace it with one that's closer to the correct length.
- Put on gloves. Position and drape the patient if necessary.
- Clean the injection site with an alcohol sponge, starting at the center of the site and moving outward in a circular motion. Let the skin dry before injecting the drug to avoid a stinging sensation from introducing alcohol into subcutaneous tissue.

Injecting the drug

- Grasp the skin firmly. This elevates the subcutaneous tissue and prevents the needle from entering the wrong skin layer.

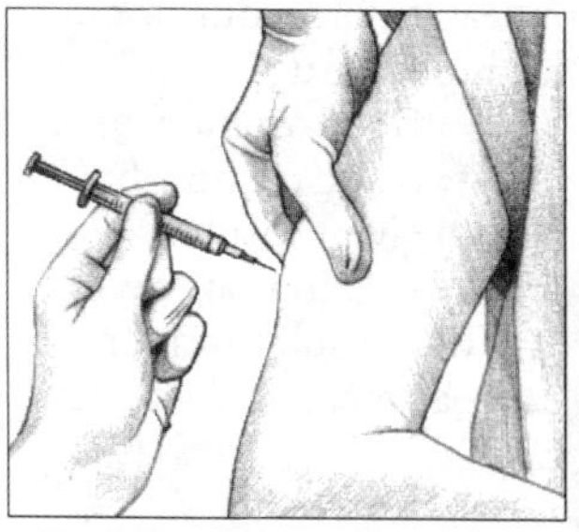

- Position the needle with the bevel facing up. If you're using a ⅝″ or longer needle, hold it at a 45-degree angle. If you're injecting the drug with a ½″ needle, hold it at a 90-degree angle. Insert the

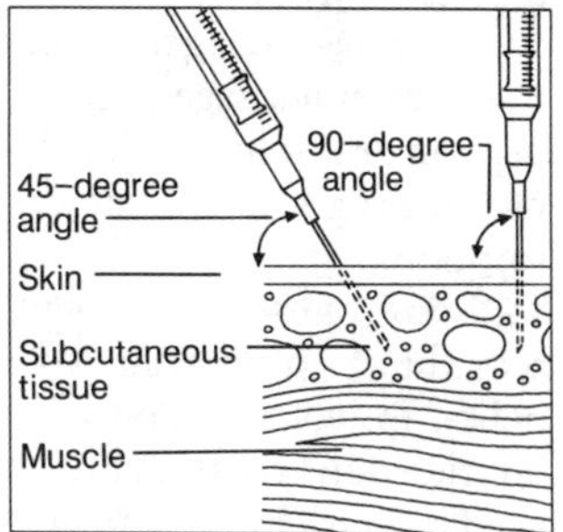

needle with one quick motion; then release your grasp on the patient's skin. If you don't, you'll inject the drug into the compressed tissue, which will irritate nerve fibers and cause the patient discomfort.

- Pull back slightly on the plunger to check needle placement. If no blood flows back into the syringe, begin injecting the drug slowly. If blood appears upon aspiration, withdraw the needle, prepare another syringe, and repeat the procedure for injecting the drug.

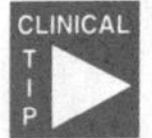

Don't aspirate for blood return when giving insulin or heparin. Aspiration isn't necessary with insulin and can cause a hematoma with heparin.

Aftercare

- After injection, remove the needle gently, but quickly, at the same angle used for insertion.
- Cover the site with an alcohol sponge. Then massage the site gently (unless you have injected a drug that contraindicates massage, such as heparin or insulin) to distribute the drug and facilitate absorption.
- Dispose of used equipment according to your facility's policy. To avoid needle-stick injuries, don't resheath the needle. Finish by documenting the procedure.

Special considerations

- Avoid giving S.C. injections at sites that are inflamed, edematous, scarred, or covered by a mole, a birthmark, or another lesion. Such injections may also be contraindicated in patients with coagulation defects.
- When injecting heparin and insulin subcutaneously, which are commonly given at least once daily, you'll need to rotate injection sites. To ensure consistent blood levels, use specific sites because the absorption rate varies from one anatomic region to another.

When giving S.C. heparin, for instance, the designated administration site is the lower abdominal fat pad just below the umbilicus. ■

Should I aspirate before giving an S.C. injection?

Traditionally, you'd aspirate for blood before giving an S.C. drug to avoid inadvertently injecting some of it into a vein. Clinicians believed this would help prevent serious side effects caused by certain drugs, such as insulin or morphine.

Heparin was the exception to this rule: If you injured the area during aspiration, heparin could cause a hematoma.

Current thinking

For two reasons, some clinicians now believe that aspiration is unnecessary with any drug:

- First, some needles are made specifically for S.C. injections, and they're shorter than the needles you may have used in the past. If you have a needle of the correct length and the right site, hitting a vein would be anatomically impossible; the needle just wouldn't penetrate that far.
- Second, today's needle tips have sharper edges and more sharply angled bevels so that they're less likely to lodge in a vein. Even if a vein were inadvertently pierced when the needle was inserted, this design would minimize the risk of the drug actually entering it.

Most of the time, you don't need to aspirate for blood before injecting insulin. But you should consider doing so in children, thin adults, or any patient who has many superficial blood vessels at the injection site or well-developed underlying muscle (which is common among diabetic athletes).

The best approach is to discuss this issue with your nurse-manager as a first step toward developing practice standards within the nursing department. ■

What's the safest way to inject S.C. drugs?

The S.C. injection route uses adipose and connective tissue under the skin and above skeletal muscles to promote systemic drug action. The best sites yield a 1" (2.5-cm) fat fold when pinched and have relatively few sensory nerve endings.

Several factors determine how well medication is absorbed from a given site: the patient's cardiovascular and fluid status, his physical build, the condition of his subcutaneous tissue, and your injection skills.

Preventing absorption problems

Absorption after an S.C. injection occurs by relatively slow diffusion into the capillaries. The rate is 1 to 2 ml/hour per injection site. So when a drug is given by the S.C. rather than the I.M. route, initial blood concentrations of the drug will be lower, but the drug's effects will persist longer.

Be aware that the S.C. route's slow absorption rate, as well as the drug's effects, could markedly and dangerously increase if the patient exercises or if he warms or elevates the site after an injection. For example, an insulin-dependent diabetic could develop acute hypoglycemia from previously unabsorbed insulin if he jogs 2 miles (3.2 km).

Preventing tissue damage
To prevent subcutaneous tissue damage, irritating or concentrated drugs are usually given I.M. An irritating solution that's mistakenly given subcutaneously can cause tissue ischemia and necrosis. Also, concentrated drug solutions injected S.C. can cause sterile abscesses.

Sterile and nonsterile abscesses, cysts, granulomas, and nodules are common among drug abusers who inject suspensions made from capsules and tablets. These immunologic reactions can be caused by injecting irritating solutions, solutions containing invisible microcrystals (such as talc and cellulose found in oral forms), or more than 1 ml of a drug per site. Overusing a site can also cause these immunologic reactions. ■

How can I correct glucose levels with an infusion pump?

Changes in food consumption, problems with an insulin infusion pump, and other factors can contribute to abnormally high or low blood glucose levels. In some cases, reactions can be corrected by adjusting the amount of insulin delivered by the infusion pump.

High blood glucose levels
Consider the patient's blood glucose level to be high if it's greater than 240 mg/dl in two consecutive readings.

This condition may result from such causes as increased food intake, illness, stress, menses, or decreased exercise. High blood glucose levels may also stem from a bolus dose of insulin delivered too soon (or not at all). High blood glucose levels can result if the pump settings are incorrectly programmed, if the syringe is empty, or if the infusion set or syringe is leaking. Air bubbles or an obstruction in the infusion set or syringe, or irritation at the infusion site can also increase blood glucose levels.

Correcting high levels
To correct high blood glucose levels, follow these guidelines:
- Check all pump settings, including those for routine insulin dosage or bolus doses, profiles, insulin concentration, and total insulin delivered; then reprogram settings as needed.
- Also check the syringe, and replace it if it's empty. Tighten the connection between

the syringe and infusion set, or change the syringe and infusion set.

- Change the infusion site.
- If you can find no reasonable explanation for the patient's increased blood glucose level, test his urine for ketone bodies. If test results are positive, call the doctor; if they're negative, change the infusion set.

Low blood glucose levels

A low blood glucose level (below 60 mg/dl) may stem from reduced food intake or increased exercise or activity. Below-normal blood glucose levels may also occur if pump settings are incorrectly programmed or if the infusion set is incorrectly disconnected from the syringe. A patient's blood glucose level will also decrease if he has consumed alcohol in the past 12 hours.

Correcting low levels

To correct low blood glucose levels, follow these guidelines:

- Reprogram the insulin dosage as ordered. Decrease basal or bolus doses before exercise if indicated.
- Check pump settings, including bolus doses, profiles, insulin concentration, and total insulin delivered; then reprogram insulin settings as needed. Review correct disconnection procedures to prevent excessive insulin infusion.
- Check with the doctor regarding the hypoglycemic effect of alcohol. Reprogram the insulin dosage as ordered.
- If no reason can be found for the drop in blood glucose level, correct hypoglycemia, reprogram the insulin dosage as ordered, and monitor pump settings. ■

What's the safest way to inject heparin?

When injecting heparin, your goal is to avoid local bleeding and irritation. Follow these guidelines:

- Locate the preferred site for heparin injection in the lower abdominal fat pad, about 2″ (5 cm) beneath the umbilicus and between the right and left iliac crests. Injecting heparin into this area, which doesn't have muscular activity, reduces the risk of local capillary bleeding. Always rotate the sites from one side of the lower abdominal fat pad to the other.
- Don't administer any injections within 2″ of a scar, a bruise, or the umbilicus.
- Don't aspirate to check for blood return because this may cause bleeding into the tissues at the site.
- Don't rub or massage the site after the injection. Rub-

bing can cause localized minute hemorrhages or bruises.
- If the patient bruises easily, apply ice to the site for the first 5 minutes after the injection to minimize local hemorrhage, and then apply pressure. ■

How do I combine NPH and regular insulin?

NPH and regular insulin in combination are commonly administered simultaneously. When you receive an order for this combination of drugs, draw them up into the same syringe, following this procedure.

Getting ready
- Read the insulin order carefully.
- Read the vial labels carefully, noting the type, concentration, source, and expiration date of the drugs.
- Roll the NPH vial between the palms of your hands to mix it properly.
- Choose a needle of the appropriate gauge and length.
- Clean the tops of both vials with alcohol sponges.

Drawing up the insulins
- Inject air into the NPH vial equal to the amount of insulin you need to administer. Withdraw the needle and syringe, but don't withdraw any NPH insulin.
- Now inject into the regular insulin vial the amount of air equal to the dose of regular insulin. Then invert or tilt the vial and withdraw the ordered amount of regular insulin into the syringe. (Regular insulin is drawn up first to avoid contamination by the addition of longer-acting insulin.)
- Clean the top of the NPH vial again. Then insert into this vial the needle of the syringe containing the regular insulin and withdraw the ordered amount of the NPH insulin.
- Mix the insulins in the syringe by pulling back slightly on the plunger and tilting the syringe back and forth.
- Recheck the drug orders, and administer and chart the medications immediately. ■

INTRAMUSCULAR ADMINISTRATION

Giving an I.M. injection

An I.M. injection is recommended for a patient who's uncooperative or who can't take medication orally, and for drugs that are altered by digestive juices. Because muscle tissue has few sensory nerves, an I.M. injection allows less painful administration of irritating drugs.

Choose the method and site of an I.M. injection carefully, taking into account your patient's build, his age, and the purpose of the injection. (See *Locating I.M. injection sites*, pages 400 and 401.)

Getting ready

- Begin by gathering the necessary equipment, including the prescribed medication, the patient's medication administration record (MAR), a 3- to 5-ml syringe and a 20G to 25G 1″ to 3″ needle, gloves, and alcohol sponges.
- Verify the order on the patient's MAR by checking it against the doctor's order. Also check the patient's allergy history, his name, and bed and room number, and verify his identity.
- Inspect the prescribed drug for color, clarity, and expiration date. Never use an expired, cloudy, or precipitated solution unless the manufacturer's instructions allow it. Remember also that some drugs (such as suspensions) normally contain particles.
- Provide privacy, and explain the procedure to the patient. Position and drape him appropriately, making sure that the injection site is well-lit and exposed. Put on gloves.
- Loosen the protective needle sheath, but don't remove it. After selecting the injection site, gently tap it to stimulate nerve endings and minimize pain when you insert the needle.
- Next, clean the skin at the site with an alcohol sponge. Move the sponge outward in a circular motion to a circumference of about 2″ (5 cm) from the injection site. Allow the skin to dry to avoid introducing alcohol into the nearby tissue, which causes pain.

Injecting the drug

- With the thumb and index finger of your nondominant hand, gently stretch the skin taut at the injection site.

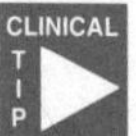

Always encourage the patient to relax the muscle you'll be injecting, because injections into tense muscles are more painful and cause more bleeding.

- Holding the syringe in your dominant hand, remove the needle sheath by slipping it between the free fingers of your nondominant hand and then removing the syringe from the sheath.
- Position the syringe at a 90-degree angle to the skin, with the needle a couple of inches from the skin. Tell the patient that he'll feel a prick as you insert the needle.
- Then quickly and firmly thrust the needle through the

Locating I.M. injection sites

An I.M. injection deposits medication deep into muscle tissue, where a large network of blood vessels can absorb it quickly. Choose the site carefully, taking into account the patient's physical build and the purpose of the injection. Don't give I.M. injections at inflamed, edematous, or irritated areas, or those containing scar tissue or other lesions. I.M. injections may also be contraindicated in impaired coagulation, occlusive peripheral vascular disease, edema, suspected acute MI, and shock conditions that impair absorption.

Deltoid

- To locate the densest area of muscle and avoid major nerves and blood vessels, find the lower edge of the acromial process and the point on the lateral arm in line with the axilla.

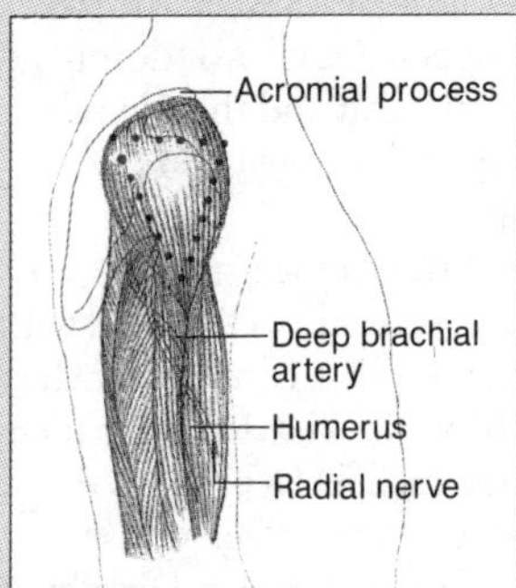

- Insert the needle 1″ to 2″ (2.5 to 5 cm) below the acromial process, usually two to three fingerbreadths, at a 90-degree angle or angled slightly toward the acromial process.
- Standard injection: 0.5 to 2 ml.

Dorsogluteal (upper outer corner of the gluteus maximus)

- Restrict injections to the area above and outside the diagonal line drawn from the posterior superior iliac spine to the greater trochanter of the femur. Or divide the buttock into quadrants, and inject into the upper outer quadrant, about 2″ to 3″ (5 to 7.6 cm) below the iliac crest.

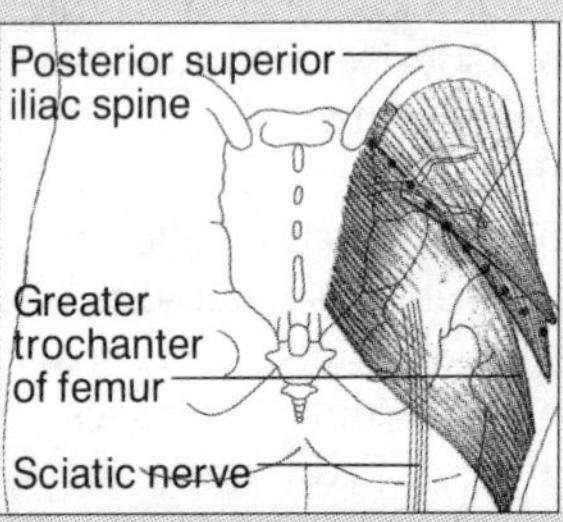

- Insert the needle at a 90-degree angle to the muscle.
- Standard injection: 1 to 5 ml.

Locating I.M. injection sites *(continued)*

Ventrogluteal (gluteus medius and gluteus minimus)

- Locate the greater trochanter of the femur with the heel of your hand. Then spread your index and middle fingers to form a "V" from the anterior superior iliac spine to the farthest point along the iliac crest that you can reach.

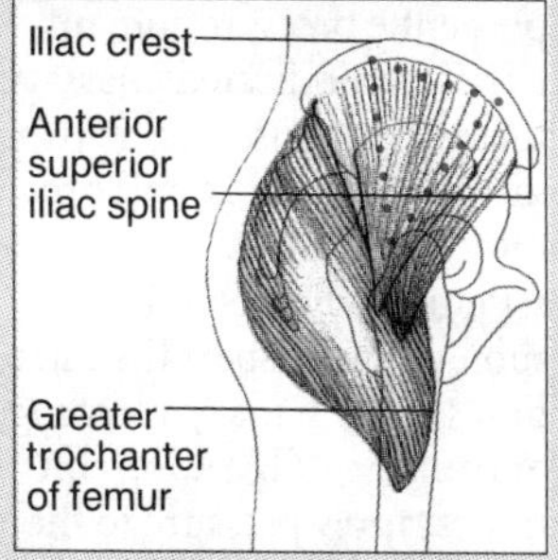

- Insert the needle into the area between the two fingers at a 90-degree angle to the muscle. Remove your hand before inserting the needle.
- Standard injection: 1 to 5 ml.

Vastus lateralis

- Use the lateral muscle of the quadriceps group, along that length of the muscle from one handbreadth below the greater trochanter to one handbreadth above the knee.

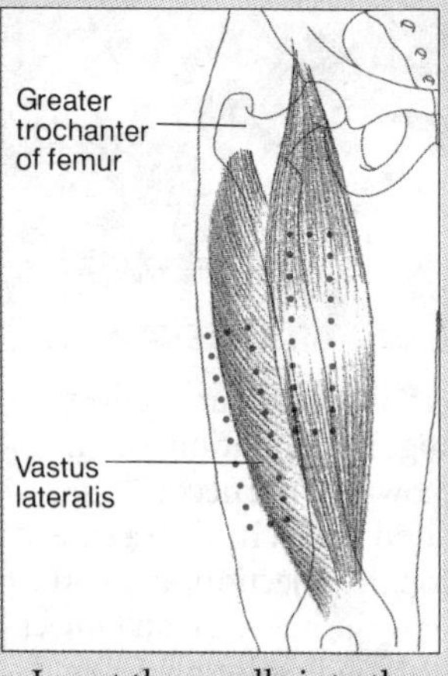

- Insert the needle into the middle third of the muscle on a plane parallel to the surface on which the patient is lying. You may have to bunch the muscle before inserting the needle.
- Standard injection: 1 to 5 ml; 1 to 3 ml for infants.

skin and subcutaneous tissue, deeply into the muscle.

▪ Because you won't resheath the needle, discard the sheath. Then support the syringe with your nondominant hand if desired. Pull back slightly on the plunger with your dominant hand to aspirate for blood.

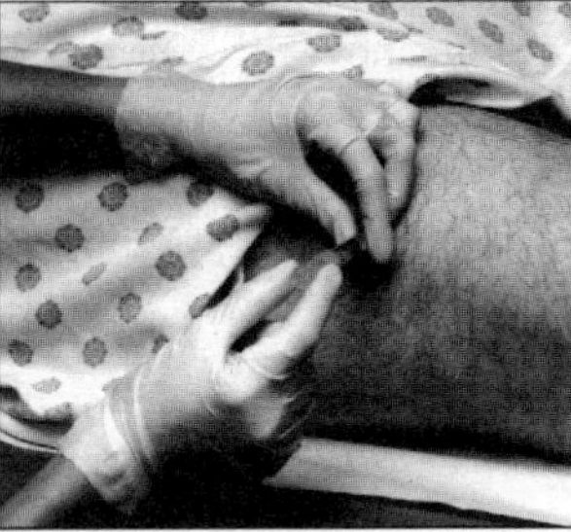

▪ If blood appears in the syringe on aspiration, you'll know that the needle is in a blood vessel. In such a case, stop the injection, and withdraw the needle. Don't inject the bloody solution. Instead, prepare another injection with new equipment, and use another injection site.

▪ If no blood appears in the syringe, proceed. Place your thumb on the plunger rod. Slowly and steadily inject the medication into the muscle, allowing the muscle to distend gradually and draw in the medication under minimal pressure. You should feel little or no resistance against the force of the injection.

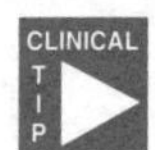

If the patient experiences pain or anxiety with repeated injections, use ice to numb the area before cleaning it. Hold the ice in place for several seconds. If you must inject more than 5 ml of solution, divide the solution, and inject it at two separate sites.

Aftercare

▪ After the injection, gently but quickly remove the needle at a 90-degree angle. Using a gloved hand, cover the injection site immediately with an alcohol sponge. Apply gentle pressure and, unless contraindicated, massage the relaxed muscle to help distribute the drug and promote absorption.

▪ Remove the alcohol sponge, and inspect the injection site for signs of bleeding or bruising. If bleeding continues, apply pressure to the site; if bruising occurs, you may apply ice.

▪ Watch for side effects at the site for 30 minutes after the injection. Discard all equipment according to your facility's policy. ■

What must I consider when giving I.M. injections?

The Z-track method for I.M. injection prevents leakage, or tracking, of injected medication into the subcutaneous tissue. You may need to use this method if your patient is an older adult and has reduced muscle mass or if you're injecting an irritating medication. (See *Using the Z-track method*, pages 404 and 405.)

Choosing the injection site

- If your patient is a healthy adult, the gluteal muscles (gluteus medius, gluteus minimus, and the upper outer corner of the gluteus maximus) are the sites most commonly used. The deltoid muscle may be used for a small-volume injection (2 ml or less).
- If your patient is an infant or a young child, however, using the gluteal muscles isn't appropriate. The rule of thumb in this age-group is that the younger the child, the less developed is the muscle. In a child under age 3 (or a child who hasn't been walking for at least 1 year), the gluteal muscles aren't developed enough to receive an I.M. injection safely — and without injury to the sciatic nerve. In this age-group, the thigh's vastus lateralis muscle is the most common site for an I.M. injection because it's usually better developed than the gluteal muscles and has no large nerves or blood vessels. These factors minimize the risk of injury. Other appropriate sites are the deltoid muscle in older children, if it's sufficiently developed, and the rectus femoris muscle in infants.
- An elderly patient usually has less subcutaneous tissue and muscle mass (especially in the buttocks and deltoid muscles), so you may need to use a shorter needle. Also, an older adult patient typically has more fat around the hips, abdomen, and thighs. This makes the vastus lateralis muscle and ventrogluteal area (gluteus medius and minimus, but not gluteus maximus muscles) primary injection sites.
- Rotate injection sites if your patient requires repeated injections.

Injection tips

- If your older adult patient is extremely thin, pinch the muscle gently to elevate it and to avoid inserting the needle completely through the muscle. Never give an I.M. injection in an immobile limb because of poor drug absorption and the risk of sterile abscess.
- Because of age-related vascular changes, elderly patients are also at greater risk for hematomas. To control bleeding, you may need to apply direct pressure over the puncture site for longer than usual. Gently massage the injection site to aid drug absorption and distribution. However, avoid site massage when giving certain drugs by

Using the Z-track method

If you're administering an irritating drug, such as iron dextran, or giving an injection to an older adult patient with decreased muscle mass, you'll need to vary the standard I.M. procedure by using the Z-track method. By staggering the needle pathway after injection, this technique allows I.M. drug delivery while minimizing the risk of subcutaneous staining and irritation from certain drugs.

With this method, you'll inject the drug into the patient's buttock — but never inject more than 5 ml into a single site. Before the procedure begins, the skin, subcutaneous fat, fascia, and muscle lie in their normal positions, as shown.

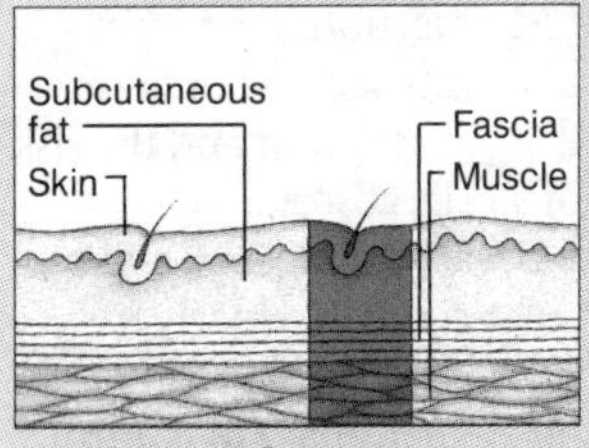

Getting ready

- Gather the necessary equipment, including the prescribed medication; the patient's medication administration record, a 3- to 5-ml syringe, a 20G to 25G 1″ to 3″ needle, gloves, and alcohol sponges.,
- After drawing up 0.3 to 0.5 cc of air into the syringe, replace the needle with a sterile one that's 3″ long. Put on gloves.
- Then place your finger on the skin surface, and pull the skin and subcutaneous layers out of alignment with the underlying muscle (see below). Move the skin about 1″ (2.5 cm). This ensures entry of the injected medication into the muscle tissue.

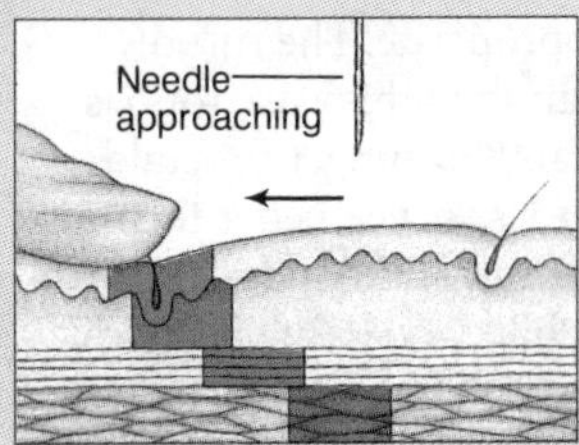

Injecting the drug

- After cleaning the site, insert the needle at a 90-degree angle in the site where you initially placed your finger (see below). Inject

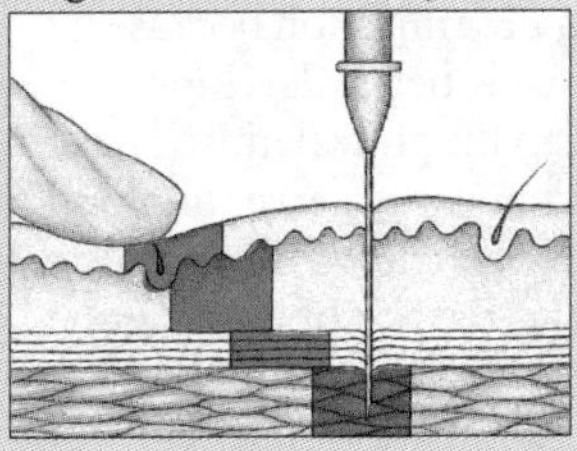

Using the Z-track method *(continued)*

the drug slowly. When you're finished, wait 10 seconds before withdrawing the needle. This keeps the medication from seeping out of the site.

- After withdrawing the needle, allow the retracted skin to resume its normal position. The needle track (shown by the broken line) is now broken at the junction of each tissue layer, trapping the drug in the muscle.

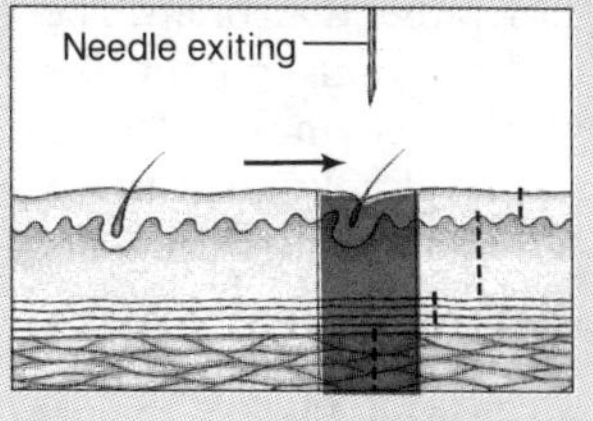

Special considerations

Never massage the site or allow the patient to wear a tight-fitting garment over the site. Either action could force the medication into the subcutaneous tissue and cause irritation. To increase the rate of absorption, encourage physical activity such as walking. For subsequent injections, alternate buttocks.

the Z-track method, such as iron dextran or hydroxyzine hydrochloride.

- Also remember that I.M. injections require sterile technique to maintain the integrity of muscle tissue. The prescribed medication also must be sterile. The needle may be packaged separately or already attached to the syringe.
- Needles used for I.M. injections are longer than those used for S.C. injections because they must reach deep into the muscle. Needle length depends on the injection site, the patient's build, and the amount of fat covering the muscle. The needle gauge for I.M. injections should be larger than that used for S.C. injections to accommodate viscous solutions and suspensions. ■

How can I improve I.M. drug absorption?

Absorption rates from muscle tissue may vary from site to site. For example, absorption is faster from the arms than the thighs, and faster from the thighs than the buttocks.

In fact, research studies have shown that blood flow in the deltoid muscle is 7% greater than that in the vastus lateralis and 17% greater than that in the gluteal muscles. Thus, injections into the deltoid muscle provide the fastest and highest peak serum concentrations of such drugs as haloperidol, lorazepam, and chlordiazepoxide.

Proper injection technique
Poor injection technique can impede absorption from any I.M. site. In a classic study, researchers measured serum levels of diazepam in one group of patients after a team of health care professionals injected 10 mg of a drug into their patients' buttocks. Then, diazepam levels in another group of patients were measured after injections by a second team of professionals. The result? Serum levels were two-and-a-half times higher in the patients injected by the first group.

Technique seemed to account for the difference. The first group of health care professionals routinely used 1½″ needles; the second group used smaller 1¼″ needles, probably to save their patients from unnecessary pain.

As you know, needles are usually inserted to three-fourths of their length. So the second group, who used the shorter needles, probably injected the diazepam into their patients' subcutaneous tissue instead of muscle. Undoubtedly, the poor blood supply and high fat content of subcutaneous tissue limited the bioavailability of the diazepam, which tends to collect in fatty tissue anyway.

Proper drug choice
Compared with oral drugs, I.M. drugs are generally absorbed faster. But that doesn't always hold true. Chlordiazepoxide, diazepam, digoxin, and phenytoin are less dependable when given I.M. rather than orally. Their I.M. solutions contain 10% alcohol (ethanol), 40% propylene glycol, and nearly 50% water. These drugs are rapidly diluted with tissue fluid, making them temporarily insoluble. ■

How can I make I.M. injections less painful?

You can reduce the pain of I.M. injections with expert patient preparation and skillful injection technique and aftercare.

Patient preparation
- Encourage the patient to relax the muscle you'll be injecting. An injection into a tense muscle causes more bleeding and pain. Using the techniques that follow will relax the appropriate muscles.

- For gluteal injections, the patient should lie facedown, stand with his toes pointed inward, or lie on his side with the uppermost leg drawn up in front of the lower one.
- For a vastus lateralis injection, the patient's toes should point inward so that the hip rotates internally.
- For a deltoid muscle injection, the patient should flex his elbow and support the lower arm.
- Avoid especially sensitive areas. When you choose an injection site, roll the muscle mass with your fingers and watch for twitching, an indication that the area is too sensitive.
- If the patient is very apprehensive about the injection, numb the site briefly by holding ice on it or by spraying an anesthetic coolant on it before you clean the site with an alcohol sponge. Then wait until the alcohol is dry. If you don't, the alcohol may cling to the needle and cause pain when you insert it.

Injection technique

Follow these guidelines to help minimize I.M. injection pain:

- After you draw up the drug, change needles. A needle's point and bevel can be dulled when you puncture the drug vial's stopper, and dull needles hurt. By changing needles, you eliminate another source of pain — medication that clings to the outside of the needle when you draw medication out of the vial or ampule.
- Insert the needle smoothly and rapidly to minimize puncture pain. As you're doing so, try to distract the patient's attention away from the injection.
- If the needle is properly placed, proceed to inject the drug gradually to prevent creating high pressure in the muscle.
- Remember to withdraw the needle smoothly and rapidly.

Aftercare

- Unless contraindicated by the medication (iron dextran, for example), gently massage the muscle to distribute the drug better and increase absorption. This helps reduce pain, which is caused by tissue stretching from a large-volume injection. (Lightly exercising the injected muscle accomplishes the same thing: increased absorption.) ■

INTRA-ARTICULAR ADMINISTRATION

Giving an intra-articular injection

An intra-articular injection delivers drugs directly into the synovial cavity of a joint to relieve pain and helps to preserve function, prevent contractures, and delay muscle atrophy. Before intra-articular injection, synovial fluid may be withdrawn to relieve pressure or to be tested in the laboratory.

Drugs commonly administered intra-articularly include corticosteroids, anesthetics, and lubricants. Rarely, antiseptics, analgesics, and counterirritants may be injected by this administration route.

Usually performed by a doctor with a nurse assisting, intra-articular injection requires sterile technique. This technique is contraindicated in patients with joint infection, joint instability or fracture, or systemic fungal infection.

Getting ready

- Begin by gathering the necessary equipment, including the prescribed medication, the patient's medication administration record (MAR) and chart, 3-ml and 5- or 10-ml syringes, labels, a sterile towel, sterile gloves, sterile cotton balls or gauze pads (or sterile povidone-iodine sponges), pillows, a sterile emesis basin, an antiseptic cleaning agent, a sterile fenestrated drape, local anesthetic, 25G ⅝″ and 18G 1½″ needles, and an adhesive bandage.
- Optional equipment for giving an intra-articular injection includes sterile test tubes for synovial fluid aspiration, with appropriate additives and specimen labels, and a 10- or 20-ml syringe for aspirating a specimen of synovial fluid.
- Verify the order on the patient's MAR by checking it against the doctor's drug order.
- Wash your hands thoroughly.
- Draw the prescribed amount of medication into the 5- or 10-ml syringe before entering the patient's room.
- Label the syringe with the name of the medication and the amount. Take the container from which you drew the medication with you so the doctor can verify the syringe contents.
- Confirm the patient's identity, explain the procedure and its purpose, and provide privacy while the injection is administered.

- Position the patient comfortably. The joint to be injected should be stabilized, supported (with pillows, if necessary), and fully exposed.
- Employing strict aseptic technique, open the sterile towel and place it on the bedside stand to create a sterile field.
- Using aseptic technique, open the packages of syringes, needles, and cotton balls or gauze pads, and drop these supplies onto the sterile field.
- After putting on the sterile gloves, the doctor picks up sterile cotton balls or gauze pads and holds them over the emesis basin.
- Pour the antiseptic cleaning agent over the cotton balls or gauze pads.
- The doctor cleans the injection site with the saturated cotton balls or gauze pads. After draping the site, he checks the label on the local anesthetic while you hold the bottle. Turn the bottle upside down so the doctor can fill the 3-ml syringe.
- The doctor anesthetizes the skin and subcutaneous tissue at the injection site, using the 25G ⅝″ needle.

Aspirating synovial fluid

- Position the sterile test tubes in the correct sequence.
- The doctor withdraws synovial fluid with the 18G 1½″ needle, using the 10-ml or 20-ml syringe. He leaves the needle in the joint for the subsequent injection of medication. (The syringe containing the synovial fluid can be set aside until after the procedure.)
- The doctor will then attach a needle to the specimen syringe and insert the appropriate amount of synovial fluid into the test tubes. Label the test tubes appropriately, and send them to the laboratory.

Giving the injection

Hand the 5- or 10-ml medication syringe with an 18G 1½″ needle to the doctor, who then injects the medication into the synovial cavity. (If synovial fluid was aspirated, remove the needle, and hand the doctor the medication syringe. He attaches the syringe to the needle already in the joint and injects the medication.)

Aftercare

- After the intra-articular injection, apply pressure to the site, and (if appropriate) massage the area gently for 1 or 2 minutes to facilitate absorption.
- Apply an adhesive bandage to the site.
- Advise the patient to avoid excessive use of the affected joint because the injected

medications may mask any pain that he may have.

- Because the medication may infiltrate and initially irritate surrounding tissue, local joint pain may actually increase for 24 to 48 hours after an intra-articular injection. However, fever, persistent increased pain, redness, and swelling may indicate septic arthritis, a serious complication caused by contamination during the procedure.
- Record the injected medication, dose, date, time and site of injection, and the doctor's name in your progress notes.
- Also note the amount of synovial fluid aspirated, any laboratory studies requested, and the patient's tolerance of the injection. ■

CHAPTER 14

DELIVERING INFUSIONS

Peripheral venous therapy

Central venous therapy

PERIPHERAL VENOUS THERAPY

Infusing drugs through a secondary I.V. line

A secondary I.V. line is used for continuous or intermittent infusion. It connects to the Y-port of the patient's primary I.V. line rather than directly to the venipuncture device. A secondary setup that delivers solution intermittently is known as a *piggyback* infusion. When it supplies a solution continuously over several hours, it's known as a *continuous secondary* I.V. infusion.

Giving a piggyback infusion

- Hang the piggyback setup on the I.V. pole. Using an alcohol sponge, clean the Y-port above the roller clamp of the primary I.V. tubing. Insert the needle from the piggyback line into the Y-port of the primary line.
- Tape this connection securely, unless you're using a recessed needle that doesn't require taping. Instead, a plastic covering may lock the needle in place. To reduce the risk of needle-stick injury, use a needleless or click-lock system with any type of secondary infusion or with an intermittent infusion device.
- To infuse the piggyback medication without infusing the fluid from the primary I.V. bag or bottle, hang the primary I.V. bag or bottle below the level of the piggyback container. Use the extension hook supplied with the piggyback infusion set. To infuse the primary and secondary solutions simultaneously, hang them at the same height.
- Completely open the roller clamp on the piggyback tubing. Then adjust the roller clamp of the primary set to regulate the infusion rate of the piggyback infusion. The primary I.V. solution won't run while the piggyback medication is infusing. If the secondary I.V. solution isn't compatible with the primary I.V. solution, be sure to flush the primary line before and after infusing the incompatible solution.

Giving a continuous secondary infusion

- Adjust the roller clamp on the tubing of the secondary solution to the desired drip rate. Then adjust the roller clamp on the tubing of the primary solution to achieve the desired total infusion rate.
- If your facility's policy allows, use a pump or a time

tape on the secondary line to maintain an even flow rate.

- If you're using a continuous secondary setup and the primary and secondary solutions are incompatible, stop the primary infusion. Before beginning the secondary infusion, flush the line with 5 or 10 ml of normal saline solution. Then administer the secondary infusion. Once you complete the secondary infusion, flush the line again before resuming the primary infusion.
- If you can't interrupt the primary infusion, use a double-lumen catheter, or administer the medication through another I.V. site.
- During the infusion, frequently check that the medication in the secondary I.V. line is infusing at the desired rate and over the desired time. When a continuous secondary infusion finishes, the primary infusion will continue. Likewise, when a piggyback solution finishes infusing, the primary infusion will resume. In either case, adjust the primary I.V. solution drip rate, as needed, when the secondary infusion finishes. If you're using an infusion pump, reset the rate or volume as needed.
- If you'll be reusing the tubing from the secondary infusion set on the same patient, close the clamp on the tubing. Then replace the used needle with a new one, or leave it securely taped or locked in the injection port. Label the tubing with the time it was first used, according to facility policy. Also, leave the empty secondary solution container in place until you replace it with a new one. Change this tubing according to policy (usually every 48 to 72 hours). Inspect the injection port for leakage with each use. Change the port more often if needed.
- If you won't be reusing the tubing from the secondary line, discard it appropriately along with the empty solution container.
- Finally, record the amounts and types of drug and I.V. solution on the patient's intake and output and medication administration records. Note the date, time, duration, and rate of infusion, and the patient's responses, where applicable. ■

Giving an I.V. bolus injection

Commonly called an *I.V. push*, an I.V. bolus injection allows rapid drug delivery and a maximum (or peak) drug level in the patient's bloodstream immediately. Used in emergencies, the technique also allows administration of a drug that can't be diluted — for example, phenytoin, digoxin, furosemide, diazoxide, diazepam, many chemotherapeutic drugs, and diagnostic contrast media.

Usually, you'll give a bolus injection directly into an existing peripheral primary I.V. line, an existing intermittent infusion device, or a vein. You may also use the technique to give a drug through an existing central venous line or a vascular access port. Because a drug given by I.V. bolus takes effect rapidly, you'll need to monitor your patient carefully for such side effects as cardiac arrhythmias.

Getting ready

- Compare the order on the patient's medication administration record (MAR) with the doctor's order.
- Gather the prepared drug, flush solutions, and other necessary equipment, and take them to the patient's bedside. Explain the procedure to the patient.
- Verify the patient's identity by asking him his name and comparing the name, room number, and bed number on his identification bracelet with the same information on the MAR.

Giving an I.V. bolus through a peripheral line

- Gather the following equipment, including the prescribed drug in a syringe with an attached 20G or 22G 1″ needle, alcohol sponges, two syringes (usually 3 ml) filled with normal saline solution with attached 20G or 22G 1″ needles, and gloves. Depending on facility policy, you may need another 3-ml syringe with an attached 20G or 22G 1″ needle filled with heparin flush solution.
- Check the compatibility of the drug with the I.V. solution. If they're compatible, put on gloves, and close the flow clamp on the existing I.V. line. Clean the Y-port closest to the venipuncture site with an alcohol or a povidone-iodine sponge. Insert the syringe's needle into the Y-port, and inject the drug according to the manufacturer's recommendation.

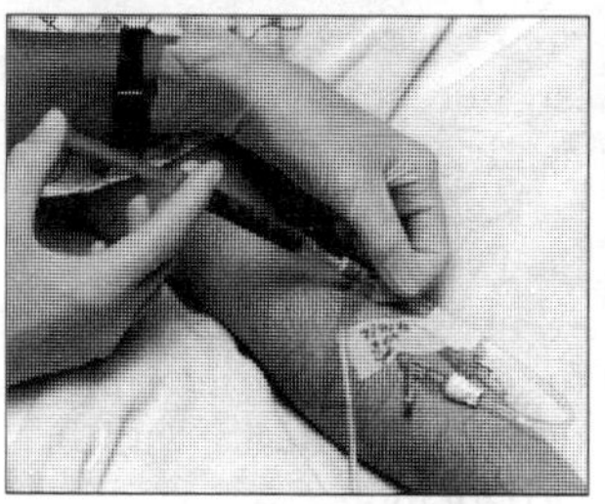

- Remove the needle from the Y-port, open the flow clamp, and read just the primary solution flow rate as prescribed.

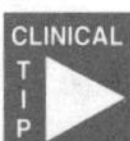

If the delivered drug is incompatible with the primary solution, consult the pharmacist or manufacturer, who may tell you to flush the line with 5 to 10 ml of normal saline solution. Then deliver the drug, reflush the line, and restart the primary solution. If the patient has only a peripheral line and is in cardiac arrest, flush the line with 20 ml of the saline solution, and elevate the site to speed drug circulation. Or, if needed, use a venipuncture device or a T-connector for drug delivery.

Giving an I.V. bolus through an intermittent infusion device

- Gather the following equipment, including a winged infusion set, a tourniquet, alcohol or povidone-iodine sponges, two syringes filled with normal saline solution, one syringe filled with the prescribed drug, 1″ hypoallergenic tape or an adhesive bandage, sterile 2″ × 2″ gauze pads, gloves, and the patient's MAR.
- Put on gloves. Clean the infusion port of the intermittent infusion device with an alcohol sponge.
- Verify the device's patency and proper placement in the vein by inserting the needle of one syringe filled with normal saline solution and aspirating for blood. If no blood appears, apply a tourniquet above the site for about 1 minute. Aspirate again. If blood still doesn't appear, remove the tourniquet and inject the saline solution slowly. Stop if you feel resistance, indicating an occlusion. In this case, insert a new intermittent infusion device.
- Once you aspirate blood, slowly inject the normal saline solution, and observe for signs of infiltration (puffiness or pain at the site). If infiltration occurs, remove and reinsert the intermittent infusion device. After flushing, withdraw the syringe and the needle.
- Insert the needle of the medication-filled syringe into the injection port of the intermittent infusion device. Inject the drug (as shown) at

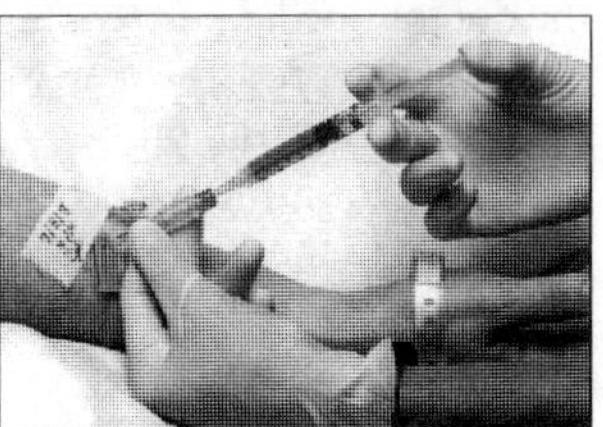

the appropriate rate; then remove this needle. Insert the needle of the other syringe filled with normal saline solution into the injection port.
- Inject the solution to flush the drug through the intermittent infusion device, and remove this needle. Document the procedure on the

patient's MAR. Record the amount of I.V. solution used to dilute the medication and to flush the line on the intake and output record.

Giving an I.V. bolus directly into a vein

- Gather the following equipment, including a winged infusion set, a tourniquet, alcohol or povidone-iodine sponges, two syringes filled with normal saline solution, one syringe filled with the prescribed medication, 1″ hypoallergenic tape or an adhesive bandage, sterile 2″ × 2″ gauze pads, gloves, and the patient's MAR.
- Select the largest vein suitable for an injection. (The larger the vein, the more the drug must be diluted to minimize vascular irritation.) Apply a tourniquet above the injection site to distend the site.
- Put on gloves. Clean the injection site with an alcohol or a povidone-iodine sponge. Work outward from the site in a circular motion to prevent recontaminating the site with skin bacteria.
- Using the winged infusion set, insert the needle, bevel side up, into the vein. Tape the wings in place with a single piece of tape. Depending on the size of the needle, you may or may not see blood in the tubing.
- Attach a syringe filled with normal saline solution to the venipuncture device. Pull back on the plunger to check for blood backflow (as shown).

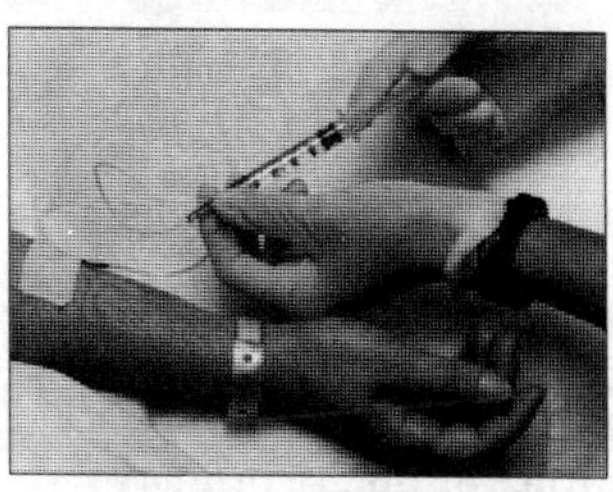

- Once blood flows back into the tubing, remove the tourniquet and slowly inject the normal saline solution into the vein, observing for signs of infiltration. Then remove this syringe from the tubing and attach the medication-filled syringe to the winged venipuncture device. Inject the drug at the appropriate rate.
- Remove the used medication syringe, and attach the second syringe filled with normal saline solution. Flush the winged device with this solution to ensure delivery of all the drug into the vein.
- Remove the winged device from the vein, and cover the site with a sterile 2″ × 2″ gauze pad. Apply pressure to the site for at least 3 minutes to prevent formation of a hematoma. After the bleeding stops, secure the gauze with tape or an adhesive bandage.
- Finally, record the type and amount of drug given and

the times of administration on the MAR. ■

Using a controlled release infusion system

IVAC Corporation's controlled release infusion system (CRIS) offers an alternative way to administer secondary drugs through a primary I.V. line. Connected to the I.V. line between the primary container and the administration set, this adapter-type device allows you to administer a drug dose without using a minibag and a piggyback administration set.

Attach a single-dose vial to the CRIS adapter's spike, and turn the valve handle toward the vial. The primary infusion flows into the vial and mixes with the drug; the mixture then flows down the line into the patient. The CRIS works with any I.V. solution container and any primary set. Use it with unvented I.V. tubing and liquid or reconstituted drugs in single-dose vials (from 5 to 20 ml).

Advantages

Besides being easy to operate, the CRIS adapter can save you time. When using it, you needn't interrupt the primary flow to administer a secondary drug, and you don't have to flush the I.V. tubing between drug deliveries. Because you don't need additional solution containers, you can modify the patient's fluid intake easily and save the time you would usually spend priming secondary sets, adjusting and readjusting flow rates, and handling secondary containers. What's more, the adapter saves the space you would need for storing minibags and secondary I.V. sets.

Getting ready

- To use the CRIS adapter, the patient must have a primary I.V. line in place. Gather the additional equipment you'll need, including the CRIS adapter, liquid or reconstituted medication in a single-dose vial (in quantities ranging from 5 to 20 ml, as ordered), alcohol sponges, and the patient's medication administration record (MAR). Depending on the situation, you may also need time tape, an infusion pump, or unvented tubing.
- Compare the order on the MAR with the doctor's order on the patient's chart. Ask the patient his name, and compare the name, room number, and bed number on the MAR with the information on the patient's identification bracelet.
- Explain the procedure to the patient.

- Check that the I.V. setup has unvented tubing. If the setup has vented tubing, replace it with the appropriate apparatus.

Installing the adapter on the I.V. line

- Push, don't twist, the spike of the administration set into the adapter's lower port.
- Pick up the single-dose vial of the drug (as ordered) and an alcohol sponge. Remove the temporary cover and clean the vial's diaphragm with the alcohol sponge.
- With a twisting motion, remove the protective cover from the spike, and insert the spike into the vial.

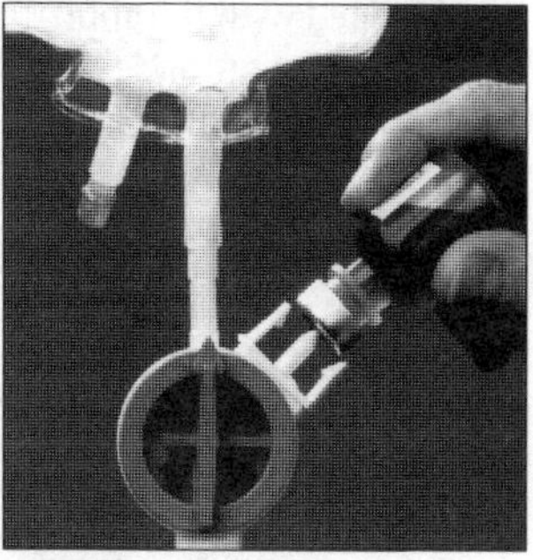

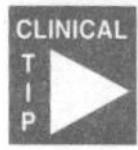

If you encounter resistance, puncture the diaphragm with a needle to release air.

Giving the infusion

- Make sure that the primary container of I.V. solution holds at least 60 ml of fluid (the volume needed to deliver the dose and flush the system).
- Then, to begin drug delivery, turn the CRIS's valve handle toward the vial until you feel resistance. Click the valve into the 2 o'clock position.

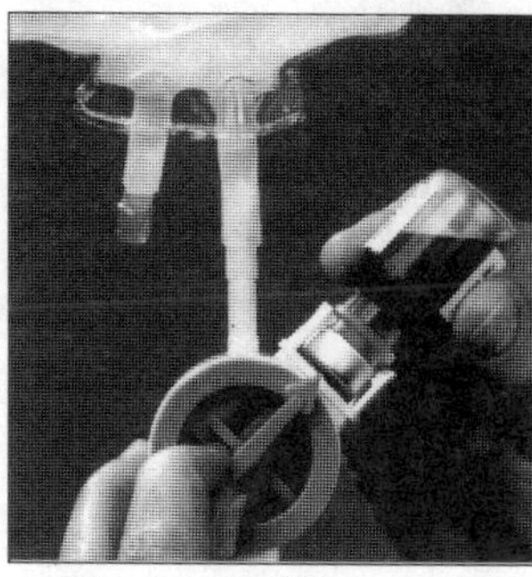

- Calculate the flow rate, and mark the primary container to indicate the amount that should be infused. Attach a time tape, or set the infusion pump appropriately.
- After the drug is delivered, leave the vial in place and keep the valve handle in the 2 o'clock position until the patient needs another dose. (*Note:* The primary infusion flows through the vial; therefore, the vial doesn't empty.) Leaving the vial in place keeps the vial's spike sterile.
- Before giving another drug dose, make sure that the primary I.V. container holds at least 60 ml of fluid. Then turn the valve handle to the 12 o'clock position. Adjust the fluid level of the drip chamber, if necessary.
- If the vial inadvertently becomes pressurized during drug reconstitution, if the

drug produces gas, or if you squeeze the drip chamber with the valve still set at 2 o'clock, the backcheck valve will prevent reflux of the drug solution into the primary container.

- Remove the used drug vial, and replace it with a new one. Turn the valve handle back to the 2 o'clock position. Adjust the flow rate, if necessary.
- Change the CRIS adapter when you change the administration set — every 48 hours or according to facility policy.

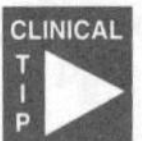

You can use the CRIS adapter on a primary I.V. line while delivering another drug through a piggyback set. ■

Delivering drugs with a syringe pump

You may find a syringe pump useful when you're administering small volumes of medication intermittently or continuously. Able to deliver fluid very slowly, the syringe pump is ideal for infants and children and for use in oncology and emergency departments and in labor and delivery settings.

Compact and portable, the syringe pump uses a disposable syringe with a 50-ml volume limit and operates on either AC power or with a rechargeable battery. Typically, a motor-driven lead screw or gear mechanism controls the syringe's plunger. The motor's speed determines how quickly the plunger moves and, in turn, the infusion rate. Keep in mind that the pump lacks an air detector, so make sure that you eliminate all air bubbles from the syringe, tubing, and needle before you start the infusion.

Getting ready

- Gather the following equipment at the patient's bedside, including the syringe pump, a sterile syringe extension set, a 50-ml syringe labeled and prefilled with the appropriate medication, a 20G 1″ needle, alcohol sponges, clean gloves, hypoallergenic tape, and the patient's medication administration record (MAR).
- Explain the procedure to the patient, and wash your hands.
- Confirm the patient's identity by asking him his name and comparing the name, room number, and bed number on his identification bracelet with the information on his MAR. Then match the label on the medication syringe with the drug ordered on the MAR.

Preparing the syringe

- Connect the prefilled syringe to the extension set, using the set's female luer-lock connector. To prime the extension set, grasp the occlusion-sensing disk between your thumb and forefinger. Hold the membrane of the disk flat, and rub your thumb over the membrane.
- With your other hand, push in the syringe's plunger. Tap the disk, and push the plunger in again to completely expel trapped air.

CLINICAL TIP Push the plunger to at least the 50 ml mark so that the syringe will fit into the clamp.

- Turn on the pump by pressing the ON/OFF control. The pump will beep to confirm that it's functioning. When "Pr 1" appears in the message display window, open the syringe clamp, and put the syringe (tip first) in the pump's cradle. Align the notch on the plunger with the track on the pump's case, and close the clamp over the end of the plunger. The next message to appear will read "Pr 2." This indicates that you may insert the occlusion-sensing disk into the disk retainer.
- Insert the occlusion-sensing disk into the disk retainer on the end of the pump's case. Set the flow rate and the volume to bc infused after the message "Pr 3" appears in the display window.
- Press the START/STOP or any of the MILLILITERS/HOUR controls to display the last rate selected. Press the appropriate MILLILITERS/HOUR controls (on the model shown below, they're up or down arrows) to enter the new flow rate. Press the MI? (volume infused) control to display the previous volume infused. Press the ML? and M/L (clear volume) controls to reset the volume infused to zero.

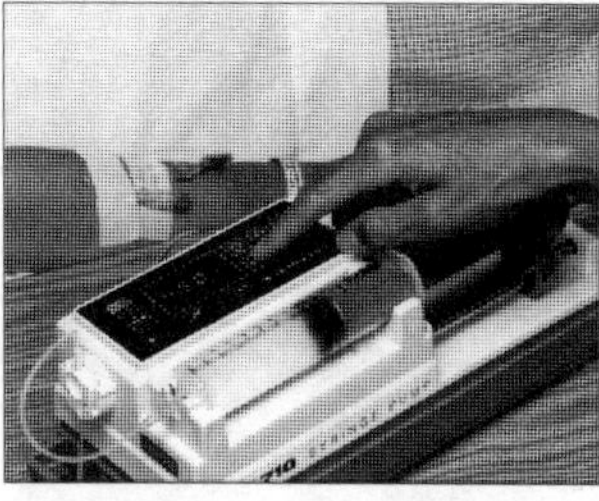

Infusing the drug

- Put the pump on the same side of the bed as the I.V. setup to avoid crisscrossing I.V. lines over the patient. Put on gloves, and attach a 20G needle to the male luer-lock connector of the I.V. extension set. Wipe the injection port with an alcohol sponge.
- Then insert the needle into the patient's I.V. port or intermittent infusion device. Secure the needle and tubing using hypoallergenic tape, according to facility policy. Then press the START/STOP control to begin the infusion. Periodically check the pa-

Correcting syringe pump problems

PROBLEM	POSSIBLE CAUSE	SOLUTION
Battery light flashing and audible alarm	The battery is losing its charge.	Plug the pump into a wall outlet, and turn the power off and on. You may have to wait several minutes before the pump will function.
Battery light flashing while operating on AC power	The pump has blown a fuse or has malfunctioned.	Check the fuses. If you replace the fuse and it blows again, call for service.
No display and audible alarm when turning pump on	The pump battery is too low.	Plug the pump into a wall outlet. You may have to wait several minutes before the pump will function.
No display and audible alarm with pump on hold	The 2-minute hold limit passed without an intervention, such as opening the clamp or changing one of the controls.	Press START/STOP once to silence the alarm and again when you're ready to restart the infusion.

tient's I.V. line for patency and the site for infiltration.
- To change the rate or temporarily stop the infusion, press START/STOP. A flashing "H" will appear on the right side of the message display window, and the pump will sound a repeated click, indicating that it has stopped infusing. The pump will stay on hold for 2 minutes. To change the rate, press the appropriate MILLILITERS/HOUR arrows. Then restart the infusion by pressing START/STOP. (See *Correcting syringe pump problems.*)
- When the syringe is almost empty, the infusion indicator (located on the right side of the message display window) will change to half-size and a repeated double click tone will sound.
- To continue the infusion, put the pump on hold and replace the syringe. When all the ordered drug has been infused, turn off the pump, and disconnect the tubing from the patient. If the patient has an intermittent infusion device, flush it according to facility policy.
- Document the procedure. ■

How can I avoid needle-stick injuries?

Currently, I.V. system technology focuses on housings that either shield (recess) the needle or slide over it. (See *Preventing needle-sticks,* page 424.) The latest trend involves needleless systems, which eliminate the steel needle. These use a plastic "needle" or a special valve to connect a syringe or piggyback tubing to I.V. tubing or into an intermittent-infusion cap to infuse solutions. You can use needleless systems for every aspect of I.V. therapy except for piercing the skin.

Because you use many more needles to give drugs and infusions than to access a vein directly, these devices greatly increase your safety. And they make connecting or disposing of I.V. components less risky. Here's a look at the latest products and how they work.

Needle-housing systems

Two types of housing systems are over-the-needle catheters and recessed-needle units.

Over-the-needle catheters

At least two manufacturers market protective over-the-needle catheters. After venipuncture, both devices enclose the sharp tip of the stylet needle with a plastic cover. With Critikon's Protectiv I.V. Catheter Safety System, a plastic chamber slides over the stylet needle. Becton Dickinson offers the Insyte Saf-T-Cath, which has a plastic shield that slides over the

Preventing needle sticks

The latest I.V. products, some of which are shown here, make it easier than ever to avoid needle sticks.

Critikon's Protectiv I.V. Catheter Safety System

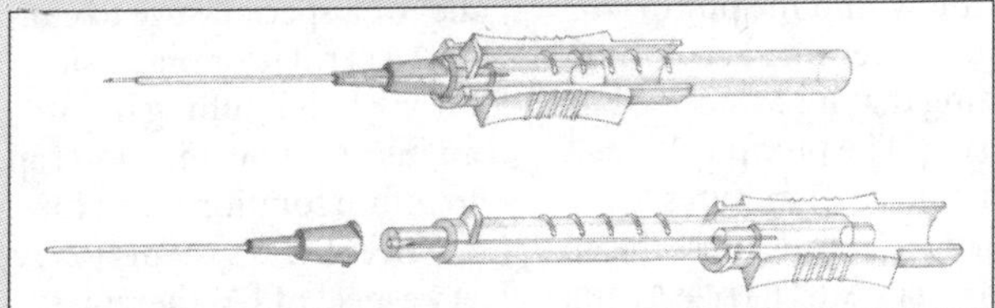

Becton Dickinson's Insyte Saf-T-Cath

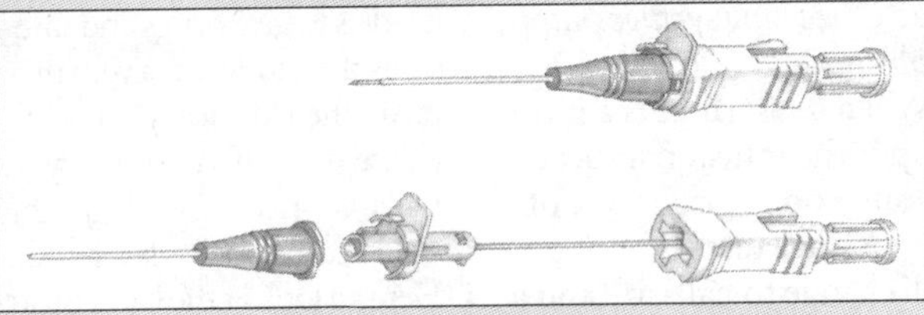

Centurion's Kleen-Needle

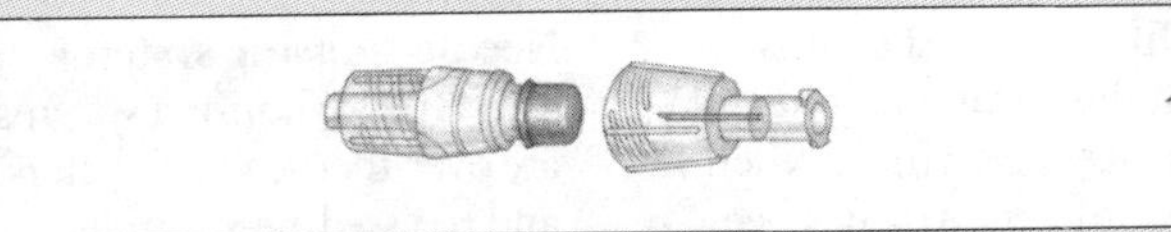

Baxter Healthcare's Lever Lock

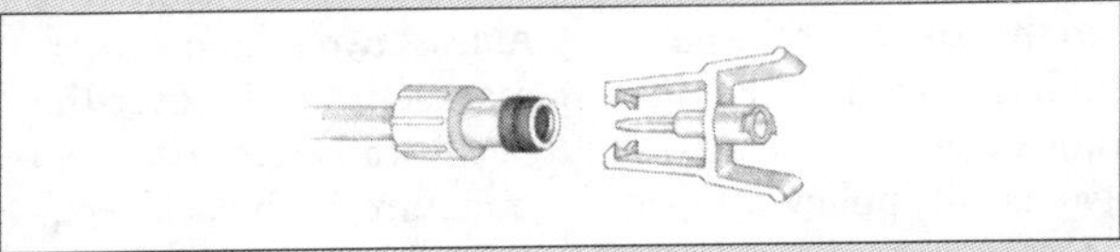

ICU Medical's Clave

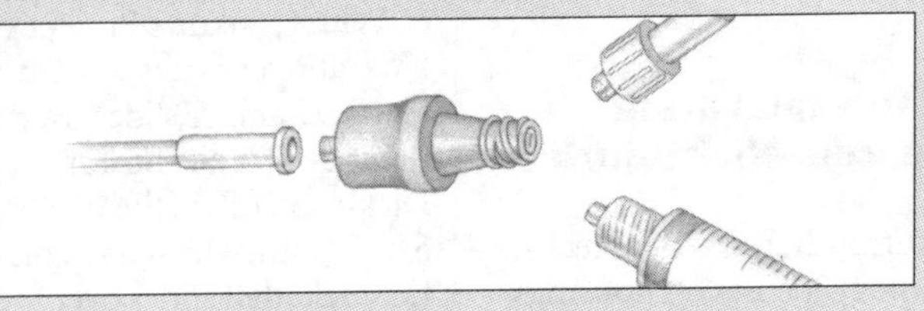

tip of the stylet when the stylet is retracted.

Recessed-needle units

You can use recessed-needle units to connect I.V. tubing to an intermittent-infusion cap or a primary Y-site. These devices consist of a housing unit with a recessed steel needle that sits inside the housing. To use the system, attach a syringe or primary or secondary tubing to the end of the device. Then insert the recessed needle into an intermittent-infusion cap or a Y-site, and lock the housing over the infusion cap or the Y-site. Centurion's Kleen-Needle and Abbott Laboratories' LifeShield are two recessed-needle systems.

Needleless systems

Such needleless systems use rubber diaphragms, valves, or connectors.

Diaphragm systems

These use a slitted rubber diaphragm that looks like a conventional intermittent-infusion cap. The diaphragm fits over the catheter hub. You can access the diaphragm in two ways. The first involves a plastic piercing needle enclosed in a plastic housing unit that resembles a clothespin, such as Baxter Healthcare's Lever Lock. The second has a plastic needle covered with a drum-type plastic housing unit. With both, you penetrate the slitted rubber septum of the diaphragm cap with the plastic needle. The plastic housing secures the device to the diaphragm.

Nondiaphragm systems

Another system involves valve technology and doesn't use a rubber diaphragm. Burron Medical's Safsite, for example, has a valve with a plastic male adapter on one end and a female adapter on the other. The male adapter screws into the hub of the catheter. The female adapter accepts a syringe or I.V. tubing. The system's two-way valve opens to allow you to aspirate or infuse fluid and closes when you remove the syringe or tubing. To maintain sterility, put a dead-end cap over the female adapter between uses. ■

When should I use a filter?

Using an in-line filter helps reduce the risk of phlebitis by removing impurities from the I.V. solution. But because in-line filters are expensive and their installation cumbersome and time-consuming, they're not yet routinely used. Many health care facilities require a filter only for administration of an admixture. If you're unsure of whether or not to use a filter, check the policy of your health care facility.

When to use a filter

Expect to use an in-line I.V. filter when:

- administering solution to an immunocompromised patient.
- providing total parenteral nutrition.
- using additives comprising many separate particles, such as antibiotics requiring reconstitution or when administering several additives.
- repeatedly using rubber injection sites or plastic diaphragms.

Special considerations

- Be sure to change the in-line filter according to the manufacturer's recommendations (typically every 24 to 96 hours). If you don't, bacteria trapped in the filter release an endotoxin, a pyrogen small enough to pass through the filter into the bloodstream.
- When infusing lipid emulsions and albumin mixed with nutritional solutions, use an add-on filter with a larger pore size (1 to 1.2 microns).

When not to use a filter

Don't use an in-line filter when:

- administering solutions with large particles that will clog a filter — for example, blood and its components, suspensions, lipid emulsions, and high-molecular volume plasma expanders.
- administering 5 mg or less of a drug because the filter may absorb the drug.

When to use a filter needle

Use a filter needle when:

- mixing and drawing up drugs in powder form.
- removing a reconstituted drug from a vial to filter out any glass or undissolved particles (injecting foreign particles into a patient's peripheral vein could cause an embolism).
- withdrawing drugs from a glass ampule (if the top of the ampule breaks off, microscopic slivers of glass could fall into the drug solution). Before withdrawing a drug from an ampule, place the filter needle on the syringe. Remove and discard it before injecting the drug into the diluent. ■

How do I choose the right venipuncture device?

The venipuncture device you choose hinges on several factors, including your patient's age, weight, and condition. Select the device with the shortest length and the smallest diameter that allows for proper administration of the solution. Selection also depends on the solution to be infused, the frequency and duration of the infusion, and the types of veins available. (See *Comparing peripheral venipuncture devices*, page 428.)

Choose from among three types of venipuncture devices: an over-the-needle catheter, a through-the-needle catheter, and a winged infusion set.

Over-the-needle catheter

- This is the most commonly used device for peripheral I.V. therapy.
- It's indicated mainly for long-term therapy for the active or agitated patient.
- An over-the-needle catheter consists of a plastic outer catheter and an inner needle that extends just beyond the catheter; the needle is withdrawn after insertion, leaving the catheter in place.
- It's available in lengths of 1", 1¼", and 2" and diameters of 14G to 26G.

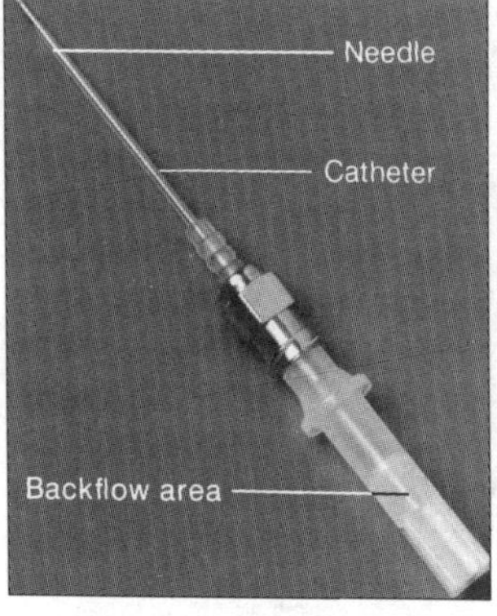

Through-the-needle catheter

- This device is used for placement in long arm veins.
- It's used if venous access is poor and for giving caustic drugs or hypotonic solutions.
- It consists of a long, plastic radiopaque catheter whose tip lies inside the cannula of an 1½" to 2" introducer needle.
- A plastic sleeve protects the catheter from surface contamination when the catheter is gently pushed into the vein after the needle is in place.
- Then the needle is withdrawn and secured outside the skin with a plastic bevel cover.
- Catheter placement is confirmed by chest X-ray.
- It's available in 8" to 12" lengths and 14G to 19G diameters.

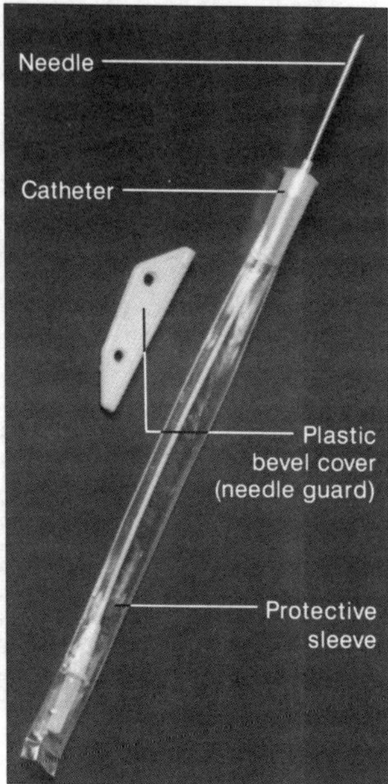

Comparing peripheral venipuncture devices

DEVICE	ADVANTAGES	DISADVANTAGES
Over-the-needle catheter	▪ Accidental vein puncture less likely than with a needle. ▪ Needle can be removed after insertion, reducing the risk of catheter embolus. ▪ Once in place, catheter is more comfortable than a needle. ▪ Device holds a radiopaque thread for easy location by X-ray.	▪ Insertion is more difficult than with other devices. ▪ Device is prone to surface contamination.
Through-the-needle catheter	▪ Accidental puncture of the vein is less likely than with a needle. ▪ Once in place, catheter is more comfortable than a needle. ▪ Tubing holds a radiopaque thread for easy location by X-ray.	▪ Leakage may occur at the insertion site. ▪ If a needle guard isn't used, the catheter may break. ▪ Catheter embolus can occur if the catheter is withdrawn through the needle.
Winged infusion set	▪ Device is easy to insert. ▪ Device is ideal for delivering medication by I.V. push. ▪ Patient feels little discomfort on insertion. ▪ Winged inserter reduces the risk of touch contamination.	▪ Patient is at higher risk for infiltration with this device. ▪ Device isn't suitable for delivery of highly viscous liquids or for long-term therapy.

Winged infusion set

- This device is indicated when using the patient's hand veins for infusion.
- It consists of a winged, over-the-needle catheter, with short, small-bore tubing between the catheter and the hub.
- Flexible wings can be grasped to ease insertion.
- It's available in a ¾″ length with narrow-gauge needles and a 1″ length with wider gauge needles.
- Types include heparin lock, butterfly needle, and the Intima.

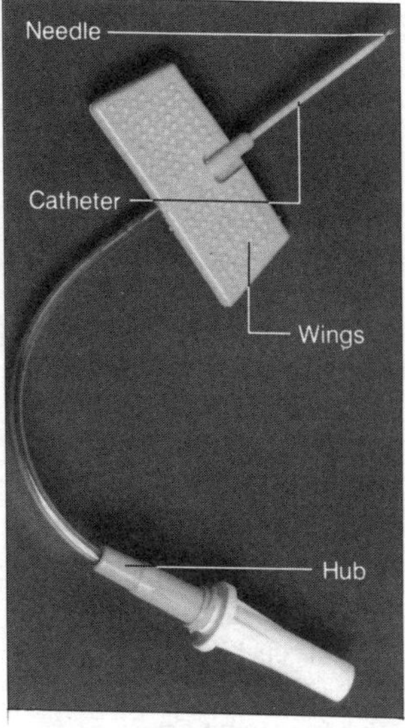

Heparin lock

- This intermittent infusion device consists of a steel needle and tubing, which ends in a resealable, rubber injection port.
- The needle remains in the patient's vein — a plastic catheter isn't used.

Butterfly needle

- Originally designed for children and elderly patients, this device can be used for any patient who's in stable condition, has adequate veins, and requires short-term I.V. therapy.
- A butterfly needle consists of a thin-walled device with no hub, which lies flat on the skin.
- It's available in ¾″ length and diameters ranging from 16G to 27G.
- A butterfly needle is also called a winged steel needle.

Intima

- This device allows continuous and intermittent therapy or simultaneous infusion of two compatible solutions.
- It consists of a Y-shaped device with a latex cap.
- The Intima is available in diameters ranging from 16G to 24G. ■

How do I choose the best venipuncture site?

Successful I.V. therapy depends on selecting the best possible venipuncture site. Consider the vein's location and condition, the purpose of the infusion, and the duration of the therapy. Also assess whether the patient can cooperate and determine which site he prefers. (See *Comparing venipuncture sites,* pages 431 to 433.)

Selecting a vein

- If possible, choose a vein in the patient's nondominant arm or hand. The best sites are the cephalic and basilic veins in the lower arm and the veins in the dorsum of the hand.
- Choose antecubital veins if no other veins are available, if you need to accommodate a large-bore needle, or if you must administer drugs requiring large volume dilution.
- If a patient will require long-term I.V. therapy, get maximum use from his arm veins by starting therapy in a hand vein and then moving to sites farther up his arm as necessary.

Special considerations

- The least favored venipuncture sites are leg and foot veins because of the increased risk of thrombophlebitis.
- Some conditions contraindicate insertion of a peripheral I.V. line. These include a sclerotic vein, an edematous or impaired arm or hand, the arm on the affected side of a mastectomy patient, burns in the area, or an arteriovenous fistula.
- When you're performing a venipuncture in an arm or leg previously used for I.V. therapy — or in a previously injured vein — take care to insert the line proximal to the former site. ■

How can I locate hard-to-find veins?

Sometimes, palpation and visualization techniques aren't enough to help you find an appropriate peripheral vein for I.V. therapy. The Landry Vein Light Venoscope helps you locate veins that otherwise aren't easily seen or palpated. It illuminates the subcutaneous tissue while freeing your hands to perform venipuncture.

This device, which has two fiber-optic probes that rest on the skin a few inches apart, shines intense beams into the patient's subcutaneous tissue. Veins absorb the light and appear as dark lines against the pinkish, illuminated skin, thus giving you easy targets for venipuncture.

Disadvantages and advantages

- Using the Landry Venoscope is less convenient than palpation and visualization techniques in some patients.

(Text continues on page 434.)

Comparing venipuncture sites

SITE	ADVANTAGES	DISADVANTAGES
Basilic veins Run along ulnar side of forearm and upper arm	▪ Straight, strong veins suitable for large-gauge devices	▪ Is uncomfortable position for patient during insertion. ▪ Penetration of dermal layer, where nerve endings are, causes pain. ▪ Veins tend to roll during insertion.
Cephalic veins Run along radial side of forearm and upper arm	▪ Large veins that readily accept large-gauge needles ▪ Don't impair mobility	▪ Veins tend to roll during insertion. ▪ Proximity to elbow may decrease joint mobility.
Antecubital veins Located in antecubital fossa (median cephalic, on radial side, median basilic on ulnar side, and median cubital in front of elbow)	▪ Large veins that facilitate drawing blood ▪ Often visible or palpable in children when other veins won't dilate ▪ May be used in an emergency or as a last resort	▪ Is difficult to splint elbow area with arm board. ▪ Median cephalic vein crosses in front of brachial artery. ▪ Veins may be small and scarred if blood is drawn frequently from same site.

Comparing venipuncture sites *(continued)*

SITE	ADVANTAGES	DISADVANTAGES
Accessory cephalic veins Run along radial bone as a continuation of metacarpal veins of the thumb	▪ Large veins that readily accept large-gauge needles ▪ Don't impair mobility ▪ Veins don't require arm board in older child or adult	▪ Sometimes it's difficult to position catheter flush with skin. ▪ Device is placed at bend of wrist, so movement is uncomfortable.
Median antebrachial veins Begin at the palm and run along ulnar side of forearm	▪ Veins that hold winged needles well ▪ A last resort when no other site is available	▪ Many nerve endings in area may cause painful insertion. ▪ Infiltration occurs easily in this area, which increases the risk of nerve damage.
Metacarpal veins Located on dorsum of hand; formed by union of digital veins between knuckles	▪ Easily accessible veins that lie flat on back of hand ▪ In adult or large child, bones of hand act as splint	▪ Wrist mobility is decreased unless a short catheter is used. ▪ Many nerve endings in the hand may cause painful insertion. ▪ Site becomes inflamed easily.

Comparing venipuncture sites *(continued)*

SITE	ADVANTAGES	DISADVANTAGES
Digital veins Run along lateral and dorsal surfaces of fingers	▪ May be used for brief therapy ▪ May be used when other sites aren't available	▪ Fingers must be splinted with a tongue blade, impairing hand mobility. ▪ Is uncomfortable for patient. ▪ Infiltration occurs easily. ▪ Can't be used if metacarpal veins have already been used.
Great saphenous veins Located at internal malleolus	▪ Large veins that are excellent for venipuncture	▪ May impair lower leg circulation. ▪ Walking is difficult with device in place. ▪ Is increased risk of deep-vein thrombosis.
Dorsal venous network Located on dorsal surface of foot	▪ Suitable for infants and toddlers	▪ Veins may be difficult to see if edema is present. ▪ Walking is difficult with device in place. ▪ Is heightened risk of deep-vein thrombosis.

- It must be used in a dimly lit or dark environment, which can make it hard to see.
- The Venoscope helps you see peripheral veins that aren't readily visible or are hard to detect by palpation.
- The device is useful for critically ill and elderly patients who require multiple attempts for successful venipuncture.
- The Venoscope makes veins easier to see, and it secures the vessels and prevents them from rolling.
- The Venoscope reveals the vein's size, the presence of bifurcations, and unusual angles, which helps you choose the right size catheter.
- It can be used on patients of any age or size and on virtually any part of the body.

Getting ready
First, attach disposable tips, or skids, to the fiber-optic arms. Replace the skids for each patient to prevent spreading infection.

Locating a vein
- Turn off the lights or dim them to the lowest level. Draw the shades or pull the curtains to block out sunlight.
- Apply a tourniquet in the usual manner.
- Put the Venoscope on its brightest setting, and position the adjustable fiber-optic probes a finger's length apart, tilted toward each other. Run the probes across the skin. Veins will appear as dark lines.

Verifying a vein
- Push the probes down on each side of the vein you intend to use. You'll know it's a vein if it collapses and disappears, then reappears when you relieve the pressure. Keep in mind that a vein that doesn't collapse and refill may be thrombosed from previous unsuccessful venipuncture attempts or long-term I.V. therapy. Try finding another one.
- Once you've verified a vein, use the twin beams to track it proximally to ensure a path for the I.V. catheter.

Securing the Venoscope
Use the Velcro straps to secure the Venoscope at the planned puncture site. Tighten it enough to slightly depress the skin — but not so much that the vein collapses.

Performing venipuncture
- Besides the twin beams, the Venoscope has a tiny spotlight to guide you while you prepare the skin for venipuncture and assess needle bevel position.
- Pull the skin back, away from the insertion site. Insert the catheter at a point just beyond the spot between the

probes, angling the catheter down slightly as you begin the insertion, as shown.

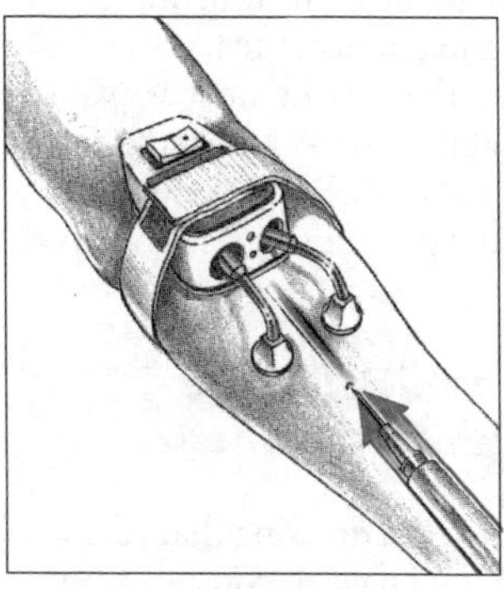

Threading the catheter
After you've penetrated the vein, use the spotlight while you check for blood return. Reduce the angle of approach before advancing the catheter farther; then thread the catheter, and complete the procedure as you normally would. Now you can turn the room lights back on. ■

How can I prevent veins from rolling?

Prevent the vein from rolling by maintaining it in a taut, stable, distended position. Because the wrist and hands are flexible, hand veins are generally easier to immobilize than arm veins. Hand veins may also be easier to cannulate because they're usually surrounded with less fatty tissue. And they enlarge with age as they lose their elasticity, providing a bigger target. Use these techniques to immobilize hand and arm veins:

- To immobilize a hand vein, grasp the patient's hand with your nondominant hand. Place your fingers under his palm and fingers and your thumb on top of his fingers below the knuckles. Pull his hand downward to flex his wrist, creating an arch. To maintain the proper angle, make sure his elbow remains on the bed. Use your thumb to stretch the skin over the knuckles to stabilize the vein. Grip the patient's hand firmly throughout the venipuncture.
- To stabilize the cephalic vein along the thumb side of the arm, ask the patient to clench his fist. Grasp his fist and pull it laterally downward. Although this maneuver may make the vein harder to see, it keeps it stable, which is crucial. ■

What's the easiest way to cannulate a vein?

Although a deep arm vein is a challenge to cannulate, sometimes you have no choice because it's the only vein that's available. However, cannulating an arm vein has the virtue of freeing the patient's hand so that he can move around freely. An arm vein is also less likely to become phlebitic.

When you stretch a deep arm vein to immobilize it, it may seem to disappear because stretching flattens it slightly. So you must be able to "see" it by palpating it with your fingers.

Cannulating a deep vein

To cannulate a deep vein that is palpable but hard to see, follow these steps:

- Ask the patient to clench his fist. Stretch the extremity and vein while placing the fingers of your nondominant hand on top of the vein where the shaft of the catheter will lie. Using moderate pressure, retract the skin away from the insertion site to stabilize the vein.
- Grasp the catheter with your fingers, while touching only the hub, so that you can easily see the blood return. Aim the catheter tip at the vein you feel under your fingers, and insert it in one smooth, aggressive motion.
- Use your nondominant hand to continue stretching the vein. Decrease the angle of insertion, and continue advancing the catheter until you see blood return in the hub, indicating that the tip has entered the vein.
- Place a protective pad under the hub; then remove the stylet. Blood will flow into the backflow chamber. If the vein or catheter is large, the chamber may fill very rapidly.
- Remove the tourniquet and connect the I.V. tubing to the hub. Remove your gloves; apply a dressing, tape, and a label; and document the procedure. ■

Which I.V. site dressing is better?

Select a dressing that you won't have to constantly manipulate to check the site — such handling can lead to contamination.

Several studies have shown that transparent dressings tend to keep an I.V. device more stable and, in the long run, are less costly to maintain than gauze dressings. Because you can see the insertion site through a transparent dressing, you'll save time checking it as well.

Although all I.V. site dressings should be changed at least once every 48 hours, one study suggests that transparent dressings can be worn for a longer time than gauze dressings without increasing the risk of contamination. The study found that a transparent dressing worn for up to 7 days was comparable to a gauze dressing worn for an average of 2½ days — in terms of incidence of infections and phlebitis. ■

Which flushing solution should I use?

Recommended practices for maintaining patency of a heparin lock vary, depending on your health care facility's policy. According to results of a nationwide practice survey, 40% of the respondents use 100 units/ml of heparin to flush heparin locks; 37%, 10 units/ml of heparin; and 18%, normal saline solution.

If you are giving a bolus injection of a drug that's incompatible with D_5W, such as diazepam or phenytoin, flush the device with normal saline solution. ■

Is it all right to irrigate a peripheral I.V. line?

The possibility of pulmonary emboli and infection makes peripheral I.V. line irrigation a controversial issue. Pulmonary emboli can occur if irrigation pushes a clot into the pulmonary vasculature. Infection may occur if bacteria colonizes the occluding clot.

However, some clinicians argue that pulmonary emboli aren't likely to occur because clots typically originate in the legs' deep veins — not in the veins normally used for I.V. insertion. What's more, the likelihood of infection is low because a clot in an I.V. catheter typically isn't established long enough to colonize bacteria. Those in favor of I.V. irrigation consider the risks slight when compared with the alternative of restarting the I.V.

Aspiration and irrigation

All clinicians, however, agree that you should never risk forcing a blood clot into the bloodstream by using high irrigation pressure. So, if you observe an occlusion in your patient's I.V. line, use the aspiration and irrigation procedure. If you're still unable to irrigate the line, discontinue it. ■

How can I prevent uncontrolled I.V. flow?

Let's suppose that you're caring for a patient who's receiving a drug through an electronic infusion device. His gown needs changing, but it doesn't have sleeve snaps. So you have to deactivate the infusion device, clamp and remove the tubing, remove the fluid bag from the I.V. pole, and pull the I.V. bag and tubing through the sleeve — a tiresome job.

Actually, the task is more than tiresome — it's dangerous. In one documented case, a nurse deactivated an

I.V. infusion device, and her patient died. Either she didn't secure the roller clamp correctly or it malfunctioned, causing rapid, uncontrolled drug flow into the patient.

No safety standards
Standards are nonexistent for I.V. infusion devices and sets, so many systems don't have a free-flow safety mechanism. Because safer infusion systems are typically more expensive, some facilities may use them only in labor and delivery units or critical care areas or to give drugs with narrow therapeutic windows. This increases your risk for error because you may get accustomed to using the safer equipment and consequently mistake a safe system for an unsafe one.

To protect your patient and yourself, be extremely careful when using infusion devices — especially if you're unfamiliar with a facility's equipment because you're on a temporary assignment. Your caution is essential until free-flow protected equipment becomes the standard in all facilities. ■

How can I prevent clotted I.V. lines?

Here are some helpful hints to avoid clotted I.V. lines.

Insert the catheter correctly
When starting an I.V. line, insert the catheter with its tip away from the extremity's joints. This helps prevent catheter kinking and stasis of blood at its tip.

Use heparin locks
Use heparin locks instead of slow keep-vein-open I.V. lines as much as possible. If your patient must have a keep-vein-open I.V. line, open the clamp wide for a fast flush for 3 to 4 seconds every few hours (providing the medication in the I.V. fluid would produce no ill effects).

Flush immediately
Flush I.V. lines or heparin locks with either heparin or normal saline immediately after infusion of any solution or drug, especially drugs which tend to precipitate, such as phenytoin, diazepam, or antibiotics.

Elevate the solution
To prevent blood from backing up and clotting in the catheter or tubing, keep the I.V. solution elevated at least 36″ (91 cm) above the cathe-

ter's insertion site. If your patient is active, he's especially vulnerable to blood backup because activity increases peripheral venous pressure. Also, movement may cause the catheter tip to lodge against the vein wall, preventing I.V. flow.

Retract the catheter

If the I.V. rate is sluggish despite efforts to improve it, try this: Remove the tape and dressing from the catheter insertion site; then pull the catheter out about ¼″ (5 mm). This helps if the catheter is lodged against a vein wall or located in a valve or narrow section of a vein.

Never attempt to push the catheter farther into the vein because doing so will introduce bacteria into the bloodstream. ■

How can I prevent I.V. tubing contamination?

Constant manipulation of an I.V. device may cause contamination as well as separation of the I.V. tubing from the catheter hub. Multiple I.V. boluses (or pushes) and tubing changes also increase the risk of in-line contamination. You can reduce that risk by following these guidelines:

- Use strict aseptic technique when changing I.V. tubing, particularly when connecting (or disconnecting) the tubing to the solution container or catheter hub. Because the catheter can easily shift during this procedure, extravasation often occurs.
- Change the catheter and primary tubing simultaneously whenever possible.
- When piggybacking a solution into the injection port, wipe the port with an alcohol sponge before inserting the needle.
- When a piggyback solution is discontinued (and before starting a new infusion), take precautions in removing the I.V. needle and extension set, which may harbor contaminants. Dispose of them properly to protect other personnel and equipment from contact with solutions or contaminated blood.
- Change I.V. tubing every 48 hours, as recommended by the Intravenous Nurses Society. This procedure is often neglected because of rotating staffing practices, use of agency nurses, random accountability for performing this task, and failure to label tubing.
- Never leave a contaminated needle or I.V. dressing attached to I.V. tubing that's not being used; doing so may cause upward contamination of the entire tubing set and the solution.

- Never let I.V. tubing touch the floor; contamination may occur through microscopic pores in the tubing. ■

How can I ensure patient safety when giving a bolus injection?

For certain drugs, the manufacturer supplies specific administration directions, such as the appropriate injection rate. If you don't have such directions, keep the following precautions in mind:

- Don't give an I.V. bolus when you need to dilute a drug — an antibiotic or a vitamin, for example — in a large volume parenteral solution before it enters the bloodstream.
- Avoid giving an I.V. bolus whenever the rapid administration of a drug, such as potassium chloride, could be life-threatening.
- Finish each bolus injection by recording the type and amount of drug given and the administration times on the patient's medication administration record. Record all I.V. solutions used to dilute the drug and to flush the line on the patient's intake and output record.
- Keep in mind that drug tolerance declines in patients with decreased cardiac output, diminished urine output, pulmonary congestion, or generalized edema. To compensate, you may need to administer the drug at a slower rate. ■

How can I piggyback an incompatible drug safely?

If you are delivering a piggyback drug that's incompatible with the primary I.V. solution, consult the pharmacist, and read the manufacturer's directions. You should be able to flush the line with 5 to 10 ml of normal saline solution, administer the drug, flush the line again, and then restart the flow of the primary I.V. solution.

If you were told by the pharmacist not to do this, insert a venipuncture device to deliver the medication or use a T-connector. ■

CENTRAL VENOUS THERAPY

Giving drugs through a VAP

Surgically placed beneath a patient's skin, an implanted vascular access port (VAP) permits intermittent long-term delivery of medications (including chemotherapeutic agents), I.V. fluids, total parenteral nutrition, or blood products through a central venous line.

Getting ready

- Gather the following equipment, including a non-coring needle of appropriate type and gauge (usually a straight or right-angle Huber needle), extension tubing with clamp (this equipment may already be attached to the Huber needle), gloves, two masks, alcohol sponges, povidone-iodine swabs, two 10-ml syringes prefilled with normal saline solution, a 5-ml syringe prefilled with heparin flush solution, a local anesthetic (such as 1% or 2% lidocaine), a tuberculin syringe, sterile drapes, sterile 2″ × 2″ gauze pads, and the patient's medication administration record (MAR).
- Take the equipment to the patient's bedside. Identify the patient by asking his name and checking his identification bracelet. Explain the procedure, and wash your hands. Put on a mask, and have the patient wear one too. Also put on gloves.
- Inspect the area around the port for signs of infection and skin breakdown.
- Clean the area with an alcohol sponge. Start at the center of the port and work outward for 4″ to 5″ (10 to 13 cm), using a firm, circular motion. Repeat this procedure two more times, using a new alcohol sponge each time.
- Then clean the area the same way with the povidone-iodine swabs. Remove any excess povidone-iodine by dabbing the area with a sterile gauze pad.
- If your facility's policy calls for a local anesthetic, check the patient's MAR for possible allergies. As indicated and as ordered, numb the insertion site by injecting 0.1 ml of lidocaine (without epinephrine), using a tuberculin syringe.
- Place a sterile drape around the patient. Attach one of the 10-ml prefilled syringes containing normal saline solution to the end of the extension tubing attached to the non-coring needle. Fill the tubing with the solution and close the clamp.

Using a top-entry VAP

- To use a top-entry VAP, palpate the area over the port to locate the septum. Anchor the port between the thumb and first two fingers of your nondominant hand. Use your dominant hand to aim the non-coring needle at the center of the VAP, and insert it perpendicular to the port's septum. Push the needle through the skin and septum until you reach the bottom of the reservoir.

- Check for correct needle placement by aspirating for blood return. If you see a blood return, inject 5 ml of heparin flush solution. If you don't see a blood return, remove the needle and aspirate again.

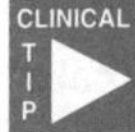

Inability to obtain blood suggests that the catheter leading from the VAP is lodged against the vessel wall. Ask the patient to change his position, such as raising his arms, to free the catheter.

- Flush the VAP with the other syringe containing normal saline solution. Then clamp the extension tubing. If you notice swelling or if the patient reports pain at the site, remove the needle and notify the doctor.

Using a side-entry VAP

- To use a side-entry VAP, follow the same procedure as you did with a top-entry VAP. However, you should insert the needle parallel to the reservoir instead of perpendicular to it.

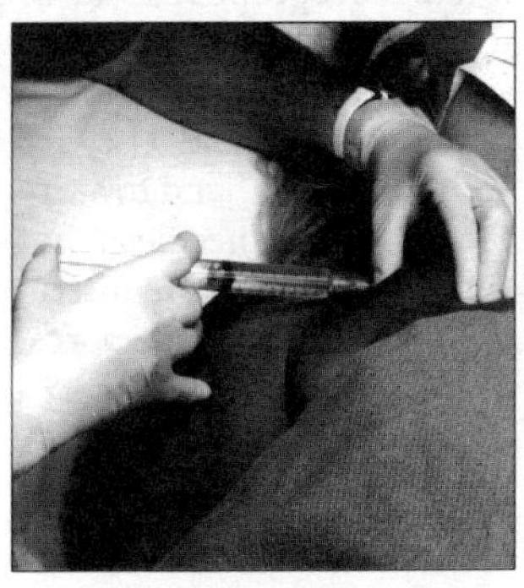

Giving a bolus injection through a VAP

- In addition to the equipment required to use the VAP, you'll need a syringe containing the prescribed medication, two 10-ml syringes prefilled with normal saline solution, a 5-ml syringe prefilled with heparin flush solution, and the patient's MAR.
- Verify the medication order on the patient's MAR and chart. If you haven't already done so, attach a syringe filled with normal saline to the extension set. Flush the set and the VAP. Then connect the medication syringe to the extension set.
- Open the clamp and inject the drug as ordered. Examine the skin surrounding the needle for signs of infiltration, such as swelling or tenderness. If you note these signs, stop the injection and notify the doctor.

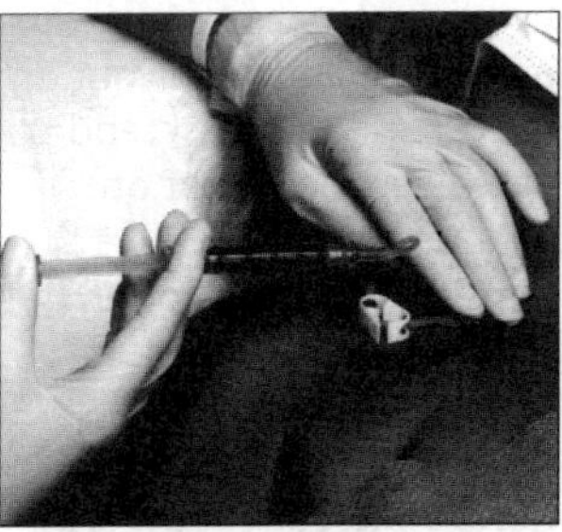

- After completing the injection, clamp the extension set and remove the medication syringe. Attach the other syringe with normal saline solution, and flush the set and the VAP with 5 ml of the solution. Perform this step after each drug injection to minimize possible drug incompatibility reactions. Also use a heparin flush solution if your facility's policy requires it. After flushing, remove the needle, and document the procedure.

Giving a continuous infusion through a VAP

- In addition to the equipment required to use the VAP, you'll need the prescribed I.V. solution or medication, an I.V. administration set, a 10-ml syringe filled with normal saline solution, povidone-iodine ointment, and the patient's MAR. You'll also need a transparent semipermeable dressing and, possibly, a filter.
- Verify the medication order against the patient's MAR. Connect the administration set, and secure the connections with sterile tape, if necessary. Unclamp the extension set, open the clamp on the administration set, and begin the infusion.
- Depending on your facility's policy, you may apply a small amount of povidone-iodine ointment to the insertion site; then apply a transparent semipermeable dressing over the entire site.

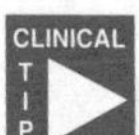

If the needle hub isn't flush with the skin, place a folded, sterile 2″ × 2″ gauze pad under the hub. Then apply Steri-Strips across it. Secure the needle and tubing, using the chevron-taping method.

- Examine the site carefully for infiltration. If you note infiltration or if the patient complains of stinging, burning, or pain at the site, clamp the extension tubing, discontinue the infusion, and notify the doctor. Dispose of all soiled supplies and used equipment appropriately. Wash your hands and document the procedure. ■

How soon after placement can I use a VAP?

A vascular access port (VAP) can be used immediately after placement, although some edema and tenderness may persist for about 72 hours. This makes the device initially difficult to palpate and slightly uncomfortable for the patient. Place an ice pack over the area for several minutes to alleviate discomfort from the needle puncture. ■

What if I can't flush or withdraw fluid from a VAP?

To handle common problems associated with a vascular access port (VAP), follow these guidelines:

- Inability to get a blood return could mean that the catheter leading from the VAP is lodged against the vessel wall. Ask the patient to raise his arms, perform Valsalva's maneuver, or change position to free the catheter.
- If this doesn't work, consider other possible causes. Check the I.V. tubing for kinks and the pump for malfunction. Also check the needle for proper placement. If the needle is placed incorrectly, reposition the needle, and advance the tip up to the bottom of the reservoir. Verify that the needle is positioned correctly by aspirating for blood.
- If none of these measures corrects the problem, a fibrin sleeve on the distal end of the catheter may be occluding the opening. Flush the catheter with 3 ml of sterile normal saline solution, and repeat if necessary.
- If clots are occluding the port, use a declotting or fibrinolytic agent such as urokinase as ordered.
- If the problem stems from a kinked catheter or port rotation, contact the doctor. ■

Which drugs should always be given through a CV line?

Experts generally agree on which drugs should always be administered through a central venous (CV) line. Make sure that you know your facility's policy. Consider these general guidelines:

- Most hospitals require CV therapy for delivering highly osmolar fluids, such as hypertonic saline solution, dextrose 50% in water (often used in total parenteral nutrition), and certain chemotherapeutic agents.
- Many facilities require CV administration of amphotericin B because peripheral administration increases the likelihood of thrombophlebitis and local inflammation.
- Many facilities also specify that dopamine must be given only through a CV line because of the risk of extravasation with a peripheral line. ■

What's involved in maintaining a CV catheter?

While your patient has a central venous (CV) catheter,

you'll care for the insertion site and maintain the setup to prevent complications. Routine care involves changing the dressing, changing the injection cap, and flushing the catheter at regular intervals.

Changing the CV catheter dressing

- In general, hospital infection-control practices and the Intravenous Nurses Society (INS) standards of practice require you to change the catheter's dressing every 48 hours or whenever it becomes soiled, moist, or loose.
- When you change the dressing, use sterile technique, and select the type of dressing your facility recommends for catheter insertion sites. Recent studies show that transparent dressings may increase the risk of infection because they allow moisture to accumulate under the dressing. In light of these findings, some hospitals elect to use gauze and tape dressings.

Changing the injection cap

- Guidelines on changing the catheter's injection caps also vary among hospitals (although INS standards specify injection cap changes at least weekly).
- Generally, the more often you puncture an injection cap, the more often it should be changed; repeated punctures increase the risk of infection. Besides, pieces of the rubber stopper may break off after repeated punctures, placing the patient at risk for an embolus.

Flushing the catheter

- As a general rule, flush all lumens of a multilumen CV catheter regularly. (Most experts recommend daily flushing.) However, flushing isn't necessary for a single-lumen CV catheter in use for a continuous infusion.
- Facility policies vary widely regarding flush solutions. Most hospitals use a heparin flush solution that's available in premixed 10-ml multidose vials.
- Recommended heparin concentrations range from as little as 10 units/ml to as much as 100 units/ml. However, some facilities don't use heparin. They rely instead on normal saline solution because some studies show that heparin isn't always needed to keep the CV line open.
- The recommended amount of flush solution can vary. (See *How much flush solution should I use in a CV catheter?* page 446.) Keep in mind, too, that different catheters require different amounts of solution. A catheter that's been cut to fit the patient, for

How much flush solution should I use in a CV catheter?

The amount and the strength of heparin to flush a CV catheter varies with the patient's body size. Follow these guidelines:

- For pediatric patients weighing less than 11 lb (5 kg), infuse 1 ml of a 10 units/ml solution every 12 hours.
- For pediatric patients weighing more than 11 lb, infuse 1 ml of a 10 units/ml solution every 12 hours.
- For adults, infuse 1.5 ml of a 10 units/ml solution every 12 hours.

example, needs less flush solution.

- Whatever the flush solution volume, use a 10-ml catheter to reduce the risk of rupturing the catheter. ■

How often should I change a Huber needle?

Commonly, the needle is left in place for several days for continuous I.V. infusions. For intermittent or cycled infusions, you may also leave the needle in the port, and you may heparinize the injection cap, I.V. extension tubing, needle, and port between uses. For most infusions, the needle will be changed every 3 to 7 days.

Some home care patients receiving cycled total parental nutrition infusions prefer to insert a new needle every day. They remove the needle after the infusion so that they can participate in certain activities. The skin over the port may become irritated if the needle is left in place between infusions or if the patient is very active. Using the muscles of the upper body may also cause the needle to move, resulting in an ulcerated or craterlike appearance around the needle. ■

When should I change a PICC line dressing?

Determining when to change the dressing over a peripherally inserted central catheter (PICC) really depends on your health care facility's policy. Every 3 days is typical for transparent film dressings; every 24 to 48 hours, for dry sterile dressings.

Make sure that you use a sterile dressing and sterile technique. On the dressing, record the type and length of the line, the insertion date, the date of the dressing change, and the date of the next dressing change. ■

Can I take blood pressure readings or draw blood from a PICC?

Don't take the patient's blood pressure or draw blood from the arm where the peripherally inserted central catheter (PICC) line is inserted; the blood pressure cuff could damage the catheter, or the needle could puncture the catheter. ■

How can I manage PICC line problems?

When caring for a patient with a peripherally inserted central catheter (PICC) line, you can anticipate such complications as occlusion; a damaged, broken, or disconnected catheter; inability to infuse fluid; and inability to draw blood. Here's how to intervene appropriately.

Occlusion

This problem may indicate thrombus formation, improper flushing, precipitate formation, or improper positioning.

- If thrombus formation has occluded the line, try repositioning the patient; then check for flow. If the line hasn't been flushed properly, attempt to aspirate the clot, taking care not to force it.
- If these measures don't work, notify the doctor; he may wish to increase the flow rate.
- Occlusion also may be caused by precipitate that forms when incompatible substances are infused through the line. Infusing thrombolytic agents, such as streptokinase or urokinase, may correct the problem.
- Finally, occlusion may occur if the catheter is improperly positioned in the vein or if the catheter tip is lodged against the vessel wall. A possible solution is to remove the catheter. (It may be repositioned in the vein with verification by a chest X-ray.) Be sure to document your interventions.

Damaged or broken catheter

- To detect pinholes, leaks, or tears in the catheter, examine for drainage after flushing. Follow the recommended clamping procedure, and remove the catheter if ordered.
- To prevent this problem, avoid using sharp objects near the catheter, and avoid injecting needles longer than 1″ through the injection cap.

Inability to infuse fluid

- First check the infusion system and clamps, and make sure that none of the clamps are closed.

- If this doesn't work, try changing the patient's position: The catheter may be displaced or kinked.
- Finally, inability to infuse fluid may indicate thrombus formation. Have the patient cough, breathe deeply, or perform Valsalva's maneuver. Remove the dressing, and examine the external portion of the catheter. If a kink isn't apparent, obtain a chest X-ray order. Try to withdraw blood. Also try a gentle flush with saline solution.

Inability to draw blood
- Inability to draw blood may result from a closed clamp, a displaced or kinked catheter, a thrombus, or a catheter lodged against the vessel wall.
- To intervene, first check the infusion system and clamps. Then change the patient's position. Have the patient cough, breathe deeply, or perform Valsalva's maneuver.
- Remove the dressing, and examine the external portion of the catheter. Finally, obtain a chest X-ray order.

Disconnected catheter
- This problem can result from patient movement or from the catheter's not being securely connected to the tubing.
- To intervene, apply a catheter clamp if one is available. Place a sterile syringe or catheter plug in the catheter hub. Change the extension set. Do not reconnect contaminated tubing. Clean the catheter hub with alcohol or povidone-iodine. Do not soak the hub. Connect clean I.V. tubing or a heparin lock plug to the site. Then restart the infusion. ■

How can I spot complications of CV therapy?

Complications can occur at any time during central venous (CV) therapy. Generally, though, traumatic complications such as a punctured subclavian artery occur during CV catheter insertion; systemic complications such as infection occur later during infusion therapy. Here are some common complications, their possible causes, and characteristics. (For interventions, see *Managing complications of CV therapy.*)

Air embolism
- This may be caused by air introduced into the CV circulation during catheter insertion or tubing changes.
- Suspect an air embolism if your patient develops low blood pressure; a weak, rapid pulse; and loss of consciousness.
- To help prevent an air embolism, have the patient per-

Managing complications of CV therapy

Complications that occur during central venous (CV) therapy demand prompt, assured intervention. To manage common problems effectively, follow these guidelines.

Air embolism

- Clamp the catheter immediately.
- Administer 100% oxygen through a nonrebreather face mask to improve oxygen concentration in the blood.
- Place the patient on his left side with his head down. This position displaces air to the apex of the heart, where it can be reabsorbed or aspirated.
- Ask another nurse to put the crash cart outside the room, and have someone else call the doctor immediately.
- Place a pressure dressing over the original dressing to prevent more air from entering the circulation.
- Be sure to reassure the patient and explain what you're doing; he's probably frightened.

Catheter embolism

- Stop the procedure.
- Prepare the patient for fluoroscopy, as ordered, to locate and retrieve the foreign object.
- Monitor the patient's ECG.
- Administer oxygen and turn the patient on his left side with his head down. This position displaces air traveling with the foreign body to the apex of the heart, where the air can be reabsorbed or aspirated.

Clotted catheter

- Clamp the catheter immediately.
- Have the patient change position, or attempt to reposition the catheter by having the patient raise his arms and cough.
- Obtain a doctor's order to use urokinase to dissolve the clot.

Hydrothorax

- Stop the insertion procedure.
- Apply ointment and a dressing over the insertion site.
- Obtain a chest X-ray (and possibly contrast studies).
- Set up equipment and assist with insertion of chest tubes.
- Administer oxygen as ordered.

(continued)

Managing complications of CV therapy *(continued)*

Infection
- Frequently monitor vital signs, including temperature, to detect infection as soon as possible.
- Obtain a blood sample for culture according to your facility's policy.
- Provide antibiotic therapy as ordered.

Pneumothorax
- Stop the insertion procedure.
- Apply ointment and a dressing over the insertion site.
- Obtain a chest X-ray.
- Set up equipment and assist with insertion of chest tubes.
- Administer oxygen as ordered.

Punctured subclavian artery
- Remove the cannulation needle.
- Apply digital pressure over the site for 10 minutes.

Venous thrombosis
- Prepare the patient for venography to verify thrombosis.
- Avoid using or removing the catheter.
- Use a peripheral line to begin a continuous heparin infusion as needed or ordered.
- Don't use the limb on the affected side for subsequent venipunctures.
- Apply warm, moist compresses locally.
- Obtain a doctor's order to use urokinase to dissolve the clot.

form Valsalva's maneuver during catheter insertion and removal.

Catheter embolism
- This is caused by a dislodged piece of catheter.
- A catheter embolism may cause cardiac arrhythmias, chest pain, cyanosis, weak pulse, decreased blood pressure, and altered level of consciousness or loss of consciousness.

Clotted catheter
- This results from blood coagulating in the lumen.
- Suspect a clotted catheter if you meet resistance when attempting to flush the catheter, or if you're unable to infuse I.V. solutions or medications.

Hydrothorax
- This complication may result if the catheter punctures the lung during insertion or

exchange over a guide wire. It may also result from a punctured lymph node and leaking lymphatic fluid or from I.V. solution infiltrating the chest.

- Suspect hydrothorax if your patient develops sudden, sharp, needlelike chest pain; a wet cough; and shortness of breath.
- Auscultation may reveal decreased breath sounds on the affected side.

Infection

- Infection may be caused by failure to maintain aseptic technique during catheter insertion or maintenance, or failure to comply with dressing change protocol. It may also be caused by immunosuppression, a contaminated catheter or I.V. solution, frequent opening of the catheter, or long-term use of a single I.V. access site.
- You'll recognize infection by its classic signs and symptoms such as fever, chills, and malaise along with nausea and vomiting.
- Inspection may reveal tenderness, redness, warmth, or swelling at the insertion site.
- You may also detect drainage at the site and local rash or pustules.

Pneumothorax

- This complication may occur if the lung is punctured by the catheter during catheter insertion or exchange over a guide wire.
- Suspect pneumothorax if your patient develops sudden, sharp, needlelike chest pain; cough; and shortness of breath.
- Auscultation may reveal decreased breath sounds on the affected side.

Punctured subclavian artery

- This occurs when the cannulation needle punctures the artery.
- A punctured artery is heralded by bright red blood pulsating from the insertion site. Later, hemorrhage, tracheal compression, and respiratory distress may develop.

Venous thrombosis

- Thrombosis may stem from a sluggish flow rate, preexisting limb edema, infusion of irritating solutions, or preexisting cardiovascular disease.
- It produces unilateral edema on the side of catheter insertion, beginning at the fingers and progressing to the neck.
- It may also cause difficulty in maintaining the infusion flow rate and occlusion, signaled by the infusion pump's alarm. ■

INTRAOSSEOUS THERAPY

Assisting with an intraosseous infusion

During intraosseous infusion, the bone marrow serves as a noncollapsible vein; thus, fluid infused into the marrow cavity rapidly enters the circulation via an extensive network of venous sinusoids.

Getting ready

- Gather the following equipment at the patient's bedside, including a bone marrow biopsy needle or specially designed intraosseous infusion needle (catheter and obturator), povidone-iodine sponges, sterile gauze pads, sterile gloves, sterile drape, bone marrow set, heparinized saline flush solution, the appropriate I.V. fluids and tubing, 1% lidocaine, and a 3- to 5-ml syringe.
- If the patient is conscious, explain the procedure to allay his fears and promote his cooperation. Ensure that the patient or a responsible family member understands the procedure and has signed a consent form.
- Check the patient's history for hypersensitivity to the local anesthetic. With an adult, explain which bone site will be infused. Inform the patient that he'll receive a local anesthetic and feel pressure from needle insertion.

Preparing the patient

- Provide a sedative, if ordered, before the procedure.
- Position the patient based on the selected puncture site.
- Using sterile technique, clean the puncture site with a povidone-iodine sponge, and allow it to dry. Then cover the area with a sterile drape.

Administering the infusion

- After anesthetizing the insertion site, the doctor inserts the catheter and obturator through the skin and into the bone at a 10- to 15-degree angle. He advances it with a to-and-fro rotary motion through the periosteum until the needle penetrates the marrow cavity. The needle should "give" suddenly when it enters the marrow and should stand erect when released.
- Then the doctor removes the obturator from the catheter and attaches a 5-ml syringe. He aspirates some bone marrow to confirm needle placement.
- The doctor replaces this syringe with a syringe containing 5 ml of heparinized saline flush solution and then flushes the catheter to confirm needle placement and

clear the catheter of clots or bone particles.

▪ Next, the doctor removes the syringe of flush solution and attaches the I.V. tubing to the catheter to allow infusion of medications and I.V. fluids.

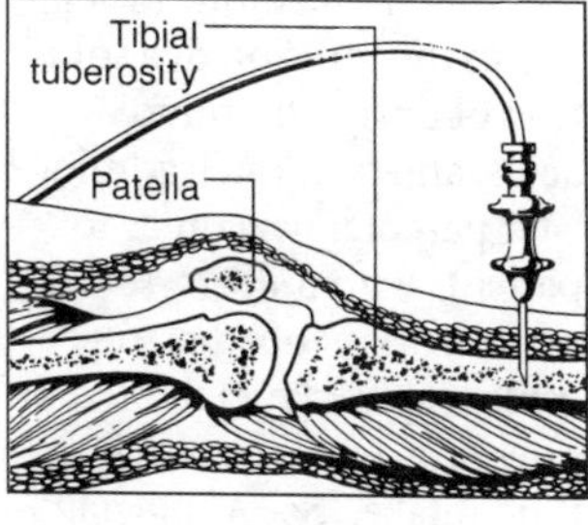

▪ Put on sterile gloves, and clean the infusion site with povidone-iodine sponges, and then secure the site with tape and a sterile gauze dressing.

▪ Monitor the patient's vital signs, and check the infusion site for bleeding, extravasation, and infection.

▪ After the needle is removed, place a sterile dressing over the injection site, and apply firm pressure to the site for 5 minutes.

Special considerations

▪ Intraosseous flow rates are determined by needle size and flow through the bone marrow. Fluids should flow freely if needle placement is correct. Normal saline solution has been administered intraosseously at a rate of 600 ml/minute and up to a rate of 2,500 ml/hour when delivered under pressure of 300 mm/Hg through a 13G needle.

▪ Intraosseous infusion should be discontinued as soon as conventional vascular access is established (within 2 to 4 hours, if possible). Prolonged infusion significantly increases the risk of infection. ■

When is an intraosseous infusion used?

When rapid venous infusion is difficult or impossible, intraosseous infusion allows delivery of fluids, medications, or whole blood into the bone marrow. Performed on infants and children, this technique is used in such emergencies as cardiopulmonary arrest or circulatory collapse, hypokalemia from traumatic injury or dehydration, status epilepticus, status asthmaticus, burns, near-drowning, and overwhelming sepsis.

Any drug that can be given by the I.V. route can be given by intraosseous infusion; drug absorption and effectiveness are comparable. Intraosseous infusion has been used as an acceptable alternative for infants and children.

Intraosseous infusion is commonly undertaken at the

anterior surface of the tibia. Alternate sites include the iliac crest, spinous process, or (rarely) the upper anterior portion of the sternum. Only personnel trained in this procedure should perform it. Usually, a nurse will assist.

Contraindications

Intraosseous infusion is contraindicated in patients with osteogenesis imperfecta, osteopetrosis, and ipsilateral fracture because of the potential for subcutaneous extravasation. Infusion through an area with cellulitis or an infected burn increases the risk of infection.

Complications

Common complications of intraosseous infusion include extravasation of fluid into subcutaneous tissue, resulting from incorrect needle placement; subperiosteal effusion, resulting from failure of the fluid to enter the marrow space; and clotting in the needle, resulting from delayed infusion or failure to flush the needle after placement. Other complications include subcutaneous abscess, osteomyelitis, and epiphyseal injury. ■

PARENTERAL NUTRITION

Administering a parenteral feeding

Parenteral nutrition (PN) involves the infusion of a solution of dextrose, amino acids, and fats. You'll administer parenteral feedings to patients with mild-to-severe malnutrition, normal to severely elevated metabolic rates and, possibly, restricted fluid intake. (See *Managing complications of PN.*) Here's how to proceed.

Getting ready

- Gather the necessary equipment, including the solution for total parenteral nutrition (TPN), peripheral parenteral nutrition (PPN), or lipids; an infusion pump; sterile pump tubing; two 20G 1″ needles; alcohol sponges; and adhesive tape.
- Because infusing a chilled solution can cause pain, hypothermia, venous spasm, and venous constriction, let the solution warm to room temperature before you infuse it.

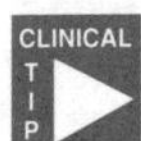

Never use a microwave oven to warm the solution — the nutrients may decompose, and the glucose may caramelize.

(Text continues on page 459.)

Managing complications of PN

Patients receiving parenteral nutrition (PN) risk developing certain metabolic, mechanical, and other problems. Use this chart to review common problems associated with PN, their characteristics, and the appropriate interventions.

COMPLICATIONS	SIGNS AND SYMPTOMS	INTERVENTIONS
Metabolic problems		
Hepatic dysfunction	Elevated serum AST, alkaline phosphatase, and bilirubin levels	Reduce total caloric and dextrose intake, making up lost calories by administering lipid emulsion. Change to cyclical infusion. Use specific hepatic formulations only if the patient has encephalopathy.
Hypercapnia	Heightened oxygen consumption, increased carbon dioxide production, measured respiratory quotient of 1 or greater	Reduce total caloric and dextrose intake, and balance dextrose and fat calories. Decrease carbohydrate calories.
Hyperglycemia	Fatigue, restlessness, confusion, anxiety, weakness, polyuria, dehydration, elevated serum glucose levels and, in severe hyperglycemia, delirium or coma	Restrict dextrose intake by decreasing either the rate of infusion or the dextrose concentration. Compensate for calorie loss with administration of lipid emulsion. Begin insulin therapy.

(continued)

Managing complications of PN *(continued)*

COMPLICATIONS	SIGNS AND SYMPTOMS	INTERVENTIONS
Hyper-osmolarity	Confusion, seizures, lethargy, hyperosmolar nonketotic syndrome, hyperglycemia, dehydration, and glycosuria.	Discontinue dextrose infusion. Administer insulin and 0.45% saline solution with 10 to 20 mEq/L of potassium to rehydrate the patient.
Hypo-calcemia	Polyuria, dehydration, and elevated blood and urine glucose levels	Increase calcium supplements.
Hypo-glycemia	Diaphoresis, tremor, and irritability after the infusion has stopped	Increase dextrose intake, or decrease exogenous insulin intake.
Hypokalemia	Muscle weakness, paralysis, paresthesia, and arrhythmias	Increase potassium supplements.
Hypo-magnesemia	Tingling around the mouth, paresthesia in fingers, mental changes, and hyperreflexia	Increase magnesium supplements.
Hypo-phosphatemia	Irritability, weakness, paresthesia, coma, and respiratory arrest	Increase phosphate supplements.

Managing complications of PN *(continued)*

COMPLICATIONS	SIGNS AND SYMPTOMS	INTERVENTIONS
Metabolic acidosis	Elevated serum chloride and reduced serum bicarbonate levels	Increase acetate, and decrease chloride in PN solution.
Metabolic alkalosis	Decreased serum chloride and, elevated serum bicarbonate levels	Decrease acetate, and increase chloride in PN solution.
Zinc deficiency	Dermatitis, alopecia, apathy, depression, taste changes, confusion, poor wound healing, and diarrhea	Increase zinc supplements.
Mechanical problems		
Clotted I.V. catheter	Interrupted flow rate, resistance to flushing and blood withdrawal	Attempt to aspirate the clot. If unsuccessful, instill urokinase to clear the catheter lumen as ordered.
Cracked or broken tubing	Fluid leaking from the tubing	Apply a padded hemostat above the break to prevent air from entering the line. Replace the tubing.
Dislodged catheter	Catheter out of the vein	Apply pressure to the site with a sterile gauze pad. Remove the catheter.

(continued)

Managing complications of PN *(continued)*

COMPLICATIONS	SIGNS AND SYMPTOMS	INTERVENTIONS
Too-rapid infusion	Nausea, headache, and lethargy	Adjust the infusion rate and, if applicable, check the infusion pump.
Other problems		
Air embolism	Apprehension, chest pain, tachycardia, hypotension, cyanosis, seizures, loss of consciousness, and cardiac arrest	Clamp the catheter. Place the patient in a steep, left lateral Trendelenburg's position. Administer oxygen as ordered. If cardiac arrest occurs, begin cardiopulmonary resuscitation. When the catheter is removed, cover the insertion site with a dressing for 24 to 48 hours.
Extravasation	Swelling and pain around the insertion site	Stop the infusion. Assess the patient for cardiopulmonary abnormalities; a chest X-ray may be required.
Phlebitis	Pain, tenderness, redness, and warmth	Apply moist heat at 105° F (40.5° C) to the area, and elevate the insertion site if possible.
Pneumothorax and hydrothorax	Dyspnea, chest pain, cyanosis, and decreased breath sounds	Assist with chest tube insertion, and apply suction as ordered.

Managing complications of PN *(continued)*

COMPLICATIONS	SIGNS AND SYMPTOMS	INTERVENTIONS
Septicemia	Red and swollen catheter site, chills, fever, and leukocytosis	Remove the catheter and culture the tip. Obtain a blood culture if the patient has a fever. Give appropriate antibiotics.
Thrombosis	Erythema and edema at the insertion site; ipsilateral swelling of the arm, neck, face, and upper chest; pain at the insertion site and along the vein; malaise; fever; and tachycardia	Remove the catheter promptly. If not contraindicated, systemic thrombolytic therapy may be used. Apply warm compresses to the insertion site, and elevate the affected extremity. Venous flow studies may be done.

- Compare the label on the bottle with the doctor's order. Most hospitals have a specific PN order form that the doctor completes. Set up as a grid, the form provides a checklist of the solution, additives, bottle numbers, and flow rate.
- Inspect the solution for cloudiness, turbidity, and particles. Inspect the container for cracks and other defects. If you find any defects, return the solution to the pharmacy immediately.
- If you're using a lipid solution, inspect the bottle for an oily separation of the emulsion; don't use the bottle if this occurs.
- Explain the procedure to the patient, and wash your hands. Prepare the solution container and the tubing as you would set up a primary I.V. Attach the needle to the end of the tubing. Then prime the tubing. Invert the filter at the distal end of the tubing, and open the roller clamp, letting the solution completely fill the tubing and the filter.
- Remember that you won't use tubing with a filter for lipid solutions because the

large molecules of the lipids may clog the filter.

- Once the tubing fills, close the roller clamp and inspect the pump chamber, filter, and Y-ports for air bubbles.
- If you see air bubbles in the tubing after priming it, open the roller clamp, remove the cap to the sterile needle, and let the air bubbles and a small amount of fluid escape. Close the roller clamp, and put a new 20G needle on the tip of the tubing.
- Insert the tubing into the infusion pump. Open the clamps, and set the pump to the prescribed rate, following the manufacturer's directions. Don't start the pump yet.
- Clean the rubber diaphragm on the catheter injection cap with an alcohol sponge.

Infusing the solution

- If you're infusing a lipid solution, uncap the 20G needle, which is attached to the end of the lipid tubing and, using aseptic technique, insert the needle into the Y-port of the TPN tubing below the filter. Because lipids are compatible with TPN, the lipid solution can be given by an I.V. piggyback setup that's hung below the filter of the TPN solution.
- Tape the needle securely, and label the tape "TPN" or "PPN." Now start the pump. If you're infusing a lipid solution, tape the connection securely, and label the tape "Lipids."
- Write the date on another piece of tape, and place it near the drip chamber so that it's clearly visible. Change the tubing every 24 hours to prevent growth of microorganisms.
- Finally, document the procedure. ■

Should I use a peripheral or central vein for PN?

Parenteral nutrition (PN), given through a peripheral vein, is indicated for patients who have interrupted enteral intake, but can probably resume enteral feedings in 5 to 10 days. This route is also indicated for patients with mild-to-moderate malnutrition, normal or mildly elevated metabolic rate, and no fluid restrictions. You'll need to supplement enteral feedings as ordered.

Use a central venous (CV) line to administer the solution if the patient is unable to tolerate enteral intake for more than 10 days. Also use a CV line for patients with moderate-to-severe malnutrition that can't be corrected with enteral feedings, moderately or severely elevated metabolic rates, and restricted fluid intake. Finally, use this route if the patient has poor or inaccessible peripheral veins and an accessible central vein. ■

How long does PN solution remain stable?

Some doctors send patients home on a three-in-one parenteral nutrition (PN) mixture. The patient or pharmacist must then mix all three components (fat, carbohydrates, and amino acids) in one bag. This procedure significantly lowers the cost of home PN and, because the solution isn't premixed, the patient knows exactly what it contains.

If the three-in-one solution is mixed by the pharmacist, it should remain stable for 7 days. But if the patient is preparing the solution, he should mix only 1 day's supply at a time. This helps limit the growth of bacteria in case the solution is inadvertently contaminated. It also helps cut down on medication errors. ■

How often should the PN line site dressing be changed at home?

A dressing made of semipermeable membrane can stay in place for 7 days, whereas one made of gauze and tape should be changed two to three times a week. Some home parenteral nutrition (PN) programs advocate using no dressing at all.

Changing the dressing

- Change the dressing over the catheter according to the policy at your health care facility — usually every 24 to 72 hours or whenever the dressing becomes wet, soiled, or nonocclusive. Always use strict aseptic technique.
- When performing dressing changes, watch for signs of phlebitis or catheter retraction from the vein.
- Measure the catheter's length from the insertion site to the hub for verification.
- Change the tubing and filters every 24 to 72 hours or according to your health care facility's policy.
- Always document the times of the dressing, filter, and solution changes; the condition of the catheter insertion site; your observations of the patient's condition; and any complications and resulting treatments. ■

Can I use a PN line for other functions?

Exercise caution when using the parenteral nutrition (PN) line for other purposes. If you're using a single-lumen central venous (CV) catheter, don't use the line to:

- infuse blood or blood products
- give a bolus injection
- administer simultaneous I.V. solutions
- measure CV pressure
- draw blood for laboratory tests.

In addition to these safety measures, observe the following precautions:

- Never add medication to a PN solution container.
- Don't use a three-way stopcock, if possible, because add-on devices increase the risk of infection.
- Don't administer PN solution through a pulmonary artery catheter because of the high risk of phlebitis.
- After infusion, flush the catheter with heparin or normal saline solution, according to the policy at your health care facility. ■

PATIENT-CONTROLLED ANALGESIA

Providing PCA

A patient-controlled analgesia (PCA) system delivers a medication — usually a narcotic — with the press of a button on an infusion pump. Especially effective for postoperative and intractable pain, a PCA system controls both acute and chronic pain by delivering small amounts of medication at a slow, continuous rate. Here's how to proceed.

Getting ready

- Take a PCA pump (such as the IVAC Corporation's PCA infuser model 310) to the patient's bedside. Assemble the rest of the equipment at the patient's bedside, including a 60-ml syringe prefilled by the pharmacist with the ordered medication, special extension tubing with needle, alcohol sponges, the patient's medication administration record (MAR), and the PCA information sheet. You may also need an I.V. pole and four D batteries.
- Wash your hands. Then explain the procedure to the patient.
- Match the doctor's order on the patient's MAR to the medication-filled syringe, and verify his identity. The doctor's orders should include the drug to be administered; the continuous dose, rate, and volume; the lockout interval; and the volume limit of the bolus dose.
- Before giving a narcotic analgesic, review the patient's MAR. Find out whether he has allergies or takes other CNS depressants. Using two CNS depressants together may cause drowsiness, oversedation, disorientation, and anxiety.

- Check the patient's I.V. site for infiltration or redness. Ensure that the venipuncture device is patent.

Preparing the equipment

- Next, prepare the PCA pump. For this particular model, insert the key into the lock and turn it to the unlocked position. Then open the syringe compartment door.
- Turn on the pump by pressing the ON button that's located inside the syringe compartment. The pump will perform a self-test as the indicator lights on the front of the pump light up in sequence.
- Using sterile technique, attach the special extension tubing to the 60-ml prefilled syringe.
- Open the syringe driver on the PCA pump, and slide the driver away from the syringe housing.
- Then place the syringe into the syringe holder.
- Slide the syringe driver until it aligns with the top of the plunger. Then close the syringe driver, capturing the top of the syringe plunger.
- With the syringe in place, you should select the syringe size by pressing the corresponding PCA DOSE key. The adjacent display window will blink to verify the syringe size.
- Then press the CLEAR MEMORY key four times to enter the selection.
- Or, instead of pressing the CLEAR MEMORY key, you may enter an access code. You can use this code instead of the CLEAR MEMORY key to display and clear memory information and to review and change programming information.
- To remove a stop condition, you should press the code button inside the PCA pump and press the three unit keys, pushing 10, 1, or 0.1, which convert to A, B, and C, respectively. Then press the code button to enter the code.
- Prime the I.V. infusion system by pressing the patient control button. Allow the solution to flow through the extension tubing until a droplet appears at the end of the infusion line. Then press the STOP button. Priming takes about 3 minutes.

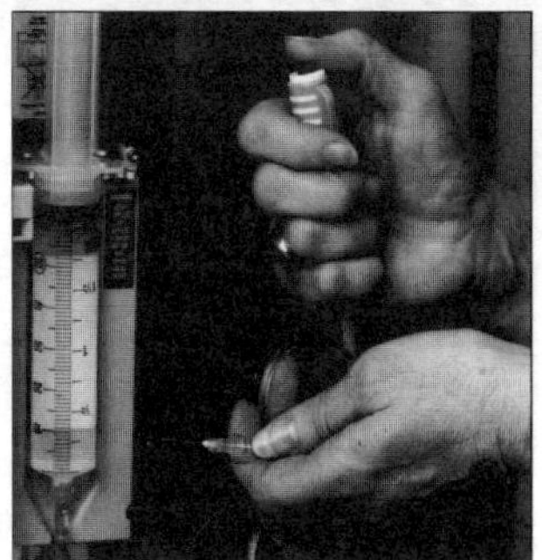

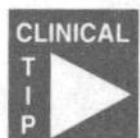
Never prime the infusion system with the infuser connected to the patient.

Programming the infuser

- First press the corresponding keys as well as the appropriate unit keys to enter the ordered concentration, ordered PCA or bolus dose, lock-out interval (interval between doses), and prescribed loading dose. If you don't program an interval, the infuser will default to a lockout interval of 5 minutes. The loading dose is administered once at the beginning of PCA therapy. It establishes an initial plasma concentration for the drug. The amount entered shouldn't exceed four times the PCA dose.
- Adjust the unit on the I.V. pole so that the pump is level with, or just below, the patient's venipuncture device.

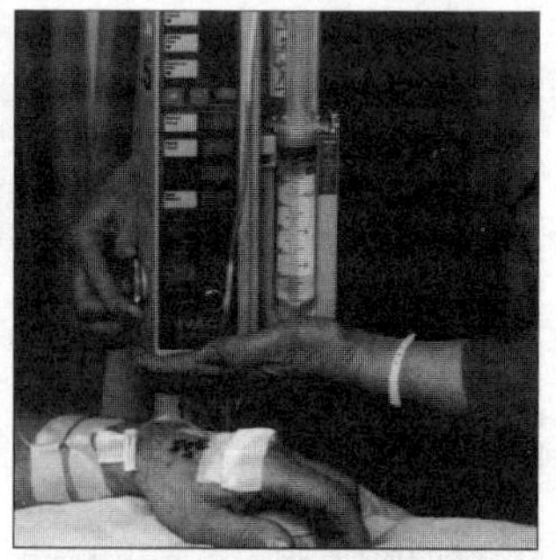

- Close the syringe compartment door. Then turn the key to the locked position.

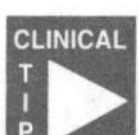
An audible alarm will sound to alert you to a programming error. In such a situation, turn the key to the unlocked position before trying to correct the problem.

Starting the infusion

- Wipe the administration set's Y-port with an alcohol sponge, and then attach the extension tubing and needle to the patient's venipuncture device.
- Double-check the settings for accuracy, and check the syringe compartment door to make sure that it's locked. Then press the patient control button to deliver the loading dose.
- Once the infusion starts, teach the patient how to use the PCA pump and when to administer bolus doses. (Give him a prepared information sheet if available.) Evaluate his understanding by observing how he uses the pump.
- Finally, document the procedure on the patient's MAR and the amount of medication administered on a PCA flowsheet. Make a note of your patient teaching, the patient's understanding of PCA, and the effectiveness of therapy. ■

Is my patient a good candidate for PCA?

Patients receiving patient-controlled analgesia (PCA) therapy must be mentally alert and able to understand and comply with instructions and procedures. Patients with limited respiratory reserve, a history of drug abuse, or a psychiatric disorder are ineligible for PCA. ■

What should I teach my patient about PCA?

Your patient must understand how patient-controlled analgesia (PCA) works in order for therapy to succeed. Often, you're in the best position to teach him and his family about PCA. And you may have to reinforce your teaching several times.

When your patient plans to receive PCA therapy at home, make sure that he and his family fully understand this method. Explain how the pump works and precisely how he can increase or decrease his dose. Also, make sure that he and his caregivers know when to notify the doctor.

Managing doses

- Explain to the patient that a narcotic analgesic relieves pain best when taken *before* the pain becomes intense.
- Stress that the patient shouldn't increase the frequency of administration.
- If he misses a dose, he should take it as soon as he remembers. But, if it's almost time for the next dose, tell him to skip the missed dose. Advise the patient never to double-dose.

Using caution

- Advise the patient to get up slowly from his bed or a chair because the drug may cause postural hypotension.
- Instruct him to eat a high-fiber diet, to drink plenty of fluids, and to take a stool softener if one has been prescribed.
- Caution him against drinking alcohol because this may enhance CNS depression.

Calling the doctor

- Your patient should notify his doctor if the drug loses it effectiveness.
- His family should report signs of an overdose: slow or irregular breathing, pinpoint pupils, or loss of consciousness. Teach family members how to maintain respirations until help arrives. ■

How do I select bolus doses and lock-out intervals?

Follow these suggestions for determining bolus doses for bolus-only patient-controlled analgesia pumps and lock-out intervals in bolus-only or bolus plus continuous infusion devices.

Bolus doses

If the patient has only intermittent pain, simply estimate a dose, and increase or decrease it until you determine the amount that relieves pain. Calculate the number of milligrams per dose and the total dose (or number of boluses) that he may receive per hour.

Lock-out intervals

For I.V. boluses (whether bolus only or bolus plus continuous infusions), set the lock-out interval for 6 minutes or more. Typically, pain relief following an I.V. narcotic bolus takes 6 to 10 minutes.

For S.C. boluses (whether bolus only or bolus plus continuous infusions), set the lock-out interval for 30 minutes or more. Typically, pain relief following an S.C. bolus takes 30 to 60 minutes.

For epidural boluses (bolus only or bolus plus continuous infusions), set the lock-out interval for 60 minutes or more. Typically, pain relief after an epidural bolus takes 30 to 60 minutes. ■

What should I do if an epidural catheter disconnects from the PCA tubing?

A catheter that becomes disconnected from the patient-controlled analgesia (PCA) tubing is a potential conduit for microorganisms to migrate into the epidural space, so your main concerns are preventing an epidural infection and relieving the patient's pain.

Immediate interventions

- Don't reconnect the catheter. While you explain to the patient what happened, cover the tip of the catheter with a heparin lock adapter or a sterile dressing, and tape the catheter securely to his back.
- Have another nurse notify the doctor and get another analgesic for the patient. (Make sure the dosage is an equianalgesic one.)

Catheter repair or removal

- Some facilities permit only certified nurses to repair or remove epidural catheters. If a repair is ordered and if you're qualified, put on sterile gloves and, using sterile scissors, cut 1″ (2.5 cm) off the catheter's distal end. Attach a new sterile connector tightly on the end.

- Flush the air out of the new PCA pump catheter tubing; then connect the tubing to the epidural catheter. Tape the catheter tubing to the patient's back.
- If removal is ordered and if you're qualified to do it, put on clean gloves. After carefully removing the butterfly bandages, grasp the catheter close to the insertion site, and slowly pull it straight toward you.
- If the catheter doesn't come out easily and stretches instead, ask the patient to bend forward at the waist. (This increases the distance between the spinous processes and makes catheter removal easier.) If the catheter still doesn't come out, stop pulling and notify the anesthesiologist.

Aftercare

- Once the catheter is removed, check its proximal tip for a black dot or a similar marking. This indicates that you've removed all of it. Send the tip for culture and sensitivity testing, and discard the catheter in the sharps container.
- Assess the site for redness, swelling and exudate. Apply antimicrobial ointment to the site, and cover it with an adhesive bandage.
- Document the amount of drug remaining in the infusion device, and discard the remaining drug according to facility protocol. ■

How can I manage complications of PCA?

The primary complication of patient-controlled analgesia (PCA) is respiratory depression. Other complications include anaphylaxis, nausea, vomiting, constipation, postural hypotension, and drug tolerance. Infiltration into the subcutaneous tissue and catheter occlusion may also occur, and these can cause the drug to back up into the primary I.V. tubing.

Respiratory depression

Watch for respiratory depression during administration. If the patient's respiratory rate declines to 10 or fewer breaths per minute, call his name and shake him gently. Tell him to breathe deeply. If he can't be aroused or is confused or restless, notify the doctor and prepare to administer oxygen. If ordered, give a narcotic antagonist such as naloxone.

Respiratory depression during PCA therapy is uncommon, because if a patient receives too much narcotic, he usually falls asleep and isn't able to press the bolus button. Make sure that family or staff members don't give extra doses of the narcotic when a patient hasn't requested them.

Anaphylaxis
In case of anaphylaxis, treat the patient's symptoms, and give another drug for pain relief as ordered.

Nausea and vomiting
If a patient has persistent nausea and vomiting during therapy, the doctor may change the medication. If ordered, give an antiemetic such as chlorpromazine.

Constipation
- To prevent constipation, give the patient a stool softener and, if necessary, a senna-derivative laxative. Provide a high-fiber diet, and encourage the patient to drink fluids. Regular exercise may also help.
- In case of urine retention, monitor the patient's intake and output.

Postural hypotension
- Guard against accidents. Keep the side rails up on the patient's bed. If the patient is mobile, help him out of bed, and assist him in walking.
- Encourage him to practice coughing and deep breathing to promote ventilation and prevent pooling of secretions, which could lead to respiratory difficulty.

Drug intolerance
- Evaluate the effectiveness of the drug at regular intervals. Is the patient getting relief? Does the dosage need to be increased because of persistent or worsening pain? Is the patient developing a tolerance to the drug?
- Although you should give the smallest effective dose over the shortest time period, narcotic analgesics shouldn't be withheld or given in ineffective doses. Psychological dependence on narcotic analgesics occurs in fewer than 1% of hospitalized patients. ■

■ CHAPTER 15

GIVING DRUGS BY OTHER ROUTES

ENTERAL TUBE ADMINISTRATION

Giving a drug through an NG tube

If your patient has a nasogastric (NG) tube, you may use the tube to administer medications. Here's how to proceed.

Getting ready

- Gather the following equipment, including the patient's medication administration record, the prescribed medication, a linen-saver pad, a stethoscope, gloves, tissues, a glass of water, and a 60-ml piston-type, catheter-tipped syringe.
- Place the patient in semi-Fowler's position. Wash your hands and put on gloves. To protect the patient from spills, cover him with a towel or linen-saver pad.

Confirming proper tube position

- Next, remove the clamp from the NG tube, and check the tube's position. To do this, insert a catheter-tipped syringe into the distal end of the tube, and aspirate a small amount of stomach contents. If no stomach contents return, place the diaphragm of your stethoscope over the patient's stomach. Then, while listening with the stethoscope, instill about 10 to 30 cc of air with the syringe. If the tube is in the stomach, you'll hear a loud gurgle when you inject the air.

Administering the drug

- Once you've confirmed the tube's proper position, remove the syringe from the NG tube. Then remove the piston from the syringe. Insert the catheter tip into the NG tube port, making sure it fits snugly.
- Hold the syringe attached to the NG tube upright, slightly above the level of the patient's nose.
- Slowly pour the medication into the syringe, which acts as a funnel. Allow the medication to flow slowly through the tube. If the medication flows too slowly, raise the syringe slightly. As the syringe empties, add the rest of the medication.
- To prevent air from entering the stomach, avoid letting the syringe drain completely during administration.
- After giving all of the medication, pour 30 to 50 ml of water into the syringe. Let the water flow through the tube to rinse it and to ensure that all of the medication reaches the stomach.
- Next, clamp the tube and remove the syringe. Clean

and store the equipment, or dispose of it, as appropriate.

- Have the patient remain in semi-Fowler's position, or allow him to lie on his side, for at least 30 minutes to prevent esophageal reflux. ■

Giving a drug through a gastrostomy tube

To deliver a drug through a gastrostomy tube, prepare the medication as you would for nasogastric (NG) tube delivery. Follow these guidelines.

Getting ready

- Gather the following equipment, including the patient's medication administration record, the prescribed medication, a 60-ml piston-type, catheter-tipped syringe, gloves, tissues, and a glass of water.
- Put on gloves. Remove the dressing covering the tube, if necessary, as well as the dressing or plug at the distal tip of the tube.
- Remove the piston from the catheter-tipped syringe, and insert the catheter tip into the gastrostomy tube.

Checking tube patency

Release the clamp on the tube, and check the tube's patency by instilling about 10 ml of water. If the water flows freely, the tube is patent.

Administering the drug

- Then pour up to 30 ml of medication into the syringe. Regulate the flow rate by lowering the syringe. After giving all the medication, instill about 30 ml of water to rinse the tube.
- Remove the syringe from the tube and tighten the clamp. Replug the gastrostomy tube opening. Keep the patient in semi-Fowler's position for at least 30 minutes to prevent esophageal reflux. ■

Giving a drug through a gastrostomy button

To give a drug through a gastrostomy button, prepare the medication as you would for nasogastric (NG) tube instillation.

Getting ready

- Gather the following equipment, including gloves, a feeding tube sized to fit the patient's gastrostomy button, a catheter-tipped syringe, the prescribed medication, the patient's medication administration record, and a glass of water.
- Put on gloves. Remove the safety plug on the gastrostomy button, and attach the

feeding tube to the button (as shown).

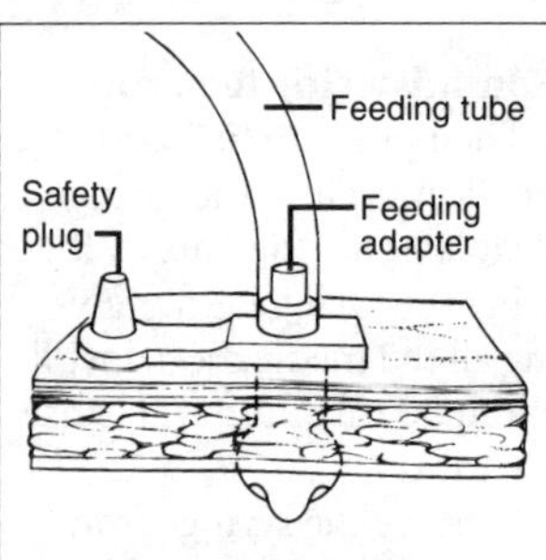

Administering the drug

- Remove the piston from the catheter-tipped syringe, and insert the catheter tip into the distal end of the feeding tube.
- Pour the prescribed medication into the syringe, and allow it to flow into the stomach.
- After instilling all of the medication, pour 30 to 50 ml of water into the syringe, and allow it to flow through the tube.
- When all of the water has been delivered, remove the feeding tube and replace the safety plug. Have the patient remain in semi-Fowler's position for at least 30 minutes to prevent esophageal reflux. ■

Which drugs can I crush or dissolve?

If a drug for enteral administration is available in both tablet and liquid form, give the liquid whenever practical. Digoxin and acetaminophen, for example, are available as elixirs. But many oral drugs are available only as tablets or capsules. Some can be crushed (or, in the case of capsules, opened), mixed with water, and delivered by tube.

Crushing tablets

- You can always crush simple compressed tablets, which are designed to dissolve immediately in the GI tract. Crushing the tablet allows it to enter the bloodstream slightly faster than it would if swallowed whole, but the difference is clinically insignificant.
- You can also crush tablets with sugar coatings, such as cimetidine and conjugated estrogen. The coating is intended to mask the bitter taste, not to delay tablet dissolution.
- Always confirm the type of coating with the pharmacist because sugar coatings resemble enteric coatings, and enteric-coated tablets shouldn't be crushed.

Dissolving capsule contents

Although capsules shouldn't be crushed, you can open these types of capsules and mix the contents with water.

Hard gelatin capsules

Each capsule's hard gelatin envelope contains the drug in powder form. Pull the capsule open (it's designed to separate in the middle), and mix the powder thoroughly in water. Ampicillin and doxycycline are two drugs available in this form.

Sustained-release capsules

- Like sustained-release tablets, these capsules are designed to release the active drug slowly, over time. Feosol Spansules (a brand name for ferrous sulfate) and Slo-Bid Gyrocaps (a brand name for theophylline) are common examples. The coated beads or pellets inside these capsules are designed to dissolve in the GI tract at different rates, prolonging the drug's duration of action. Obviously, crushing the capsules or their contents destroys their timed-release mechanism.
- If the doctor orders a sustained-release capsule, the best option is to ask him to order a liquid preparation of the drug instead. Theophylline, for example, is available in an elixir as well as a sustained-release capsule. Or the drug may be available as a simple compressed tablet that you can crush.
- When changing to a formulation that isn't sustained-release, make sure the dosage is adjusted appropriately.
- As an alternative, some capsules can be opened and their contents mixed with fluid or sprinkled on applesauce to ease swallowing. As long as the protective coatings aren't disturbed, the medication will retain its sustained-release properties. Ask the pharmacist for advice.

Soft gelatin capsules

- Drugs available in this form include chloral hydrate and various vitamin preparations. You can administer these drugs through a feeding tube by poking a pinhole in one end of the capsule and squeezing out the liquid contents or by drawing up the contents in a syringe.
- Don't use either of the above methods if delivering an exact dose is important. No matter how careful you are, the drug can never be completely expressed from the capsule.
- If you want to make sure the patient gets the total dose, dissolve the capsule in warm water (15 to 30 ml for adults and 5 to 10 ml for children); then administer the drug and water mixture. Al-

low up to 1 hour for the capsule to dissolve. ■

Can I combine drugs and enteral formulas?

Avoid adding medications to enteral formulas in a feeding bag. Doing so not only can alter the drug's therapeutic effect, but also may disrupt the integrity of the formula, causing it to curdle.

If the doctor orders the addition of a nonnutrient (such as sodium or potassium chloride) to the feeding bag, check with the pharmacist first to make sure the solutions are compatible. If so, shake the feeding bag thoroughly after adding any medication. Label the bag with the name and amount of the medication added, and watch the formula for precipitation or other changes. ■

Which drugs require special care when given by tube?

Here are some common examples of medications that must be handled carefully when given by tube.

Antacids

- Antacid liquids should be delivered only to the stomach, so don't give them through a tube that's placed beyond the pylorus.
- Don't administer antacids through a tube that's smaller in diameter than a #10 French for adults (#6 to 8 French for children), or the tube may clog.
- Ideally, you should give any other medications 15 minutes before an antacid dose to avoid potential interactions.

Antibiotics

- Some antibiotics should be given with food, others on an empty stomach. Check with the pharmacist or in a drug reference for guidelines applying to specific drugs.
- If the drug should be given on an empty stomach, stop continuous tube feedings for 15 to 30 minutes before giving the drug, and wait 15 to 30 minutes before resuming the feeding. Adjust the feeding schedule appropriately to meet the patient's nutritional needs over each 24-hour period.

Bulk-forming agents

Avoid giving a psyllium preparation (such as Metamucil) and other similar drugs through a feeding tube, if possible. Because they quickly congeal when mixed with water or juice, they can clog the tube. Check with the pharmacist for alternatives.

Phenytoin

- Because the therapeutic range is so narrow for phenytoin, maintaining an adequate blood level of this drug is difficult when it's given through a tube. The patient may need much higher doses than usual.
- Discontinue tube feedings for 1 to 2 hours before and after giving phenytoin to enhance absorption. Because of these lengthy interruptions in the feeding routine, you'll need to adjust the patient's schedule to meet his nutritional needs over each 24-hour period.
- Carefully monitor phenytoin blood levels and patient response, especially after any changes in the tube-feeding regimen — the dosage may need adjustment.

Theophylline

This drug may be poorly absorbed when given with continuous tube feedings. Monitor theophylline levels closely, and alter the dosage as needed after tube feedings are discontinued.

Warfarin

Tube-feeding solutions contain vitamin K, and warfarin and vitamin K are pharmacologically antagonistic. Any change in the patient's feeding or medication regimen could cause side effects, such as bleeding. Monitor the patient's PTs closely, and adjust warfarin dosages as indicated. ■

EPIDURAL ADMINISTRATION

Providing epidural drugs in bolus doses

To prevent or relieve moderate-to-severe acute pain or to manage chronic pain, your patient may receive analgesics epidurally. A drug delivered by this route provides rapid, regional relief because it diffuses directly into the pain site.

To administer a drug epidurally, a catheter is placed in the epidural space — the compartment between the dura mater and the bony and ligamentous walls of the spinal cord. Inserted for temporary or permanent use, an epidural catheter allows direct injection or infusion.

The doctor may order bolus doses of medication in addition to the patient's continuous infusion of the same drug. (See *Epidural drugs: Doses and effects*, page 476.) You may provide such doses by an I.V. pump or by injection. Here's how to proceed.

Epidural drugs: Doses and effects

The most commonly prescribed epidural analgesics and their doses appear below. In some cases, the drug may be combined with an anesthetic agent, such as bupivacaine, to potentiate the analgesic's effect. The onset of pain relief varies, depending on the drug. For example, lipophilic (fat-soluble) drugs, such as meperidine and methadone, begin acting in about 5 minutes; hydrophilic (water-soluble) drugs, such as morphine, in 30 to 60 minutes. The peak and duration of the effect also vary, as described below.

EPIDURAL DRUG AND DOSE	PEAK EFFECT (min)	DURATION OF EFFECT (hr)
fentanyl 50 to 100 mcg	10 to 15	2 to 4
meperidine (usually combined with low-dose bupivacaine) 25 to 50 mg	15	4 to 6
methadone 3 to 10 mg	10 to 30	6 to 8
morphine and fentanyl 3 to 5 mg morphine and 50 mcg fentanyl	10	6 to 24
morphine sulfate 3 to 10 mg	15 to 60	8 to 24
sufentanil 25 to 50 mcg	10	3 to 5

Providing a bolus dose by I.V. pump

- Wash your hands, and explain the procedure to the patient.
- Reset the volume to be infused on the I.V. pump to the amount of solution in the bolus dose. For example, if the doctor orders a 2-mg bolus dose of morphine and the solution contains 100 mg of morphine in 50 ml of solution, then 1 ml of solution contains 2 mg of morphine.

- Increase the pump rate to deliver the bolus dose. Stay with the patient while the bolus dose infuses. Then reset the pump rate to the ordered infusion rate, and reset the volume to be infused as ordered.
- Evaluate the patient's response to the medication, and check his blood pressure and respiratory rate 10, 20, and 30 minutes after giving the bolus dose.
- Finally, document the procedure.

Providing a bolus dose by injection

If the patient has a capped epidural catheter, you may inject bolus doses of medication through it, as ordered, after the doctor gives the first dose.

- Gather the needed equipment, including clean gloves, an alcohol sponge, two syringes, the ordered drug, and a new catheter cap.
- Wash your hands, and fill a syringe with the prescribed medication. Make sure that the preparation is preservative-free.

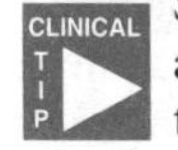

Some practitioners add about 1 cc of air to the syringe to completely clear the syringe of medication.

- Put on clean gloves, and clean the connection site between the catheter and the cap with an alcohol sponge.
- Disconnect the cap, connect the empty syringe to the catheter, and pull back on the plunger. If you aspirate blood, the catheter may be in the epidural blood vessels. If you aspirate clear fluid (which is probably CSF), the catheter may be in the subarachnoid space. In either case, withhold the drug, and inform the doctor.
- If you aspirate nothing, remove the empty syringe, attach the syringe with the medication, and slowly inject the drug.

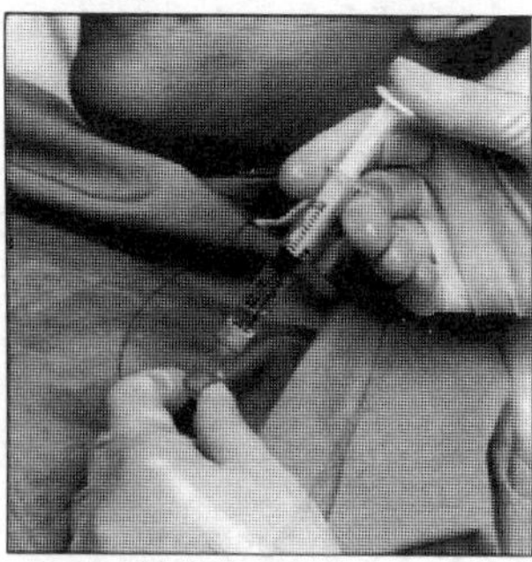

- Fully depress the plunger to empty the syringe of all medication. Disconnect the syringe, and recap the catheter. Dispose of the syringe and other supplies according to facility policy. Then remove your gloves and wash your hands.
- Check the patient's blood pressure and respiratory rate 10, 20, and 30 minutes after the injection.
- Document the procedure and the patient's response. ■

What's my role in epidural drug administration?

Epidural drugs are delivered through a thin catheter that the anesthesiologist inserts into the narrow epidural space in the patient's spinal cord. Your role in this procedure will vary, depending on your state's nurse practice act and your facility's policy.

- You'll need to understand spinal cord anatomy and physiology, the pharmacokinetics of the medications used, catheter and patient care measures, and possible side effects of the drug as well as appropriate interventions.
- When administering an epidural infusion, inspect the drug label for evidence that the drug solution is preservative-free and concentrated. Drugs with preservatives irritate the spinal cord. Concentrated solutions reduce the drug volume needed.
- Make sure that the patient's signed consent form is on file.
- Also make sure that the patient has a patent I.V. line or venous access device in place (for delivery of emergency drugs if necessary). If he'll receive a temporary epidural catheter, the venous access device will stay in place for the duration of therapy. If he'll receive a permanent catheter, I.V. access may be maintained until his response to the medication has stabilized and the correct maintenance dosage has been determined.
- Thoroughly assess the patient for pain, using a standard pain scale. This serves as a baseline for evaluating the effectiveness of subsequent therapy.
- When the patient's epidural catheter is in place, administer analgesics through it by infusion pump or injection. Familiarize yourself with equianalgesic dosing, and learn to convert the patient's other medications into equivalent epidural doses if appropriate. ■

ENDOTRACHEAL TUBE ADMINISTRATION

Giving a drug through an ET tube

When an I.V. line isn't available in a life-threatening emergency, you can administer drugs safely and effectively through an endotracheal (ET) tube. You'll use this route only until an I.V. line can be established.

Getting ready

- Calculate the drug dose if you haven't already done so.

Then dilute the drug with 5 to 10 ml of sterile distilled water or sterile normal saline solution, as directed.

- Note that the absorption of a drug diluted by water exceeds that of a drug diluted by normal saline solution. However, a drug diluted by water tends to lower the patient's partial pressure of arterial oxygen.

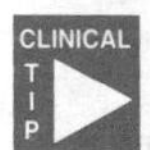

According to the American Heart Association's guidelines for Advanced Cardiac Life Support, the drug dose given through an ET tube should be two to two-and-one-half times the usual recommended dose. (See *Reviewing ET drugs and doses,* pages 480 and 481.)

- Move the patient into a supine position with his head level with or slightly higher than his trunk. Put on clean gloves. Then auscultate the patient's lungs while you ventilate him to check the ET tube's placement.

Instilling the drug

- After confirming that the ET tube is properly positioned, provide three to five ventilations with the handheld resuscitation bag. Then, remove the bag from the ET tube.
- Next, remove the needle from the syringe, and insert the tip of the syringe into the ET tube. Rapidly instill the drug into the tube.

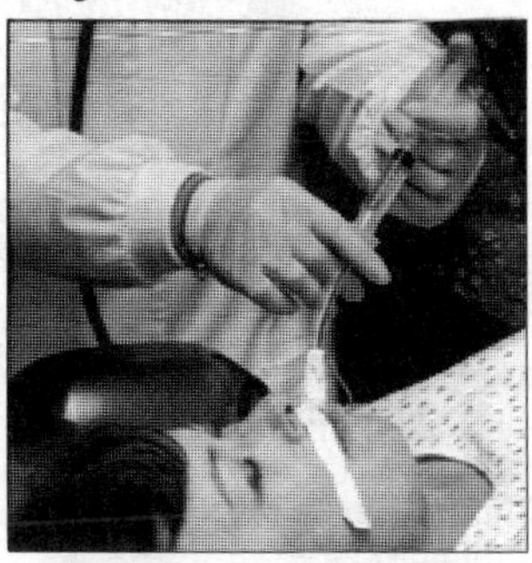

- Place your thumb briefly over the ET tube after instilling the drug. This helps to minimize drug reflux.
- Reattach the resuscitation bag to the ET tube, and provide five or six brisk ventilations. Doing so will propel the drug into the lungs, provide the patient with additional oxygen, and clear the ET tube.
- Monitor the patient's response to the medication.
- Document the procedure.

Special considerations

- Endotracheally delivered drugs take effect rapidly because the pulmonary alveoli provide a large surface area for drug absorption. Pulmonary circulation propels blood to the left side of the heart, ensuring rapid, dissemination of the drug through the central circulation. However, only a few drugs, such as atropine, epinephrine, and lidocaine, can

Reviewing ET drugs and doses

Use this chart to help determine endotracheal (ET) drug doses in an emergency. Keep in mind that ET doses are calculated by multiplying the usual I.V. dose by 2 to 2½, and that the drug should be diluted in 10 ml of sterile normal saline solution or sterile distilled water, as prescribed. The ET dose is provided below with the usual I.V. dose indicated in parentheses.

DRUG AND INDICATION	E.T. DOSE	SPECIAL CONSIDERATIONS
atropine Symptomatic bradycardia or asystole	1 to 2.5 mg diluted in 10 ml of sterile normal saline solution or sterile distilled water (0.5 to 1 mg I.V.)	▪ Monitor the patient's ECG continuously. ▪ Atropine may cause tachycardia. Use cautiously in patients with cardiac ischemia or MI because tachycardia increases myocardial oxygen consumption. ▪ Full vagolytic doses (0.04 mg/kg) should be reserved for patients with asystole because of the risk of tachycardia.
epinephrine Cardiac arrest	2 to 2.5 mg diluted in 10 ml of sterile normal saline solution or sterile distilled water (1 mg I.V.)	▪ Epinephrine has good bioavailability following ET administration, but the optimal dose is unknown. ▪ High doses (5 mg I.V.) are not more efficacious than standard doses. As ordered, administer high-dose regimens only after standard doses have failed.

Reviewing ET drugs and doses *(continued)*

DRUG AND INDICATION	E.T. DOSE	SPECIAL CONSIDERATIONS
lidocaine (4%) Ventricular tachycardia or ventricular fibrillation	2 to 3.75 mg/kg diluted in 10 ml of sterile normal saline solution or sterile distilled water (1 to 1.5 mg/kg I.V.)	▪ Lidocaine is usually given by I.V. bolus followed by continuous I.V. infusion; only bolus therapy should be used in cardiac arrest. ▪ Watch for signs of toxicity, such as metallic taste, somnolence, confusion, and seizures.

adequately penetrate the pulmonary surface.

▪ The duration of action is usually longer with ET tube delivery than with I.V. administration because the alveoli sustain absorption — called the *depot effect.* Therefore, you'll need to adjust subsequent doses and monitor I.V. infusions to guard against side effects. ■

INTRAPLEURAL ADMINISTRATION

Assisting with an intrapleural injection

Drugs may be injected through the chest wall via a catheter that's been inserted into the pleural space or through a chest tube that's been placed intrapleurally for drainage. Intrapleural administration (which causes pleural sclerosis) provides superior chemotherapeutic effects, reduces drug toxicity, and maintains higher and longer-lasting pleural drug concentrations. (See *Reviewing intrapleural drugs and doses,* pages 482 and 483.)

Indications

Increasingly, intrapleural administration is used to promote analgesia, treat spontaneous pneumothorax, resolve pleural effusions, and deliver chemotherapeutic drugs.

(Text continues on page 484.)

Reviewing intrapleural drugs and doses

Increasingly, intrapleural drug administration is used to promote analgesia, treat spontaneous pneumothorax, resolve pleural effusions, and deliver chemotherapeutic drugs. This chart lists commonly ordered drugs, their indications, doses, and special considerations.

DRUG AND INDICATION	INTRAPLEURAL DOSE	SPECIAL CONSIDERATIONS
bleomycin Pleural effusions and lung cancer	One-time dose of 60 to 150 units; lifetime dosage shouldn't exceed 400 units (to prevent pulmonary toxicity)	▪ Assess respiratory function carefully before each treatment, especially in patients at high risk for pulmonary toxicity, such as those with dyspnea, bibasilar crackles, and a nonproductive cough. ▪ Monitor the patient for 1 hr after treatment. ▪ Monitor BUN level, creatinine clearance, and pulmonary function. ▪ Arrange for chest X-rays before and during drug treatment. ▪ Monitor the patient with lymphoma for possible allergic reactions.

Reviewing intrapleural drugs and doses *(continued)*

DRUG AND INDICATION	INTRAPLEURAL DOSE	SPECIAL CONSIDERATIONS
bupivacaine Postoperative pain from cholecystectomy, renal surgery, breast surgery, rib fractures, chest metastasis, or pancreatic cancer	Dosage shouldn't exceed 175 mg when administered alone or 225 mg when administered with epinephrine. Usually, dose shouldn't be repeated more than once q 3 hr. Daily dosage shouldn't exceed 400 mg.	▪ Observe the patient for adverse CNS effects, including dizziness, disorientation, blurred vision, drowsiness, and seizures. ▪ Administer cautiously to patients with hepatic dysfunction.
doxycycline Prevention of recurrent spontaneous pneumothorax and pleural effusion	One-time dose of 500 mg	▪ Inform the patient that this drug causes severe discomfort, so he may receive a local anesthetic along with it. ▪ Tell the patient that the doctor injects this drug.
talc Prevention of recurrent spontaneous pneumothorax and pleural effusion	One-time dose of 4 to 10 g	▪ Explain that the doctor administers this drug after the patient undergoes general anesthesia. ▪ Monitor the patient for fever, severe pain, hypertension, and tachycardia.

Usually, drug delivery through a chest tube is indicated for patients with empyema, pleural effusion, or pneumothorax; delivery by intrapleural catheter is indicated for all other patients.

Drugs that are commonly administered by intrapleural injection include bleomycin, bupivacaine, doxycycline, and talc.

Complications and contraindications

- Intrapleural injection can cause complications, such as pneumothorax or tension pneumothorax, if air accidentally enters the pleural cavity.
- Additional serious complications include chemical irritation of the pleurae and subsequent neutropenia or thrombocytopenia (or both) as well as pain and infection at the insertion site. However, meticulous skin preparation, strict aseptic technique, and sterile dressings usually prevent infection.
- Drugs aren't given intrapleurally to a patient with fibrosis or adhesions (which impede drug infusion to the intended site), pleural inflammation, sepsis, or infection at the insertion site.
- Intrapleural administration isn't suitable for a patient with bullous emphysema or one who needs respiratory therapy with positive end-expiratory pressure, because this type of drug therapy may sometimes exacerbate an already compromised pulmonary condition.

Getting ready

- Take the following equipment to the patient's bedside, including the prescribed medication, a 60-ml syringe, the patient's medication administration record (MAR), a rubber-tipped clamp (for clamping the chest tube), a face shield, a gown, sterile gloves, and a sterile drape.
- Explain the procedure to the patient. If required by facility policy, make sure that he has given his informed consent.
- If the doctor prescribes a narcotic analgesic, put on gloves and administer it 30 minutes before the procedure.
- Verify the drug by comparing it with the patient's MAR.

Assisting with drug injection

- If the drug isn't already prepared, calculate the drug dose and dilute it with the correct amount of normal saline solution or another diluent. Draw up the drug into the 60-ml syringe.
- Position the patient on his side, with the affected side up. Clamp the chest tube. Then put on a gown and face shield. Using aseptic tech-

nique, the doctor will place a sterile drape under the chest tube connection and disconnect the chest tube from the drainage system.

- The doctor will attach the medication-filled syringe to the chest tube, remove the clamp, and administer the medication.

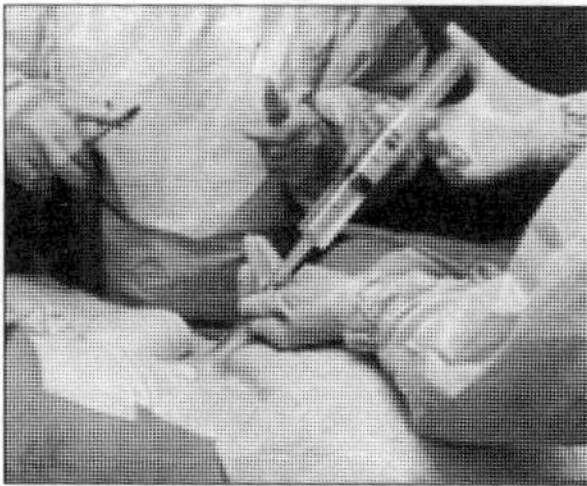

Aftercare

- After drug administration, you'll clamp the chest tube with the rubber-tipped clamp. Then close the clamp on the drainage tubing. Next, reconnect the chest tube to the drainage system (for added security).
- Ensure that the patient is as comfortable as possible. Have him remain on his unaffected side for 10 to 30 minutes, as tolerated, to help ensure that the medication circulates between the pleurae. (The longer the patient can maintain this position, the better.) However, the intense pain experienced by most patients usually makes this impossible.
- When the prescribed time has elapsed, help the patient into a supine position. Have him stay in this position for 10 to 30 minutes, as tolerated.
- Next, help the patient into a prone position. Have him stay in this position for 10 to 30 minutes, as tolerated.
- Help the patient into a sitting position. Have him stay in this position for 10 to 30 minutes, as tolerated. If he can't tolerate sitting, put the head of the bed in an elevated position that he can tolerate for 10 to 30 minutes.
- Now help the patient into Trendelenburg's position. Have him stay in this position for 10 to 30 minutes, as tolerated.
- Position the patient on the affected side for another 10 to 30 minutes. If he reports pain during position changes, the doctor may order another dose of a narcotic analgesic.
- Finally, help the patient into a comfortable position (usually semi-Fowler's position). Remove the clamp from the chest tube.
- Unclamp the drainage tube, and allow it to drain for 12 to 24 hours. If ordered, connect the drainage container to continuous wall suction.
- Document the procedure, including the medication injected and the patient's tolerance of it. ■

PART FOUR

DRUG THERAPY

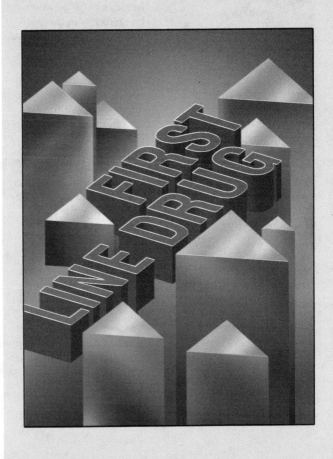

■ CHAPTER 16

IDENTIFYING DRUG THERAPY IN COMMON DISORDERS

Infectious disorders

Immune disorders

Cardiovascular disorders

Respiratory disorders

Neurologic disorders

Musculoskeletal disorders

GI disorders

Renal and urologic disorders

Endocrine disorders

Fluid and electrolyte disorders

INFECTIOUS DISORDERS

Amebiasis

Caused by *Entamoeba histolytica*, this liver or intestinal infection can be prevented by boiling drinking water and avoiding uncooked fruits and vegetables. Therapy varies with disease severity. Patients with hepatic abscesses may require surgical drainage as well as antiparasitic drugs.

For asymptomatic disease

▼FIRST-LINE DRUG

iodoquinol

Adult dosage

650 mg P.O. q 8 hours for 20 days

Points to remember

- Iodoquinol may cause nausea and vomiting.
- Because of the risk of optic neuritis, don't exceed recommended dose.

diloxanide furoate

Adult dosage

500 mg P.O. q 8 hours for 10 days

Points to remember

- This is a second-line drug.
- Diloxanide must be obtained from the CDC.

paromomycin

Adult dosage

25 to 30 mg/kg/day P.O. in three divided doses for 7 days

Point to remember

- This is a second-line drug.

For mild to moderate intestinal infection

▼FIRST-LINE DRUG

metronidazole

Adult dosage

750 mg P.O. q 8 hours for 10 days, followed by 650 mg of iodoquinol P.O. q 8 hours for 20 days, or 25 to 30 mg/kg/day of paromomycin in three divided doses for 7 days

Point to remember

- Because of the risk of optic neuritis, don't exceed recommended iodoquinol dose.

For severe intestinal disease

▼FIRST-LINE DRUG

metronidazole

Adult dosage

750 mg P.O. q 8 hours for 10 days, followed by 650 mg of iodoquinol P.O. q 8 hours for 20 days, or 25 to 30 mg/kg/day of paromomycin in three divided doses for 7 days

Point to remember

- Because of the risk of optic neuritis, don't exceed recommended iodoquinol dose.

dehydroemetine

Adult dosage

1 to 1.5 mg/kg/day I.M. for 5 days (maximum dose: 90

mg/day), followed by 650 mg of iodoquinol P.O. q 8 hours for 20 days

Point to remember

- This is a second-line drug.
- Because of the risk of optic neuritis, don't exceed recommended iodoquinol dose.

For hepatic abscess

▼FIRST-LINE DRUG

metronidazole

Adult dosage

750 mg P.O. q 8 hours for 10 days, followed by 650 mg of iodoquinol P.O. q 8 hours for 20 days, or 25 to 30 mg/kg/day of paromomycin in three divided doses for 7 days

Point to remember

- Because of the risk of optic neuritis, don't exceed recommended iodoquinol dose.

dehydroemetine

Adult dosage

1 to 1.5 mg/kg/day I.M. for 5 days (maximum dose: 90 mg/day), followed by 650 mg of iodoquinol P.O. q 8 hours for 20 days plus 600 mg/day (base) of chloroquine phosphate for 2 days, then 300 mg/day (base) of chloroquine phosphate

Points to remember

- This is a second-line drug.
- Dehydroemetine must be obtained from the CDC.
- Because of the risk of optic neuritis, don't exceed recommended iodoquinol dose. ■

Blastomycosis

This infectious disease is caused by a yeastlike fungus, *Blastomyces dermatitidis.* Acute pulmonary infection usually is self-limiting and requires no treatment. However, severe or progressive disease requires antifungal therapy.

▼FIRST-LINE DRUG

ketoconazole

Adult dosage

400 mg/day P.O. for at least 6 months

Points to remember

- This is a first-line drug for mild infections.
- Don't administer with antacids, H_2-receptor antagonists, or omeprazole (drug absorption requires gastric acid).
- Patients who respond poorly may require 600 to 800 mg/day.
- This drug isn't indicated for CNS infections because it doesn't enter CSF.

▼FIRST-LINE DRUG

amphotericin B

Adult dosage

0.3 to 0.5 mg/kg/day to a total cumulative dose of 1.5 to 2.5 g

Points to remember

- Drug is for moderate to severe infections, CNS infections, and patients who don't respond to ketoconazole.

- Administer 1-mg I.V. test dose before giving first dose.
- Infuse over 4 to 6 hours.
- Drug isn't stable in electrolyte solutions.

itraconazole
Adult dosage
200 to 400 mg/day P.O.
Points to remember
- This drug is an alternative to amphotericin and ketoconazole.
- Administer with food to increase bioavailability.
- This drug isn't indicated for CNS infections because it doesn't enter CSF. ■

Candidiasis

Most candidal infections are caused by *Candida albicans.* Drug therapy varies with the infection site and must be adjusted for the specific species. The regimens described below apply to *C. albicans.*

For thrush

▼FIRST-LINE DRUG
clotrimazole
Adult dosage
Oral troche: 10 mg P.O. three to five times daily for 10 to 14 days
Points to remember
- Instruct patient to suck on troche.
- AIDS patients usually don't respond significantly to this topical therapy; fluconazole or ketoconazole therapy may be necessary.

▼FIRST-LINE DRUG
nystatin
Adult dosage
500,000 units of oral suspension swished and swallowed three to five times daily for 10 to 14 days
Point to remember
- AIDS patients usually don't respond significantly to this topical therapy; fluconazole or ketoconazole therapy may be necessary.

fluconazole
Adult dosage
200 mg P.O. loading dose on day 1, followed by 50 to 100 mg/day P.O. for 5 to 7 days
Points to remember
- This is an alternative drug for patients who don't respond to topical therapy.
- AIDS patients may require prolonged therapy.

ketoconazole
Adult dosage
200 mg P.O. q 12 hours for 5 to 7 days
Points to remember
- This is an alternative drug for patients who don't respond to topical therapy.
- Don't administer with antacids, H_2-receptor antagonists, or omeprazole (drug absorption requires gastric acid).
- AIDS patients may require prolonged therapy.

For cutaneous infection

▼FIRST-LINE DRUG

nystatin cream

Adult dosage

Apply cream to affected area b.i.d.

Points to remember

- Powder form may be preferable for moist areas.
- Miconazole or clotrimazole cream may be substituted.

For esophageal candidiasis

▼FIRST-LINE DRUG

fluconazole

Adult dosage

100 to 400 mg/day P.O. for 10 to 21 days

Point to remember

- AIDS patients may require prolonged therapy and higher doses.

▼FIRST-LINE DRUG

ketoconazole

Adult dosage

200 mg P.O. q 12 hours for 10 to 21 days

Points to remember

- Don't administer with antacids, H_2-receptor antagonists, or omeprazole (drug absorption requires gastric acid).
- AIDS patients may require prolonged therapy.

amphotericin B

Adult dosage

0.2 to 0.4 mg/kg/day I.V. for 7 to 14 days

Points to remember

- This drug is reserved for patients with severe or unresponsive infections.
- Administer 1-mg I.V. test dose before giving first dose.
- Infuse over 4 to 6 hours.
- Monitor serum creatinine, magnesium, and electrolyte levels closely.

For disseminated candidiasis or candidemia

▼FIRST-LINE DRUG

amphotericin B

Adult dosage

0.3 to 0.8 mg/kg/day I.V. to total cumulative dose of 0.5 to 1 g (given with or without flucytosine)

Points to remember

- Administer 1-mg I.V. test dose before giving first dose.
- Infuse drug over 4 to 6 hours.
- Amphotericin B isn't stable in electrolyte solutions.
- Monitor serum creatinine, magnesium, and electrolyte levels carefully; about 80% of patients receiving 1 g or more of amphotericin B experience nephrotoxicity.
- In candidemia, remove or change I.V. lines.

fluconazole

Adult dosage

400 mg I.V. loading dose, then 200 to 400 mg/day I.V.

Points to remember

- This is an alternative drug.
- Duration of therapy depends on patient's response.

flucytosine
Adult dosage
100 to 150 mg/kg/day P.O. divided in four doses
Points to remember
- Adjust dosage in renal dysfunction.
- Therapeutic serum drug level is 25 to 100 mcg/ml.

For candiduria

▼FIRST-LINE DRUG
amphotericin B
Adult dosage
Continuous bladder irrigant: 50 mg in 1 liter of sterile water infused into bladder via triple-lumen catheter over 24 hours for 5 days
Clamped bladder irrigant: 5 to 10 mg in 1 liter of sterile water; infuse 200 to 300 ml into bladder; clamp for 60 to 90 minutes and drain; repeat q 6 to 8 hours for 5 days
Point to remember
- Check inflow and outflow lines periodically for kinks to make sure solution runs freely. Catheter outflow obstruction can cause bladder distention.

fluconazole
Adult dosage
200 mg P.O. loading dose, followed by 100 mg/day P.O. for 3 to 5 days
Point to remember
- This is an alternative drug.

For vaginal candidiasis

▼FIRST-LINE DRUG
miconazole nitrate
Adult dosage
Insert 1 applicatorful of 2% vaginal cream h.s. for 7 days
Points to remember
- This is a first-line drug.
- Butoconazole, clotrimazole, or terconazole vaginal cream or ticonazole ointment may be substituted.
- Three-day regimen with vaginal suppository (200 mg miconazole nitrate) may be substituted.

fluconazole
Adult dosage
One-time dose of 150 mg P.O.
Points to remember
- This is an alternative drug.
- Relapse rate may be higher than with topical regimens.

itraconazole
Adult dosage
200 mg/day P.O. for 3 days
Point to remember
- This is an alternative drug. ■

Cholera

This acute bacterial infection is caused by *Vibrio cholerae.* Aggressive fluid and electrolyte replacement is the mainstay of therapy and can help avert death. Antibiotics are given to relieve diarrhea and decrease fluid and electrolyte loss.

▼FIRST-LINE DRUG

doxycycline

Adult dosage

One-time dose of 300 mg P.O.

Points to remember

- Contraindicated during pregnancy and in patients with hypersensitivity to tetracycline.
- Don't use in children under age 8 because drug discolors the teeth.

▼FIRST-LINE DRUG

tetracycline

Adult dosage

500 mg P.O. q 6 hours for 3 to 5 days

Point to remember

- Don't administer with antacids or dairy products.

co-trimoxazole (sulfamethoxazole-trimethoprim)

Adult dosage

One double-strength tablet (containing 800 mg sulfamethoxazole and 160 mg trimethoprim) P.O. q 12 hours for 3 days

Point to remember

- This is an alternative drug.

furazolidone

Adult dosage

100 mg P.O. q 6 hours for 3 days

Point to remember

- This is an alternative drug. ■

CMV infection

In this viral infection, duration of therapy depends on the patient's immune status and the infection site. AIDS patients with cytomegalovirus (CMV) retinitis require lifelong antiviral maintenance therapy after an induction course. Associated pneumonitis and colitis are treated for 14 to 21 days with either ganciclovir or foscarnet. Bone marrow transplant recipients usually receive CMV prophylaxis (ganciclovir) for 100 days after transplantation and may also receive I.V. gamma globulin therapy. Solid organ transplant recipients requiring CMV prophylaxis usually receive an antiviral agent (ganciclovir) for 28 days; CMV immunoglobulin may be added to the regimen in liver transplant recipients.

▼FIRST-LINE DRUG

foscarnet

Adult dosage

Induction therapy: 60 mg/kg I.V. q 8 hours for 14 to 21 days

Maintenance therapy: 90 to 120 mg/kg/day I.V. infused over 2 hours

Points to remember

- Foscarnet may cause nephrotoxicity; adjust dosage in renal dysfunction.

- Monitor serum electrolyte levels closely.
- Maintenance therapy is necessary for AIDS patients with CMV retinitis; most patients with CMV-associated colitis or pneumonitis need only 14- to 21-day induction therapy.
- In AIDS patients, foscarnet has been associated with an increased survival of approximately 3 months, compared with ganciclovir.

▼FIRST-LINE DRUG

ganciclovir

Adult dosage

Induction therapy: 5 mg/kg I.V. q 12 hours for 21 days
Maintenance therapy: 5 mg/kg/day I.V.

Points to remember

- Adjust dosage in renal dysfunction.
- Monitor WBC counts closely; severe neutropenia may warrant dosage reduction or drug discontinuation.
- Oral ganciclovir capsules recently were approved for maintenance therapy in CMV retinitis (1,000 mg P.O. q 8 hours) for patients who can't tolerate I.V. ganciclovir.
- Oral ganciclovir is associated with faster relapse rate than I.V. ganciclovir.
- Efficacy of oral ganciclovir in treating CMV infections other than retinitis hasn't been established.
- Maintenance therapy is needed for AIDS patients with CMV retinitis; AIDS patients with CMV-associated colitis or pneumonitis need only 14- to 21-day induction therapy. ■

Coccidioidomycosis

This infectious fungal disease is caused by inhaling spores of the bacterium *Coccidioides immitis.* In about 60% of cases, it's self-limiting, causing no symptoms. Antifungal therapy is needed when the infection has spread beyond the lungs or when symptoms last more than 6 weeks.

▼FIRST-LINE DRUG

amphotericin B

Adult dosage

Pulmonary or extrapulmonary disease: 0.6 mg/kg/day I.V. to total cumulative dose of 2.5 g or more (longer therapy needed if remission doesn't occur)
Meningitis: 0.6 mg/kg/day I.V. to total cumulative dose of 2.5 g or more (longer therapy needed if remission doesn't occur); some patients may require intrathecal as well as I.V. administration

Points to remember

- Administer 1-mg I.V. test dose before giving first dose.
- Infuse over 4 to 6 hours.
- Drug isn't stable in electrolyte solutions.

- Monitor serum creatinine, magnesium, and electrolyte levels carefully; about 80% of patients receiving 1 g or more experience nephrotoxicity.
- Pulmonary infection with associated cavitary lesions may necessitate surgery.

itraconazole
Adult dosage
400 mg/day P.O. for 6 to 18 months
Points to remember
- This is an alternative drug.
- Administer with food to increase drug bioavailability.
- Don't use to treat meningitis; drug doesn't penetrate blood-brain barrier.

ketoconazole
Adult dosage
400 to 800 mg/day for 6 to 18 months
Points to remember
- This is an alternative drug.
- Don't use to treat meningitis; drug doesn't penetrate blood-brain barrier.
- Don't administer with antacids, H_2-receptor antagonists, or omeprazole (drug absorption requires gastric acid). ■

Common cold

The common cold is treated symptomatically with analgesics, cough suppressants, and decongestants. Gargling with warm saline solution helps relieve sore throat.

aspirin
Adult dosage
325 to 650 mg P.O. q 4 to 6 hours p.r.n.
Points to remember
- This drug is an analgesic and antipyretic.
- An NSAID may be substituted.

codeine
Adult dosage
10 to 20 mg P.O. q 4 to 6 hours p.r.n.
Points to remember
- This drug is a cough suppressant.
- Don't exceed 60 mg/day.
- Don't use for cough associated with excessive respiratory secretions.

dextromethorphan
Adult dosage
Lozenges or syrup: 10 to 30 mg P.O. q 4 to 8 hours p.r.n.
Sustained-action liquid: 60 mg P.O. q 12 hours
Points to remember
- This drug is a cough suppressant.
- Don't exceed 120 mg/day.
- Don't use for cough associated with excessive respiratory secretions.

ibuprofen
Adult dosage
400 mg P.O. q 4 to 6 hours p.r.n.

Points to remember
- This drug is an analgesic and antipyretic.
- Another NSAID may be substituted.

pseudoephedrine
Adult dosage
30 to 60 mg P.O. q 6 hours p.r.n.
Points to remember
- This drug is a decongestant.
- Don't exceed 240 mg/day.
- Other decongestants may be substituted.
- Use cautiously in patients with acute angle-closure glaucoma or uncontrolled hypertension. ■

Enterobacteriaceae infections

These local and systemic infections are caused by enterobacteriaceae, a group of mostly aerobic, gram-negative bacilli that are part of the normal flora of the GI tract. Antibiotic selection depends on the causative organism, infection site, and results of culture and sensitivity testing. Empiric drug therapy is described below.

gentamicin
Adult dosage
Based on patient's weight and renal function (usually a loading dose of 1.8 to 2 mg/kg, with maintenance dose of 1.3 to 1.5 mg/kg at intervals based on creatinine clearance); given with or without one of the following drugs

cefotaxime
Adult dosage
1 to 2 g I.V. q 8 hours

ciprofloxacin
Adult dosage
400 mg I.V. q 12 hours

imipenem
Adult dosage
500 mg I.V. q 6 hours

piperacillin
Adult dosage
3 g I.V. q 4 to 6 hours

ticarcillin disodium/ clavulanate
Adult dosage
3.1 g I.V. q 4 to 6 hours
Points to remember for all infections caused by Enterobacteriaceae
- Recommended dosages are for patients with normal renal function; decrease dosage in renal dysfunction.
- Another aminoglycoside may be substituted for gentamicin.
- Other third-generation cephalosporins, penicillins, or fluoroquinolones may be substituted for cefotaxime, piperacillin, or ciprofloxacin, respectively.
- Anaerobic coverage (using cefoxitin, metronidazole, clindamycin, imipenem, or

ticarcillin/clavulanate) should be included if intra-abdominal disease is suspected. ■

Herpes simplex

Drug dosages for this viral infection vary with the infection site and the patient's immune status.

For patients with normal immune status

▼FIRST-LINE DRUG

acyclovir

Adult dosage

Mucocutaneous infection: 5 mg/kg I.V. q 8 hours, or 200 to 400 mg P.O. five times daily for 10 to 14 days

Disseminated disease: 10 to 12.4 mg/kg I.V. q 8 hours for 7 days

Herpes encephalitis: 10 to 12.4 mg/kg I.V. q 8 hours for 7 to 14 days

Points to remember

- Drug resistance may occur; foscarnet is a second-line drug for such patients.
- Adjust dosage in renal dysfunction.

For immunocompromised patients

▼FIRST-LINE DRUG

acyclovir

Adult dosage

5 to 12.4 mg/kg q 8 hours for 7 to 14 days

Points to remember

- Drug resistance may occur; foscarnet is a second-line drug for such patients.
- Adjust dosage in renal dysfunction.

foscarnet

Adult dosage

40 mg/kg I.V. q 8 hours for 7 to 14 days

Points to remember

- Foscarnet is an alternative drug for patients with acyclovir-resistant herpes strains.
- Monitor serum electrolyte levels.
- Adjust dosage in renal dysfunction; drug may cause nephrotoxicity. ■

Herpes zoster

Herpes zoster (also called shingles) is caused by the varicella-zoster virus. Drug dosages vary with the infection site and the patient's immune status. Mild infection in patients with normal immune status may not require antiviral therapy.

For patients with normal immune status, mild pneumonia, or dermatomal infection

▼FIRST-LINE DRUG

acyclovir

Adult dosage

800 mg P.O. five times daily for 7 to 10 days

Points to remember

- Drug resistance may occur.
- Adjust dosage in renal dysfunction.
- AIDS patients may require long-term immunosuppressant therapy.
- Varicella-zoster immune globulin may be given as prophylaxis to exposed and susceptible immunocompromised patients.

For severe disseminated disease or immunocompromised patients

▼FIRST-LINE DRUG

acyclovir

Adult dosage

10 to 12.4 mg/kg I.V. q 8 hours for 7 to 10 days

Points to remember

- Drug resistance may occur.
- Adjust dosage in renal dysfunction.
- AIDS patients may require long-term immunosuppressant therapy.
- Varicella-zoster immune globulin may be given as prophylaxis to exposed and susceptible immunocompromised patients.

foscarnet

Adult dosage

40 mg/kg I.V. q 8 hours for 7 to 14 days

Points to remember

- Foscarnet is an alternative drug for patients with acyclovir-resistant herpes strains.
- Monitor serum electrolyte levels.
- Adjust dosage in renal dysfunction; drug may cause nephrotoxicity. ■

Histoplasmosis

This disease is caused by inhaling spores of the fungus *Histoplasma capsulatum.* Most pulmonary infections produce no symptoms and are self-limiting. However, immunocompromised patients are most likely to have severe or disseminated disease that requires antifungal therapy.

For acute or severe pulmonary infections

▼FIRST-LINE DRUG

amphotericin B

Adult dosage

0.6 mg/kg/day I.V. to total cumulative dose of 500 mg (over 2 to 3 weeks)

Points to remember

- This is a first-line drug for severe infections.

- Administer 1-mg test dose before giving first dose.
- Infuse over 4 to 6 hours.
- Drug isn't stable in electrolyte solutions.
- Oral suppressant antifungal therapy may be needed after I.V. therapy.
- Monitor serum creatinine and electrolyte levels carefully; about 80% of patients receiving 1 g or more of amphotericin B experience nephrotoxicity.
- Chronic pulmonary or cavitary infections may require higher cumulative doses of 2 to 2.5 g.

For chronic infections or disseminated disease in immunocompromised patients without CNS involvement

▼FIRST-LINE DRUG

itraconazole

Adult dosage

200 mg P.O. q 12 hours for 6 to 12 months

Points to remember

- Administer with food to increase bioavailability.
- Itraconazole isn't indicated for meningitis because it doesn't cross blood-brain barrier.

ketoconazole

Adult dosage

400 mg/day P.O. for 6 to 12 months

Points to remember

- This is an alternative drug.
- Ketoconazole isn't indicated for meningitis because it doesn't cross blood-brain barrier.
- Don't administer with antacids, H_2-receptor antagonists, or omeprazole (drug absorption requires gastric acid).

For disseminated disease in immunocompromised patients with CNS involvement

▼FIRST-LINE DRUG

amphotericin B

Adult dosage

0.6 mg/kg/day I.V. to cumulative dose of 30 to 40 mg/kg

Points to remember

- This is a first-line drug for severe infections.
- Administer 1-mg I.V. test dose before giving first dose.
- Infuse over 4 to 6 hours.
- Drug isn't stable in electrolyte solutions.
- Monitor serum creatinine and electrolyte levels carefully; about 80% of patients receiving 1 g or more of amphotericin experience nephrotoxicity.
- In AIDS patients, itraconazole oral suppressant therapy (400 mg/day P.O.) is recommended after amphotericin therapy. ■

Hookworm disease

This disease is caused by infection with the nematodes *Necator americanus* or *Ancylostoma duodenale.* Treatment requires anthelmintic therapy to eradicate the parasite (mebendazole is 90% effective in eradication). Anemia is treated with iron supplementation.

▼FIRST-LINE DRUG

mebendazole

Adult dosage

100 mg P.O. q 12 hours for 3 days

Point to remember

- Tablets may be chewed, swallowed, or crushed.

pyrantel pamoate

Adult dosage

11 mg/kg/day P.O. for 3 days; maximum daily dose 1 g

Points to remember

- This is an alternative drug.
- Oral suspension may be mixed with milk or juice. ■

Lassa fever

A highly contagious disease caused by a virulent arenavirus, Lassa fever may be fatal. Currently, no approved treatment exists; ribavirin is being used investigationally.

ribavirin

Investigational adult dosage

1 g I.V. loading dose, followed by 1 g I.V. q 6 hours for 4 days; then 0.5 g I.V. q 8 hours for 6 days

Points to remember

- Drug is FDA-approved for administration by aerosol only.
- Ribavirin isn't FDA-approved for this indication or for administration by the I.V. route. ■

Lyme disease

This multisystemic disorder is caused by *Borrelia burgdorferi,* a spirochete transmitted by *Ixodes dammini* or another tick. Treatment depends on the stage of Lyme disease. Erythema chronicum migrans, which occurs in 80% to 90% of patients with the disease, is confirmed when tests isolate the spirochete in body fluids. This is evidenced by the presence of immunoglobulins M and G in CSF or serum or when changes in antibody levels are linked to symptoms.

For early Lyme disease (indicated by the skin lesion erythema chronicum migrans)

▼FIRST-LINE DRUG
doxycycline
Adult dosage
100 mg P.O. b.i.d. or t.i.d. for 10 to 30 days
Point to remember
- Doxycycline is contraindicated in pregnant patients.

amoxicillin
Adult dosage
250 to 500 mg P.O. q 8 hours for 10 to 30 days
Points to remember
- This is an alternative drug.
- It's safe for use in pregnant patients.

erythromycin (base, estolate, or stearate)
Adult dosage
250 mg P.O. q 6 hours for 10 to 30 days
Point to remember
- Erythromycin is used as an alternative drug; it's less effective than doxycycline or amoxicillin.

For late Lyme disease (indicated by carditis, arthritis, or neurologic disorders)

▼FIRST-LINE DRUG
ceftriaxone
Adult dosage
2 g/day I.V. for 14 to 21 days
Point to remember
- Drug may be used during pregnancy, although penicillin G (2 million units/day) is the preferred treatment. ■

Malaria

This disease is caused by four species of the protozoan genus *Plasmodium (P. ovale, P. falciparum, P. vivax,* and *P. malariae)*. Treatment and prophylactic drug regimens vary geographically because of chloroquine-resistance patterns. Check with the CDC for the latest recommendations.

For prophylaxis against malaria

▼FIRST-LINE DRUG
chloroquine phosphate
Adult dosage
300 mg (base) P.O. once a week
Points to remember
- This is a first-line prophylactic drug for chloroquine-susceptible *P. falciparum.*
- Prophylaxis should begin 1 to 2 weeks before entering endemic area and should continue for 4 weeks after leaving the area.
- This drug may cause serious hemolytic anemia; patients should be tested for G6PD deficiency before ther-

apy starts. Monitor CBC and heart rate.
- Use this drug with caution in patients with liver disease.

▼FIRST-LINE DRUG
mefloquine
Adult dosage
228 mg (base) P.O. once a week
Points to remember
- This is a first-line prophylactic drug for chloroquine-resistant *P. falciparum.*
- Prophylaxis should begin 1 to 2 weeks before entering endemic area and should continue for 4 weeks after leaving the area.
- Mefloquine is contraindicated in pregnant women and children; chloroquine is the recommended alternative.
- Drug may cause significant side effects, including nausea, vomiting, seizures, psychosis, and cardiac arrhythmias. Drug is contraindicated in patients with history of epilepsy, who are at increased risk for seizures.
- Don't administer with beta blockers because this combination increases the risk of cardiac arrest.

hydroxychloroquine sulfate
Adult dosage
310 mg (base) P.O. once a week
Points to remember
- This is an alternative drug for patients who can't tolerate chloroquine.
- Prophylaxis should begin 1 to 2 weeks before entering endemic area and should continue for 4 weeks after leaving the area.

doxycycline
Adult dosage
100 mg/day P.O.
Points to remember
- This drug is an alternative to mefloquine; it's a first-line drug for travelers to Thailand.
- Prophylactic therapy should begin 1 to 2 weeks before entering endemic area and should continue for 4 weeks after leaving the area.
- Doxycycline is contraindicated in pregnant women and children; chloroquine is the recommended alternative.

primaquine phosphate
Adult dosage
15 mg/day (base) P.O. for 14 days (during last 2 weeks of prophylactic regimen)
Points to remember
- This drug prevents relapses caused by *P. vivax* and *P. ovale.*
- It's given to all at-risk patients during last 2 weeks of prophylactic regimen.
- Administer with food if GI upset occurs.

- This drug may cause hemolytic anemia; patients should be tested for G6PD deficiency before drug therapy starts. Monitor CBC.

For treatment of malaria

▼FIRST-LINE DRUG
chloroquine
Adult dosage
One-time dose of 600 mg (base) P.O., then 300 mg (base) P.O. 6 hours later, followed by another 300-mg dose 24 hours and 48 hours later
Points to remember
- Drug is first-line therapy for chloroquine-susceptible *P. falciparum.*
- Quinidine gluconate can be substituted if parenteral therapy is necessary.
- This drug may cause serious hemolytic anemia; patients should be tested for G6PD deficiency before starting therapy. Monitor CBC and heart rate.
- Use with caution in patients with liver disease.

▼FIRST-LINE DRUG
primaquine phosphate
Adult dosage
15 mg/day (base) P.O. for 14 days
Points to remember
- Drug is first-line therapy for *P. ovale* and *P. vivax* only.
- It may cause hemolytic anemia; patients should be tested for G6PD deficiency before starting therapy. Monitor CBC.
- Administer with food if GI upset occurs.

▼FIRST-LINE REGIMEN
quinine sulfate
Adult dosage
650 mg P.O. q 8 hours for 3 to 7 days, with or without one of the following

clindamycin
Adult dosage
900 mg P.O. q 8 hours for 3 days

pyrimethamine with sulfadoxine
Adult dosage
One-time dose of 3 tablets P.O. (75 mg pyrimethamine and 1,500 mg sulfadoxine)

tetracycline
Adult dosage
250 mg P.O. q 6 hours for 7 days
Points to remember
- This regimen is first-line therapy for chloroquine-resistant strains of *Plasmodium.*
- Tetracycline and pyrimethamine with sulfadoxine are contraindicated in pregnant patients.
- Quinidine gluconate can be substituted if parenteral therapy is necessary.
- Administer pyrimethamine with sulfadoxine with 8 oz (240 ml) of fluid.
- This regimen may cause serious hemolytic anemia; pa-

tients should be tested for G6PD deficiency before starting therapy. Monitor CBC.

mefloquine
Adult dosage
One-time dose of 1,250 mg P.O.
Points to remember
- This is an alternative drug for patients with chloroquine-resistant strains of *Plasmodium.*
- It's contraindicated in pregnant patients and children.
- Drug may cause significant side effects, including nausea, vomiting, seizures, psychosis, and cardiac arrhythmias. It's contraindicated in patients with history of epilepsy, who are at increased risk for seizures.
- Don't administer with beta blockers because this combination increases the risk of cardiac arrest. ■

Plague

This potentially lethal disease is caused by the bite of a flea infected by a rat infected with the bacillus *Yersinia pestis.* Besides antibiotic therapy, the patient may need supportive therapy to manage dehydration and shock.

▼FIRST-LINE DRUG
streptomycin
Adult dosage
30 mg/kg I.M. in two divided doses q 10 days
Point to remember
- Therapy may be shortened to 3-day course to decrease risk of toxicity in pregnant patients and in those with renal or auditory disorders.

chloramphenicol
Adult dosage
25 mg/kg I.V. loading dose, followed by 60 mg/kg I.V. in four divided doses q 10 days
Points to remember
- This is an alternative drug for patients with meningitis or for those in whom I.M. injections are contraindicated or not well absorbed.
- Chloramphenicol may cause bone marrow suppression and, rarely, aplastic anemia; monitor CBC.

tetracycline
Adult dosage
500 to 1,000 mg P.O. q 6 hours for 10 days
Points to remember
- This is an alternative drug for patients who are allergic to streptomycin.
- Don't administer with antacids or dairy products.
- Tetracycline is contraindicated in pregnant patients and children. ■

Pseudomonas aeruginosa infections

Double antibiotic coverage is recommended in most of these infections to prevent rapid development of drug resistance. Because organism susceptibility varies widely, antibiotic selection is based on results of culture and sensitivity tests. Empiric therapy is described below.

tobramycin
Adult dosage
Based on patient's weight and renal function (usually a loading dose of 1.8 to 2 mg/kg, with a maintenance dose of 1.3 to 1.5 mg/kg at intervals based on creatinine clearance); given with or without one of the following drugs

aztreonam
Adult dosage
1 g I.V. q 6 to 8 hours

ceftazidime
Adult dosage
1 to 2 g I.V. q 8 hours

ciprofloxacin
Adult dosage
400 mg I.V. q 12 hours

imipenem
Adult dosage
500 mg I.V. q 6 hours

piperacillin
Adult dosage
3 g I.V. q 4 to 6 hours

ticarcillin disodium/clavulanate
Adult dosage
3.1 g q 4 to 6 hours
Points to remember
- Recommended dosages are for patients with normal renal function. Decrease dosage in renal dysfunction.
- Another aminoglycoside may be substituted for tobramycin. ■

Rocky Mountain spotted fever

This infectious disease is caused by *Rickettsia rickettsii*, a rod-shaped bacterium transmitted by ticks. Patients with pulmonary edema and other severe symptoms require supportive therapy in addition to antibiotics. Antibiotic therapy should be given to all patients and should continue until the patient's body temperature has been normal for at least 2 days.

▼FIRST-LINE DRUG
doxycycline
Adult dosage
100 mg P.O. or I.V. q 12 hours for at least 7 days
Point to remember
- Doxycycline is contraindicated in pregnant patients.

▼FIRST-LINE DRUG
tetracycline
Adult dosage
25 to 50 g/kg/day P.O. in four divided doses for at least 7 days
Points to remember
- Don't administer with antacids or dairy products.
- Tetracycline is contraindicated in pregnant patients.

chloramphenicol
Adult dosage
50 to 75 mg/kg/day P.O. in four divided doses for at least 7 days
Point to remember
- This is an alternative drug used in pregnant patients.

ciprofloxacin
Adult dosage
250 to 750 mg P.O. q 12 hours for at least 7 days
Points to remember
- This is an alternative drug.
- It's contraindicated in pregnant patients. ■

Salmonellosis

This infection is caused by ingesting food contaminated with *Salmonella typhi* or another *Salmonella* species. For most patients with enterocolitis, fluid and electrolyte replacement is the mainstay of therapy; few need antibiotic therapy. However, severe symptoms (such as those occurring with the typhoid variant of salmonellosis) call for antibiotics. Drug-resistant bacterial strains are common; therapy is based on culture and sensitivity testing. Empiric therapy is described below.

▼FIRST-LINE DRUG
ampicillin
Adult dosage
100 mg/kg/day P.O. or I.V. in four divided doses for at least 2 weeks
Points to remember
- Don't use this drug in patients with a penicillin allergy.
- Common side effects include rash and diarrhea.

▼FIRST-LINE DRUG
chloramphenicol
Adult dosage
50 mg/kg/day P.O. in four divided doses for at least 2 weeks
Points to remember
- Dosage must be decreased in patients with hepatic dysfunction.
- Rarely, drug may cause bone marrow suppression and aplastic anemia; monitor CBC, particularly platelet and reticulocyte counts.

co-trimoxazole (sulfamethoxazole-trimethoprim)
Adult dosage
One or two double-strength tablets (containing 800 mg sulfamethoxazole and 160

mg trimethoprim) P.O. q 12 hours for at least 2 weeks
Point to remember
- This is an alternative drug; it may be less effective than first-line drugs. ■

Scarlet fever

This acute contagious disease is caused by a toxin-producing strain of *Streptococcus pyogenes.* Antibiotic therapy is used to prevent complications, such as sinusitis, otitis media, and acute rheumatic fever.

▼FIRST-LINE DRUG
penicillin G benzathine
Adult dosage
One-time dose of 1.2 million units
Points to remember
- Administer by deep I.M. injection into the upper outer quadrant of the buttocks.
- Drug may cause pain at the insertion site.

▼FIRST-LINE DRUG
penicillin V potassium
Adult dosage
250 mg P.O. q 8 hours for 10 days
Point to remember
- One-time dose of penicillin G benzathine may be preferred by patients unwilling or unable to comply with 10-day course required in penicillin V therapy.

erythromycin (base, stearate, or estolate)
Adult dosage
250 mg P.O. q 6 hours for 10 days
Point to remember
- This is an alternative drug for patients who are allergic to penicillin. ■

Sepsis

Sepsis is defined as bacteremia with accompanying tachycardia, hyperthermia or hypothermia, and tachypnea. Patients in septic shock may need supportive therapy, such as vasopressors and I.V. fluids, as well as antibiotics. Antibiotic selection is based on results of culture and sensitivity testing. The regimen below describes empiric therapy.

gentamicin
Adult dosage
Based on patient's weight and renal function (usually a loading dose of 1.8 to 2 mg/kg, with a maintenance dose of 1.3 to 1.5 mg/kg at intervals based on creatinine clearance); given with or without one of the following drugs

cefotaxime
Adult dosage
1 to 2 g I.V. q 6 to 8 hours

imipenem
Adult dosage
500 mg I.V. q 6 hours

piperacillin
Adult dosage
3 g I.V. q 4 to 6 hours

ticarcillin disodium/ clavulanate
Adult dosage
3.1 g q 4 to 6 hours
Points to remember
- Recommended dosages are for patients with normal renal function; decrease dosages in renal dysfunction.
- Another aminoglycoside may be substituted for gentamicin.
- Other third-generation cephalosporins or penicillins may be substituted for cefotaxime and piperacillin, respectively.
- Vancomycin should be added if methicillin-resistant *Staphylococcus aureus* is suspected.
- Anaerobic coverage (with cefoxitin, metronidazole, clindamycin, imipenem, or ticarcillin disodium/clavulanate) should be included if intra-abdominal disease is suspected. ■

Shigellosis

This acute bacterial bowel infection may call for fluid and electrolyte management in addition to antibiotics. Antibiotic selection is based on results of culture and sensitivity testing. Empiric therapy is described below.

▼FIRST-LINE DRUG
ciprofloxacin
Adult dosage
500 mg P.O. q 12 hours for 3 to 5 days
Point to remember
- Other fluoroquinolones may be substituted.

▼FIRST-LINE DRUG
co-trimoxazole (sulfamethoxazole-trimethoprim)
Adult dosage
One double-strength tablet (containing 800 mg sulfamethoxazole and 160 mg trimethoprim) P.O. q 12 hours for 3 to 5 days
Points to remember
- Monitor for side effects, such as sore throat, fever, chills, pale skin, yellowing of skin or eyes, rash, or unusual bleeding or bruising.
- Don't give to patients with allergy to sulfa drugs.

ampicillin
Adult dosage
500 mg P.O. q 6 hours for 3 to 5 days
Point to remember
- This is a second-line drug. ■

Toxic shock syndrome

This severe, acute disease is caused by toxin-producing strains of *Staphylococcus aureus* or *Streptococcus.* Initial therapy focuses on aggressive management of hypotension with fluid replacement, colloids, or both. Also, the infection source (such as a tampon) should be found and eliminated. Patients with significant desquamation may need continued fluid replacement and aggressive skin care. Antibiotic therapy doesn't alter the course of the acute syndrome but can prevent recurrences.

▼FIRST-LINE DRUG

nafcillin

Adult dosage

1 to 2 g I.V. q 4 to 6 hours

Point to remember

- Oxacillin may be substituted.

cefazolin

Adult dosage

1 to 2 g I.V. q 8 hours

Point to remember

- This is a second-line drug. ■

Toxoplasmosis

This infection is caused by *Toxoplasma gondii,* a protozoan intracellular parasite. Antiparasitic therapy typically eliminates symptoms in 90% of affected patients after 2 weeks of therapy. AIDS patients, however, must receive maintenance therapy to prevent symptom recurrence.

For acute infection

▼FIRST-LINE DRUG REGIMEN

pyrimethamine

Adult dosage

100 mg P.O. loading dose, followed by 25 to 100 mg/day P.O., plus 1 to 2 g of sulfadiazine P.O. q 6 hours

Points to remember

- Give folinic acid (10 mg/day P.O.) with pyrimethamine to decrease risk of bone marrow suppression.
- AIDS patients with encephalitis should be treated with this regimen for 6 weeks after resolution of symptoms and then maintained on lifelong therapy.
- This regimen may cause serious hemolytic anemia; patients should be tested for G6PD deficiency before starting therapy.
- Administer with food.

clindamycin

Adult dosage

600 mg I.V. or 300 to 450 mg P.O. q 6 hours, plus 25 to 100 mg/day of pyrimethamine P.O. for 6 weeks

Points to remember

- This is an alternative regimen.
- Give folinic acid (10 mg/day P.O.) along with pyrimethamine to decrease risk of bone marrow suppression.
- Administer with food.
- This regimen may cause serious hemolytic anemia; patients should be tested for G6PD deficiency before starting therapy.
- Therapy consisting of azithromycin or atovaquone plus pyrimethamine is under investigation.

For maintenance therapy for AIDS patients

▼FIRST-LINE DRUG

co-trimoxazole (sulfamethoxazole-trimethoprim)

Adult dosage

One double-strength tablet (containing 800 mg sulfamethoxazole and 160 mg trimethoprim) P.O. daily for life

Points to remember

- This drug is also effective as prophylaxis against *Pneumocystis carinii* pneumonia.
- Primary prophylaxis is also recommended for patients with $CD4^+$ T-cell counts below 100 cells/µl and positive immunoglobulin G (IgG) *Toxoplasma* serology.

dapsone

Adult dosage

50 mg/day P.O. alone or in combination with 50 mg (or less) of pyrimethamine and 25 mg of folinic acid every week

Points to remember

- This is an alternative drug.
- It's roughly as effective as co-trimoxazole.
- Dapsone may cause serious hemolytic anemia; patients should be tested for G6PD deficiency before starting therapy.
- Primary prophylaxis is also recommended for patients with $CD4^+$ T-cell counts below 100 cells/µl and positive IgG *Toxoplasma* serology. ■

Trichinosis

This disease is caused by infestation with *Trichinella spiralis*, a parasitic roundworm transmitted in raw or undercooked pork. It can be prevented by cooking pork adequately. Trichinosis rarely causes symptoms and typically involves only a small number of roundworms. Treatment is usually ineffective.

mebendazole

Adult dosage

200 to 400 mg P.O. q 8 hours for 3 days, followed by 400 to

500 mg P.O. q 8 hours for 10 days

Points to remember

- Tablets may be swallowed, chewed, or crushed and mixed with food.
- This drug may be given concomitantly with corticosteroids for severe infections.
- This drug isn't FDA-approved for treating trichinosis; its efficacy in this disease hasn't been clearly established. ■

Varicella

More commonly called chickenpox, this acute, contagious disease may be treated with antiviral drugs; dosages vary with the infection site and the patient's immune status. Patients with normal immune systems who have mild infections may not require antiviral therapy.

▼FIRST-LINE DRUG

acyclovir

Adult dosage

800 mg P.O. five times daily for 7 to 10 days

Severe disseminated disease or immunocompromised patients: 10 to 12.4 mg/kg I.V. q 8 hours for 7 to 10 days

Points to remember

- To ensure effective treatment, drug therapy must begin within 24 hours of lesion formation.
- Adjust dosage in renal dysfunction.
- AIDS patients may require long-term suppressant therapy.
- Drug resistance may occur.
- Varicella-zoster immune globulin may be given prophylactically to exposed immunocompromised patients.
- Infection is typically self-limiting in nonimmunocompromised children, so antiviral therapy is not indicated.

foscarnet

Adult dosage

40 mg/kg I.V. q 8 hours for 7 to 14 days

Points to remember

- This is an alternative drug used for acyclovir-resistant varicella strains.
- Monitor serum electrolyte levels.
- Adjust dosage in renal dysfunction; drug may cause nephrotoxicity.
- Although this infection may be life-threatening in adults, in children it's typically self-limiting and usually not treated. Foscarnet is rarely given to children. ■

Whooping cough

Also called pertussis, this acute, contagious respiratory disease is caused by *Bordetella pertussis.* Antibiotic therapy must include a drug that penetrates respiratory tissue. Erythromycin appears to be effective in reducing the infection's severity and preventing relapses.

▼FIRST-LINE DRUG

erythromycin (base)

Adult dosage

500 mg P.O. q 6 hours for 14 days

Points to remember

- Nausea and diarrhea are common side effects.
- Drug should be given with food to prevent GI upset. ■

IMMUNE DISORDERS

AIDS

Drugs are used as first-line therapy in patients with AIDS. Although they don't cure the disease, they may delay its progression. Unfortunately, side effects often limit the duration and aggressiveness of drug therapy.

▼FIRST-LINE DRUG

zidovudine

Adult dosage

100 mg P.O. q 4 hours (six times daily); 200 mg P.O. q 8 hours (when given with zalcitabine); or 1 mg/kg I.V. q 4 hours (six times daily)

Points to remember

- Dosage listed above is for patients with symptomatic infection; asymptomatic patients require oral or I.V. doses q 4 hours while awake.
- Dilute intermittent I.V. doses with D_5W to a concentration not exceeding 4 mg/ml; administer over 1 hour.
- Discard discolored I.V. solutions or those containing particulates.
- Reduce dosage in renal dysfunction.

didanosine

Adult dosage

Patients weighing over 60 kg: 200 mg P.O. (chewable tablet) q 12 hours

Patients weighing less than 60 kg: 125 mg P.O. (chewable tablet) q 12 hours

Points to remember

- This is a second-line drug, typically used in patients who don't respond to or can't tolerate zidovudine.
- Administer 1 hour before or 2 hours after a meal.
- Instruct patient to chew tablets thoroughly, crush them manually, or disperse them in water before swallowing. For dispersion, instruct patient to dissolve in water only.

zalcitabine

Adult dosage

750 mcg (0.75 mg) P.O. q 8 hours

Points to remember

- This is a second-line drug.

- Zalcitabine is currently used in combination with zidovudine in patients with advanced HIV infection who don't respond to zidovudine alone.
- Reduce dosage in severe renal impairment.

stavudine
Adult dosage
Patients weighing over 60 kg: 40 mg P.O. q 12 hours
Patients weighing less than 60 kg: 30 mg P.O. q 12 hours
Points to remember
- This is a third-line drug, typically used in adults who don't respond to or can't tolerate zidovudine, didanosine, or other antiviral agents.
- Reduce dosage in renal impairment. ■

Anaphylaxis

Drug therapy is the primary treatment for anaphylaxis. Early recognition and treatment of this life-threatening condition is essential.

▼FIRST-LINE DRUG
epinephrine
Adult dosage
0.2 to 0.5 ml of 1:1,000 dilution S.C.; may repeat twice at 3- to 20-minute intervals in severe reactions
Point to remember
- Monitor patient's heart rate and blood pressure.

aminophylline
Adult dosage
I.V. loading dose: 5 to 6 mg/kg over 20 to 30 minutes (not to exceed 20 mg/minute) in patients who have never received this drug before; 2.5 mg/kg in patients who have received this drug previously
I.V. maintenance infusion: 0.5 mg/kg/hour
Oral: 200 to 400 mg P.O. q 8 to 12 hours (sustained-release capsule)
Points to remember
- This drug typically is used in patients with bronchospasm.
- If I.V. theophylline is used in place of aminophylline, the dose must be reduced to 20% of the ordered dose of aminophylline.
- Maintenance infusion usually is administered by large-volume parenteral solution.
- Maintenance dose requirements vary.
- Monitor serum drug levels.
- This drug may interact with many other drugs; drug action is also affected by smoking, CHF, and liver disease.

diphenhydramine
Adult dosage
50 to 80 mg I.V. or I.M.; repeat q 4 to 6 hours
Points to remember
- This second-line drug is indicated for patients with urticaria and angioedema.

- It may cause sedation or delirium.
- Diphenhydramine may aggravate prostatism, uncontrolled glaucoma, or constipation.
- Reduce dosage in elderly patients.

methylprednisolone
Adult dosage
0.5 to 4 mg/kg by direct I.V. injection, repeated q 4 to 6 hours as needed, or as continuous I.V. infusion
Points to remember
- This drug is used for persistent bronchospasm and hypotension; it doesn't have an immediate effect.
- For life-threatening anaphylactic shock, you may give up to 30 mg/kg q 4 to 6 hours as needed. ■

Ankylosing spondylitis

Drugs can't cure this chronic inflammatory disease. However, they can relieve symptoms, allowing the patient to perform exercises that help maintain a functional posture and range of motion.

▼FIRST-LINE DRUG
indomethacin
Adult dosage
75 mg P.O. b.i.d. (sustained-release capsules)
Points to remember
- Administer with food.
- This drug is associated with a high incidence of side effects, especially in elderly patients. Other NSAIDs can be substituted and may be just as effective and cause fewer side effects.
- Monitor patient for GI bleeding, hypertension, psychotic episodes, renal insufficiency, and headache. ■

Atopic dermatitis

Drugs are used as first-line therapy for this disease. However, they can only relieve symptoms, not provide a cure. Topical corticosteroids, emollients, and systemic antihistamines are used not only to relieve symptoms but also to prevent secondary skin infections and lichenification. Symptoms of atopic dermatitis wax and wane with the seasons and with the patient's emotions and age; drug therapy may be stepped up or down, depending on disease severity.

▼FIRST-LINE DRUG
diphenhydramine
Adult dosage
25 to 50 mg P.O. t.i.d. or q.i.d.
Points to remember
- This is a first-line drug for relief of itching.
- Reduce dosage in elderly patients.

- Diphenhydramine may cause dizziness or drowsiness and may aggravate uncontrolled glaucoma, constipation, prostatic hyperplasia, or dementia.

▼FIRST-LINE DRUG

hydrocortisone ointment (various strengths)

Adult dosage

Apply topically in a thin layer b.i.d. or t.i.d.

Points to remember

- This is a first-line drug for relief of itching and inflammation.
- Instruct patient to apply ointment sparingly after bathing.

▼FIRST-LINE DRUG

Eucerin cream

Adult dosage

Apply topically in liberal amounts once or twice daily.

Points to remember

- This is a first-line emollient.
- It contains no perfumes or dyes.
- Instruct patient to apply the drug after bathing. ■

Cancer-related immunosuppression

Bone marrow growth factors are the latest advances in treating immunosuppression caused by chemotherapy. They're usually administered between courses of myelosuppressive chemotherapy. Alternative treatments include bone marrow transplant and frequent blood transfusions.

▼FIRST-LINE DRUG

filgrastim (granulocyte colony-stimulating factor; G-CSF)

Adult dosage

Highly individualized

Points to remember

- This drug is used to stimulate granulocyte production.
- It may be administered by S.C. injection or by continuous I.V. or S.C. infusion.
- Store in refrigerator; discard room-temperature solutions after 24 hours.
- Don't shake single-dose vials.
- Inspect for particulate matter and discoloration.

epoetin alfa (erythropoietin, recombinant human)

Adult dosage

- 150 units/kg S.C. three times weekly for 8 weeks

Points to remember

- This drug is used to treat chemotherapy-induced anemia.
- Monitor patient's hematocrit weekly.
- Don't shake vial before use.
- Inspect for particulate matter and discoloration.

sargramostim (granulocyte-macrophage colony-stimulating factor; GM-CSF)
Adult dosage
Highly individualized
Points to remember
- Administer by I.V. infusion.
- Powder for I.V. infusion contains no preservatives; administer as soon as possible after reconstitution.
- Inspect for particulate matter and discoloration.
- Potency varies with manufacturer; don't substitute one product for another.
- This drug comes in single-dose vials; don't reuse. ■

Common variable immunodeficiency

To treat this inherited disorder, I.V. immune globulin is administered monthly to prevent complications—especially infection.

▼FIRST-LINE DRUG
immune globulin intravenous (IGIV)
Adult dosage
- Gamimune N 10%: 100 to 200 mg/kg I.V. once monthly
- Gammagard SD or SD Polygam: 200 to 400 mg/kg I.V. once monthly
- Gammar-IV: 100 to 200 mg/kg I.V. q 3 to 4 weeks
- Iveegam: 200 mg/kg I.V. once monthly
- Sandoglobulin: 200 mg/kg I.V. once monthly
- Venoglobulin-I or Venoglobulin-S: 200 mg/kg I.V. once monthly

Points to remember
- Dosage and administration instructions vary with product; products are not interchangeable.
- Dosage is based on patient's immunoglobulin G levels. ■

Hashimoto's disease

Patients who have a small goiter or no symptoms may not require treatment for this autoimmune disease of the thyroid gland. Surgery is rarely indicated; however, drug therapy may be required for accompanying hypothyroidism.

levothyroxine sodium (T_4)
Adult dosage
0.1 to 0.25 mg/day P.O.
Point to remember
- To help suppress thyroid-stimulating hormone and allow goiter regression, levothyroxine dosage is slightly higher than normal physiologic replacement dosage. ■

Mucocutaneous candidiasis, chronic

Local therapy for candidiasis of the nails and skin typically includes 1% ciclopirox cream, nystatin cream, miconazole, ketoconazole, or clotrimazole cream or lotion applied three or four times daily. Local therapy for vulvar and anal mucous membranes may include miconazole cream, clotrimazole suppositories, terconazole vaginal cream or suppositories, or nystatin for 7 days. The patient should keep affected body parts dry and expose them to air as much as possible. If possible, systemic antibiotics should be discontinued because they worsen candidiasis and may even precipitate the disorder.

▼FIRST-LINE DRUG

ciclopirox

Adult dosage

1% cream or lotion gently massaged into affected area and surrounding skin b.i.d., morning and evening.

Points to remember

- Improvement usually occurs within first week of treatment.
- If no improvement occurs after 4 weeks, the diagnosis should be reevaluated.

▼FIRST-LINE DRUG

clotrimazole

Adult dosage

1% cream or lotion gently massaged into affected area and surrounding skin b.i.d.

Points to remember

- Improvement usually occurs within first week of treatment.
- If no improvement occurs after 4 weeks, the diagnosis should be reevaluated.

▼FIRST-LINE DRUG

fluconazole

Adult dosage

200 mg P.O. on the first day, followed by 100 mg/day for 2 weeks

Point to remember

- Adjust dosage in renal dysfunction.

▼FIRST-LINE DRUG

miconazole

Adult dosage

2% lotion or cream applied to affected area b.i.d.; or 2% spray or powder sprayed or sprinkled over affected area b.i.d, in morning and evening

Point to remember

- Notify doctor if no improvement occurs after 2 weeks.

▼FIRST-LINE DRUG

nystatin

Adult dosage

Apply cream (100,000 units/g) to affected area b.i.d. or t.i.d.

Point to remember
- Clean affected area before applying cream.

ketoconazole
Adult dosage
200 mg b.i.d. for 5 days
Point to remember
- Monitor patient's liver function.

Polymyositis and dermatomyositis

Patients with one of these conditions may require therapy for several years; relapses can occur at any time. Bed rest is recommended during acute disease; however, physical therapy is beneficial in long-term care.

azathioprine
Adult dosage
1 to 3.5 mg/kg/day P.O. in divided doses
Points to remember
- Azathioprine commonly is used in combination with corticosteroid therapy.
- Monitor CBC weekly.
- Administer in divided doses after meals to minimize GI upset.
- Tell patient to avoid people with bacterial or viral infections and to avoid vaccinations containing live viruses.
- Warn patient that drug therapy may reactivate herpes zoster.
- Patients who are pregnant or breast-feeding shouldn't take this drug.
- Patients on concurrent allopurinol therapy and those with hepatic impairment require decreased dosage.

cyclophosphamide
Adult dosage
1 to 2 mg/kg/day P.O.; adjust dosage based on patient's WBC count
Points to remember
- Tell patient to avoid people with bacterial or viral infections and to avoid vaccinations containing live viruses.
- Warn patient that drug therapy may reactivate herpes zoster.
- This drug is contraindicated in pregnant and breast-feeding patients.
- Patients with renal or hepatic impairment may require a lower dosage.
- Keep patient well hydrated before drug administration and for up to 72 hours afterward to minimize risk of hemorrhagic cystitis. Encourage patient to void frequently.
- High-dose or long-term therapy may cause hemorrhagic cystitis, pulmonary interstitial fibrosis, or acute myopericarditis. Monitor patient for fever, tachycardia, shortness of breath, painful urination, and bloody urine.

prednisone

Adult dosage

1 to 2 mg/kg/day (or equivalent dosage) P.O. initially; then titrate dosage to lowest effective level

Points to remember

- Improvement may occur after several weeks of therapy.
- To minimize chronic side effects, decrease daily dosage by 5 mg weekly to lowest effective level, or use alternate-day regimen. Be aware that decreasing dosage too quickly can cause relapse of symptoms or hypoadrenalism.
- Combined use of prednisone with cytotoxic drugs (azathioprine, methotrexate, or cyclophosphamide) may allow reduction of prednisone dosage.
- Total-body radiation has been used in patients unresponsive to combination therapy with corticosteroids and cytotoxic agents. ■

Psoriatic arthritis

Physical and occupational therapy helps maintain the patient's muscle strength and joint function. Orthotics and intra-articular corticosteroids are used to treat acutely inflamed joints.

▼FIRST-LINE DRUGS

NSAIDs (various)

Adult dosage

Ibuprofen: 400 to 800 mg P.O. t.i.d., not to exceed 3.2 g/day
Naproxen: 250 to 500 mg P.O. b.i.d., not to exceed 1.5 g/day
Piroxicam: 20 to 40 mg/day P.O.
Sulindac: 150 to 200 mg P.O. b.i.d.

Points to remember

- NSAIDs are first-line drugs for pain management.
- Don't administer to patients with aspirin sensitivity, bleeding disorders, active bleeding, or peptic ulcer disease.
- Use cautiously in patients with a history of peptic ulcers and in those receiving heparin, warfarin, or thrombolytic agents.
- Give these drugs with food or antacids to minimize GI upset.
- Instruct patient to avoid alcoholic beverages.

gold salts

Adult dosage

Auranofin: 6 mg/day P.O. or 3 mg P.O. b.i.d. to maximum of 9 mg/day
Aurothioglucose and gold sodium thiomalate: 10 mg I.M. during week 1, 25 mg during weeks 2 and 3, then 25 to 50 mg weekly until total of 800 mg to 1 g has been given;

then gradually decrease to 25 mg q 2 to 4 weeks

Points to remember

- Gold salts have been effective in some patients who don't respond to NSAIDs.
- During initiation of gold salt therapy, NSAIDs usually are continued for symptomatic relief.
- Reassure patient that it may take several weeks before improvement occurs.
- Patients shouldn't breastfeed during gold salt therapy.

azathioprine

Adult dosage

1 to 2 mg/kg/day P.O. initially; may increase by 0.5 mg/kg/day to maximum of 2.5 mg/kg/day

Points to remember

- Azathioprine is often used in patients who don't respond to gold salt therapy.
- Patients typically receive 12-week trial of azathioprine to check efficacy. If drug is effective, dosage is decreased to lowest effective level.
- Give in divided doses after meals to minimize GI upset.
- Monitor CBC weekly.
- Decrease dosage in patients taking allopurinol and those with hepatic impairment.
- Instruct patient to avoid people with bacterial or viral infections.
- Advise patient to avoid vaccinations containing live viruses.
- Inform patient that drug may reactivate herpes zoster.
- This drug is contraindicated in pregnant and breastfeeding patients.

methotrexate

Adult dosage

2.5 to 5 mg P.O. q 12 hours for three doses per week

Points to remember

- This drug is indicated for severe psoriatic arthritis unresponsive to other therapy.
- Caution patient to avoid alcoholic beverages and excessive sunlight.
- Instruct patient to avoid vaccinations containing live viruses.
- Warn patient that this drug may reactivate chickenpox or herpes simplex.
- Adjust dosage in renal impairment. ■

Reiter's syndrome

Patients with Reiter's syndrome require physical therapy and long-term monitoring for complications. Because the infection that triggers this disorder is sexually transmitted, instruct patients to avoid sexual promiscuity and to use condoms.

NSAIDs typically are prescribed to treat symptoms of Reiter's syndrome. Be aware that certain drugs used to treat rheumatoid arthritis are ineffective in Reiter's syndrome; they include systemic corticosteroids, antimalarial agents, gold salts, and penicillamine.

NSAIDs

Adult dosage

Indomethacin: 75 to 100 mg/day P.O. in divided doses
Phenylbutazone: 100 mg P.O. t.i.d. or q.i.d.

Points to remember

- These drugs are used to treat symptoms.
- Phenylbutazone usually is prescribed for patients who experience side effects from other NSAIDs.
- Instruct patient to take drug with food or antacids and to avoid alcoholic beverages to minimize GI upset.
- Don't administer these agents to patients with aspirin sensitivity, bleeding disorders, active bleeding, or peptic ulcer disease.
- Use caution when administering to patients with a history of peptic ulcers and to those also receiving heparin, warfarin, or thrombolytic agents.

azathioprine

Adult dosage

1 to 2 mg/kg/day P.O.

Points to remember

- Azathioprine is often used in patients who don't respond to NSAIDs.
- To minimize GI upset, give in divided doses after meals.
- Tell patient to avoid people with bacterial or viral infections.
- Instruct patient to avoid vaccinations containing live viruses.
- Warn patient that drug may reactivate herpes zoster.
- Decrease dosage in patients taking allopurinol and those with hepatic impairment.
- Monitor CBC weekly.
- Azathioprine is contraindicated in pregnant and breast-feeding patients.

methotrexate

Adult dosage

7.5 to 15 mg P.O. weekly

Points to remember

- This drug is indicated for patients who don't respond to NSAIDs.
- Once an adequate response occurs, decrease dosage to lowest effective level.
- Caution patient to avoid alcoholic beverages and excessive sunlight.
- Instruct patient to avoid vaccinations containing live viruses.
- Warn patient that drug may reactivate chickenpox or herpes simplex.
- Adjust dosage in renal impairment. ■

Rheumatoid arthritis

Therapy for rheumatoid arthritis aims to decrease pain

and joint destruction and to prevent disease progression. Physical therapy can help prevent joint weakness and limit range-of-motion loss. Because excessive strain on joints may exacerbate rheumatoid arthritis, restricting the motion of inflamed joints with splints or braces may help decrease pain and support the joint. Synovectomy may be performed to relieve pain. Patients with severely damaged weight-bearing joints may require joint replacement.

▼FIRST-LINE DRUGS

NSAIDs

Adult dosage

Ibuprofen: 400 to 800 mg P.O. t.i.d., not to exceed 3.2 g/day
Naproxen: 250 to 500 mg P.O. b.i.d., not to exceed 1.5 g/day
Piroxicam: 20 to 40 mg/day P.O.
Sulindac: 150 to 200 mg/day P.O.

Points to remember

- NSAIDs are first-line drugs for relieving pain and inflammation; however, they may not affect the natural course of the disease.
- Patients vary in their response to different NSAIDs. Another NSAID may be tried if patient doesn't respond to initial drug used. However, patient shouldn't take more than one NSAID at a time.
- Instruct patient to take drug with food or antacids to minimize GI upset or to take an enteric-coated product. Patients at high risk for serious GI toxicity may receive misoprostol concurrently.
- Instruct patient to avoid alcoholic beverages.
- Don't administer to patients with aspirin sensitivity, bleeding disorders, active bleeding, or peptic ulcer disease.
- Use cautiously in patients with a history of peptic ulcers and those receiving heparin, warfarin, or a thrombolytic agent (such as streptokinase).

▼FIRST-LINE DRUG

gold salts

Adult dosage

Auranofin: 6 mg/day P.O. or 3 mg P.O. b.i.d. to maximum of 9 mg/day
Aurothioglucose and gold sodium thiomalate: 10 mg I.M. during week 1, 25 mg during weeks 2 and 3, then 25 to 50 mg weekly until total of 800 mg to 1 g has been given; then decrease gradually to 25 mg I.M. q 2 to 4 weeks

Points to remember

- Patient may receive a trial of gold salts if NSAIDs prove ineffective. During initiation of gold salt therapy, NSAIDs usually are continued for symptomatic relief.

- Administer injections into gluteal muscle.
- Metallic taste may be an early sign of toxicity.
- Tell patient that improvement may take 3 to 6 months.
- Patients shouldn't breastfeed during gold salt therapy.

▼FIRST-LINE DRUG

hydroxychloroquine

Adult dosage

200 mg P.O. b.i.d.

Points to remember

- Patient may receive trial of this drug if NSAIDs prove ineffective. During initiation of hydroxychloroquine therapy, NSAIDs usually are continued for symptomatic relief.
- Tell patient to take drug with meals or milk to minimize GI upset.
- Because of possible retinopathy, patient should undergo ophthalmologic examination when therapy starts and have eyes examined every 6 months during therapy.
- Inform patient that 4 to 6 weeks of therapy may be required before response occurs. If no improvement occurs in 6 months, therapy should be discontinued.
- Patients with hepatic impairment may require decreased dosage.

▼FIRST-LINE DRUG

methotrexate

Adult dosage

2.5 to 5 mg P.O. q 12 hours for three doses a week; don't exceed 20 mg/week

Points to remember

- Methotrexate is an alternative drug used in patients who don't respond adequately to NSAIDs and in those with erosive joint disease or persistent pain.
- Once an adequate response occurs, decrease dosage to lowest effective level.
- Caution patient to avoid alcoholic beverages and excessive sunlight.
- Instruct patient to avoid vaccinations containing live viruses.
- Warn patient that drug may reactivate chickenpox or herpes simplex.
- Adjust dosage in renal impairment.

azathioprine

Adult dosage

1 to 2 mg/kg/day P.O. initially; may increase by 0.5 mg/kg to maximum of 2.5 mg/kg/ day

Points to remember

- Azathioprine is an alternative treatment for patients who don't respond to or can't tolerate gold therapy, methotrexate, or hydroxychloroquine.
- Many patients receive a 12-week trial of azathioprine to check its efficacy. If drug is effective, dosage should be de-

creased to lowest effective level.

- Give medication in divided doses after meals to minimize GI upset.
- Monitor CBC weekly.
- Instruct patient to avoid people with bacterial or viral infections.
- Advise patient to avoid vaccinations containing live viruses.
- Warn patient that drug may reactivate herpes zoster.
- Decrease dosage in hepatic impairment.
- This drug is contraindicated in pregnant and breast-feeding patients.

corticosteroids

Adult dosage

5 to 7.5 mg/day P.O. of prednisone or equivalent

For intra-articular therapy: 200 mcg to 6 mg of dexamethasone, 3 to 48 mg of triamcinolone, or 1.5 to 12 mg of betamethasone

Points to remember

- These drugs are used only to treat acute flare-ups of rheumatoid arthritis. Intra-articular injections may be used when a single joint is involved.
- Corticosteroids don't alter natural disease course.
- Give lowest dose needed to control inflammation.
- To minimize adrenal suppression, administer dose in morning or on alternate-day regimen.
- Patients shouldn't receive intra-articular injections in same joint more than three times in 1 year to minimize potential for degenerative arthritis in that joint.
- Long-term complications of corticosteroid therapy include osteoporosis, cataracts, glaucoma, and adrenal suppression. With shorter regimens, psychoses, glucose intolerance, potassium wasting, and immunosuppression may occur.

cyclophosphamide

Adult dosage

50 to 100 mg/day P.O. to a maximum of 1 to 2 mg/kg/day

Points to remember

- Cyclophosphamide is an alternative treatment for patients who don't respond to or can't tolerate gold therapy, methotrexate, or hydroxychloroquine.
- Because of its serious side effects, this drug usually is reserved for patients with severe disease. High-dose or long-term therapy may cause hemorrhagic cystitis, pulmonary interstitial fibrosis, or acute myopericarditis. Monitor for fever, tachycardia, shortness of breath, painful urination, and bloody urine.
- To minimize risk of hemorrhagic cystitis, keep patient well hydrated and encourage frequent voiding.

- Instruct patient to avoid people with bacterial or viral infections.
- Advise patient to avoid vaccinations containing live viruses.
- Warn patient that drug may reactivate herpes zoster.
- Patients with renal or hepatic impairment and those who have undergone radiation therapy may require lower dosages.
- This drug is contraindicated in pregnant and breast-feeding patients.

misoprostol
Adult dosage
100 to 400 mcg P.O. q.i.d.
Points to remember
- This drug is used for long-term prevention of gastric ulcers caused by NSAIDs. It is not indicated for short-term or long-term treatment of peptic ulcers.
- Misoprostol is contraindicated in pregnancy. Tell women of childbearing years to use adequate contraceptive.

penicillamine
Adult dosage
125 to 250 mg/day P.O.; may increase by 250 mg/day q 2 to 3 months to maximum of 1 to 1.5 g/day or until maximum response occurs
Points to remember
- Penicillamine is an alternative drug for patients who don't respond to or can't tolerate gold therapy, methotrexate, or hydroxychloroquine.
- Tell patient to take drug on empty stomach to maximize absorption.
- Dosages over 500 mg/day should be given in divided doses.
- This drug may cause allergic reactions in patients who are allergic to penicillin.
- Discontinue drug if no response occurs after 3 to 4 months.
- Patient requires increased amounts of pyridoxine during therapy. If diet is poor, patient should receive supplementation.
- Elderly patients should receive no more than 750 mg/day. ■

Systemic lupus erythematosus

No cure for systemic lupus erythematosus (SLE) exists, and remissions are rare. Patients may receive anticoagulants or psychotropic drugs for symptomatic relief. Instruct the patient to use a sunscreen with an SPF of 15 or higher to treat rashes.

NSAIDs
Adult dosage
Ibuprofen: 400 to 800 mg P.O. t.i.d., not to exceed 3.2 g/day

Naproxen: 250 to 500 mg P.O. b.i.d., not to exceed 1.5 g/day
Piroxicam: 20 to 40 mg/day P.O.
Sulindac: 20 to 40 mg/day P.O.

Points to remember

- NSAIDs are used for symptomatic treatment of fever, mild serositis, and arthralgia in patients with mild disease.
- Individual patients respond differently to various NSAIDs. Patient should show some response to drug within 2 to 4 weeks.
- To minimize GI upset, tell patient to take NSAID with food or antacids or to take an enteric-coated product. Patients at high risk for serious GI toxicity may receive misoprostol concurrently.
- Instruct patient to avoid alcoholic beverages.
- Don't administer to patients with aspirin sensitivity, bleeding disorders, active bleeding, or peptic ulcer disease.
- Use caution when administering to patients with a history of peptic ulcers and to those receiving heparin, warfarin, or thrombolytic agents.
- SLE patients who are taking NSAIDs are at increased risk for elevated liver enzyme levels, aseptic meningitis, and renal impairment.

hydroxychloroquine

Adult dosage

200 mg P.O. b.i.d.

Points to remember

- Hydroxychloroquine is an alternative treatment for rash, serositis, and arthritis in patients who don't respond to NSAIDs. It may also be prescribed to treat pericarditis and pleuritis.
- Because of risk of retinopathy, patients should have baseline ophthalmologic evaluation before starting therapy and then have eyes examined every 6 months.
- To minimize GI upset, tell patient to take drug with meals or milk.
- Inform patient that several weeks of therapy may be required before response occurs.
- Patients with hepatic impairment may require lower dosage.

cyclophosphamide

Adult dosage

10 to 15 mg/kg I.V. q 4 weeks; or 1.5 to 2.5 mg/kg/day P.O. to maximum of 4 mg/kg

Points to remember

- Cyclophosphamide is used to control active SLE, reduce frequency of flare-ups, and decrease corticosteroid requirement. Patients with glomerular nephritis may receive trial therapy, but this form of disease is less responsive to the drug.

- Once patient responds to drug, reduce dosage to lowest effective level.
- High-dose or long-term therapy may cause hemorrhagic cystitis, pulmonary interstitial fibrosis, or acute myopericarditis. Monitor for fever, tachycardia, shortness of breath, painful urination, or bloody urine.
- To help minimize risk of hemorrhagic cystitis, keep patient well hydrated and encourage frequent voiding.
- Caution patient to avoid people with bacterial or viral infections.
- Instruct patient to avoid vaccinations containing live viruses.
- Warn patient that drug may reactivate herpes zoster.
- Patients with renal or hepatic impairment and those who have undergone radiation therapy may require lower dosage.
- This drug is contraindicated in pregnant and breast-feeding patients.

azathioprine

Adult dosage

2 to 3 mg/kg/day P.O.

Points to remember

- Azathioprine may be used as an alternative to cyclophosphamide.
- Patients often receive a 12-week trial of azathioprine to check its efficacy. If drug is effective, decrease dosage to lowest effective level.
- Give in divided doses after meals to minimize GI upset.
- Instruct patient to avoid people with bacterial or viral infections.
- Advise patient to avoid vaccinations containing live viruses.
- Warn patient that drug may reactivate herpes zoster.
- Monitor CBC weekly.
- This drug is contraindicated in pregnant and breast-feeding patients.

glucocorticoids

Adult dosage

1 to 2 mg/kg/day P.O. of prednisone or equivalent, or apply topical form one to four times daily p.r.n.

Points to remember

- Topical applications and intralesional injections may be used for skin lesions.
- Apply topical forms sparingly, and don't use in or around the eyes. Potency varies by drug and form (lotion, cream, or ointment). Applying an occlusive dressing may increase drug efficacy.
- Systemic glucocorticoids should be reserved for severe disease unresponsive to other therapy.
- Use lowest dose needed to control inflammation. Active disease may require higher (divided) doses.
- To minimize adrenal suppression, give single daily doses in morning or use alternate-day regimen.

- Long-term complications include osteoporosis, cataracts, glaucoma, weight gain, and adrenal suppression. With shorter regimens, psychoses, glucose intolerance, potassium wasting, hypertension, acne, irritability, insomnia, and immunosuppression can occur.
- Supplemental calcium and vitamin D may be given to minimize osteoporosis risk. Estrogen replacement should also be considered for postmenopausal patients and for those who have undergone hysterectomy. ■

Systemic sclerosis (scleroderma)

No cure for systemic sclerosis exists, and no therapy has been clearly shown to suppress or reverse the disease process. (Aspirin, dipyridamole, colchicine, and chlorambucil haven't been shown to be effective.) However, treatment can ease symptoms and improve the patient's functional level. Monitor the patient's renal and pulmonary function, blood pressure, urinalysis, and blood counts. The patient may also require symptomatic treatment of Raynaud's disease. (See "Raynaud's disease" in Cardiovascular disorders.)

azathioprine

Adult dosage

2 to 3 mg/kg/day P.O.

Points to remember

- Azathioprine is indicated for life-threatening or rapidly progressing disease.
- Patients often receive a 12-week trial to check drug's efficacy. If drug is effective, decrease dosage to lowest effective level.
- Give in divided doses after meals to minimize GI upset.
- Instruct patient to avoid people with bacterial or viral infections.
- Instruct patient to avoid vaccinations containing live viruses.
- Warn patient that drug may reactivate herpes zoster.
- Monitor CBC weekly.
- Decrease dosage in hepatic impairment.
- Azathioprine is contraindicated in pregnant and breast-feeding patients.

glucocorticoids

Adult dosage

Acute symptoms: 40 to 60 mg/day P.O. of prednisone or equivalent glucocorticoid

Chronic arthritis: 10 mg/day P.O. of prednisone or equivalent glucocorticoid

Points to remember

- Glucocorticoids are used to treat myositis, pericarditis, and chronic arthritis in patients who don't respond to NSAIDs. Except in arthritis, these agents are rarely used as long-term therapy.

- These drugs have been associated with precipitation of acute renal failure.
- Patient should receive lowest dose needed to control disease. Active disease may require higher dosage, which should be divided daily.
- Give single daily doses in morning or on an alternate-day regimen to minimize adrenal suppression.
- Complications of long-term therapy include osteoporosis, cataracts, glaucoma, weight gain, and adrenal suppression. With shorter regimens, psychoses, glucose intolerance, potassium wasting, hypertension, acne, irritability, insomnia, and immunosuppression may occur.
- Patient should receive calcium and vitamin D supplements to minimize osteoporosis risk. Estrogen replacement should also be considered for postmenopausal patients and for those who have had a hysterectomy.

penicillamine
Adult dosage
250 mg/day P.O. initially; increase at 1- to 3-month intervals by 125 to 150 mg/day to 1.5 g/day, as tolerated
Points to remember

- Penicillamine may help reduce skin thickening and prevent organ involvement.
- Tell patient to take drug on empty stomach to maximize absorption.
- Divide daily dosages above 500 mg.
- Discontinue drug if no response occurs after 3 to 4 months.
- Be aware that this drug may cause allergic reactions in patients who are allergic to penicillin.
- Patient requires increased amounts of pyridoxine during therapy. If diet is poor, patient should receive pyridoxine supplementation.
- Elderly patients should receive no more than 750 mg/day. ■

Vasculitis

Therapy for this inflammatory blood vessel condition aims to treat the primary disease, such as systemic lupus erythematosus, rheumatoid arthritis, or Sjögren's syndrome. Vasculitis also may occur as part of a serum sickness–like reaction to drugs such as penicillins and sulfa drugs. In that case, simply discontinuing the drug may resolve the vasculitis.

cyclophosphamide
Adult dosage
2 mg/kg/day P.O.

Points to remember

- This drug often is used in combination with glucocorticoids to treat Wegener's granulomatosis. It may also be used as a single agent to treat hypersensitivity vasculitis that fails to respond to corticosteroids.
- Adjust dosage to maintain patient's WBC count over 3,000/µl.
- When treating Wegener's granulomatosis, therapy continues for 1 year after complete remission and then gradually is tapered down and stopped. Shorter regimens may be used for other vasculitis syndromes.

glucocorticoids

Adult dosage

1 mg/kg/day P.O. of prednisone or equivalent

Points to remember

- Glucocorticoids are used in combination with cyclophosphamide to treat Wegener's granulomatosis, or they may be used alone to treat hypersensitivity vasculitis.
- When treating Wegener's granulomatosis, regimen gradually is converted to alternate-day therapy and then tapered down and stopped. Therapy usually lasts 6 to 12 months. Shorter regimens may be used for other vasculitis syndromes. ■

CARDIOVASCULAR DISORDERS

Abdominal aortic aneurysm, dissecting

Surgery is the first-line therapy for this disorder. Preoperatively, the patient receives emergency I.V. drugs to reduce the surgical risk. Long-term oral drug therapy aims to reduce blood pressure and maintain cardiac output.

▼FIRST-LINE DRUG

labetalol hydrochloride

Adult dosage

Oral: 200 mg initially, then additional dose of 200 to 400 mg in 6 to 12 hours; usual dose is 200 to 400 mg b.i.d.
Emergencies: 20 to 80 mg by slow I.V. push q 10 minutes, or 2 mg/minute by continuous I.V. infusion until desired blood pressure is achieved or maximum of 300 mg is given

Points to remember

- Administer I.V. with patient in supine position.
- Reduce dosage in elderly patients and those with hepatic dysfunction.
- Provide continuous blood pressure monitoring during I.V. therapy.

- This drug may exacerbate asthma, heart failure, second- and third-degree heart block, and bradycardia.

▼FIRST-LINE DRUG

nitroprusside sodium
Adult dosage
0.25 to 0.3 mcg/kg/minute I.V.; may titrate upward every few minutes to maximum dosage of 10 mcg/kg/minute
Points to remember
- Lower dosage may be adequate in elderly patients, patients receiving other antihypertensives, and patients with renal, hepatic, or thyroid dysfunction.
- Don't add other drugs to I.V. infusion line.
- Protect reconstituted I.V. solutions from light.
- Discard unused portion or cloudy or discolored solutions.
- Monitor patient's blood pressure continuously.

propranolol hydrochloride
Adult dosage
Oral: 160 to 480 mg in three or four divided doses
I.V.: 0.5 to 3 mg initially; may give second dose after 2 minutes and additional doses at intervals of no less than 4 hours
Points to remember
- This is a second-line drug used as an alternative to labetalol.
- Dosage must be individualized because of variable patient response.
- Monitor patient's blood pressure and pulse before each I.V. dose; withhold dose if pulse rate is less than 50 beats/minute.
- This drug may exacerbate asthma, heart failure, second- or third-degree heart block, bradycardia, or Raynaud's disease. ■

Accelerated idioventricular rhythm

The underlying cause of this disorder, such as electrolyte imbalance or MI, must be treated to prevent recurrences. The patient may require atrial pacing.

▼FIRST-LINE DRUG

atropine sulfate
Adult dosage
0.4 to 0.6 mg by I.V. push; repeat q 4 to 6 hours
Points to remember
- Drug effect may be more pronounced in elderly patients.
- This drug may exacerbate uncontrolled glaucoma, hiatal hernia with reflux esophagitis, intestinal obstruction, and severe constipation.

▼FIRST-LINE DRUG

isoproterenol
Adult dosage
I.V. bolus: 0.02 to 0.06 mg (1 to 3 ml of 1:50,000 dilution),

followed by 0.01 to 0.2 mg (0.05 to 10 ml of 1:50,000 dilution)
I.V. infusion: 5 mcg/minute (1.25 ml of 1:250,000 dilution), followed by 2 to 20 mcg/minute
Points to remember
- Elderly patients and those with renal dysfunction may require dosage reduction.
- Monitor patient's ECG continuously during I.V. therapy.
- This drug may exacerbate hypertension, coronary insufficiency, angina, degenerative heart disease, and diabetes. ■

Accelerated junctional rhythm

Patients with this rhythm disturbance rarely require drug therapy because their ventricular rate is usually normal. Alternative treatments include a temporary pacemaker if symptoms of decreased cardiac output occur.

▼FIRST-LINE DRUG
atropine sulfate
Adult dosage
0.4 to 0.6 mg I.V. (range: 0.3 to 1.2 mg); repeat q 4 to 6 hours
Points to remember
- Elderly patients may require dosage reduction.
- This drug may exacerbate obstructive uropathy, uncontrolled glaucoma, hiatal hernia with reflux esophagitis, intestinal obstruction, or severe constipation. ■

Aortic insufficiency

Surgical valve replacement is the treatment of choice for this disorder. Drug therapy aims to relieve symptoms of secondary complications, including CHF, angina, MI, and pulmonary edema.

captopril
Adult dosage
25 mg P.O. t.i.d.
Points to remember
- Captopril commonly is given with digoxin and a diuretic to manage symptomatic CHF.
- Patient response to this drug varies greatly.
- Reduce dosage in elderly patients and those with renal dysfunction.
- This drug may aggravate renal impairment, hyperkalemia, and cough.

(For information on digoxin, furosemide, nitroglycerin, and isosorbide, see "Aortic stenosis," which follows.) ■

Aortic stenosis

Surgical valve replacement or reconstruction is the treatment of choice for aortic stenosis. Drugs are used mainly to relieve symptoms in patients who can't undergo surgery.

digoxin
Adult dosage
0.125 to 0.25 mg/day P.O. (dosage is highly individualized)
Points to remember
- Digoxin is used to treat CHF in symptomatic patients.
- Withhold dose if patient's pulse rate is less than 50 beats/minute.
- Monitor serum digoxin level to minimize toxicity risk. Therapeutic blood drug level is 1 to 2 ng/ml.
- Hypokalemia and decreased renal function increase the risk of digoxin toxicity.

furosemide
Adult dosage
20 to 80 mg P.O. or I.V. in single or divided doses q 6 to 24 hours
Points to remember
- This is a first-line drug for treating CHF with edema.
- Give I.V. infusion over 1 to 2 minutes.
- Discard injectable preparation if it has yellow discoloration.
- Shield injectable preparation from light.
- Monitor patient's serum electrolyte levels and fluid volume status regularly.

isosorbide dinitrate
Adult dosage
10 to 20 mg P.O. t.i.d. or q.i.d.; alternatively, 20 to 40 mg sustained-release capsules q 6 to 12 hours
Points to remember
- This drug is used to control symptoms of heart failure.
- Administer on empty stomach.
- Sustained-release form may reduce headache.

isosorbide mononitrate
Adult dosage
30 to 240 mg P.O. q 4 hours (extended-release tablets) beginning in morning; or 20 mg P.O. b.i.d. (12-hour release tablets)
Points to remember
- This drug is used to control symptoms of heart failure.
- Instruct patient not to crush or chew tablets.
- Initial dose usually is given first thing in morning.
- Nitrate-free interval of 8 to 12 hours overnight is recommended.

nitroglycerin
Adult dosage
Ointment: apply ½″ to 2″ to skin q 6 to 8 hours, or one transdermal patch (0.1 to 0.6 mg/ hour) q 24 hours
Lingual: give 1 to 2 sprays (0.4 to 0.8 mg) to the tongue; repeat q 3 to 5 minutes for two additional doses p.r.n.
Sublingual/buccal: 0.15 to 0.6 mg S.L. or in buccal pouch; repeat two times p.r.n.
Points to remember
- Apply nitroglycerin ointment to applicator paper in prescribed amount; using paper (not fingers), gently spread on hairless skin area in thin, uniform layer.
- This drug form is used mainly for acute episodes. Patient usually is switched to transdermal patch for long-term maintenance.
- To prevent tolerance, patient should have nitroglycerin-free interval of 8 to 12 hours each night.
- Instruct patient to apply a transdermal patch at the same time each day to clean, dry, hairless skin area on the upper arm or body.
- Tell patient to rotate application sites to prevent skin irritation, to remove patch before showering, and to maintain nitroglycerin-free period of 8 to 12 hours each night.
- Remove transdermal patch before defibrillation or cardioversion.
- Topical preparations are first-line drugs for angina prevention.
- Lingual and S.L. forms are first-line drugs for managing acute angina symptoms.
- Titrate dosage to patient response.
- Keep tablets and extended-release formulations in original glass containers. ■

Arterial occlusive disease

Surgery is the definitive therapy for this disease. Drugs help control symptoms only in patients with mild to moderate disease. Adjunctive drug therapy aims to control hypertension and reduce serum cholesterol levels to slow disease progression.

pentoxifylline
Adult dosage
400 mg P.O. t.i.d.
Points to remember
- This drug reduces blood viscosity.
- Give with meals.
- Reduce dosage if GI upset, dizziness, or headache occurs. ■

Asystole

This condition is a medical emergency that calls for defibrillation with cardiopulmonary resuscitation. The patient should be intubated if possible to allow for endotracheal drug administration. Drug therapy is the first line of treatment to restore cardiac rhythm.

▼FIRST-LINE DRUG

epinephrine

Adult dosage

0.5 to 1 mg of 1:10,000 dilution by I.V. push; repeat q 5 minutes

Point to remember

- If blood pressure rises sharply, vasodilators (such as nitrates or alpha-adrenergic blockers) should be given to counteract the pressor effect of epinephrine.

atropine sulfate

Adult dosage

1 mg by I.V. push; repeat in 5 minutes

Point to remember

- This is a second-line drug.

sodium bicarbonate

Adult dosage

1 mEq/kg by I.V. push; then 0.5 mEq/kg q 10 minutes

Points to remember

- This is a third-line drug.
- It's not recommended for routine use early in resuscitation but is reserved for patients with hyperkalemia or preexisting metabolic acidosis.
- Don't administer into same I.V. site as that used for calcium or catecholamine preparations. ■

Atrial fibrillation

Drug therapy is the preferred treatment for this arrhythmia. An alternative treatment is cardioversion. Adjunctive anticoagulant therapy may be used, especially before cardioversion or in patients with valvular heart disease.

▼FIRST-LINE DRUG

digoxin

Adult dosage

1 mg I.V. loading dose given in three divided doses over 24 hours; maintenance dose is 0.125 to 0.5 mg/day I.V. or P.O.

Points to remember

- This drug is a first-line treatment for controlling the heart rate in patients with reduced ventricular function.
- Administer only if digoxin toxicity isn't the cause of atrial fibrillation.
- Withhold dose if patient's pulse rate is less than 50 beats/minute.
- Dosages are highly individualized.
- Drug has a narrow therapeutic range (0.8 to 2 ng/ml). Monitor patient's serum digoxin level.
- Reduce dosage in elderly patients and in patients with

renal failure or hepatic compromise.

▼FIRST-LINE DRUG

diltiazem hydrochloride

Adult dosage

Oral: 90 to 360 mg/day P.O. as single dose (sustained-release tablet) or divided in three or four daily doses (standard tablet)
I.V.: 0.25 mg/kg by slow I.V. push over 2 minutes (average 20 mg); if ineffective, repeat in 15 minutes; or 10 to 15 mg/hour by I.V. infusion for up to 24 hours

Points to remember

- This drug is used as a first-line treatment for controlling the heart rate in patients with good ventricular function.
- Withhold dose if patient's pulse rate is less than 50 beats/minute.
- Monitor patient's ECG and blood pressure continuously during I.V. therapy.
- Monitor for dizziness and CHF.
- Dosage may need to be reduced in elderly patients.

▼FIRST-LINE DRUG

quinidine sulfate

Adult dosage

Oral: 300 to 400 mg of quinidine sulfate q 6 hours or 324 to 600 mg of quinidine gluconate (sustained-release) q 8 to 12 hours
I.M.: 600 mg initially, then up to 400 mg q 2 hours, based on patient's response
I.V.: 800 mg diluted in 40 ml of D_5W and infused I.V. at 16 mg (1 ml)/minute

Points to remember

- This drug is a first-line antiarrhythmic.
- Administer 200-mg test dose I.M. before initiating I.M. or I.V. therapy.
- Monitor patient's ECG and blood pressure continuously during I.V. therapy.
- Before initiating therapy, patient should be digitalized to control ventricular rate and prevent ventricular tachycardia.
- Reduce dosage in hepatic and renal dysfunction.

▼FIRST-LINE DRUG

verapamil

Adult dosage

I.V.: 0.075 to 0.15 mg/kg (5 to 10 mg) by slow I.V. push over 2 minutes (3 minutes in elderly patients); may give additional 0.15 mg/kg (average of 10 mg) in 15 to 30 minutes
Oral: 240 to 320 mg/day P.O. in three or four divided doses (standard tablet) or once daily (sustained-release)

Points to remember

- This drug is a first-line treatment for controlling heart rate in patients with adequate ventricular function.

- Withhold dose if patient's pulse rate is less than 50 beats/minute.
- Monitor patient's ECG and blood pressure continuously during I.V. therapy.
- Monitor patient for dizziness and CHF.
- Decrease the I.V. infusion rate in elderly patients.

procainamide hydrochloride
Adult dosage
Oral: 1.25 g initially, followed by 750 mg 1 hour later, with additional doses of 500 mg to 1 g q 2 hours (conventional tablets); after patient is stabilized, give 500 mg to 1 g (conventional tablets) q 4 to 6 hours or 1 g (sustained-release) q 6 hours
I.M.: 50 mg/kg in divided doses q 3 to 6 hours
I.V.: 50 to 100 mg by I.V. bolus q 5 minutes to maximum dose of 500 mg; alternatively, infuse at rate not exceeding 25 to 50 mg/minute; or 500 to 600 mg by I.V. bolus over 25 to 30 minutes, followed by continuous infusion of 1 to 6 mg/minute
Points to remember
- This drug is a second-line antiarrhythmic after quinidine.
- As ordered, administer a digitalis glycoside before starting procainamide.
- Dosage is highly individualized, based on serum drug levels.
- Reduce dosage in patients with renal or hepatic dysfunction, those over age 50, and those with severe CHF or hypotension.
- Monitor patient's ECG and blood pressure continuously during I.V. therapy.

flecainide acetate
Adult dosage
50 to 150 mg P.O. q 12 hours
Points to remember
- This drug is a second- or third-line agent used to prevent disabling supraventricular arrhythmias only in patients without structural heart disease.
- Monitor patient's ECG when initiating therapy.
- Reduce dosage in renal and hepatic dysfunction.
- Titrate dosage upward on individual basis. ■

Atrial flutter

Cardioversion and drug therapy are first-line treatments for this arrhythmia. The goal of therapy is to convert atrial flutter to atrial fibrillation and to keep the heart rate below 100 beats/minute. (For specific drug therapy, see the entry "Atrial fibrillation" in this section.) ■

Atrial tachycardia

Only symptomatic patients or those with underlying heart disease require treatment for this arrhythmia. In emergencies, carotid sinus massage, Valsalva's maneuver, or cardioversion may be attempted before drug therapy begins.

▼FIRST-LINE DRUG

digoxin

Adult dosage

1-mg I.V. loading dose in three divided doses over 24 hours, usually given as 0.5 mg first, 0.25 mg 8 hours after the first dose, then 0.25 mg 16 hours after the first dose; maintenance dose is 0.125 to 0.5 mg/day I.V. or P.O.

Points to remember

- This is a first-line treatment for patients with reduced ventricular function.
- Use only if digoxin toxicity isn't the cause of atrial tachycardia.
- Dosages are highly individualized; digoxin has a narrow therapeutic range (0.8 to 2 ng/ml).
- Withhold dose if patient's pulse rate is less than 50 beats/minute.
- Monitor serum digoxin levels.
- Reduce dosage in elderly patients and in those with renal failure or hepatic compromise.
- Digoxin may interact with various drugs.

▼FIRST-LINE DRUG

diltiazem hydrochloride

Adult dosage

Oral: 90 to 360 mg/day P.O. as a single dose (sustained-release tablet) or divided into three or four daily doses (standard tablet)

I.V.: 0.25 mg/kg by slow I.V. push over 2 minutes; if ineffective, repeat in 15 minutes; or give 10 to 15 mg/hour by I.V. infusion for up to 24 hours

Points to remember

- This is a first-line drug used in patients with good ventricular function.
- Withhold dose if patient's pulse rate is less than 50 beats/minute.
- Monitor patient for dizziness and CHF.
- With I.V. administration, monitor patient's ECG and blood pressure continuously.
- Elderly patients may require reduced dosage.

▼FIRST-LINE DRUG

verapamil

Adult dosage

I.V.: 0.075 to 0.15 mg/kg by slow push over 2 minutes (over 3 minutes in elderly patients); may give additional 0.15 mg/kg in 15 to 30 minutes

Oral: 240 to 320 mg/day P.O. divided in three or four doses

Points to remember

- This is a first-line drug used in patients with adequate ventricular function.
- Withhold dose if patient's pulse rate is less than 50 beats/minute.
- With I.V. administration, monitor patient's ECG and blood pressure continuously.
- Slow I.V. administration rate in elderly patients.
- Monitor patient for dizziness and CHF.

adenosine

Adult dosage

6 mg by I.V. push over 1 to 2 seconds; if necessary, give 12-mg I.V. bolus 1 or 2 minutes later

Points to remember

- This is a second-line drug.
- Monitor patient's ECG and blood pressure continuously.

esmolol

Adult dosage

500 mcg/kg I.V. over 1 minute, then 50 mcg/kg/minute for 4 minutes; if optimal response doesn't occur in 5 minutes, repeat loading dose, and increase maintenance I.V. infusion to 100 mcg/kg/minute for 4 minutes; if necessary, repeat loading dose, and increase infusion rate by 50 mcg/kg/minute to maximum of 200 mcg/kg/minute for 4 minutes

Points to remember

- This is a first- or second-line drug; it brings a rapid response in critical situations.
- Use I.V. controller to infuse.
- Dilute concentrate for injection with compatible I.V. solution to final concentration of 10 mg/ml.
- Drug extravasation may cause skin irritation or necrosis.
- Monitor patient's ECG and blood pressure continuously.

propranolol hydrochloride

Adult dosage

I.V.: 0.5 to 3 mg (don't exceed 1 mg/minute); may repeat in 2 minutes

Oral: 10 to 30 mg P.O. t.i.d. or q.i.d., or one dose as sustained-release tablet daily

Points to remember

- This is a third-line drug.
- It may cause serious side effects.
- Dosages are highly individualized.
- Withhold oral dose if patient's pulse rate is less than 50 beats/minute.
- Dilute oral solution concentrate, or mix with semisolid food just before administration.
- Give oral doses before meals and at bedtime.
- With I.V. administration, monitor patient's ECG and central venous pressure. ■

Atrial tachycardia, multifocal

Although benign in healthy people, this arrhythmia usually occurs in patients with chronic pulmonary disease or elevated atrial pressure. Immediate treatment, if necessary, is similar to that used for atrial tachycardia. Cardiac pacing may be used if conventional therapy fails. (For specific drug therapy, see "Atrial tachycardia" in this section.) ■

Atrial tachycardia, paroxysmal

This arrhythmia is benign in healthy persons, requiring no treatment. In patients with reduced cardiac function, or if the arrhythmia is sustained, treatment options resemble those used for atrial tachycardia; the patient may require quinidine or procainamide with digoxin (see "Atrial fibrillation" in this section) or esmolol, verapamil, or adenosine (see "Atrial tachycardia" in this section).

▼FIRST-LINE DRUG

digoxin

Adult dosage

1 mg I.V. as loading dose in three divided doses over 24 hours; maintenance dosage is 0.125 to 0.5 mg/day I.V. or P.O.

Points to remember

- This drug is a first-line treatment for patients with reduced ventricular function.
- Withhold dose if patient's pulse rate is less than 50 beats/minute.
- Dosages are highly individualized.
- Digoxin has narrow therapeutic range (0.8 to 2 ng/ml); monitor serum drug levels.
- Reduce dosage in elderly patients and those with renal failure or hepatic compromise.
- Use only if digoxin toxicity isn't the cause of the arrhythmia.

▼FIRST-LINE DRUG

quinidine

Adult dosage

Oral: 300 to 400 mg P.O. of quinidine sulfate q 6 hours or 324 to 600 mg of quinidine gluconate (sustained-release) q 8 to 12 hours
I.M.: 600 mg initially, then up to 400 mg q 2 hours based on patient's response
I.V.: 800 mg diluted in 40 ml of D_5W infused at 16 mg (1 ml) per minute

Points to remember

- Before starting I.M. or I.V. therapy, administer 200-mg test dose I.M.
- Before initiating therapy, patient should receive a digitalis glycoside to control ven-

tricular rate and prevent ventricular tachycardia.
- Monitor patient's ECG and blood pressure continuously during I.V. therapy.
- Reduce dosage in hepatic and renal impairment.

▼FIRST-LINE DRUG
verapamil
Adult dosage
I.V.: 0.075 to 0.15 mg/kg (5 to 10 mg) by slow I.V. push over 2 minutes (3 minutes in elderly patients); may give additional 0.15 mg/kg (10 mg) in 15 to 30 minutes
Oral: 240 to 320 mg/day P.O. in three or four divided doses (standard tablet) or once daily (sustained-release)
Points to remember
- This is a first-line drug used in patients with adequate ventricular function.
- Withhold dose if patient's pulse rate is less than 50 beats/minute.
- Monitor patient's ECG and blood pressure continuously during I.V. therapy.
- Slow I.V. administration rate in elderly patients.
- Monitor patient for dizziness and CHF.

adenosine
Adult dosage
6 mg by I.V. push over 1 to 2 seconds; if necessary, give bolus of 12 mg 1 to 2 minutes later
Points to remember
- This is a second-line drug after verapamil or diltiazem.
- Monitor patient's ECG and blood pressure continuously.

esmolol hydrochloride
Adult dosage
500 mcg/kg I.V. loading dose over 1 minute, followed by 50 mcg/kg/minute for 4 minutes; if optimal response doesn't occur in 5 minutes, repeat loading dose and increase maintenance infusion to 100 mcg/kg/minute for 4 minutes. If needed, repeat loading dose, and increase infusion rate by 50 mcg/kg/minute to maximum of 200 mcg/kg/minute for 4 minutes.
Points to remember
- This is a first- or second-line alternative drug that achieves a rapid response in critical situations.
- Use I.V. controller to infuse.
- Dilute concentrate for injection with compatible I.V. solution to final concentration of 10 mg/ml.
- Monitor patient's ECG and blood pressure continuously.
- Extravasation may cause skin irritation or necrosis.

procainamide hydrochloride
Adult dosage
I.M.: 50 mg/kg I.M. in divided doses q 3 to 6 hours
I.V.: 50 to 100 mg by I.V. bolus q 5 minutes to total of

500 mg or alternatively by I.V. infusion, not exceeding 25 to 50 mg/minute; or give 500- to 600-mg I.V. bolus over 25 to 30 minutes, followed by continuous infusion of 1 to 6 mg/minute
Oral: 1.25 g, followed by 750 mg 1 hour later, with additional doses of 500 mg to 1 g q 2 hours (standard tablets); when patient is stabilized, give 500 mg to 1 g (standard tablets) q 4 to 6 hours or 1 g (sustained-release tablets) q 6 hours

Points to remember

- This drug is a second-line antiarrhythmic after quinidine.
- Dosage is highly individualized, based on patient's serum procainamide levels.
- Patient should receive a digitalis glycoside before starting procainamide.
- Reduce dosage in patients with renal or hepatic dysfunction, those over age 50, and those with severe CHF or hypotension.
- Monitor patient's ECG and blood pressure continuously during I.V. therapy. ■

AV dissociation

This heart problem isn't a primary disturbance but a symptom of an underlying disorder. Its significance varies with the cause. No treatment is necessary if the patient's heart rate and rhythm are acceptable. Drug therapy aims to correct the primary cause. Alternative treatments include cardioversion and pacemaker insertion.

isoproterenol
Adult dosage
I.V.: 0.02 to 0.06 mg (1 to 3 ml of 1:50,000 dilution) by I.V. bolus initially, then 0.01 to 0.2 mg (0.5 to 10 ml of 1:50,000 dilution) for subsequent doses; or by I.V. infusion at 5 mcg/minute (1.25 ml of 1:250,000 dilution/minute) initially
Intracardiac injection: 0.02 mg (0.1 ml of 1:5,000 dilution)
I.M. or S.C.: 0.2 mg (1 ml of 1:5,000 dilution), then 0.02 to 1 mg (0.1 to 5 ml of 1:5,000 dilution) I.M.; or 0.15 to 0.2 mg (0.75 to 1 ml of 1:5,000 dilution) S.C. p.r.n.
S.L.: 10 to 30 mg four to six times daily
P.R.: 5 mg initially, then 5 to 15 mg p.r.n.

Points to remember

- This drug, an alternative to atropine, is used for nonspecific therapy.
- Monitor patient's ECG during I.V. therapy.

atropine sulfate
Adult dosage
1 mg by I.V. push; repeat in 5 minutes

Point to remember
- This is a second-line drug after isoproterenol. ■

Bradycardia, symptomatic

Pacemaker insertion is the primary definitive treatment. Drugs are used as adjunctive therapy.

atropine sulfate
Adult dosage
0.5 to 1 mg I.V.; repeat q 3 to 5 minutes
Points to remember
- Total dose shouldn't exceed 0.03 mg/kg for mild bradycardia or 3 mg for severe bradycardia.
- Monitor patient's ECG continuously. ■

Buerger's disease

Smoking cessation is the most important treatment for this disease. Drug therapy is adjunctive and proves effective only in mild to moderate cases. Calcium channel blockers, such as nifedipine, may be prescribed to dilate arterioles. Local infection or gangrene may warrant antibiotics.

nifedipine
Adult dosage
10 to 30 mg P.O. t.i.d. (standard tablets); or 30 to 90 mg/day (sustained-release)
Points to remember
- This drug dilates the arterioles.
- Instruct patient not to chew, crush, or break sustained-release tablets.
- Use cautiously in patients with CHF or aortic stenosis. ■

Cardiac tamponade

The treatment of choice for this disorder is surgery, which usually involves removal of excess pericardial fluid. Drug therapy is adjunctive.

dopamine hydrochloride
Adult dosage
1 to 5 mcg/kg/minute I.V. initially; increase by 1 to 4 mcg/kg/minute at intervals of 10 to 30 minutes until desired response occurs
Points to remember
- This drug is used in conjunction with fluids and albumin to maintain cardiac output.
- Preferably, administer by I.V. infusion pump in antecubital vein.
- Discard darkened solution.
- Monitor patient's ECG, blood pressure, urine flow, cardiac output, and pulmo-

nary wedge pressure continuously. ■

Cardiogenic shock

This life-threatening condition may occur in patients who have suffered large ventricular wall MIs or other conditions that result in severe left ventricular dysfunction. Drug therapy is the treatment of choice. Aggressive intensive care management is essential for survival.

▼FIRST-LINE DRUG

dobutamine hydrochloride

Adult dosage

2 to 5 mcg/kg/minute I.V. initially; titrate to achieve desired hemodynamic effect (typically 5 to 15 mcg/kg/minute)

Points to remember

- This is a first-line inotropic agent used to improve myocardial contractility in patients with severely diminished cardiac output.
- Administer by I.V. infusion pump.
- Monitor patient's heart rate, blood pressure, urine flow, central venous or pulmonary wedge pressure, and cardiac output continuously.
- Use solutions diluted for I.V. administration within 24 hours.

amrinone lactate

Adult dosage

0.75 mg/kg by direct I.V. injection over 2 to 3 minutes; may repeat in 30 minutes; then give 5 to 10 mcg/kg/minute by I.V. infusion as a maintenance dosage

Points to remember

- This drug is used to increase myocardial contractility.
- It's an alternative to dobutamine in patients with severe cardiogenic low-output syndrome.
- Monitor cardiac output, pulmonary wedge pressure, and central venous pressure.
- Watch for signs and symptoms of CHF.
- Monitor patient's renal and hepatic function and platelet counts.
- Dilute with saline solution only.

dopamine hydrochloride

Adult dosage

1 to 5 mcg/kg/minute I.V. initially; increase by 1 to 4 mcg/kg/minute at intervals of 10 to 30 minutes until desired response occurs

Points to remember

- This drug is used in conjunction with fluids and albumin to maintain cardiac output, blood pressure, and renal blood flow.
- Preferably, administer by I.V. infusion pump in an antecubital vein.

- Discard darkened solutions.
- Monitor patient's ECG, blood pressure, urine flow, cardiac output, and pulmonary wedge pressure continuously.

nitroprusside sodium
Adult dosage
0.25 to 0.3 mcg/kg/minute I.V. initially; titrate upward to 3 mcg/kg/minute (dosage range is 0.3 to 10 mcg/kg/minute)
Points to remember
- This drug is used with amrinone or dobutamine to improve cardiac output by reducing peripheral vascular resistance and left ventricular end-diastolic pressure.
- Monitor patient's blood pressure to prevent severe hypotension. Diastolic pressure should be lowered and maintained at about 30% to 40% below pretreatment level.
- If patient doesn't respond adequately at maximum dosage of 10 mcg/kg/minute within 10 minutes, discontinue drug.
- Reduce dosage in elderly patients and those with renal or hepatic dysfunction.
- Protect solution from light.

norepinephrine bitartrate
Adult dosage
8 to 12 mcg/minute; titrate to achieve desired response
Points to remember
- This drug is used for a more potent vasoconstrictor effect in patients who don't respond to volume replacement.
- Monitor patient's heart rate, blood pressure, cardiac output, and central venous or pulmonary wedge pressure continuously.
- Take precautions to prevent extravasation; check for free flow and blanching of infused vein.
- Use I.V. solution immediately after preparation.
- Discard pink, dark yellow, or brown solutions and those containing precipitate. ■

Cardiomyopathy, dilated

In this disorder, the goal of therapy is to correct the underlying cause and improve the heart's pumping ability. Heart transplantation is the only definitive treatment; however, many patients are not eligible for this procedure. Drug therapy is directed toward treating CHF, arrhythmias, and volume overload.

captopril
Adult dosage
6.25 to 50 mg P.O. t.i.d.

Points to remember

- This drug may cause hyperkalemia; monitor serum potassium levels closely.
- Monitor patient's renal function and blood pressure closely.
- This drug may cause cough or diminished taste.
- Reduce dosage in renal dysfunction.

digoxin

Adult dosage

0.125 to 0.25 mg/day P.O. or I.V.

Points to remember

- This drug is used to increase myocardial contractility and prevent heart failure.
- Dosages are highly individualized.
- This drug has a very narrow therapeutic range (1 to 2 ng/ml); monitor serum digoxin levels.
- Withhold dose if patient's pulse rate is less than 50 beats/minute.
- Reduce dosage in elderly patients and those with renal or hepatic dysfunction.

enalapril maleate

Adult dosage

2.5 to 20 mg/day P.O.

Points to remember

- This drug may cause hyperkalemia; monitor serum potassium levels closely.
- Monitor patient's renal function and blood pressure closely.
- This drug may cause cough or diminished taste sensation.
- Reduce dosage in renal dysfunction.

furosemide

Adult dosage

20 to 120 mg/day P.O. or I.V. in single or divided doses

Points to remember

- This drug is used to reduce fluid overload.
- Titrate dosage to achieve desired response without causing dehydration.
- Monitor serum electrolyte levels closely, especially potassium.
- Patient may require potassium supplement.
- Reduce dosage in elderly patients.

nitroglycerin ointment

Adult dosage

Apply ½″ to 2″ of 2% ointment to applicator paper; using paper (not fingers), gently spread on hairless area in thin, uniform layer q 6 to 8 hours

Points to remember

- To prevent tolerance, patient should have nitrate-free interval of 8 to 12 hours overnight.
- This drug is used primarily in acute disease episodes; for long-term maintenance, patients usually are switched to nitroglycerin patch or a long-acting oral nitrate.

nitroglycerin transdermal patch

Adult dosage

Apply one patch (0.1 to 0.6 mg/hour) to clean, dry, hairless area on upper arm or body q 24 hours

Points to remember

- This drug is used to reduce cardiac preload and afterload.
- Instruct patient to apply patch at same time each day.
- Tell patient to rotate application sites to prevent skin irritation.
- Instruct patient to remove patch each day before showering.
- To prevent tolerance, patient should maintain nitrate-free interval of 8 to 12 hours overnight. ■

Cardiomyopathy, hypertrophic

In patients with severe symptoms, surgical excision of part of the myocardial septum has been successful. Drug therapy aims to treat dyspnea, angina, and arrhythmias.

atenolol

Adult dosage

25 to 100 mg/day P.O.

Point to remember

- This is typically the first drug given to symptomatic patients, especially those with dynamic outflow obstruction.

metoprolol

Adult dosage

50 to 100 mg/day P.O.

Point to remember

- This drug may be the first drug given to symptomatic patients, especially those with dynamic outflow obstruction.

verapamil

Adult dosage

240 mg/day P.O. in three divided doses

Point to remember

- This drug may cause constipation. ■

Cardiomyopathy, restrictive

Few drugs have been adequately studied for this form of cardiomyopathy, which is rare in the United States. Because the causes of this disease are varied and hard to treat, therapy focuses on relieving symptoms of CHF. Diuretics and vasodilators may be helpful; digoxin usually isn't. Patients also may benefit from a low-sodium diet and long-term anticoagulation therapy. Rarely, surgery or immunosuppressant therapy (with corticosteroids or antimetabolites) brings improvement.

hydralazine hydrochloride
Adult dosage
10 mg P.O. q.i.d. initially; then titrate to 50 mg q.i.d. as tolerated; continue to titrate to lowest effective dosage
Points to remember
- Hydralazine is used only to relieve symptoms of CHF.
- Some patients can't tolerate this drug. Monitor carefully for worsening of heart failure.

loop diuretics
Adult dosage
Bumetanide: 0.5 to 2 mg/day P.O. to maximum dosage of 10 mg/day
Furosemide: 20 to 80 mg/day P.O.; increase in 20- to 40-mg increments to achieve optimum response with the lowest effective dosage
Points to remember
- These drugs are used only to relieve symptoms of CHF.
- Some patients may experience worsened symptoms from excessive diuretic doses.

prazosin hydrochloride
Adult dosage
1 to 2 mg P.O. t.i.d.
Points to remember
- This drug is used only for symptomatic treatment of CHF.
- Advise patient to avoid alcohol.

warfarin sodium
Adult dosage
2 to 10 mg/day P.O.
Points to remember
- This drug is used only for patients at high risk for thromboembolism.
- Adjust dosage to maintain international normalized ratio between 2 and 3.
- Instruct patient to consume adequate amounts of vitamin K.
- Overdose may be treated with vitamin K_1.
- This drug is contraindicated after recent lumbar puncture, trauma, childbirth or surgery and in severe hepatic or renal impairment, endocarditis, pregnancy, thrombocytopenia, severe uncontrolled hypertension, pericarditis, active bleeding, or cerebrovascular accident.
- Elderly patients may be more susceptible to bleeding during therapy.
- Advise patient to notify other health care professionals if he's taking warfarin long-term and to carry identification indicating such therapy. ■

Coarctation of the aorta

Surgery is the definitive treatment for this disorder. Drug therapy is an interim measure used to manage symptoms of CHF.

digoxin
Adult dosage
1 mg I.V. loading dose in three divided doses over 24 hours; maintenance dosage is 0.125 to 0.5 mg/day I.V. or P.O.
Points to remember
- This drug is a first-line alternative in patients with reduced ventricular function.
- Dosages are highly individualized.
- Withhold dose if patient's pulse is below 50 beats/minute.
- Monitor patient's serum drug level.
- Reduce dosage in elderly patients and those with renal failure or hepatic compromise.

furosemide
Adult dosage
40 to 240 mg/day P.O. or I.V. in single or divided doses
Points to remember
- This drug is used as a first-line diuretic to prevent or treat symptomatic volume overload.
- Monitor patient's blood pressure, fluid balance, serum electrolyte levels, BUN, and creatinine level. ■

Coronary artery disease

Therapy for this disease must be individualized. Treatment measures may include surgery, drug therapy, or both. Behavior modification also is important. Drug therapy aims to reduce angina symptoms and prevent coronary occlusion, thereby helping to avert MI.

amlodipine besylate
Adult dosage
5 to 10 mg/day P.O.
Points to remember
- This drug is used to reduce cardiac preload.
- Titrate to effective dosage gradually with intervals of 7 to 14 days between increases.
- Monitor patient's blood pressure and check for peripheral edema frequently.
- Elderly patients may need dosage reduction.

atenolol
Adult dosage
25 to 100 mg/day P.O.
Points to remember
- This drug is used to reduce cardiac preload and heart rate.
- Individualize dosage based on patient's response; titrate upward gradually.
- This drug may exacerbate asthma and CHF. It may mask hypoglycemia in patients with diabetes.
- When discontinuing drug, reduce dosage gradually over 2 weeks.
- Reduce dosage in elderly patients.

heparin

Adult dosage

5,000 units S.C. q 8 to 12 hours, or 1 unit/kg/hour I.V.

Points to remember

- This drug is used to prevent further occlusion of the coronary arteries.
- Monitor patient's platelet count.
- Use with caution in patients at increased risk for hemorrhage; if hemorrhage occurs, stop drug immediately.

isosorbide dinitrate

Adult dosage

10 to 20 mg P.O. t.i.d. or q.i.d.; alternatively, 20- to 40-mg sustained-release capsule q 6 to 12 hours

Points to remember

- This drug is used to reduce cardiac preload and afterload.
- Instruct patient to take drug on empty stomach.
- Using sustained-release preparation may reduce headache.

isosorbide mononitrate

Adult dosage

30 to 240 mg/day P.O. (24-hour extended-release tablets) given in morning; or 20 mg P.O. (12-hour extended-release tablets) b.i.d. given 7 hours apart

Points to remember

- This drug is used as a long-acting oral alternative to the transdermal patch.
- Instruct patient not to crush or chew tablets.
- First dose is usually given in the morning.
- Nitrate-free interval of 8 to 12 hours overnight is recommended.

metoprolol

Adult dosage

50 to 200 mg P.O. b.i.d.

Points to remember

- This drug is used to reduce cardiac preload and heart rate.
- Individualize dosage based on patient's response; titrate upward gradually.
- This drug may exacerbate asthma and CHF. It masks hypoglycemia in patients with diabetes.
- When discontinuing drug, reduce dosage gradually over 2 weeks.
- Reduce dosage in elderly patients.

nadolol

Adult dosage

40 to 80 mg/day P.O.

Points to remember

- This drug is used to reduce cardiac preload and heart rate.
- Individualize dosage based on patient's response; titrate upward gradually.
- This drug may exacerbate asthma and CHF. It may mask hypoglycemia in diabetics.

- When discontinuing drug, reduce dosage gradually over 2 weeks.
- Reduce dosage in elderly patients.

nifedipine
Adult dosage
10 to 20 mg P.O. t.i.d., or 60 to 90 mg/day P.O. sustained-release tablets
Points to remember
- This drug is used to reduce cardiac preload.
- Instruct patient not to chew or crush sustained-release preparations.
- Titrate dosage gradually as needed with intervals of 7 to 14 days between increases.
- Monitor patient's blood pressure and check for peripheral edema frequently.
- Elderly patients may require dosage reduction.

nitroglycerin ointment
Adult dosage
Apply ½″ to 2″ of 2% ointment to applicator paper; using paper (not fingers), gently spread on hairless area in thin, uniform layer q 6 to 8 hours
Points to remember
- Ointment is used mainly for acute symptoms. For long-term maintenance, patients usually are switched to nitroglycerin patch or a long-acting oral nitrate.
- To prevent tolerance, patient should have nitrate-free interval of 8 to 12 hours overnight.

nitroglycerin transdermal patch
Adult dosage
Apply one patch (0.1 to 0.6 mg/hour) to clean, dry, hairless area on upper arm or body q 24 hours
Points to remember
- Instruct patient to apply patch at same time each day.
- Tell patient to rotate application sites to prevent skin irritation.
- Instruct patient to remove patch each day before showering.
- To prevent tolerance, patient should have nitrate-free interval of 8 to 12 hours overnight. ■

Endocarditis

Drugs are the treatment of choice for this abnormal condition of the heart's interior lining. Many patients must undergo surgical replacement of damaged heart valves. Drug therapy is directed toward eradicating the infectious organism that causes valve damage.

When the causative organism is unknown, the choice of empiric antibiotic depends on whether the patient has acute or subacute disease. In acute disease, the antibiotic should provide coverage for *Staphylococcus aureus*, streptococcal organisms, and gram-negative bacilli. In subacute disease, antibiotic therapy is directed empirically toward most streptococci, including *Streptococcus faecalis*.

Once the causative agent is identified, antibiotic coverage should be narrowed appropriately. Most patients require 4 to 8 weeks of antibiotic therapy. Many patients complete uncomplicated courses of treatment with home I.V. therapy.

ampicillin

Adult dosage

2 g I.V. q 4 hours

Points to remember

- This drug is used to treat streptococcal infections.
- It's used in combination with nafcillin and gentamicin for acute endocarditis and in combination with gentamicin for subacute endocarditis.
- Reduce dosage in severe renal dysfunction.

gentamicin

Adult dosage

1 mg/kg (60 to 80 mg) I.V. q 8 hours

Points to remember

- This drug is used empirically in combination with ampicillin and nafcillin in acute endocarditis and in combination with ampicillin in subacute endocarditis. It provides gram-negative coverage and synergistic gram-positive effect when used in combination with ampicillin, nafcillin, or both.
- This drug has a narrow therapeutic index. Monitor patient's serum gentamicin levels.
- Dosages are highly individualized, especially when drug is used long-term.
- Reduce dosage in renal insufficiency.

nafcillin sodium

Adult dosage

2 g I.V. q 4 hours

Points to remember

- This drug is active against staphylococcal organisms. It is used in combination with ampicillin and gentamicin.
- Reduce dosage in severe renal dysfunction. ■

Heart failure

Any reversible causes of heart failure should be treated, and the patient's sodium intake should be limited to 2 g/day. Drug therapy is aimed at eliminating the symptoms of heart failure, such as fluid retention and arrhythmias.

▼FIRST-LINE DRUGS

ACE inhibitors

Adult dosage

Captopril: initially 6.25 or 12.5 mg P.O. t.i.d.; increase to 25 to 100 mg P.O. t.i.d.
Enalapril maleate: 5 to 40 mg P.O. once or twice daily
Lisinopril: 5 to 40 mg/day P.O.
Quinapril hydrochloride: 10 to 80 mg P.O. once or twice daily

Points to remember

- These drugs may cause significant hypotension; use cautiously at first.
- Discontinue other vasodilators and reduce or withhold diuretic doses for 24 hours before therapy starts.
- These drugs may increase serum potassium level; discontinue any potassium-sparing agents before starting therapy.

▼FIRST-LINE DRUGS

diuretics

Adult dosage

Bumetanide: 1 to 8 mg/day P.O. or I.V.
Furosemide: 20 to 320 mg/day P.O. or I.V. in single or divided doses
Hydrochlorothiazide: 25 to 100 mg/day P.O. (only for mild fluid retention)
Metolazone: 2.5 to 10 mg/day P.O.
Torsemide: 10 to 20 mg/day P.O. or I.V.

Points to remember

- Thiazide diuretics are indicated only for mild fluid retention; generally, they're ineffective when glomerular filtration rate falls below 30 ml/minute.
- Potassium-sparing agents (triamterene, amiloride, and spironolactone) are often used in combination with thiazide or loop diuretics.
- Monitor serum electrolyte levels.

digoxin

Adult dosage

I.V.: 0.5 mg over 10 to 20 minutes; may give additional doses of 0.125 to 0.25 mg after 3 hours to maximum of 1 to 1.25 mg
Oral: 1 to 1.25 mg in divided doses over first 24 hours (daily oral maintenance dosage ranges from 0.125 to 0.5 mg P.O.)

Points to remember

- This agent may serve as a first- or second-line drug, depending on the patient's condition.
- Monitor serum drug levels, and adjust therapy accordingly.
- Adjust dosage in renal dysfunction.

dobutamine hydrochloride

Adult dosage

2.5 to 10 mcg/kg/minute by I.V. infusion

Points to remember

- Adjust dosage to patient's individual needs and desired clinical response.
- Don't administer through same I.V. line as heparin, hydrocortisone sodium succinate, cefazolin, cefamandole, cephalothin, or penicillin.

hydralazine hydrochloride

Adult dosage

200 to 400 mg/day P.O. in divided doses q 6 to 12 hours

Point to remember

- Combination of nitrates and oral hydralazine produces greater hemodynamic and clinical effects.

nitrates

Adult dosage

Isosorbide dinitrate: 20 to 80 mg P.O. three times daily

Nitroglycerin ointment: 12.5 to 50 mg applied topically q 8 hours

Nitroprusside sodium: 0.25 to 0.3 mcg/kg/minute by I.V. infusion; titrate to 0.3 to 10 mcg/kg/minute during acute decompensation

Points to remember

- Nitrate therapy is generally well tolerated, but headaches and hypotension may limit dosages.
- Tolerance may occur but can be minimized by enforcing a nitrate-free interval of 8 to 12 hours overnight.

positive inotropic agents

Adult dosage

Amrinone lactate: initially 0.75 mg/kg I.V. bolus over 2 to 3 minutes, followed by 5 to 10 mcg/kg/minute; may give additional bolus of 0.75 mg/kg 30 minutes after therapy starts (maximum daily dose is 10 mg/kg)

Milrinone: initial loading dose of 50 mcg/kg I.V. over 10 minutes, followed by 0.375 to 0.75 mcg/kg/minute by I.V. infusion (titrate to therapeutic response)

Points to remember

- These drugs are used for acute management of severe heart failure.
- Avoid injecting furosemide into an I.V. line containing amrinone or milrinone because an immediate chemical interaction may occur, as indicated by precipitate formation.
- Amrinone precipitates in solutions containing dextrose. ■

Hyperlipidemia

This disease calls for weight reduction and dietary restriction of total fats, saturated fatty acids, and cholesterol. Drug therapy and other medical measures are based on the patient's serum cholesterol and triglyceride levels.

▼FIRST-LINE DRUG

cholestyramine

Adult dosage

4 g t.i.d. P.O.; then increase to four to six times daily

Points to remember

- This drug is used mainly to treat type IIA hypercholesterolemia.
- It may interact with warfarin, digitoxin, thyroxine, and fat-soluble vitamins.

▼FIRST-LINE DRUG

colestipol

Adult dosage

5 g P.O. once or twice daily, increased gradually up to 30 g/day in two to four divided doses.

Point to remember

- This drug is used mainly to treat type IIA hypercholesterolemia.

▼FIRST-LINE DRUG

niacin

Adult dosage

1 to 2 g P.O. t.i.d.

Points to remember

- This drug is used mainly to treat types IIA, IIB, III, IV, and V hypertriglyceridemia or hypercholesterolemia.
- It may cause flushing and headache.

clofibrate

Adult dosage

500 to 1,000 mg P.O. b.i.d. to q.i.d.

Points to remember

- This drug is used mainly to treat types IIB, III, IV, and V hypertriglyceridemia.
- It may increase the risk of gallstones, heart disease, and cancer; monitor patient for signs and symptoms.

gemfibrozil

Adult dosage

600 mg P.O. b.i.d.

Points to remember

- This drug is used mainly to treat types IIB, III, and IV hypertriglyceridemia.
- Discontinue drug if liver function test results rise significantly or suggest worsening abnormalities.

lovastatin

Adult dosage

5 to 40 mg P.O. b.i.d.

Points to remember

- This drug is used mainly to treat type IIA hypercholesterolemia.
- Monitor for myositis; instruct patient to report muscle aches and pains.
- Liver function tests should be performed frequently when therapy begins and periodically thereafter.

pravastatin sodium

Adult dosage

10 to 40 mg/day P.O.

Points to remember

- This drug is used mainly to treat type IIA hypercholesterolemia.

- Watch for signs and symptoms of myositis.
- Discontinue drug temporarily in patients with acute condition that suggests developing myopathy or in those with risk factors that may predispose them to renal failure secondary to rhabdomyolysis.

probucol
Adult dosage
500 mg P.O. b.i.d. with meals
Points to remember
- This drug is used mainly to treat types IIA and IIB hypercholesterolemia.
- Don't exceed 1 g/day.
- Monitor patient's ECG periodically during therapy.

simvastatin
Adult dosage
20 to 40 mg/day P.O.
Points to remember
- This drug is used mainly to treat type IIA hypercholesterolemia.
- Liver function tests should be performed frequently when therapy starts and periodically thereafter. ■

Hypertension

Nondrug approaches to treating hypertension include losing weight, reducing alcohol and salt consumption, getting regular exercise, and reducing stress. If these measures fail to reduce blood pressure, therapy with various antihypertensives should proceed in a stepwise manner. Drug therapy is highly individualized.

▼FIRST-LINE DRUGS
ACE inhibitors
Adult dosage
Benazepril: 5 to 40 mg/day P.O., divided in one or two doses
Captopril: 50 to 300 mg/day P.O., divided in two or three doses
Enalapril maleate: 5 to 40 mg/day P.O., divided in one or two doses
Fosinopril sodium: 10 to 80 mg/day P.O., divided in one or two doses
Lisinopril: 5 to 40 mg/day P.O.
Quinapril hydrochloride: 10 to 80 mg/day P.O., divided in one or two doses
Ramipril: 2.5 to 20 mg/day P.O., divided in one or two doses
Points to remember
- These first-line drugs are preferred in patients with insulin-dependent diabetes.
- These drugs may be used in combination with diuretics or calcium channel blockers.

▼FIRST-LINE DRUGS
beta blockers
Adult dosage
Atenolol: 25 to 50 mg/day P.O.; may be increased to 100

mg/day to achieve optimum response
Labetalol hydrochloride: 200 to 1,200 mg/day P.O. in two doses
Metoprolol: 100 mg in a single dose or in divided doses
Pindolol: 10 to 30 mg P.O., divided in two doses
Propranolol hydrochloride: 40 to 320 mg/day P.O., divided in two doses

Point to remember

- These drugs are contraindicated in CHF, symptomatic bronchospasm, and insulin-dependent diabetes.

▼FIRST-LINE DRUGS

calcium channel blockers

Adult dosage

Amlodipine besylate: 5 to 10 mg/day P.O.
Diltiazem hydrochloride: 18 to 360 mg/day P.O., divided in three doses; or 260 mg in two doses (sustained-release form); or 18 to 360 mg/day (controlled-delivery form)
Felodipine: 5 to 20 mg/day P.O.
Isradipine: 5 to 10 mg/day P.O., divided in two doses
Nifedipine: 30 to 120 mg/day P.O., divided in three doses; or 30 to 120 mg/day P.O. (sustained-release form)
Verapamil: 240 mg/day P.O., divided in three doses

Points to remember

- These agents apparently are effective in all demographic groups and all grades of hypertension.
- Use cautiously when combining with beta blockers; this combination may depress AV conduction and sinus node automaticity.

▼FIRST-LINE DRUGS

diuretics

Adult dosage

Bumetanide: 0.5 to 10 mg P.O., divided in two or three doses
Furosemide: 40 to 320 mg P.O., divided in two or three doses
Hydrochlorothiazide: 12.5 to 50 mg/day P.O.
Metolazone: 1.25 to 50 mg/day P.O.

Points to remember

- Thiazide diuretics are indicated only for mild fluid retention; generally, they're ineffective when glomerular filtration rate falls below 30 ml/minute.
- Thiazide or loop diuretics often are used in combination with potassium-sparing agents (such as triamterene, amiloride, and spironolactone).
- Monitor serum electrolyte levels.

alpha-adrenergic receptors

Adult dosage

Doxazosin mesylate: 1 to 16 mg/day P.O.
Prazosin hydrochloride: 2 to 20 mg/day P.O., divided in two or three doses

Terazosin hydrochloride: 1 to 20 mg/day P.O., divided in one or two doses

Points to remember

- These drugs are sometimes effective as single-drug therapy; however, tachyphylaxis may occur during long-term therapy, and side effects are common.
- In less responsive patients, these drugs are most useful when given in combination with another antihypertensive agent.

central sympatholytics

Adult dosage

Clonidine: 0.2 to 0.6 mg/day P.O., divided in two doses; or 0.1- to 0.3-mg/day patch weekly
Guanabenz acetate: 8 to 64 mg/day P.O., divided in two doses
Guanfacine: 1 to 3 mg/day P.O.
Methyldopa: 500 to 2,000 mg/day P.O., divided in two doses

Point to remember

- These drugs usually are used as second- or third-line drugs because of high incidence of drug intolerance.

direct vasodilators

Adult dosage

Hydralazine hydrochloride: 50 to 300 mg/day P.O., divided in two to four doses
Minoxidil: 5 to 40 mg/day P.O.

Point to remember

- These drugs are usually given in combination with diuretics and beta blockers to patients who are unresponsive to vasodilators alone.

reserpine

Adult dosage

0.05 to 0.25 mg/day P.O.

Point to remember

- This drug is used mainly in patients with refractory hypertension. ■

Hypertensive emergencies and malignant hypertension

Parenteral drug therapy is indicated for these conditions, especially if encephalopathy is present. Nitroprusside is the agent of choice. However, in patients with myocardial ischemia, I.V. nitroglycerin or an I.V. beta blocker is preferred.

▼FIRST-LINE DRUG

nitroprusside sodium

Adult dosage

0.25 to 10 mcg/kg/minute I.V.

Points to remember

- Dosages must be individualized.
- Drug is used with a beta blocker in patients with aortic dissection.

▼FIRST-LINE DRUG

esmolol hydrochloride

Adult dosage

I.V. loading dose of 500 mcg/kg over 1 minute, then maintenance I.V. infusion of 25 to 200 mcg/kg/minute

Point to remember

- This drug is contraindicated in CHF and asthma.

▼FIRST-LINE DRUG

hydralazine hydrochloride

Adult dosage

5 to 20 mg I.V.; may repeat after 20 minutes

Point to remember

- This drug is contraindicated in coronary artery disease and aortic dissection.

▼FIRST-LINE DRUG

labetalol hydrochloride

Adult dosage

20 to 40 mg I.V. q 10 minutes to a maximum dose of 300 mg

Points to remember

- This drug is contraindicated in CHF and asthma.
- It may be continued as oral therapy.

▼FIRST-LINE DRUG

nifedipine

Adult dosage

10 mg P.O.; may repeat once after 30 minutes

Points to remember

- This drug may also be given by sublingual or buccal route.
- It may precipitate angina.

▼FIRST-LINE DRUG

nitroglycerin

Adult dosage

0.25 to 5 mcg/kg/minute I.V.

Points to remember

- This drug is useful in patients with myocardial ischemia.
- Dosages must be individualized.
- Patient may develop drug tolerance.

clonidine hydrochloride

Adult dosage

0.1 to 0.2 mg P.O. initially, then 0.1 mg P.O. q hour to maximum of 0.8 mg/day

Points to remember

- Sedation is a common side effect.
- Rebound hypertension may occur when the drug is stopped.

enalaprilat

Adult dosage

1.25 mg I.V. q 6 hours

Points to remember

- This agent causes additive effects when given with a diuretic.
- Enalaprilat may be continued as oral therapy.

furosemide

Adult dosage

10 to 80 mg I.V. over 1 to 2 minutes

Points to remember

- Dosages must be individualized.
- This drug is used as an adjunct to vasodilator therapy.

nicardipine hydrochloride
Adult dosage
5 mg/hour I.V.; may increase by 1 to 2.5 mg/hour q 15 minutes to maximum of 15 mg/hour
Point to remember
- This drug may precipitate myocardial ischemia. ■

Junctional tachycardia

Treatment focuses on terminating this arrhythmia quickly, but without using measures more dangerous than the arrhythmia itself. Mechanical measures, such as Valsalva's maneuver, may prove effective. Synchronized electrical cardioversion may be tried in patients who require immediate arrhythmia termination but who don't respond to adenosine or verapamil. Drugs serve as first-line therapy.

▼FIRST-LINE DRUG
adenosine
Adult dosage
6 mg by rapid I.V. bolus (over 1 to 2 seconds); if this fails to halt the arrhythmia in 1 or 2 minutes, give 12 mg by rapid I.V. push; repeat 12-mg dose if needed
Points to remember
- Drug is used to terminate junctional tachycardia during an acute attack.
- Single doses of more than 12 mg aren't recommended.
- For I.V. administration, use proximal port and follow with rapid saline flush to make sure drug reaches systemic circulation rapidly.

▼FIRST-LINE DRUG
digoxin
Adult dosage
0.5 to 0.75 mg I.V., increased in increments of 0.125 to 0.25 mg q 2 to 4 hours to maximum of 1 to 1.25 mg
Points to remember
- Oral digoxin is therapy of choice for prophylaxis of junctional tachycardia.
- Tailor dosage to patient's serum digoxin level.

esmolol hydrochloride
Adult dosage
500 mcg/kg I.V. over 1 minute, followed by infusion of 25 to 200 mcg/minute
Point to remember
- This drug is used in acute attacks.

verapamil
Adult dosage
I.V.: 2.5 mg by I.V. bolus, followed by additional doses of 2.5 to 5 mg q 1 to 3 minutes to maximum of 20 mg (if patient's blood pressure and rhythm are stable)
Oral: 80 to 120 mg P.O. q 4 to 6 hours (if patient is stable and can tolerate junctional tachycardia)

Points to remember
- Oral verapamil is second choice for prophylaxis of junctional tachycardia.
- Verapamil increases serum digoxin levels. ■

Myocardial infarction

Patients typically receive I.V. morphine to relieve pain associated with MI. Those with ventricular fibrillation (VF) may receive I.V. lidocaine. Bed rest is another important measure. Thrombolytic therapy reduces mortality and may limit the size of the infarct. Nitrates are the drug of choice for treating recurrent ischemic pain. Beta blockers reduce the duration of ischemic pain and the incidence of VF.

▼FIRST-LINE DRUGS
beta blockers
Adult dosage
Atenolol: 5 mg I.V. initially, followed by another 5 mg I.V. 10 minutes later; start oral therapy 10 minutes after a second dose in patients who can tolerate full I.V. dose.
Metoprolol: three 5-mg I.V. boluses q 2 minutes; 15 minutes after last I.V. dose, give 50 mg P.O. and continue giving this dose q 6 hours for 48 hours (maintenance dose: 100 mg P.O. twice daily)

Point to remember
- Beta blockers are most effective when given immediately after onset of MI symptoms.

▼FIRST-LINE DRUG
nitroglycerin
Adult dosage
0.25 to 5 mcg/kg/minute I.V.
Point to remember
- Individualize dosage to control ischemic pain.

▼FIRST-LINE DRUGS
thrombolytics
Adult dosage
Alteplase (tissue plasminogen activator [t-PA]): 10 mg I.V., then an additional 50 mg I.V. over first hour, followed by 10 mg/hour for next 4 hours
Anistreplase: 30 units I.V. infused over 2 to 5 minutes
Streptokinase: 750,000 units infused I.V. over 20 minutes, followed by 750,000 units infused I.V. over 40 minutes
Points to remember
- Thrombolytics are contraindicated in known bleeding diatheses, cerebrovascular disease, uncontrolled hypertension, pregnancy, and recent trauma or surgery.
- Arterial reocclusion rates are higher with alteplase; I.V. heparin is recommended for at least 24 hours.
- Streptokinase is more likely to cause allergic reactions and should be avoided if pa-

tient has received it previously.

- Experts recommend thrombolytic therapy in patients up to age 80 with ST-segment elevation or Q waves on ECG who are admitted within 6 to 12 hours of pain onset.

anticoagulants
Adult dosage
Aspirin: 325 mg/day P.O.
Heparin: dosage of I.V. infusion tailored to patient's PTT; or 5,000 units S.C. q 8 to 12 hours
Point to remember

- Anticoagulation therapy remains controversial except in patients undergoing thrombolysis. ■

Myocarditis

Specific antimicrobial therapy is indicated if an infecting agent can be identified. Treatment is directed toward manifestations of heart failure and arrhythmias. Immunosuppressant therapy with corticosteroids may be beneficial if myocardial biopsy suggests ongoing inflammation.

ampicillin
Adult dosage
2 g I.V. q 4 hours
Points to remember

- Ampicillin is effective against streptococcal infections.
- Reduce the dosage in severe renal dysfunction.
- Ampicillin is used in combination with nafcillin and gentamicin in acute disease and in combination with gentamicin in subacute disease.

digoxin
Adult dosage
I.V.: 0.5 mg over 10 to 20 minutes; additional doses of 0.125 to 0.25 mg may be administered after 3 hours to a total of 1 to 1.25 mg
Oral: 1 to 1.25 mg P.O. in divided doses over the first 24 hours (maintenance dosage ranges from 0.125 to 0.5 mg/day P.O.)
Points to remember

- Monitor serum digoxin levels, and adjust therapy accordingly.
- Adjust dosage in patients with renal impairment.

diuretics
Adult dosage
Bumetanide: 1 to 8 mg/day P.O. or I.V.
Furosemide: 20 to 320 mg/day P.O. or I.V. in single or divided doses
Hydrochlorothiazide: 25 to 100 mg/day P.O. (only for mild fluid retention)
Metolazone: 2.5 to 10 mg/day P.O.

Torsemide: 10 to 20 mg/day P.O. or I.V.

Points to remember

- Thiazides are only indicated for mild fluid retention; they're generally ineffective when the glomerular filtration rate falls below 30 ml/minute.
- Potassium-sparing agents (triamterene, amiloride, or spironolactone) are often used in combination with thiazide or loop diuretics.
- Monitor serum electrolyte levels during therapy.

gentamicin

Adult dosage

1 mg/kg (60 to 80 mg) I.V. q 8 hours

Points to remember

- This drug has a narrow therapeutic index; monitor blood levels (peak levels 4 to 8 mcg/ml and trough levels 1 to 2 mcg/ml).
- Gentamicin has highly individualized dosage requirements, especially when therapy is long-term.
- This drug may cause renal or ototoxicity.
- Reduce dosage in renal insufficiency.
- Gentamicin is used empirically in combination with ampicillin and nafcillin in acute disease and in combination with ampicillin in subacute disease.
- Gentamicin is effective against gram-negative organisms and has a synergistic effect on gram-positive organisms when combined with ampicillin, nafcillin, or both.

heparin

Adult dosage

5,000 units S.C. q 8 to 12 hours; or 1 unit/kg/hour by I.V. infusion

Points to remember

- Monitor platelet count.
- Use with caution in patients with increased risk of hemorrhage; if hemorrhage occurs, stop the drug immediately.

nafcillin

Adult dosage

2 g I.V. q 4 hours

Points to remember

- This antibiotic treats staphylococcal infections.
- It's used in combination with ampicillin and gentamicin. ■

Pericarditis

Pericarditis that follows MI is treated with bed rest and measures to relieve pain and reduce fever. Any contributing causes, such as infection, uremia, or rheumatoid arthritis, also are treated. Partial pericardiectomy may be performed for recurrent disease. If possible, drugs that may contribute to pericarditis (such as hydralazine or procainamide) should be discontinued.

aspirin and NSAIDs
Adult dosage
Aspirin: 325 to 1,000 mg P.O. q 3, 4, or 6 hours
Ibuprofen: 400 to 800 mg P.O. t.i.d., not to exceed 3.2 g/day
Naproxen: 250 to 500 mg P.O. b.i.d., not to exceed 1.5 g/day
Piroxicam: 20 to 40 mg/day P.O.
Sulindac: 20 to 40 mg/day P.O.
Points to remember
- These drugs are used as needed to relieve pain and reduce fever.
- Give with food or antacids to minimize GI upset.
- Instruct patient to avoid alcoholic beverages.
- Don't administer to patients with aspirin sensitivity, bleeding disorders, active bleeding, or peptic ulcer disease.
- Use caution when administering these drugs to patients with a history of peptic ulcers and to those receiving heparin, warfarin, or thrombolytic agents.

corticosteroids
Adult dosage
Varies with agent used; administer equivalent of 40 to 60 mg/day of prednisone
Points to remember
- These agents are used only for severe pain that does not respond to NSAIDs.
- Once symptoms diminish, taper dosage slowly over several weeks to avoid hypoadrenal symptoms and then discontinue. Don't stop therapy abruptly. ■

Premature atrial contractions, frequent

Premature atrial contractions warrant therapy when they cause palpitations or trigger paroxysmal supraventricular tachycardias. Drug therapy is the same as that used for paroxysmal atrial tachycardia. Treatment includes eliminating precipitating factors, such as use of tobacco, alcohol, or adrenergic stimulants.

▼FIRST-LINE DRUG
digoxin
Adult dosage
1 mg I.V. as loading dose in three divided doses over 24 hours; maintenance dosage is 0.125 to 0.5 mg/day I.V. or P.O.
Points to remember
- This drug is a first-line treatment in patients with reduced ventricular function.
- Withhold dose if patient's pulse rate is less than 50 beats/minute.

- Dosages are highly individualized.
- Digoxin has narrow therapeutic range (0.8 to 2 ng/ml); monitor serum drug levels.
- Reduce dosage in elderly patients and those with renal failure or hepatic compromise.
- Use only if digoxin toxicity isn't the cause of the arrhythmia.

▼FIRST-LINE DRUG

diltiazem hydrochloride

Adult dosage

Oral: 90 to 360 mg/day P.O. as a single dose (sustained-release tablets) or divided into three or four daily doses (standard tablet)
I.V.: 0.25 mg/kg by slow I.V. push over 2 minutes; if ineffective, repeat in 15 minutes, or give 10 to 15 mg/hour by I.V. infusion for up to 24 hours

Points to remember

- This is a first-line drug used in patients with good ventricular function.
- Withhold dose if patient's pulse rate is less than 50 beats/minute.
- Monitor patient for dizziness and CHF.
- With I.V. administration, monitor patient's ECG and blood pressure continuously.
- Elderly patients may require reduced dosage.

▼FIRST-LINE DRUG

quinidine

Adult dosage

Oral: 300 of 400 mg P.O. of quinidine sulfate q 6 hours or 324 to 600 mg of quinidine gluconate (sustained-release) q 8 to 12 hours
I.M.: 600 mg initially, then up to 400 mg q 2 hours based on patient's response
I.V.: 800 mg diluted in 40 ml of D_5W infused at 16 mg (1 ml) per minute

Points to remember

- Before starting I.M. or I.V. therapy, administer 200-mg test dose I.M.
- Before initiating therapy, patient should be digitalized to control ventricular rate and prevent ventricular tachycardia.
- Monitor patient's ECG and blood pressure continuously during I.V. therapy.
- Reduce dosage in hepatic or renal impairment.

▼FIRST-LINE DRUG

verapamil

Adult dosage

0.075 to 0.15 mg/kg (5 to 10 mg) by slow I.V. push over 2 minutes (3 minutes in elderly patients); may give additional 0.15 mg/kg (10 mg) in 15 to 30 minutes; or give 240 to 320 mg/day P.O. in three or four divided doses (standard tablet) or once daily (sustained-release form)

Points to remember
- This is a first-line drug used in patients with adequate ventricular function.
- Withhold dose if patient's pulse rate is less than 50 beats/minute.
- Monitor patient's ECG and blood pressure continuously during I.V. therapy.
- Decrease I.V. administration rate in elderly patients.
- Monitor patient for dizziness and CHF.

adenosine
Adult dosage
6 mg by I.V. push over 1 to 2 seconds; if necessary, give bolus of 12 mg 1 to 2 minutes later
Points to remember
- This is a second-line drug after verapamil or diltiazem.
- Monitor patient's ECG and blood pressure continuously.

esmolol hydrochloride
Adult dosage
500 mcg/kg I.V. as loading dose over 1 minute, followed by 50 mcg/kg/minute for 4 minutes; if optimal response doesn't occur in 5 minutes, repeat loading dose and increase maintenance infusion to 100 mcg/kg/minute for 4 minutes. If needed, repeat loading dose and increase infusion rate by 50 mcg/kg/minute to maximum of 200 mcg/kg/minute for 4 minutes.

Points to remember
- This is a first- or second-line drug that achieves a rapid response in critical situations.
- Use I.V. controller to infuse.
- Dilute concentrate for injection with compatible I.V. solution to final concentration of 10 mg/ml.
- Monitor patient's ECG and blood pressure continuously.
- Extravasation may cause skin irritation or necrosis.

procainamide hydrochloride
Adult dosage
I.M.: 50 mg/kg I.M. in divided doses q 3 to 6 hours
I.V.: 50 to 100 mg by I.V. bolus q 5 minutes to total of 500 mg or alternatively by I.V. infusion, not exceeding 25 to 50 mg/minute; or give 500 to 600 mg by I.V. bolus over 25 to 30 minutes, followed by continuous infusion of 1 to 6 mg/minute
Oral: 1.25 g P.O., followed by 750 mg 1 hour later, with additional doses of 500 mg to 1 g q 2 hours (standard tablets); when patient is stabilized, give 500 mg to 1 g (standard tablets) q 4 to 6 hours or 1 g (sustained-release tablets) q 6 hours
Points to remember
- This drug is a second-line antiarrhythmic after quinidine.

- Dosage is highly individualized, based on patient's serum procainamide levels.
- Patient should receive a digitalis glycoside before starting procainamide.
- Reduce dosage in patients with renal or hepatic dysfunction, those over age 50, and those with severe CHF or hypotension.
- Monitor patient's ECG and blood pressure continuously during I.V. therapy.

propranolol hydrochloride
Adult dosage
I.V.: 0.5 to 3 mg (don't exceed 1 mg/minute); may repeat in 2 minutes
Oral: 10 to 30 mg P.O. t.i.d. or q.i.d., or give one dose as sustained-release tablet daily
Points to remember
- This is a third-line drug.
- It may cause serious side effects.
- Dosages are highly individualized.
- Withhold oral dose if patient's pulse is less than 50 beats/minute.
- Dilute oral solution concentrate, or mix with semisolid food just before administration.
- Give oral doses before meals and at bedtime.
- With I.V. administration, monitor patient's ECG and central venous pressure. ■

Premature ventricular contractions, frequent

Premature ventricular contractions (PVCs) don't always require treatment. Those that cause impaired ventricular function are more likely to warrant treatment. Few patients receive long-term treatment for PVCs because the benefit is questionable and significant side effects may occur.

▼FIRST-LINE DRUG
lidocaine
Adult dosage
1 mg/kg I.V. loading dose, given at rate of 25 to 50 mg/minute; repeat after 5 minutes. Then give maintenance I.V. infusion of 1 to 4 mg/minute.
Point to remember
- Lidocaine is a first-line drug for suppressing PVCs in patients with acute MI.

beta-adrenergic blockers
Adult dosage
Metoprolol: 100 to 400 mg/day P.O., divided in two doses; or 5 mg I.V. for three doses at 2-minute intervals, followed by oral doses
Nadolol: 20 to 40 mg/day P.O., divided in two doses
Propranolol: 10 to 30 mg P.O. t.i.d. or q.i.d.; or 0.5 to 3 mg I.V. t.i.d.

Points to remember

- These drugs are useful for treating PVCs that occur during stressful situations or during the day, or in patients with mitral valve prolapse or thyrotoxicosis.
- These agents may also be used after acute MI.
- If the patient has angina, don't discontinue these drugs abruptly because doing so may precipitate an anginal attack. Taper long-term therapy gradually over 1 to 2 weeks.
- I.V. doses may be considerably smaller than oral ones.

procainamide hydrochloride

Adult dosage

Loading dose: 100 mg I.V. given at maximum rate of 50 mg/minute; repeat q 5 minutes until arrhythmia is controlled, until a total of 1 g is given, or until QRS interval (on ECG) widens.
Maintenance dosage: 50 mcg/kg P.O. of extended-release tablets divided in four doses; or 500 mg to 1 g of immediate-release tablets P.O. q 4 to 6 hours

Points to remember

- Procainamide is an alternative drug used to suppress PVCs in patients with acute MI.
- Adjust dosage in renal impairment and CHF.
- Drug is absorbed best on an empty stomach but may be administered with food to decrease GI upset.
- When switching from I.V. to oral form, wait 3 to 4 hours after discontinuing I.V. infusion before giving first oral dose.
- Don't crush extended-release tablets. Inform patient that extended-release tablet matrix may appear in stool.

quinidine

Adult dosage

Quinidine gluconate: 325 to 650 mg P.O. q 6 hours, or 324 to 660 mg P.O. of extended-release tablets q 6 to 12 hours
Quinidine sulfate: 200 to 300 mg P.O. t.i.d. or q.i.d., or 300 to 600 mg P.O. of extended-release tablets q 8 to 12 hours

Points to remember

- Quinidine may be used when beta blockers aren't effective.
- Tell patient not to break, crush, or chew extended-release tablets.
- Drug is absorbed best on an empty stomach but may be administered with food to decrease GI upset.
- Adjust dosage in renal or liver impairment. ■

Pulmonary edema

Pulmonary edema may be cardiogenic in origin (resulting from heart failure) or noncardiogenic (resulting from capillary membrane damage of the alveoli due to aspiration or infection). Treatment for cardiogenic pulmonary edema parallels therapy for heart failure, which includes drugs, bed rest, and sodium restriction. Drug therapy for the noncardiogenic type is aimed at treating the underlying aspiration or infection.

▼FIRST-LINE DRUG

furosemide

Adult dosage

0.5 to 1 mg/kg I.V.

Points to remember

- Give slowly over 1 to 2 minutes, to a maximum dosage of 4 mg/minute.
- Monitor serum electrolyte levels for an abnormal sodium or potassium level.

▼FIRST-LINE DRUG

morphine sulfate

Adult dosage

1 to 3 mg I.V.

Point to remember

- Give by slow I.V. push.

▼FIRST-LINE DRUG

nitroglycerin

Adult dosage

S.L.: 0.4 mg q 5 to 10 minutes until desired effect occurs

I.V.: Start with 10 to 20 mcg/minute and titrate until desired response occurs.

Points to remember

- Sublingual dosage is a first-line treatment if systolic pressure exceeds 100 mm Hg.
- I.V. dosage is a second-line treatment if systolic pressure exceeds 100 mm Hg.

dobutamine hydrochloride

Adult dosage

2 to 20 mcg/kg/minute I.V.

Point to remember

- This is a second-line drug used if systolic pressure exceeds 100 mm Hg.

dopamine hydrochloride

Adult dosage

2.5 to 20 mcg/kg/minute I.V.

Point to remember

- This is a second-line drug used if systolic pressure is 70 to 100 mm Hg.

nitroprusside sodium

Adult dosage

0.1 to 5 mcg/kg/minute I.V.

Point to remember

- This is a second-line drug used if diastolic pressure exceeds 110 mm Hg.

aminophylline

Adult dosage

5 mg/kg I.V.

Point to remember

- This is a third-line drug used if severe bronchospasm occurs.

amrinone lactate

Adult dosage

0.75 mg/kg I.V. initially, then 5 to 15 mcg/kg/minute I.V.

Point to remember
- This is a third-line drug used if other drugs fail.

digoxin
Adult dosage
I.V.: 0.5 mg over 10 to 20 minutes; may give additional doses of 0.125 to 0.25 mg after 3 hours to maximum of 1 to 1.25 mg
Oral: 1 to 1.25 mg P.O. in divided doses over first 24 hours; daily maintenance dosage ranges from 0.125 to 0.5 mg P.O.
Point to remember
- This is a third-line drug used if atrial fibrillation or supraventricular tachycardia occurs. ■

Pulmonary hypertension

Therapy focuses on treating the primary disease (such as COPD) and improving oxygenation. In primary pulmonary hypertension, drug treatment is only palliative. There is no drug of choice, and various drugs may be tried. However, patients typically continue to deteriorate despite drug therapy. A heart-lung transplant may be an option for some patients.

ACE inhibitors
Adult dosage
Captopril: 6.25 to 25 mg P.O. t.i.d.; may increase to 50 mg t.i.d. in 6.25- to 25-mg increments per day over several weeks
Enalapril: 2.5 to 20 mg/day P.O., divided in one or two doses
Points to remember
- Lower initial dosage may be used if patient is also receiving diuretics.
- These drugs are contraindicated in hyperkalemia, renal artery stenosis, angioedema, kidney transplant, and asthma.

alpha-adrenergic blockers
Adult dosage
Doxazosin: 1 mg/day P.O. initially; increase in 1-mg increments q 2 weeks to maximum dosage of 16 mg
Prazosin: 0.1 mg P.O. b.i.d. or t.i.d.
Point to remember
- Minimize syncope by giving initial dose at bedtime.

calcium channel blockers
Adult dosage
Diltiazem hydrochloride: 60 to 80 mg/day P.O.
Nifedipine: 30 to 180 mg/day P.O.
Points to remember
- Advise patient to avoid crushing or chewing extended-release forms.
- Immediate-release tablets are given three times daily.

hydralazine hydrochloride
Adult dosage
10 mg P.O. q.i.d. initially; then titrate to 50 mg q.i.d. as tolerated
Points to remember
- Titrate dosage to lowest effective level.
- This drug may exacerbate angina.

warfarin
Adult dosage
2 to 10 mg/day P.O.
Points to remember
- Adjust dosage to maintain international normalized ratio between 2 and 3.
- If therapy begins within first 12 months of illness, warfarin may improve survival of patients with primary pulmonary hypertension. However, it doesn't reverse the disease process.
- Instruct patient to consume relatively stable amount of vitamin K.
- Administer vitamin K_1 to treat overdose.
- Advise patient to inform other health care professionals of long-term warfarin therapy and to carry identification indicating that he's taking warfarin.
- This drug is contraindicated in recent lumbar puncture, trauma, childbirth, or surgery and in severe liver or renal impairment, endocarditis, pregnancy, thrombocytopenia, severe uncontrolled hypertension, pericarditis, active bleeding, and cerebrovascular accident.
- Elderly patients may be more susceptible to bleeding during therapy. ■

Pulmonic insufficiency

Treatment depends on the nature and severity of symptoms. Drug therapy may control such symptoms as dyspnea on exertion, fatigue, chest pain, and syncope. As symptoms worsen, the patient may require surgical valve replacement.

For heart failure

digoxin
Adult dosage
I.V.: 0.5 mg given over 10 to 20 minutes; additional doses of 0.125 to 0.25 mg may be administered after 3 hours to a total of 1 to 1.25 mg
Oral: 1 to 1.25 mg P.O. in divided doses over the first 24 hours; maintenance dosage ranges from 0.125 to 0.5 mg/day P.O.
Points to remember
- Monitor serum digoxin levels, and adjust therapy accordingly.
- Adjust dosage in patients with renal impairment.

diuretics

Adult dosage

Bumetanide: 1 to 8 mg/day P.O. or I.V.
Furosemide: 20 to 320 mg/day P.O. or I.V. in single or divided doses
Hydrochlorothiazide: 25 to 100 mg/day P.O. (only for mild fluid retention)
Metolazone: 2.5 to 10 mg/day P.O.
Torsemide: 10 to 20 mg/day P.O. or I.V.

Points to remember

- Thiazides are generally ineffective when the glomerular filtration rate falls below 30 ml/minute; they're indicated only for mild fluid retention.
- Potassium-sparing agents (triamterene, amiloride, or spironolactone) are often used in combination with thiazide or loop diuretics.
- Monitor serum electrolyte levels.

For anticoagulant therapy

heparin

Adult dosage

5,000 units S.C. q 8 to 12 hours; or 1 unit/kg/hour by I.V. infusion

Points to remember

- Monitor platelet count.
- Use with caution in patients with increased risk of hemorrhage; if hemorrhage occurs, stop drug therapy immediately.

warfarin sodium

Adult dosage

Highly variable (2.5 to 15 mg/day P.O.)

Points to remember

- Multiple drug interactions may occur.
- Warfarin is used for long-term anticoagulation.
- Monitor PT or international normalized ratio to regulate dosage.
- Reduce dosage in elderly patients, patients with hepatic disease, and those with CHF.
- Administer dose at same time each day.

Raynaud's disease

When mild, this disease can be controlled without drugs by avoiding exposure to extreme cold and by wearing gloves or mittens in cold weather. To avoid cold-induced reflex vasoconstriction, instruct the patient to protect his head, trunk, and feet from cold. Drug therapy may be used in severe disease. If drugs fail to improve the patient's condition, sympathectomy may be performed. However, this procedure often brings only temporary improvement.

calcium channel blockers
Adult dosage
Diltiazem: 60 to 360 mg/day P.O., usually in divided doses
Nifedipine: 30 to 180 mg/day P.O., usually in divided doses
Points to remember
- Instruct patient to avoid crushing or chewing sustained-release forms.
- Side effects include hypotension, peripheral edema, and arrhythmias.
- Elderly patients may require lower dosages.
- This drug is contraindicated in heart block, sick sinus syndrome, and bradycardia.

methyldopa
Adult dosage
250 mg P.O. b.i.d. or t.i.d initially; titrate as tolerated to 500 mg to 2 g/day
Points to remember
- Advise patient to avoid alcoholic beverages and sympathomimetic drugs.
- This drug is contraindicated in hemolytic anemia, liver disease, and pheochromocytoma.
- Elderly patients may be more sensitive to sedative and hypotensive effects.

prazosin hydrochloride
Adult dosage
1 to 2 mg P.O. t.i.d
Points to remember
- Caution patient to avoid alcoholic beverages.
- Elderly patients may be more sensitive to hypotensive effects.

reserpine
Adult dosage
0.25 to 0.5 mg/day P.O.
Points to remember
- Caution patient to avoid alcoholic beverages and other CNS depressants.
- Elderly patients may be more sensitive to CNS and hypotensive effects.
- Adjust dosage in renal impairment.
- This drug is contraindicated in gallstones, peptic ulcers, and depression. ■

Rheumatic fever and rheumatic heart disease

Patients with these conditions typically require aspirin or glucocorticoid therapy for several weeks after the erythrocyte sedimentation rate normalizes. Some patients develop chorea; however, this condition usually is self-limiting and resolves without long-term complications. Bed rest and safety precautions are important aspects of care.

penicillin
Adult dosage
Acute illness: 1.2 million units of penicillin G benzathine I.M. or 600,000 units

of penicillin G procaine I.M. for 10 days
Long-term prophylaxis: 1.2 million units of penicillin G benzathine I.M. every month or 200,000 units of penicillin G procaine P.O. b.i.d.

Points to remember

- Penicillin usually is used to treat group A streptococci. It may also be used for long-term prophylaxis in patients with rheumatic heart disease or recent rheumatic fever or in areas where rheumatic fever is common.
- Duration of long-term prophylaxis varies. Patients under age 18 may receive prophylaxis continuously. Those over age 18 may take the drug for 5 years or more.
- Instruct patient to take tablets or capsules on an empty stomach.
- Stress the importance of completing the entire course of antibiotic therapy.
- Adjust dosage according to renal function.

erythromycin

Adult dosage

1 g/day P.O. in divided doses

Points to remember

- This drug is used in patients who are allergic to penicillin.
- Erythromycin-resistant strains of group A streptococci have developed in areas where this drug has been widely used instead of penicillin.
- Instruct patient to take tablets on empty stomach; however, taking them with food may decrease GI upset.
- Adjust dosage in severe renal or hepatic impairment.

aspirin

Adult dosage

6 to 8 g/day P.O. in divided doses

Points to remember

- Aspirin is used to treat acute arthritis, fever, and joint inflammation.
- Don't administer to patients with aspirin sensitivity, bleeding disorder, active bleeding, or peptic ulcer disease.
- Use with caution in patients with history of peptic ulcers and those receiving heparin, warfarin, or thrombolytic agents.
- Administer with food or antacids to minimize GI upset.
- Advise patient to avoid alcoholic beverages.
- Elderly patients may be at increased risk for renal or hepatic impairment.

chlorpromazine hydrochloride

Adult dosage

12.5 to 25 mg I.M. or 10 to 25 mg P.O. b.i.d. or t.i.d.

Points to remember

- Chlorpromazine is used as needed to sedate patients with chorea.

- Instruct patient to take drug with food to decrease GI upset.
- Advise patient to avoid chewing or crushing sustained-release tablets.
- Pregnant and breast-feeding patients shouldn't receive this drug.
- Avoid skin contact with liquid preparations because they can cause skin irritation.
- Elderly patients may require lower dosages.

diazepam
Adult dosage
2 to 10 mg P.O. t.i.d. or q.i.d.
Points to remember
- Diazepam is used as needed to sedate patients with chorea.
- Patients receiving diazepam for more than 2 weeks may experience withdrawal symptoms when this drug is discontinued.
- Elderly patients and patients with liver disease or hypoalbuminemia are more sensitive to this drug's sedative and respiratory depressant effects.

glucocorticoids
Adult dosage
60 to 120 mg P.O. of prednisone or equivalent glucocorticoid in four divided doses daily
Points to remember
- Glucocorticoids may be used when aspirin therapy isn't effective. However, they are no more effective than aspirin in treating acute carditis. Also, they cause more side effects and are linked to a greater incidence of relapse.
- Don't discontinue these drugs abruptly. Instead, taper dosage over several weeks to avoid relapse and hypoadrenalism. ■

Sick sinus syndrome

Patients with sick sinus syndrome may have both bradyarrhythmias and tachyarrhythmias. This condition is hard to treat, and the cause may never be identified. Therefore, treatment aims to control symptoms. Patients with chronic bradyarrhythmias may require pacemakers.

atropine sulfate
Adult dosage
0.4 to 1 mg I.V. p.r.n. to maximum of 2 mg
Points to remember
- This drug is indicated for acute bradyarrhythmias.
- Elderly patients may be more sensitive to CNS effects.
- Side effects are more common with long-term administration.

beta-adrenergic blockers

Adult dosage

Metoprolol: 100 to 400 mg/day P.O., divided in two doses

Nadolol: 20 to 40 mg/day P.O.

Propranolol: 0.5 to 3 mg I.V., given no faster than 1 mg/minute; may repeat in 2 minutes

Points to remember

- These drugs are used to control tachyarrhythmias.
- Use cautiously in patients who don't have pacemakers.
- Carefully check I.V. dosages, which may be much smaller than oral dosages.
- Beta blockers may worsen asthma, COPD, diabetes, depression, peripheral vascular disease, CHF, and Raynaud's disease.

digoxin

Adult dosage

I.V.: 0.5 mg given over 10 to 20 minutes; may give additional doses of 0.125 to 0.25 mg after 3 hours to maximum of 1 to 1.25 mg

Oral: 1 to 1.25 mg P.O. in divided doses over first 24 hours; daily maintenance doses range from 0.125 to 0.5 mg P.O.

Points to remember

- This drug is used to treat tachyarrhythmias.
- Use cautiously in patients who don't have pacemakers.
- Digoxin is contraindicated in patients with hypokalemia, hypocalcemia, AV block, hypomagnesemia, acute MI, PVCs, ventricular tachycardia, or Wolff-Parkinson-White syndrome.
- Elderly patients and those with renal impairment may require lower dosages and may be more susceptible to drug toxicity.

isoproterenol

Adult dosage

5 mcg/minute by I.V. infusion or 10 to 30 mg P.O. four to six times daily

Points to remember

- This drug is used to control bradyarrhythmias.
- For I.V. infusion, dilute 2 mg in 500 ml of D_5W for a concentration of 4 mcg/ml. Do not use original solution if it is discolored or has a precipitate.
- To minimize insomnia, don't give close to bedtime.
- Some preparations contain sulfites. Monitor patients with sulfite sensitivity for bronchospasm and allergic reactions.
- Patients concurrently taking digoxin or diuretics are especially prone to hypokalemia. ■

Thrombophlebitis

Treatment aims to control thrombus formation, prevent complications, relieve pain, and prevent recurrence of thrombophlebitis.

For anticoagulant therapy

heparin
Adult dosage
5,000 to 10,000 units by I.V. bolus, then 1 unit/kg/hour by I.V. infusion
Points to remember
- Monitor the platelet count.
- Use with caution in patients with increased risk of hemorrhage; if hemorrhage occurs, stop drug therapy immediately.
- Adjust dosage to maintain activated PTT of 1.5 to 2 times normal.

warfarin sodium
Adult dosage
Highly variable (2.5 to 15 mg/day P.O.)
Points to remember
- Multiple drug interactions may occur.
- Drug is used for long-term anticoagulation.
- Monitor international normalized ratio to regulate dosage.
- Reduce dosage in elderly patients and in patients with hepatic disease or heart failure.
- Administer at same time each day.

For lysis of acute, extensive deep-vein thrombosis

Thrombolytic agents
Adult dosage
Streptokinase: 250,000 units over 30 minutes, followed by 100,000 units/hour for 24 to 72 hours
Urokinase: 4,400 units/kg of body weight over 30 minutes, followed by 4,400 units/kg/hour for 12 hours
Points to remember
- Side effects may include bleeding, fever, and allergic reactions.
- Avoid nonessential moving of the patient, I.M. injections, or invasive procedures during therapy.
- Don't administer any other drugs through the same I.V. line. ■

Torsades de pointes

Treatment for this atypical ventricular tachycardia involves removing or treating precipitating factors, such as hypomagnesemia, hypokalemia, bradyarrhythmias, and use of antiarrhythmic drugs, phenothiazines, TCAs, and liquid protein diets. Acute arrhythmias require direct-current cardioversion; however, the arrhythmia often recurs. Atrial or ventricular overdrive pacing may be useful, especially in drug-induced torsades de pointes. Effective prophylactic drug therapy hasn't been determined; however, procainamide is contraindicated.

isoproterenol
Adult dosage
2 mcg/minute I.V. initially, to maximum of 10 mcg/minute
Points to remember
- This drug is indicated after direct-current cardioversion to prevent recurrence of torsades de pointes.
- To infuse, dilute 1 mg in 500 ml of D_5W (2 mcg/ml), and administer by an I.V. pump.
- Don't use if solution is discolored or contains precipitate. ■

Ventricular tachycardia

Initial therapy for this arrhythmia includes correcting associated metabolic disorders, treating ischemic heart disease, and discontinuing any drugs that could precipitate the arrhythmia. Nonsustained ventricular tachycardia (VT) that's not associated with ischemic heart disease usually isn't treated. Sustained, symptomatic VT usually is treated with beta-adrenergic blockers, such as verapamil or quinidine.

VT that doesn't respond to drug therapy may respond to direct-current cardioversion; in hemodynamically compromised patients, cardioversion should be performed before drugs are given. In stable patients, overdrive pacing may be used to terminate an arrhythmia that doesn't respond to drugs. Advanced surgical techniques may be used in chronic VT.

▼FIRST-LINE DRUG
bretylium tosylate
Adult dosage
5 to 10 mg/kg by I.V. infusion over 10 to 30 minutes; may repeat dose q 6 to 8 hours or start continuous infusion at 1 to 2 mg/minute
Points to remember
- If possible, use infusion pump to control administration.
- Therapy may continue for 3 to 5 days. For long-term treatment, oral drug must be substituted for I.V. therapy.
- Adjust dosage in renal impairment.

▼FIRST-LINE DRUG
lidocaine
Adult dosage
50 to 100 mg (or 1 to 1.5 mg/kg) as I.V. loading dose at a rate not exceeding 25 to 50 mg/minute; if no response occurs, give second loading dose 5 minutes after first. After favorable response, start maintenance infusion of 1 to 4 mg/minute (dilute 1 g in liter of D_5W [1 mg/ml]).

Points to remember

- If possible, use an infusion pump to control administration.
- Don't use if I.V. solution is discolored.
- Patients sensitive to procaine, flecainide, or tocainide may also be sensitive to lidocaine.
- Elderly patients and those with renal impairment, CHF, or impaired liver blood flow may be more sensitive to side effects and may require smaller dosages.

procainamide hydrochloride

Adult dosage

100 mg as I.V. loading dose at maximum rate of 50 mg/minute; repeat q 5 minutes, as needed and tolerated, to maximum dosage of 1 g. When indicated, start maintenance infusion of 2 to 6 mg/minute (dilute 1 g in 250 to 500 ml of D_5W [2 to 4 mg/ml]); may switch to oral dose of 50 mg/kg (sustained-release tablets) in four divided doses daily.

Points to remember

- This drug is used for acute control of the heart rate and may be used to manage chronic VT.
- To avoid hypotension, don't administer I.V. infusion faster than 50 mg/minute.
- When switching from I.V. to oral administration, wait 3 to 4 hours after discontinuing infusion before giving first oral dose.
- Dosage may be adjusted based on serum drug levels. (Therapeutic range is 4 to 10 mg/ml.)
- Instruct patient to swallow sustained-release tablets whole.
- Administering oral forms on an empty stomach increases drug absorption; however, administering with food minimizes GI upset.
- Inform patient that tablet matrix may appear in stool.
- Procainamide is contraindicated in patients with a history of systemic lupus erythematosus, myasthenia gravis, heart block, torsades de pointes, CHF, or renal or hepatic impairment.
- Elderly patients are more susceptible to hypotension, especially after parenteral administration.
- Adjust dosage for degree of renal impairment.

propafenone hydrochloride

Adult dosage

150 mg P.O. q 8 hours initially; may increase to 225 mg q 8 hours or 300 mg q 12 hours. Then adjust dosage to 300 mg P.O. q 8 hours, as tolerated.

Points to remember

- This drug is used for long-term treatment of sustained VT.

- It is contraindicated in heart block, cardiogenic shock, CHF, and sick sinus syndrome.
- Don't increase dosage more frequently than every 3 to 4 days.
- Therapy usually is initiated in the hospital to monitor for increased arrhythmia frequency. ■

RESPIRATORY DISORDERS

Acute respiratory failure in COPD

In this disorder, maintaining the patient's oxygenation and ventilation is critical. Drug therapy is adjunctive and focuses on bronchodilation. Terbutaline and epinephrine are the only parenteral sympathomimetic agents; terbutaline is preferred in elderly patients and those with cardiovascular disease.

▼FIRST-LINE DRUG

albuterol

Adult dosage

Nebulizer: 2.5 mg to 5 mg q 20 minutes for up to 6 doses (for acute bronchoconstriction); then 2.5 mg t.i.d. or q.i.d.

Points to remember

- Monitor patient's ECG and blood pressure.
- Albuterol occasionally causes paradoxical bronchoconstriction.

▼FIRST-LINE DRUG

metaproterenol sulfate

Adult dosage

Nebulizer: 2.5 ml of 0.4% to 0.6% solution q 4 to 6 hours

Point to remember

- Use with caution in patients with ischemic heart disease.

▼FIRST-LINE DRUG

terbutaline sulfate

Adult dosage

0.25 mg S.C.; may repeat once after 15 to 30 minutes

Point to remember

- Don't administer more than 0.5 mg in 4 hours.

aminophylline

Adult dosage

I.V. loading dose: 5 to 6 mg/kg over 20 to 30 minutes (not to exceed 20 mg/minute) in patients who have never taken aminophylline; 2.5 mg/kg in patients who have taken it

I.V. maintenance infusion: 0.5 mg/kg/hour

Points to remember

- When giving I.V. theophylline, reduce dosage to 20% of the ordered aminophylline dosage.
- Maintenance I.V. infusion usually is administered by

large-volume parenteral solution.
- Maintenance dosage requirements vary.
- Monitor serum drug levels.
- Aminophylline may interact with many drugs; also, its action is affected by smoking, CHF, and liver disease.

epinephrine
Adult dosage
0.3 ml of 1:1,000 solution S.C.; repeat q 20 minutes for two more doses
Points to remember
- This is a second-line parenteral drug (terbutaline is preferred in elderly patients and those with cardiovascular disease).
- It may aggravate hypertension, arrhythmias, and angina.
- Epinephrine causes additive cardiovascular stimulation in patients receiving aminophylline concurrently.

ipratropium bromide
Adult dosage
Inhaler: 2 puffs of 36-mcg spray q.i.d.
Points to remember
- Ipratropium is used to prevent acute episodes. It isn't indicated as single agent for acute therapy for bronchospasm because of slow onset of action (15 to 20 minutes).
- Use with caution in patients with acute angle-closure glaucoma, prostatic hyperplasia, or bladder neck obstruction. ■

Asbestosis

Treatment aims to limit the progression of interstitial fibrosis. Drug therapy doesn't cure asbestosis but may help relieve symptoms and delay the need for long-term oxygen administration. Patients should receive annual influenza and pneumococcal vaccines.

▼FIRST-LINE DRUG
prednisone
Adult dosage
1 mg/kg/day P.O. in single or divided doses for 8 to 12 weeks; then taper to maintenance dosage
Points to remember
- Instruct patient to take drug with food or milk.
- If given as a single daily dose, advise patient to take it in the morning.
- Caution patient not to stop taking prednisone abruptly; drug must be discontinued gradually.
- Prednisone may aggravate hypertension, peptic ulcer disease, diabetes, and uncontrolled glaucoma. ■

Asthma

Drug therapy is the primary treatment for asthma. The goal of long-term drug therapy is to reduce airway inflammation and prevent acute asthma attacks. Short-term therapy aims to relieve bronchospasm and restore oxygen transport to vital organs. Inhaled medication causes fewer side effects and is preferred over oral and parenteral drugs.

▼FIRST-LINE DRUG

albuterol

Adult dosage

Inhaler: 2 puffs of 90-mcg metered spray q 4 to 6 hours p.r.n.
Nebulizer: 2.5 mg q 4 to 6 hours p.r.n.
Oral: 2 to 4 mg P.O. t.i.d. or q.i.d. (standard); 4 to 8 mg q 12 hours (sustained-release)

Points to remember

- Albuterol may cause tachycardia, nervousness, or tremor; these effects may be additive in patients who are also taking theophylline.
- Make sure patient uses proper inhalation technique; if poor technique limits drug effectiveness, suggest use of spacer device.
- Excessive use of aerosolized products may lead to tolerance.

▼FIRST-LINE DRUG

bitolterol mesylate

Adult dosage

Inhaler: 2 puffs of 370-mcg metered spray q 4 to 6 hours p.r.n.

Points to remember

- Bitolterol may cause tachycardia, nervousness, or tremor; these effects may be additive in patients who are also taking theophylline.
- Make sure patient uses proper inhalation technique; if poor technique limits drug effectiveness, suggest use of spacer device.
- Excessive use of aerosolized products may lead to tolerance.

▼FIRST-LINE DRUG

metaproterenol sulfate

Adult dosage

Inhaler: 2 puffs of 650-mcg metered spray q 4 to 6 hours p.r.n.
Nebulizer: 2.5 ml of 0.4% to 0.6% solution q 4 to 6 hours p.r.n.
Oral: 20 mg P.O. t.i.d. or q.i.d.

Points to remember

- This drug may cause tachycardia, nervousness, or tremor; these effects may be additive in patients who are also taking theophylline.
- Make sure patient uses proper inhalation technique; if poor technique limits drug effectiveness, suggest use of spacer device.

- Excessive use of aerosolized products may lead to tolerance.

▼FIRST-LINE DRUG

terbutaline sulfate

Adult dosage

Inhaler: 2 puffs of 200-mcg metered spray q 4 to 6 hours p.r.n.
Oral: 2.5 mg P.O. t.i.d. or q.i.d.
S.C.: 0.25 mg; may repeat dose in 15 minutes if needed

Points to remember

- This drug may cause tachycardia, nervousness, or tremor; these effects may be additive in patients who are also taking theophylline.
- Make sure patient uses proper inhalation technique; if poor technique limits drug effectiveness, suggest use of spacer device.
- Excessive use of aerosolized products may lead to tolerance.

cromolyn sodium

Adult dosage

Nebulizer or Spinhaler: 20 mg q.i.d.
Inhaler: 1.6 mg (2 puffs) q.i.d.

Points to remember

- This is a second-line drug.
- Drug is used for maintenance and must be taken on a schedule; it isn't effective for acute relief of bronchospasm.
- Maximal effects may not appear for up to 6 weeks of regular administration.

nedocromil sodium

Adult dosage

Inhaler: 2 puffs (3.5 mg) q.i.d.

Points to remember

- This is a second-line drug.
- Drug is used for maintenance and must be taken on a schedule; it isn't effective for relief of acute bronchospasm.
- Maximal effects may not appear for up to 6 weeks of regular administration.

beclomethasone dipropionate

Adult dosage

Inhaler: 2 puffs of 84-mcg metered spray t.i.d. or q.i.d.

Points to remember

- This drug is a second-line alternative to cromolyn or nedocromil.
- Drug is used for maintenance and must be taken on a schedule; it isn't effective for acute relief of bronchospasm.
- Instruct patient to rinse mouth after use.

triamcinolone acetonide

Adult dosage

Inhaler: 2 puffs (200 mcg) t.i.d. or q.i.d.

Points to remember

- This drug is a second-line alternative to cromolyn or nedocromil.

- It's used for maintenance and must be taken on a schedule; it isn't effective for relief of acute bronchospasm.
- Instruct patient to rinse mouth after use.

epinephrine
Adult dosage
0.3 ml of 1:1,000 solution S.C.; may repeat q 20 minutes for two more doses
Points to remember
- This is a second-line parenteral drug (terbutaline is preferred in elderly patients and those with cardiovascular disease).
- It may aggravate hypertension, arrhythmias, and angina.
- Epinephrine causes additive cardiovascular stimulation in patients receiving concomitant aminophylline.

flunisolide
Adult dosage
Inhaler: 2 puffs (500 mcg) b.i.d.
Points to remember
- This drug is a second-line alternative to cromolyn or nedocromil.
- It's used for maintenance and must be taken on a schedule; it isn't effective for relief of acute bronchospasm.
- Instruct patient to rinse mouth after use.

pirbuterol
Adult dosage
Autoinhaler: 2 puffs of 200-mcg metered spray q 4 to 6 hours p.r.n.
Point to remember
- Teach patient the correct way to use an autoinhaler.

prednisone
Adult dosage
10 to 80 mg/day P.O. in single or divided doses
Points to remember
- This is a second-line drug for acute asthma episodes and a fourth-line drug for long-term asthma maintenance.
- Oral form is used for acute asthma episodes or long-term maintenance.
- Instruct patient to take drug with food or milk to avoid stomach irritation.
- Patients requiring long-term therapy should not stop this drug abruptly; instead, the dose should be tapered gradually to prevent adrenal insufficiency.

salmeterol xinafoate
Adult dosage
Inhaler: 2 puffs of 25-mcg metered spray q 12 hours
Points to remember
- This drug is used to prevent, not treat, acute asthma attacks.
- It must be administered regularly for maximum effectiveness.

- It isn't intended for use on an as-needed basis.
- Overuse may cause excessive cardiovascular stimulation.

theophylline
Adult dosage
I.V. loading dose: 5 to 6 mg/kg over 20 to 30 minutes (not to exceed 20 mg/minute) in patients who haven't taken this drug before; 2.5 mg/kg in patients who have taken it
I.V. maintenance infusion: 0.5 mg/kg/hour
Oral: 200 to 400 mg P.O. q 8 to 12 hours (sustained-release)
Points to remember
- When giving I.V. theophylline, reduce the dose to 20% of the ordered aminophylline dose.
- Maintenance infusion usually is administered by large-volume parenteral solution.
- Maintenance dose requirements vary.
- Monitor serum drug levels.
- Theophylline may interact with many drugs; also, drug action is affected by smoking, CHF, and liver disease.

ipratropium bromide
Adult dosage
Inhaler: 2 puffs of 18-mcg metered spray q.i.d.
Nebulizer: 500 mcg t.i.d. or q.i.d.
Points to remember
- This is a third-line drug.
- It must be taken on a schedule, not as needed.
- Ipratropium may cause throat irritation when used in conjunction with other inhaled medications. ■

Berylliosis

This form of poisoning results from inhaling fine dusts, mists, or vapors containing beryllium or beryllium compounds. Affected persons must avoid subsequent exposure. Treatment is largely symptomatic; defined courses of corticosteroids may be helpful.

prednisone
Adult dosage
60 mg/day P.O. in divided doses for 2 to 3 weeks; taper gradually over next 3 to 4 weeks to 10 to 15 mg/day P.O.
Points to remember
- This drug is used to reduce inflammation.
- To minimize GI upset, instruct patient to take drug with food or antacids.
- Prednisone may exacerbate peptic ulcer disease, hypertension, edema, and uncontrolled glaucoma. It may cause confusion in elderly patients.
- Don't stop therapy abruptly in patients receiving above doses for more than 2 weeks;

drug must be tapered slowly to avoid adrenal crisis. ■

Bronchiectasis

In this disease, bronchial wall destruction is irreversible. Drug therapy is aimed at relieving symptoms and preventing further disease progression. The most commonly prescribed drugs are antibiotics to treat active infection and bronchodilators to treat bronchospasm.

▼FIRST-LINE DRUG

albuterol

Adult dosage

Inhaler: 2 puffs of 90-mcg metered spray q 4 to 6 hours p.r.n.
Nebulizer: 2.5 mg q 4 to 6 hours p.r.n.
Oral: 2 to 4 mg P.O. t.i.d. or q.i.d.; or 4 to 8 mg q 12 hours (sustained-release)

Points to remember

- Excessive use of aerosolized products can lead to tolerance.
- Make sure patient uses proper inhalation technique; if poor technique limits drug effectiveness, suggest use of spacer device.

▼FIRST-LINE DRUG

metaproterenol sulfate

Adult dosage

Inhaler: 2 puffs of 650-mcg metered spray q 4 to 6 hours p.r.n.
Nebulizer: 2.5 ml of 0.4% to 0.6% solution q 4 to 6 hours p.r.n.
Oral: 20 mg P.O. t.i.d. to q.i.d.

Points to remember

- Excessive use of aerosolized products may lead to tolerance.
- Make sure patient uses proper inhalation technique; if poor technique limits drug effectiveness, suggest use of spacer device.

▼FIRST-LINE DRUG

terbutaline sulfate

Adult dosage

Inhaler: 2 puffs of 400-mcg metered spray q 4 to 6 hours p.r.n.
Oral: 2.5 mg P.O. t.i.d. or q.i.d.
S.C.: 0.25 mg; may repeat in 15 minutes p.r.n.

Points to remember

- Excessive use of aerosolized products may lead to tolerance.
- Make sure patient uses proper inhalation technique; if poor technique limits drug effectiveness, suggest use of spacer device.

cromolyn sodium

Adult dosage

Inhaler: 2 puffs (1.6 mg) q.i.d.

Nebulizer or Spinhaler: 20 mg q.i.d.

Points to remember

- This is a second-line drug.
- Drug is used for maintenance and must be taken on schedule; it isn't effective for relief of acute bronchospasm.
- Maximal effects may not appear until 6 weeks of regular administration.

nedocromil sodium

Adult dosage

Inhaler: 2 puffs (3.5 mg) q.i.d.

Points to remember

- This is a second-line drug.
- Drug is used for maintenance and must be taken on schedule; it isn't effective for relief of acute bronchospasm.
- Maximal effects may not appear for up to 6 weeks of regular administration.

epinephrine

Adult dosage

0.3 ml of 1:1,000 dilution S.C.; may repeat q 20 minutes for two additional doses

Points to remember

- This drug is used as second-line parenteral therapy; terbutaline is preferred in elderly patients and those with cardiovascular disease.
- This drug may aggravate hypertension, arrhythmias, and angina.

theophylline

Adult dosage

I.V. loading dose: 5 to 6 mg/kg over 20 to 30 minutes (not to exceed 20 mg/minute) in patients who haven't taken this drug previously; 2.5 mg/kg in patients who have taken it

I.V. maintenance infusion: 0.5 mg/kg/hour

Oral: 200 to 400 mg P.O. q 8 to 12 hours

Points to remember

- This is a second-line drug.
- When changing from aminophylline to theophylline, the theophylline dosage should be reduced by 20% of the aminophylline dose.
- Maintenance infusion usually is delivered by large-volume parenteral solution.
- Maintenance dosage requirements vary.
- Monitor patient's serum drug levels.

beclomethasone dipropionate

Adult dosage

Inhaler: 2 puffs (84 mcg) t.i.d. or q.i.d.

Points to remember

- This is a second-line drug used as an alternative to cromolyn or nedocromil.
- Drug is intended as maintenance treatment and must be administered on schedule; it isn't effective for relief of acute bronchospasm.
- Instruct patient to rinse mouth after use.

flunisolide
Adult dosage
Inhaler: 2 puffs (500 mcg) b.i.d.
Points to remember
- This is a second-line drug used as an alternative to cromolyn or nedocromil.
- Drug is intended as maintenance treatment and must be administered on schedule; it isn't effective for relief of acute bronchospasm.
- Instruct patient to rinse mouth after use.

triamcinolone acetonide
Adult dosage
Inhaler: 2 puffs (200 mcg) t.i.d. or q.i.d.
Points to remember
- This is a second-line drug used as an alternative to cromolyn or nedocromil.
- Drug is intended as maintenance treatment and must be administered on schedule; it isn't effective for relief of acute bronchospasm.
- Instruct the patient to rinse mouth after use.

prednisone
Adult dosage
10 to 80 mg P.O. daily in single or divided doses
Points to remember
- This is a second-line drug for acute episodes and a fourth-line drug for long-term maintenance.
- Oral form is used for acute asthmatic episodes or long-term maintenance.
- Instruct patient to take with food or milk to avoid GI upset.

ipratropium bromide
Adult dosage
Inhaler: 2 puffs of 36-mcg metered spray
Nebulizer: 500 mcg t.i.d. or q.i.d.
Points to remember
- This is a third-line drug.
- It must be taken on schedule, not on as-needed basis.
- Ipratropium may cause throat irritation when used in conjunction with other inhaled medications.

salmeterol xinafoate
Adult dosage
Inhaler: 2 puffs of 25-mcg metered spray q 12 hours
Points to remember
- This drug is used for prophylaxis of acute attacks, not for treatment of existing attacks on as-needed basis.
- It must be administered regularly for maximum effectiveness.

For associated infection

ampicillin
Adult dosage
250 to 500 mg P.O. q 6 hours
Point to remember
- Repeat drug at first sign of recurring infection.

tetracycline
Adult dosage
250 to 500 mg P.O. q 6 hours

Point to remember
- Repeat drug at first sign of recurring infection. ■

Bronchitis, acute

Acute bronchitis usually results from a virus, such as a rhinovirus, coronavirus, influenza A or B virus, an adenovirus, or *Mycoplasma pneumoniae.* The value of antibiotics in treating acute bronchitis is controversial. Therapy generally is supportive and includes such drugs as cough suppressants and expectorants.

amantadine hydrochloride
Adult dosage
100 mg P.O. q 12 hours
Points to remember
- This drug is used to treat influenza A virus; it isn't effective against influenza B virus.
- To be effective, drug therapy must begin within 48 hours of symptoms and should continue for 24 to 48 hours after symptoms disappear.
- Decrease dosage in elderly patients and those with renal dysfunction or a history of seizures.

codeine
Adult dosage
10 to 20 mg P.O. q 4 to 6 hours p.r.n.
Points to remember
- This drug is a cough suppressant.
- Don't exceed 60 mg/day.
- Don't use for cough associated with excessive respiratory secretions.

dextromethorphan hydrobromide
Adult dosage
Lozenges or syrup: 10 to 30 mg P.O. q 4 to 8 hours p.r.n.
Liquid (extended-release): 60 mg P.O. q 12 hours
Points to remember
- This agent is a cough suppressant.
- Don't exceed maximum daily dosage of 120 mg.
- Don't give for cough associated with excessive respiratory secretions.

erythromycin (base, stearate, or estolate)
Adult dosage
500 mg P.O. q 6 hours for 10 days
Points to remember
- Use of antibiotics in acute bronchitis is controversial.
- This drug's spectrum of activity includes *M. pneumoniae, Bordetella pertussis,* and *Chlamydia pneumoniae.*

guaifenesin
Adult dosage
Immediate-release tablets or syrup: 100 to 400 mg P.O. q 3 to 6 hours p.r.n.; or 600 mg P.O. q 12 hours (sustained-release)

Points to remember

- This agent is an expectorant.
- Don't exceed maximum daily dosage of 2.4 g.
- Encourage adequate fluid intake to aid removal of respiratory secretions. ■

Bronchitis, chronic

Treatment of chronic bronchitis aims to ease symptoms and eliminate the cause (such as smoking). Antibiotic therapy is controversial and usually reserved for acute exacerbations. Bronchodilators may be helpful in patients with a reversible component of bronchospasm. Short courses of corticosteroid therapy may have value in severe or refractory chronic bronchitis.

albuterol

Adult dosage

Inhaler: 2 puffs of 90-mcg metered spray q 4 to 6 hours p.r.n.

Points to remember

- This bronchodilator is used in patients with bronchospasm associated with bronchitis.
- Dosage must be individualized.
- Other bronchodilators may be substituted.

amoxicillin

Adult dosage

500 mg P.O. q 8 hours for 10 days

Points to remember

- Use of this drug in chronic bronchitis is controversial.
- Amoxicillin is effective against susceptible strains of *Streptococcus pneumoniae* but not against bacterial strains that produce beta lactamases (such as some *Haemophilus influenzae* strains).

cefuroxime axetil

Adult dosage

250 to 500 mg P.O. q 12 hours for 10 days

Points to remember

- Use of this drug in chronic bronchitis is controversial.
- Cefuroxime is effective against susceptible strains of *H. influenzae.*
- Another second- or third-generation cephalosporin may be substituted.

co-trimoxazole (sulfamethoxazole-trimethoprim)

Adult dosage

One double-strength tablet (containing 800 mg sulfamethoxazole and 160 mg trimethoprim) P.O. q 12 hours

Points to remember

- Use of this drug in chronic bronchitis is controversial.
- Co-trimoxazole is effective against susceptible strains of *H. influenzae.*

prednisone
Adult dosage
20 to 30 mg/day P.O. (tablet or oral solution), reduced gradually over 3 to 6 weeks
Points to remember
- This drug is reserved for use in patients with acute exacerbations that don't respond to other treatments.
- Dosage must be individualized.
- Other corticosteroids may be substituted.
- Give in the morning.
- Taper dosage as soon as possible to reduce risk of hypothalamic-pituitary-adrenal suppression. ■

Cor pulmonale

Primary therapy for this disorder consists of treating the underlying emphysema or chronic bronchitis that is causing the ventilation-perfusion mismatch. Drug therapy is the primary treatment. Cardiac drugs are used adjunctively to treat symptoms of CHF. Supplemental oxygen is an important adjunctive therapy.

▼FIRST-LINE DRUG
digoxin
Adult dosage
1 mg I.V. loading dose in three divided doses over 24 hours; then 0.125 to 0.5 mg/day I.V. or P.O. as a maintenance dosage
Points to remember
- This drug is used to strengthen myocardial contractility, thereby improving cardiac output and reducing pulmonary congestion.
- This is a first-line therapy for patients with reduced ventricular function.
- Dosages are highly individualized.
- This drug has a narrow therapeutic index (0.8 to 2 ng/ml). Monitor serum digoxin levels.
- Withhold dose if patient's pulse is less than 50 beats/minute.
- Reduce dosage in elderly patients and those with renal failure or hepatic compromise.

furosemide
Adult dosage
40 to 240 mg/day I.V. or P.O. in single or divided doses
Points to remember
- This drug is used to reduce fluid volume overload by promoting diuresis, thereby reducing pulmonary congestion.
- Monitor patient's fluid balance, serum electrolyte levels, blood pressure, BUN, and creatinine level. ■

Cystic fibrosis

This incurable genetic disorder requires frequent use of antibiotics for respiratory infections, pancreatic enzyme supplementation, nutritional support, and bronchodilation (see "Asthma" in this section).

▼FIRST-LINE DRUG

albuterol

Adult dosage

Inhaler: 2 puffs of 90-mcg metered spray q 4 to 6 hours p.r.n.
Oral: 2 to 4 mg P.O. t.i.d. or q.i.d. (standard); or 4 to 8 mg q 12 hours (sustained-release)
Nebulizer: 2.5 mg q 4 to 6 hours p.r.n.

Points to remember

- Excessive use of aerosolized products can lead to tolerance.
- Albuterol may cause tachycardia, nervousness, or tremor that may be additive in patients also taking theophylline.
- Proper use of inhaler is essential; if poor technique limits drug effectiveness, suggest use of a spacer device.

▼FIRST-LINE DRUG

aminophylline

Adult dosage

I.V. loading dose: 5 to 6 mg/kg over 20 to 30 minutes (not to exceed 20 mg/minute) in patients who have not previously taken aminophylline; 2.5 mg/kg in those who have taken it
I.V. maintenance infusion: 0.5 mg/kg/hour

Points to remember

- When giving I.V. theophylline, reduce the dosage by 20% of the ordered aminophylline dosage.
- Maintenance I.V. infusion usually is administered in large-volume parenteral solution.
- Monitor serum drug levels.
- Aminophylline may interact with many drugs; drug action is also affected by smoking, CHF, and liver disease.

▼FIRST-LINE DRUG

bitolterol mesylate

Adult dosage

Inhaler: 2 puffs of 370-mcg metered spray q 4 to 6 hours p.r.n.

Points to remember

- This drug may cause tachycardia, nervousness, or tremor; these effects may be additive in patients also taking theophylline.
- Teach patient proper inhalation technique; if poor technique limits drug effectiveness, suggest use of a spacer device.
- Excessive use of aerosol products may lead to tolerance.

▼FIRST-LINE DRUG

ipratropium bromide

Adult dosage

Inhaler: 2 puffs of 18-mcg metered spray q.i.d.
Nebulizer: 500 mcg t.i.d. or q.i.d.

Points to remember

- Drug must be taken on schedule, not on an as-needed basis.
- Drug may irritate throat when used with other inhaled drugs.

▼FIRST-LINE DRUG

metaproterenol sulfate

Adult dosage

Inhaler: 2 puffs of 650-mcg metered spray q 4 to 6 hours p.r.n.
Nebulizer: 2.5 ml of 0.4% to 0.6% solution q 4 to 6 hours p.r.n.
Oral: 20 mg P.O. t.i.d. or q.i.d.

Points to remember

- This drug may cause tachycardia, nervousness, or tremor; these effects may be additive in patients also taking theophylline.
- Teach patient proper inhalation technique; if poor technique limits drug effectiveness, suggest use of a spacer device.
- Excessive use of aerosol products may lead to tolerance.

▼FIRST-LINE DRUG

pirbuterol

Adult dosage

Inhaler: 2 puffs of 200-mcg metered spray q 4 to 6 hours p.r.n.

Point to remember

- Teach patient the proper use of the autoinhaler to ensure drug effectiveness.

▼FIRST-LINE DRUG

terbutaline sulfate

Adult dosage

Inhaler: 2 puffs of 400-mcg metered spray q 4 to 6 hours p.r.n.
Oral: 2.5 mg P.O. t.i.d. or q.i.d.
S.C.: 0.25 mg; may repeat dose in 15 minutes, if needed

Points to remember

- Drug may cause tachycardia, nervousness, or tremor; these effects may be additive in patients also taking theophylline.
- Teach patient proper inhalation technique; if poor technique limits drug effectiveness, suggest use of spacer device.
- Excessive use of aerosol products may lead to tolerance.

dornase alfa

Adult dosage

Single-use 2.5-mg ampule inhaled once or twice daily with recommended nebulizer

Points to remember

- Don't dilute or mix with other drugs in the nebulizer.

- Store in the refrigerator and protect from light.
- This drug reduces the frequency of respiratory infections with long-term use.
- A new treatment option, dornase alfa may enhance patient outcomes if initiated early.

pancreatin
Adult dosage
8,000 to 24,000 USP units P.O. with meals
Points to remember
- Don't use in patients with hypersensitivity to pork.
- Tell patient not to crush or chew capsules.

tobramycin
Adult dosage
Based on patient's weight and renal function (a loading dose of 1.8 to 2 mg/kg and a maintenance dose of 1.3 to 1.5 mg/kg at intervals based on the patient's creatinine clearance); given with or without one of the following

aztreonam
Adult dosage
1 g I.V. q 6 to 8 hours

ceftazidime
Adult dosage
1 to 2 g I.V. q 8 hours

ciprofloxacin
Adult dosage
400 mg I.V. q 12 hours

imipenem/cilastatin sodium
Adult dosage
500 mg I.V. q 6 hours

piperacillin sodium
Adult dosage
3 g I.V. q 4 to 6 hours

ticarcillin/clavulanate
Adult dosage
3.1 g I.V. q 4 to 6 hours
Points to remember
- Duration of therapy is usually 10 to 14 days.
- Dosage must be decreased for patients with renal dysfunction.
- Another aminoglycoside may be substituted for tobramycin. ■

Diphtheria

This acute contagious disease is caused by the bacterium *Corynebacterium diphtheriae.* Patients should remain in strict isolation until cultures are negative for 3 consecutive days. Diphtheria antitoxin is the cornerstone of therapy and should be given immediately to reduce disease severity and prevent death. Antibiotics are also given to eradicate the toxin-producing organism.

▼FIRST-LINE DRUG

diphtheria antitoxin

Adult dosage

Pharyngeal or laryngeal disease of 48 hours' duration or less: One-time dose of 20,000 to 40,000 units by I.V. infusion over 60 minutes

Nasopharyngeal disease: One-time dose of 40,000 to 60,000 units by I.V. infusion over 60 minutes

Extensive disease of 3 or more days' duration: One-time dose of 80,000 to 100,000 units by I.V. infusion over 60 minutes

Points to remember

- Drug must be given as soon as diagnosis is made.
- It must be obtained from the CDC.
- Additional doses have no benefit and may cause allergic reactions.
- Drug must be given with erythromycin or penicillin G procaine.

▼FIRST-LINE DRUG

erythromycin (base, estolate, or stearate)

Adult dosage

500 mg P.O. q 6 hours for 14 days

Points to remember

- Erythromycin is as effective as penicillin.
- It's given in conjunction with diphtheria antitoxin.

penicillin G procaine

Adult dosage

600,000 units I.M. q 12 hours until patient can swallow; then switch to 125 to 250 mg penicillin V potassium P.O. q 6 hours for total of 14 days

Points to remember

- This drug is as effective as erythromycin.
- It's given in conjunction with diphtheria antitoxin. ■

Emphysema

This chronic, progressive pulmonary condition is managed primarily by drug therapy and supplemental oxygen administration.

Alpha$_1$-antitrypsin deficiency produces a similar but treatable form of disease. Pharmacologic management is symptomatic, using bronchodilators and corticosteroids.

▼FIRST-LINE DRUG

metaproterenol sulfate

Adult dosage

Inhaler: 2 puffs of 0.65-mcg metered spray (equivalent to 1.3 mg) q 4 to 6 hours p.r.n.

Nebulizer: 2.5 ml of 0.4% to 0.6% solution q 4 to 6 hours p.r.n.

Oral: 20 mg t.i.d. or q.i.d.

Points to remember

- Excessive use of aerosol products can lead to tolerance.
- Drug may cause tachycardia, nervousness, or tremor that can be additive with theophylline products.
- Teach the patient proper use of inhaler; if poor technique limits product effectiveness, suggest use of spacer device.

albuterol

Adult dosage

Inhaler: 2 puffs of 90-mcg metered spray (equivalent to 180 mcg) q 4 to 6 hours p.r.n.
Nebulizer: 2.5 mg q 4 to 6 hours p.r.n.
Oral: 2 to 4 mg P.O. (standard) t.i.d. or q.i.d.; or 4 to 8 mg q 12 hours (sustained-release)

Points to remember

- Drug may cause tachycardia, tremor, or nervousness; these effects may be additive in patients also receiving theophylline.
- Teach the patient proper use of inhaler; if poor technique limits drug effectiveness, suggest use of spacer device.

alpha-1 proteinase inhibitor (human)

Adult dosage

60 mg/kg I.V. once weekly

Points to remember

- Administer at a rate of 0.08 ml/kg/minute within 3 hours of reconstitution.
- This drug is prepared from pooled human plasma; patients should receive hepatitis B vaccine before therapy begins.
- Drug is used only to treat inherited form of emphysema caused by alpha$_1$-antitrypsin deficiency.

beclomethasone dipropionate

Adult dosage

Inhaler: 2 puffs (84 mcg) t.i.d. or q.i.d.

Points to remember

- Drug is for maintenance and must be given on schedule, not on as-needed basis.
- Tell patient to rinse his mouth after use.

bitolterol mesylate

Adult dosage

Inhaler: 2 puffs of 370-mcg metered spray q 4 to 6 hours p.r.n.

Points to remember

- Drug may cause tachycardia, tremor, and nervousness; these effects may be additive in patients also receiving theophylline.
- Teach patient proper use of inhaler; if poor technique limits drug effectiveness, suggest use of spacer device.
- Excessive use of aerosolized products may lead to tolerance.

epinephrine
Adult dosage
0.3 ml of 1:1,000 solution or dilution; may repeat q 20 minutes for two additional doses
Points to remember
- This drug is a second-line parenteral therapy for acute exacerbations of emphysema.
- Terbutaline is preferred in elderly patients and in those with cardiovascular disease.
- Epinephrine may aggravate hypertension, arrhythmias, and angina.
- Drug provides additive cardiovascular stimulation in patients receiving aminophylline.

flunisolide
Adult dosage
Inhaler: 2 puffs (500 mcg) given b.i.d.
Points to remember
- This drug is for scheduled maintenance treatment and isn't effective for relief of acute bronchospasm.
- Tell patient to rinse mouth after use.

ipratropium bromide
Adult dosage
Inhaler: 2 puffs of 36-mcg metered spray q.i.d.
Nebulizer: 500 mcg t.i.d. or q.i.d.
Points to remember
- Drug must be taken on schedule, not on an as-needed basis.
- Drug may cause throat irritation when used in conjunction with other inhaled medications.
- Ipratropium is a third-line drug.

prednisone
Adult dosage
Must be individualized
Points to remember
- Oral product is for acute episodes or long-term maintenance.
- Drug is second-line therapy for acute episodes and fourth-line therapy for chronic maintenance.
- Give with food or milk to avoid stomach irritation.

salmeterol xinafoate
Adult dosage
Inhaler: 2 puffs of 50-mcg spray q 12 hours
Points to remember
- Drug is for prevention, not treatment, of acute attacks.
- Salmeterol must be administered on schedule for maximum effectiveness; it isn't for use on an as-needed basis.

terbutaline sulfate
Adult dosage
Inhaler: 2 puffs of 200-mcg metered spray q 4 to 6 hours p.r.n.
Oral: 2.5 mg t.i.d. or q.i.d.
S.C.: 0.25 mg; may be repeated in 15 minutes if necessary
Points to remember
- Drug may cause tachycardia, tremor, or nervousness;

these effects may be additive in patients also receiving theophylline.
- Teach patient proper use of inhaler; if poor technique limits drug effectiveness, suggest use of spacer device.
- Excessive use of aerosol products may cause tolerance.

theophylline
Adult dosage
I.V. loading dose: 5 to 6 mg/kg/minute over 20 to 30 minutes (not to exceed 20 mg/minute) if patient has not received theophylline previously; 2.5 mg/kg/minute if patient has received it previously
I.V. maintenance infusion: 0.5 mg/kg/hour
Oral: highly individualized
Points to remember
- Drug is second-line therapy for emphysema.
- When switching from aminophylline to theophylline, reduce dosage by 20% of aminophylline dose.
- For maintenance infusion, drug is diluted in 500 to 1,000 ml of fluid and given by continuous I.V. infusion; maintenance dosage varies.
- Monitor blood drug levels.
- This drug interacts with many other drugs; also, its action is affected by smoking, CHF, and liver disease.

triamcinolone acetonide
Adult dosage
Inhaler: 2 puffs of 200-mcg metered spray t.i.d. or q.i.d.
Points to remember
- Drug is for scheduled maintenance treatment and isn't meant to treat acute bronchospasm.
- Tell patient to rinse mouth after use. ■

Epiglottitis

This life-threatening disorder usually occurs in children. I.V. antibiotics and corticosteroids are the mainstays of therapy.

cefotaxime sodium
Dosage
Adults: 1 to 2 g I.V. q 6 hours
Preterm or full-term neonates less than 1 week old: 50 mg/kg I.V. q 12 hours
Neonates 1 to 4 weeks old: 50 mg/kg I.V. q 6 to 8 hours
Children ages 1 month to 12 years and weighing less than 50 kg: 50 to 200 mg/kg/day I.V., divided in three to six equal doses
Children weighing 50 kg or more: 1 to 2 g I.V. q 6 hours, not to exceed 12 g/day
Points to remember
- This drug contains 2.2 mEq of sodium per gram.
- Adjust dosage in renal dysfunction.

ceftriaxone sodium
Dosage
Adults: 1 to 2 g I.V. q 12 to 24 hours
Neonates and children age 12 and younger: 50 to 75 mg/kg/day I.V., divided in equal doses q 12 hours, not to exceed 2 g/day
Children over age 12: 1 to 2 g I.V. q 12 or 24 hours
Point to remember
- This drug contains 3.6 mEq of sodium per gram.

cefuroxime
Dosage
Adults: 750 to 1,500 mg I.V. q 8 to 12 hours
Children older than 3 months: 50 to 100 mg/kg/day I.V., divided in equal doses q 6 to 8 hours
Points to remember
- This drug contains 2.4 mEq of sodium per gram.
- Reconstituted solution remains potent for 24 hours at room temperature or for 48 hours when refrigerated.
- Adjust dosage in renal dysfunction.

dexamethasone
Dosage
Adults: 4 to 10 mg by I.V. bolus initially, then 4 mg I.V. q 6 hours
Children: dosage is highly individualized; some clinicians recommend 6 to 40 mg/kg or 0.235 to 1.25 mg/m² I.M. or I.V. once or twice daily
Point to remember
- Reduce dosage gradually after long-term therapy. ■

Influenza

Bed rest, analgesics, and cough medicine may be used to treat influenza. Amantadine is used for prophylaxis and treatment of the influenza A virus.

amantadine hydrochloride
Adult dosage
200 mg/day P.O. in a single dose or divided in two doses
Points to remember
- This drug may decrease duration of influenza signs and symptoms by approximately half.
- To prevent orthostatic hypotension, instruct patient to move slowly when changing position.
- Treatment should continue for 24 to 48 hours after symptoms disappear.
- Adjust dosage in renal dysfunction. ■

Legionnaires' disease

Tetracyclines, ciprofloxacin, and co-trimoxazole have been used to treat this disease. However, because their efficacy hasn't been proven, they should be used only if erythromycin is contraindicated.

▼FIRST-LINE DRUG
erythromycin
Adult dosage
2 to 4 g/day I.V. or P.O. for 14 to 21 days
Points to remember
- Stay alert for nausea, vomiting, diarrhea, or stomach cramps.
- Instruct patient to take oral form when stomach is empty to enhance absorption; if gastric upset occurs, allow patient to take drug with food.

rifampin
Adult dosage
300 mg P.O. b.i.d. given in combination with erythromycin
Points to remember
- This drug may have synergistic effect when given with erythromycin.
- It may be used in immunocompromised patients or those with severe illness. ■

Lung abscess

A patient with a lung abscess should receive antibiotics until a chest X-ray indicates that the abscess has healed or stabilized, which may take a month or longer. Patients with empyema usually undergo tube thoracostomy; some may require open pleural drainage.

▼FIRST-LINE DRUG
penicillin G
Adult dosage
1 to 2 million units I.V. q 4 hours
Point to remember
- Once patient improves, penicillin V (0.5 to 1 g P.O. q 6 hours) may be substituted.

clindamycin
Adult dosage
600 mg I.V. q 8 hours until patient improves; then 300 mg P.O. q 6 hours
Point to remember
- This drug is used as an alternative to penicillin for treatment of anaerobic pleuropulmonary infections; it may be more effective than penicillin in treating community-acquired anaerobic lung infections. ■

Pleurisy

Treatment of this inflammatory disease depends on the underlying cause and symptoms. Analgesics are given to manage pleuritic pain. Pleurisy associated with pneumonia is treated with anti-inflammatory agents. Severe disease may warrant an intercostal nerve block.

ibuprofen
Adult dosage
Pain relief: 400 mg P.O. q 4 to 6 hours p.r.n.
Reduction of inflammation: 600 to 800 mg P.O. q 8 hours
Points to remember
- Dosage must be individualized.
- Don't exceed maximum daily dosage of 3.2 g.

naproxen
Adult dosage
Pain relief: 250 mg P.O. q 12 hours
Reduction of inflammation: 500 mg P.O. q 12 hours
Points to remember
- Dosage must be individualized.
- Don't exceed maximum daily dosage of 1,250 mg. ■

Pneumonia, aspiration

Aspiration pneumonia results from vomiting and aspiration of gastric or oropharyngeal contents into the trachea and lungs. Antibiotic selection depends on the results of culture and sensitivity testing and whether or not the patient is hospitalized.

For nonhospitalized patients

▼FIRST-LINE DRUG
clindamycin
Adult dosage
600 mg I.V. q 8 hours for 10 to 14 days
Point to remember
- Clindamycin can be given to patients who are allergic to penicillin.

▼FIRST-LINE DRUG
penicillin G, aqueous (sodium or potassium salt)
Adult dosage
2 to 3 million units I.V. q 4 to 6 hours for 10 to 14 days
Point to remember
- Penicillin must be administered with metronidazole in dosage described below.

metronidazole
Adult dosage
500 mg I.V. q 6 to 12 hours for 10 to 14 days
Point to remember
- Metronidazole is never used alone but can be given with penicillin if penicillin-resistant bacterial infection is a concern.

For hospitalized patients

ampicillin/sulbactam
Adult dosage
1.5 to 3 g I.V. q 6 hours
Points to remember
- This is a second-line drug.
- It isn't effective against *Pseudomonas aeruginosa* or

methicillin-resistant *Staphylococcus aureus* organisms.
- Duration of therapy depends on patient's response.

cefoxitin sodium
Adult dosage
1 to 2 g I.V. q 6 hours
Points to remember
- This is an alternative drug.
- It isn't effective against *P. aeruginosa* or methicillin-resistant *S. aureus* organisms.
- Vancomycin should be added to drug regimen if methicillin-resistant *S. aureus* is suspected.
- Duration of therapy depends on patient's response.

ticarcillin/clavulanate
Adult dosage
3.1 g I.V. q 6 hours
Points to remember
- Vancomycin should be added to regimen if methicillin-resistant *S. aureus* is suspected.
- Gentamicin, tobramycin, or amikacin should also be given if *P. aeruginosa* is suspected.
- Duration of therapy depends on patient's response. ■

Pneumonia, bacterial *(Klebsiella)*

Susceptibility of *K. pneumoniae* to antibiotics varies widely. Drug selection is based on results of culture and sensitivity testing. Empiric therapy is described below.

▼FIRST-LINE DRUG
gentamicin
Adult dosage
Based on patient's weight and renal function (usually a loading dose of 1.8 to 2 mg/kg and a maintenance dose of 1.3 to 1.5 mg/kg at intervals based on creatinine clearance); given with or without one of the following drugs for severe infection

aztreonam
Adult dosage
1 g I.V. q 6 to 8 hours

cefotaxime
Adult dosage
1 to 2 g I.V. q 8 hours

ciprofloxacin
Adult dosage
400 mg I.V. q 12 hours

imipenem/cilastatin sodium
Adult dosage
500 mg I.V. q 6 hours

piperacillin
Adult dosage
3 g I.V. q 4 to 6 hours

ticarcillin/clavulanate
Adult dosage
3.1 g I.V. q 4 to 6 hours
Points to remember
- Usual duration of therapy is 10 is 14 days.

- Recommended dosages are for patients with normal renal function; decrease dosage in renal dysfunction.
- Another aminoglycoside may be substituted for gentamicin.
- Other third-generation cephalosporins, fluoroquinolones, or penicillins may be substituted for cefotaxime, ciprofloxacin, or piperacillin. ■

Pneumonia, bacterial *(Pseudomonas aeruginosa)*

Double antibiotic coverage is recommended to prevent rapid development of drug resistance in this pneumonia. Susceptibility of *P. aeruginosa* to antibiotics varies widely. Ideally, drug selection is based on results of culture and sensitivity testing. However, empiric therapy (described below) may be used.

▼FIRST-LINE DRUG

tobramycin sulfate
Adult dosage
Based on patient's weight and renal function (usually a loading dose of 1.8 to 2 mg/kg and a maintenance dose of 1.3 to 1.5 mg/kg at intervals based on creatinine clearance); given with or without one of the following drugs for severe infection

aztreonam
Adult dosage
1 g I.V. q 6 to 8 hours

ceftazidime
Adult dosage
1 to 2 g I.V. q 8 hours

ciprofloxacin
Adult dosage
400 mg I.V. q 12 hours

imipenem/cilastatin sodium
Adult dosage
500 mg I.V. q 6 hours

piperacillin
Adult dosage
3 g I.V. q 4 to 6 hours

ticarcillin/clavulanate
Adult dosage
3.1 g I.V. q 4 to 6 hours
Points to remember

- Usual duration of therapy is 10 to 14 days.
- Recommended dosages are for patients with normal renal function; decrease dosage in renal dysfunction.
- Another aminoglycoside may be substituted for tobramycin if organism is susceptible.
- Another penicillin or fluoroquinolone may be substituted for piperacillin or ciprofloxacin, respectively. ■

Pneumonia, bacterial *(Staphylococcus aureus)*

Antibiotic selection for *S. aureus* pneumonia is based on results of culture and sensitivity testing. Empiric therapy is described below.

For methicillin-susceptible S. aureus *pneumonia*

▼FIRST-LINE DRUG

cefazolin sodium

Adult dosage

1 to 2 g I.V. q 8 hours for 10 to 14 days

Point to remember

- Other first-generation cephalosporins may be substituted.

▼FIRST-LINE DRUG

nafcillin sodium

Adult dosage

1 to 2 g I.V. q 4 to 6 hours for 10 to 14 days

Points to remember

- Other penicillinase-resistant penicillins may be substituted.
- An aminoglycoside or rifampin may be added if patient doesn't respond.

For methicillin-resistant S. aureus

▼FIRST-LINE DRUG

vancomycin hydrochloride

Adult dosage

Dosage varies, based on weight and renal function.

Patients with creatinine clearance (CC) above 60 ml/minute: 1 g I.V. q 12 hours for 10 to 14 days; adjust dosage based on peak and trough levels

Patients with CC of 40 to 60 ml/minute: 1 g I.V. q 24 hours

Patients with CC below 40 ml/minute: dosage based on serum drug levels (administer 1 g I.M. for first dose, with another dose when serum CC level is equal to or less than 10 mcg/ml)

Points to remember

- Steady-state and trough serum drug levels usually are measured before fourth dose is given.
- An aminoglycoside or rifampin may be added if patient doesn't respond. ■

Pneumonia, bacterial *(Streptococcus)*

Antibiotic selection for streptococcal pneumonia is based on results of culture and sensitivity testing. Empiric therapy is described below.

For S. pneumoniae

▼FIRST-LINE DRUG

erythromycin lactobionate
Adult dosage
500 mg I.V. q 6 hours for 10 to 14 days
Points to remember
- This drug is likely to cause nausea, vomiting, and diarrhea.
- Use piggyback set to infuse I.V. over 1 hour. (Parenteral administration may cause phlebitis.)

▼FIRST-LINE DRUG

penicillin G, aqueous (sodium or potassium salt)
Adult dosage
2 to 3 million units I.V. q 4 to 6 hours for 10 to 14 days
Point to remember
- Monitor renal function closely in patients with renal impairment.

cefazolin sodium
Adult dosage
1 to 2 g I.V. q 8 hours for 10 to 14 days
Point to remember
- This is a second-line drug.

clindamycin
Adult dosage
600 mg I.V. q 8 hours for 10 to 14 days
Point to remember
- This is a second-line drug.

For group D Enterococcus

gentamicin
Adult dosage
Based on patient's weight and renal function (usually a loading dose of 1.8 to 2 mg/kg and a maintenance dose of 1.3 to 1.5 mg/kg at intervals based on creatinine clearance); given in conjunction with ampicillin (1 to 2 g I.V. q 6 hours) or vancomycin (dosage based on patient's weight and renal function)
Points to remember
- Usual duration of therapy is 10 to 14 days.
- Other aminoglycosides may be substituted for gentamicin.
- Aim for a low gentamicin peak serum level of 3 to 4 mcg/ml because gentamicin is given with ampicillin or vancomycin. ■

Pneumonia, fungal

Common causative pathogens for this type of pneumonia include *Aspergillus, Candida, Blastomyces, Histoplasma, Coccidioides,* and *Cryptococcus.* Identifying the specific pathogen guides antibiotic selection and helps determine the duration of therapy.

▼FIRST-LINE DRUG

amphotericin B

Adult dosage

0.5 to 1 mg/kg/day I.V., to total cumulative dosage of 30 to 40 mg/kg

Points to remember

- Administer 1-mg I.V. test dose before giving first dose.
- Infuse over 4 to 6 hours.
- Amphotericin isn't stable in electrolyte solutions.
- Monitor serum creatinine and electrolyte levels closely; drug causes nephrotoxicity in about 80% of patients receiving 1 g or more.

(For drugs used to treat pneumonia caused by particular organisms, see the entries "Candidiasis," "Blastomycosis," and "Coccidioidomycosis.") ■

Pneumonia, mycoplasmal

Mild cases of mycoplasmal pneumonia may be treated with oral antibiotic therapy. Severe infections may warrant I.V. antibiotic administration.

▼FIRST-LINE DRUG

erythromycin (base, estolate, stearate, or lactobionate)

Adult dosage

500 mg P.O. I.V. q 6 hours for 14 to 21 days

Points to remember

- Infuse over 1 hour, using piggyback set. (Parenteral administration may cause phlebitis.)
- Oral and parenteral administration may cause nausea, vomiting, and diarrhea.

azithromycin

Adult dosage

500 mg P.O. for 1 day, then 250 mg/day P.O. for 10 to 14 days

Points to remember

- Administer this drug 1 hour before or 2 hours after a meal.
- This is a second-line drug.

clarithromycin

Adult dosage

500 mg P.O. q 12 hours for 14 to 21 days

Point to remember

- This is an alternative drug.

doxycycline

Adult dosage

100 mg P.O. or I.V. q 12 hours for 14 to 21 days

Points to remember

- This is an alternative drug.
- Infuse over 1 to 4 hours, using piggyback set. (Parenteral administration may cause phlebitis.)
- Doxycycline is contraindicated in pregnancy. ■

Pneumonia, *Pneumocystis carinii*

This type of pneumonia warrants antibiotic therapy; sometimes, a corticosteroid, such as prednisone, is given adjunctively. Prophylaxis against *P. carinii* pneumonia is recommended for AIDS patients with CD4+ T-cell counts below 200 cells/µl or after initial *P. carinii* infection.

For treatment of P. carinii *pneumonia*

▼FIRST-LINE DRUG

co-trimoxazole (sulfamethoxazole-trimethoprim)
Adult dosage
15 to 20 mg/kg/day (based on trimethoprim dose in milligrams per kilograms) in four divided doses I.V. or P.O. for 21 days (I.V. solution contains 80 mg of sulfamethoxazole and 16 mg of trimethoprim)
Point to remember
- This drug causes a rash in about 20% of patients with AIDS.

atovaquone
Adult dosage
750 mg P.O. q 8 hours for 21 days
Points to remember
- This is a second-line drug for patients with mild to moderate *P. carinii* pneumonia who can't tolerate first-line agents.
- Administer with food to increase drug bioavailability.
- This drug causes fewer side effects than co-trimoxazole but carries a higher mortality.

pentamidine isethionate
Adult dosage
4 mg/kg/day I.V. for 21 days
Points to remember
- This is a second-line drug.
- Infuse over 1 to 2 hours to decrease risk of hypotension.
- Drug may cause rash, nephrotoxicity, and hypoglycemia.

prednisone
Adult dosage
40 mg P.O. b.i.d. for 5 days, then 20 mg P.O. b.i.d. for 5 days, followed by 20 mg/day P.O. for 11 days
Points to remember
- This drug is used adjunctively in moderate to severe infection.
- Another corticosteroid may be substituted.

trimetrexate glucuronate
Adult dosage
45 mg/m^2/day I.V. for 21 days; given in conjunction with 20 mg/m^2 of leucovorin P.O. or I.V. q.i.d. for 24 days
Points to remember
- This is a second-line drug for patients with moderate to severe *P. carinii* pneumonia who can't tolerate first-line agents.

- Administer over 60 to 90 minutes.
- This drug causes fewer side effects than co-trimoxazole but is associated with a higher relapse rate.
- Leucovorin must accompany trimetrexate therapy to decrease the risk of bone marrow suppression.

For prophylaxis against **P. carinii** *pneumonia*

▼FIRST-LINE DRUG

co-trimoxazole (sulfamethoxazole-trimethoprim)
Adult dosage
One double-strength tablet (containing 800 mg sulfamethoxazole and 160 mg trimethoprim) P.O. daily or every other day
Points to remember
- This drug causes a rash in about 20% of patients with AIDS and may need to be discontinued.
- This drug is also effective as prophylaxis against toxoplasmosis.
- Do not give to patients who are allergic to sulfonamides.

dapsone
Adult dosage
25 to 100 mg/day P.O. or 100 mg P.O. three times a week
Points to remember
- This is an alternative prophylactic drug.
- It may cause serious hemolytic anemia. Patients should be tested for G6PD deficiency before starting therapy.
- Monitor CBC every week for first month, monthly for next 6 months, then twice a year.

pentamidine isethionate
Adult dosage
300 mg by Respirgard nebulizer once a month, or 4 mg/kg I.M. or I.V. q 2 to 4 weeks
Points to remember
- This is a second-line drug.
- It may cause bronchospasm; give albuterol (or equivalent) before aerosol administration. ■

Pneumonia, viral

Common causative pathogens for viral pneumonia include influenza, varicella zoster, respiratory syncytial virus (in infants), and cytomegalovirus (in immunosuppressed patients). (For specific drugs used to treat cytomegalovirus infections, see "CMV infections" under Infections.)

For pneumonia caused by influenza A

▼FIRST-LINE DRUG

amantadine hydrochloride
Adult dosage
100 mg P.O. b.i.d. for 3 to 5 days

Points to remember
- For best results, drug therapy must start within 48 hours of onset.
- Reduce dosage to 100 mg/day P.O. if patient has history of seizures.
- Adjust dosage in elderly patients and those with renal dysfunction.
- This drug isn't effective against influenza B.
- Amantadine may cause significant CNS effects, including confusion, agitation, dizziness, and seizures.

rimantadine
Adult dosage
100 mg P.O. b.i.d. for 3 to 5 days
Points to remember
- This is an alternative drug.
- Adjust dosage in elderly patients and those with renal dysfunction.
- This drug is not effective against influenza B.
- For best results, drug therapy must start within 48 hours of symptom onset.
- Rimantadine is less likely to cause side effects than amantadine.

For pneumonia caused by varicella zoster

▼FIRST-LINE DRUG
acyclovir
Adult dosage
10 to 12.4 mg/kg I.V. q 8 hours
Point to remember
- Adjust dosage in patients with renal dysfunction. ■

Pulmonary edema, acute

Treatment of acute pulmonary edema aims to remove or treat precipitating causes, such as tachyarrhythmias, bradyarrhythmias, acute MI, severe hypertension, acute mitral or aortic regurgitation, fluid overload, pulmonary embolism, or sudden discontinuation of drugs used to treat CHF. Supportive care includes positioning the patient upright and administering 100% oxygen to achieve a partial pressure of arterial carbon dioxide above 60 mm Hg. Intubation may be necessary for persistent hypoxemia.

▼FIRST-LINE DRUGS
loop diuretics
Adult dosage
Bumetanide: 1 mg I.V.; may repeat dose in 2 to 3 hours based on patient's response
Furosemide: 40 to 100 mg I.V.; may repeat dose in 1 hour based on patient's response
Points to remember
- Loop diuretics are first-line drugs for treating pulmonary edema secondary to left-sided heart failure.

- Reduce dosage if patient doesn't take diuretics regularly.

▼FIRST-LINE DRUG

morphine sulfate

Adult dosage

2 to 5 mg I.V. p.r.n.

Points to remember

- Morphine is a first-line drug for treating pulmonary edema secondary to left-sided heart failure.
- Drug is also used to treat anxiety and dyspnea.

aminophylline/theophylline

Adult dosage

6 mg/kg (5 mg/kg of theophylline) I.V. over 20 to 40 minutes, followed by infusion of 0.2 to 0.5 mg/kg/hour (0.15 to 0.4 mg/kg/hour of theophylline)

Point to remember

- Aminophylline or theophylline may be added to drug regimen if patient doesn't respond to morphine and diuretics.

digoxin

Adult dosage

750 mcg I.V. loading dose given in two or three divided doses, followed by 125 to 250 mcg/day I.V.

Points to remember

- Digoxin may be added to drug regimen if patient doesn't respond to diuretics and morphine.
- Drug is contraindicated in hypokalemia, hypocalcemia, AV block, hypercalcemia, hyperkalemia, hypomagnesemia, acute MI, PVCs, ventricular tachycardia, sick sinus syndrome, and Wolff-Parkinson-White syndrome.
- Elderly patients and those with renal impairment may require lower doses and be more susceptible to toxicity.

nitroprusside sodium

Adult dosage

0.3 to 10 mcg/kg/minute I.V. (dilute with D_5W)

Points to remember

- This drug may be given after morphine and diuretics if patient's systolic blood pressure exceeds 100 mm Hg.
- Protect I.V. solution from light.
- Nitroprusside is contraindicated in severe renal or liver impairment, vitamin B_{12} deficiency, increased intracranial pressure, and cerebrovascular or coronary artery insufficiency.
- This drug may cause cyanide toxicity. Monitor for ataxia, blurred vision, dizziness, headache, nausea, shortness of breath, and tinnitus. ■

Pulmonary embolism and infarction

When anticoagulant or thrombolytic drug therapy fails to control these conditions, surgical embolectomy may be performed. Percutaneous transvenous filters and umbrellas may be inserted to prevent further emboli, especially in patients who cannot tolerate or have other contraindications for anticoagulant and thrombolytic drugs.

▼FIRST-LINE DRUG

heparin

Adult dosage

70 to 100 units/kg (5,000 to 10,000 units) by I.V. bolus, followed by a continuous infusion of 15 to 25 units/kg/hour; titrate dosage to maintain patient's activated partial thromboplastin time (APTT) at 1.5 to 2 times normal

Points to remember

- Heparin is initial first-line therapy for acute pulmonary embolism. It may also be started after administration of thrombolytic agent.
- Therapy typically lasts 7 to 10 days.
- Patients with acute pulmonary embolism eliminate heparin at an accelerated rate and may require larger doses.
- Minidose of heparin (5,000 units S.C. q 8 to 12 hours) or adjusted-dose heparin (in which dosage is titrated to keep APTT between 31.5 and 36 seconds) may be used prophylactically in patients at moderate to high risk for pulmonary embolism or deep-vein thrombosis (DVT).

thrombolytic agents

Adult dosage

Streptokinase: 250,000 units infused I.V. over 30 minutes, followed by 100,000 units/hour for 24 to 72 hours

Urokinase: 4,400 units/kg infused I.V. over 30 minutes, followed by 4,400 units/kg/hour for 12 hours

Points to remember

- Thrombolytic agents are used in patients with massive pulmonary embolism, patients who don't respond to heparin, and those who've suffered massive pulmonary embolism but can't tolerate hemodynamic compromise.
- Don't administer other drugs through same I.V. line.
- During thrombolytic therapy, limit patient movement, and avoid I.M. injections and invasive procedures.
- These agents are contraindicated in patients with aneurysm, active bleeding, brain tumor, cerebrovascular accident (CVA), uncontrolled hypertension, recent thoracic

or neurologic surgery, or recent trauma.

warfarin sodium
Adult dosage
2 to 10 mg/day P.O.
Points to remember
- Warfarin therapy may start on day 2 or 3 of heparin therapy and may continue for several months. Duration of therapy depends on risk factors for recurrent DVT or pulmonary embolism.
- Adjust dosage to maintain international normalized ratio between 2 and 3.
- Instruct patient to consume diet containing adequate amounts of vitamin K.
- Give vitamin K_1 in case of overdose.
- Warfarin is contraindicated in recent spinal puncture, trauma, childbirth or surgery, severe liver or renal impairment, endocarditis, pregnancy, thrombocytopenia, severe uncontrolled hypertension, pericarditis, active bleeding, and CVA.
- Advise patient to notify other health professionals of chronic warfarin therapy and to carry identification indicating such therapy.
- Elderly patients may be more susceptible to bleeding during therapy. ■

Sarcoidosis

Many patients with this chronic, progressive disease suffer respiratory, cardiac, visual, or CNS impairment. However, the impairment is often mild and remains stable. Drug therapy commonly includes corticosteroids, although there's no consensus as to when to use these drugs. Typically, patients with mild disease involving the lungs, heart, eyes, and CNS are monitored without drug therapy for 2 to 3 months to see if symptoms resolve spontaneously. Patients with more serious disease forms are treated aggressively. Such drugs as chloroquine, cyclophosphamide, methotrexate, and NSAIDs also have been used to treat sarcoidosis; however, they have limited value.

▼FIRST-LINE DRUGS

corticosteroids
Adult dosage
1 mg/kg/day P.O. of prednisone or its equivalent for 4 to 6 weeks; dosage may be tapered over several months
Points to remember
- Alternate-day regimens and inhaled corticosteroids aren't effective. Mild ocular disease may respond to corticosteroid eyedrops.

- Long-term complications of corticosteroids include osteoporosis, cataracts, glaucoma, and adrenal suppression. With shorter regimens, psychoses, glucose intolerance, potassium wasting, and immunosuppression can occur. ■

Silicosis

Therapy for this lung disorder may include oxygen administration to treat hypoxia and mechanical ventilation to treat acute respiratory failure. Adequate fluid intake and chest percussion with postural drainage may help clear secretions. To prevent respiratory depression, avoid administering sedatives and tranquilizers, if possible, and advise the patient to avoid alcoholic beverages.

Patients with silicosis are at high risk for tuberculosis (TB); those with positive tuberculin skin tests should be treated for TB. They should also be monitored and treated for other respiratory infections and cor pulmonale.

beta-adrenergic agonists (such as albuterol)
Adult dosage
Inhaler: 1 or 2 puffs q 4 to 6 hours
Nebulizer: Dosage varies with agent (drug is usually diluted with 2 to 3 ml of normal saline solution)
Points to remember
- These drugs are used to relieve bronchospasm and dyspnea.
- Patients usually tolerate inhalation therapy well.
- For metered-dose inhaler to be effective, patient must use proper administration technique. Check patient's technique, and suggest use of spacer device if necessary to improve drug delivery.
- Nebulizer therapy may be necessary for patients with marked dyspnea. ■

Tuberculosis

Active tuberculosis (TB) requires combination drug therapy for 6 to 18 months (depending on the regimen). Regimens for patients with drug-resistant organisms may include five or six drugs. Combination regimens commonly include isoniazid, rifampin, and pyrazinamide (except in drug resistance or when contraindications exist). In areas where drug-resistant TB is common, regimens for resistant organisms are initiated pending results of culture and sensitivity testing.

Patients infected with TB and those who've been exposed to persons with active

TB may receive 6 to 12 months of isoniazid (INH) prophylaxis to prevent development of active disease. Immunocompromised patients and those who've had a positive skin test within the past 2 years are at highest risk for developing TB. Prophylactic INH usually is indicated for patients younger than age 35 and some patients over age 35 who are at high risk for developing TB.

Patients must comply with therapy to prevent a relapse or development of drug-resistant organisms. After the 1st month of therapy, they typically begin a twice-weekly regimen, which may improve compliance.

▼FIRST-LINE DRUG

isoniazid (INH)

Adult dosage

300 to 600 mg/day P.O. or 900 mg P.O. per week

Points to remember

- This is a first-line drug for both prophylaxis and treatment and is usually given as part of combination therapy.
- INH is contraindicated in alcoholism and impaired liver function.
- Heptatoxicity is most common in patients over age 35. AIDS patients, persons of Asian backgrounds, patients on barbiturates, and those who consume alcoholic beverages are at higher risk for hepatotoxicity. Warn patients to avoid alcoholic beverages during therapy.
- To prevent peripheral neuropathies, pregnant patients, patients over age 65, those taking anticonvulsants, and those with a history of malnutrition, alcoholism, chronic renal failure, or diabetes should receive pyridoxine, 25 to 50 mg/day.

▼FIRST-LINE DRUG

pyrazinamide

Adult dosage

15 to 30 mg/kg/day P.O. (up to 2 g/day) or 50 to 70 mg/kg two to three times per week

Points to remember

- Pyrazinamide is used as a first-line drug in shorter regimens (those lasting 6 months). It may also be given until antibiotic sensitivities are known.
- Drug is contraindicated in alcoholism and gout.

▼FIRST-LINE DRUG

rifampin

Adult dosage

10 mg/kg/day P.O., up to 600 mg/day P.O.; or 600 mg two to three times weekly

Points to remember

- A first-line drug, rifampin is included in most treatment regimens.
- This drug may turn body secretions, (including tears) reddish orange and may stain clothes and soft contact lenses.

- Patients on birth control pills should use another form of contraception.
- This drug is contraindicated in liver impairment and alcoholism.
- Rifampin works best when taken on empty stomach with full glass of water. However, taking it with food minimizes GI upset.

aminoglycosides
Adult dosage
Capreomycin: 15 to 30 mg/kg/ day I.M. to maximum of 1 g/day
Kanamycin: 15 to 30 mg/kg/day I.M. to maximum of 1 g/day
Streptomycin: 1 g/day I.M.; may decrease to two or three times per week
Points to remember
- Streptomycin often is included initially in combination therapy, especially if drug-resistant organisms are documented or suspected. Other aminoglycosides may be substituted based on antibiotic sensitivity results.
- Inject kanamycin into upper outer quadrant of gluteal muscle.
- Adjust dosage in renal impairment.
- These drugs are contraindicated during pregnancy because they may cause fetal ototoxicity.

aminosalicylic acid (PAS)
Adult dosage
3 to 4 g P.O. q 8 hours or 5 to 6 g P.O. q 12 hours
Points to remember
- This second-line drug is included in combination therapy, especially if drug-resistant organisms are documented or suspected or if patient can't tolerate first-line drugs.
- To minimize GI upset, instruct patient to take this drug as a single daily dose with food or an antacid.
- If necessary, give smaller dosages and increase dosage gradually as tolerated.
- This drug is contraindicated in patients with a history of G6PD deficiency or liver impairment.
- PAS may exacerbate CHF and peptic ulcer disease.

cycloserine
Adult dosage
250 mg P.O. q 12 hours, increasing gradually to maximum of 250 mg q 6 to 8 hours as tolerated (based on serum drug levels)
Points to remember
- This second-line drug typically is included in combination therapy, especially if drug-resistant drugs are documented or suspected or if patient can't tolerate first-line drugs.
- Cycloserine is contraindicated in patients with a history of seizures, renal impairment, or alcoholism.

- Advise patient to take the drug with meals to avoid GI upset.
- Adjust dosage in renal impairment.

ethambutol
Adult dosage
15 to 25 mg/kg/day P.O. or 50 mg/kg (up to 2.5 g) P.O. twice a week
Points to remember
- Ethambutol may be included in combination therapy for drug-resistant organisms or for patients who have contraindications for other first-line drugs.
- This drug is contraindicated in gout, optic neuritis, and ethambutol allergy.
- Taking the drug with food may decrease GI upset.
- Patients with renal impairment should have their eyes examined periodically. They may also require dosage reductions.

ethionamide
Adult dosage
250 mg P.O. q 8 to 12 hours, to maximum of 1 g/day
Points to remember
- This second-line drug typically is included in combination therapy, especially if a drug-resistant organism is documented or suspected or if patient can't tolerate first-line drugs.
- Ideally, this drug should be taken as a single dose. However, if it causes GI upset, advise patient to take it after meals or in divided doses.
- Ethionamide is contraindicated in diabetes and liver impairment. ■

NEUROLOGIC DISORDERS

Alzheimer's disease

Therapy for Alzheimer's disease includes treating manageable contributing causes, such as hypothyroidism and alcoholism. The patient may benefit from treatment of anxiety, depression, agitation, psychotic symptoms, and insomnia. Psychotropic drugs, on the other hand, may increase the patient's confusion.

tacrine hydrochloride
Adult dosage
10 mg P.O. q.i.d. initially; increase by 40 mg/day at 6-week intervals as needed, to maximum of 160 mg/day
Points to remember
- Tacrine is used for palliative treatment of mild to moderate Alzheimer's disease.
- This drug may cause modest dose-related improvement in cognitive function, but it doesn't alter the disease process. Patient's level of functioning will continue to

decline, but perhaps at slower rate than in untreated patients.

- Discontinue drug if patient develops jaundice, if serum bilirubin level exceeds 3 mg/dl, or if liver enzymes exceed five times their normal values.
- Abrupt discontinuation may cause rapid worsening of symptoms.
- Tacrine is best absorbed on an empty stomach. However, give with meals if GI upset occurs. ■

Brain abscess

This disorder may be treated with antibiotics alone or in combination with surgical aspiration or excision. Antibiotic selection is either empiric (based on the most likely pathogen) or definitive (based on identification of the causative organism by aspirate).

metronidazole
Adult dosage
3 g/day I.V. in divided doses q 6 hours
Points to remember
- This drug is effective against *Bacteroides fragilis.*
- Metronidazole may cause vision problems; monitor results of patient's eye examinations before, during, and after therapy.

nafcillin
Adult dosage
12 g/day I.V. in divided doses q 6 hours
Points to remember
- This drug typically is added to metronidazole regimen.
- Nafcillin is effective against *Staphylococcus aureus.*
- Toxicity may occur in patients with renal dysfunction.

penicillin G
Adult dosage
24 million units/day I.V. in divided doses q 6 hours
Points to remember
- This drug is effective against streptococci and most anaerobes but not against *B. fragilis.*
- Toxicity may occur in patients with renal dysfunction. ■

Cerebral aneurysm

Surgery is the definitive treatment for cerebral aneurysm. Drug therapy is adjunctive and aims to reduce the risk of rebleeding by controlling blood pressure, maintaining sedation, minimizing straining, and decreasing vasospasm.

nimodipine
Adult dosage
60 mg P.O. (ranges from 20 to 90 mg) q 4 hours for 14 to 21 days

Points to remember
- Drug therapy should begin within 96 hours of hemorrhage.
- For patients who can't take oral drugs, administer by nasogastric (NG) tube. First, puncture capsule at both ends with 18G needle. Then empty contents into an NG tube, and flush with 30 ml normal saline solution. Don't mix capsule contents with liquids.
- Reduce dosage in renal and hepatic dysfunction. ■

Cerebral palsy

Drug therapy for cerebral palsy is directed toward relieving spasticity. However, drug therapy is adjunctive, yielding an extremely variable patient response. Also, side effects are common and may be severe; many patients can't tolerate prescribed drugs.

baclofen
Adult dosage
40 to 80 mg P.O. in divided doses t.i.d. or q.i.d.
Points to remember
- Drug is used to relieve muscle spasticity.
- Initiate therapy with 5 mg t.i.d., and titrate to lowest effective dosage at 3-day intervals. Increase dosage more slowly in elderly patients and those with psychiatric or brain disorders.
- Taper drug when reducing dosage or discontinuing drug.
- This drug may cause drowsiness, dizziness, or weakness.

dantrolene sodium
Adult dosage
25 mg/day P.O. initially; titrate up to 25 mg t.i.d. to 100 mg q.i.d.
Points to remember
- Drug is used to relieve muscle spasticity.
- Dosage requirements are highly variable.
- Increase dosage at intervals of 4 to 7 days, as tolerated.
- Discontinue drug if beneficial results don't occur within 45 days.
- This drug may cause excessive muscle weakness, drowsiness, dizziness, nausea, and fatigue.
- Drug is contraindicated in active liver disease.
- Excessive relaxation of swallowing muscles increases risk of aspiration; monitor patient at mealtimes when therapy begins. ■

Cerebrovascular accident

Treatment depends on whether cerebrovascular accident (CVA) is caused by ischemia, embolus, or hemorrhage. Reducing risk factors and thus preventing subsequent CVAs is the major goal of therapy. In ischemic or embolic CVA, drug therapy aims to prevent subsequent CVAs and limit infarction progression. In hemorrhagic CVA, drug therapy is adjunctive to surgical drainage and aims to relieve vasospasm.

heparin
Adult dosage
5,000 units S.C. q 8 to 12 hours or 1 unit/kg/hour by I.V. infusion
Points to remember
- Drug is used only for treatment of embolic or ischemic stroke to prevent ischemia extension.
- Monitor patient's platelet count.
- Use with caution in patients at increased risk for hemorrhage; if hemorrhage occurs, stop drug immediately.

nimodipine
Adult dosage
60 mg P.O. (range is 20 to 90 mg) q 4 hours for 14 to 21 days
Points to remember
- Drug is used only for treatment of hemorrhagic stroke to reduce blood pressure and coronary vasospasm.
- Drug therapy should begin within 96 hours of hemorrhage.
- For patients who can't take oral drugs, administer by nasogastric (NG) tube. First, puncture capsule at both ends with 18G needle, empty contents into NG tube, and flush with 30 ml of normal saline solution. Don't mix capsule contents with liquids.
- Reduce dosage in renal or hepatic dysfunction.

warfarin sodium
Adult dosage
2.5 to 15 mg/day P.O.
Points to remember
- This drug is used for long-term anticoagulation and prevention of subsequent CVAs in patients with acute embolic CVA.
- Monitor patient's PT or international normalized ratio to regulate dosage.
- Reduce dosage in elderly patients and those with hepatic disease or CHF.
- Administer the dose at same time each day.

For prophylaxis against CVA

aspirin
Adult dosage
80 to 975 mg/day P.O. in single or divided doses
Points to remember
- This drug is used to prevent CVA in patients with new-onset or crescendo transient ischemia attacks (TIAs), as well in those with stable, completed embolic CVAs.

- Use caution when administering aspirin to patients with peptic ulcer disease.
- Enteric-coated products may reduce GI upset.
- Reduce dosage in elderly patients.

ticlopidine hydrochloride
Adult dosage
250 mg P.O. b.i.d.
Points to remember
- This is a second-line drug for prevention of CVA and TIA in patients who are allergic to aspirin or who can't tolerate its GI side effects.
- Monitor patient's CBC regularly. ■

Encephalitis

This inflammatory brain condition usually results from viral infection. The only treatable causes are herpes simplex and varicella zoster.

▼**FIRST-LINE DRUG**
acyclovir
Adult dosage
10 to 12.4 mg/kg I.V. q 8 hours for 10 to 14 days
Point to remember
- Adjust dosage in renal dysfunction. ■

Epilepsy

Therapy for epilepsy typically involves drugs specific for the seizure type. Carbamazepine, phenytoin, valproic acid, ethosuximide, and phenobarbital are among the most commonly prescribed drugs.

▼**FIRST-LINE DRUG**
carbamazepine
Adult dosage
5 to 20 mg/kg/day P.O. divided in two or three doses
Points to remember
- Adjust dosage to patient's response and therapeutic serum drug level of 4 to 12 mcg/ml.
- Monitor CBC and differential count; carbamazepine may cause bone marrow suppression.

▼**FIRST-LINE DRUG**
ethosuximide
Adult dosage
15 to 40 mg/kg/day P.O. divided in one or two doses
Point to remember
- Therapeutic serum drug levels range from 40 to 100 mcg/ml.

▼**FIRST-LINE DRUG**
phenobarbital sodium
Adult dosage
- 20 mg/kg P.O. or I.V. as loading dose; for maintenance, 1 to 3 mg/kg/day

Point to remember
- Therapeutic serum drug levels range from 15 to 40 mcg/ml.

▼FIRST-LINE DRUG
phenytoin
Adult dosage
15 to 20 mg/kg P.O. or I.V. as loading dose; for maintenance, 5 to 7 mg/kg/day divided in one or two doses
Point to remember
- Therapeutic total serum drug levels range from 10 to 20 mcg/ml; therapeutic free serum drug levels range from 1 to 2 mcg/ml.

▼FIRST-LINE DRUG
valproic acid
Adult dosage
10 to 20 mg/kg/day P.O., divided in three or four doses
Points to remember
- Therapeutic serum drug levels range from 50 to 100 mcg/ml.
- Monitor liver function tests before starting therapy and periodically thereafter.

gabapentin
Adult dosage
900 mg/day P.O., divided in three or four doses daily
Points to remember
- This is a second-line drug.
- Adjust dosage in renal impairment.

lamotrigine
Adult dosage
50 to 100 mg/day P.O.
Points to remember
- This drug is used as adjunctive therapy for certain seizure types.
- It may cause a rash. ■

Headache

Treatment of headache depends on the type of headache present. Tension headache calls for nonnarcotic analgesics (NSAIDs or aspirin) and relaxation techniques.

Patients with migraine headache should avoid precipitating factors; they may need prophylactic or symptomatic drug therapy. During acute migraine attacks, many patients also find it helpful to rest in a dark, quiet room until symptoms subside. Patients who get more than two or three migraines per month and patients who get vascular headaches may benefit from prophylactic drugs. Drug therapy also may be indicated for cluster headaches.

ergot alkaloids
Adult dosage
Cafergot (containing ergotamine tartrate, 1 mg, and caffeine, 100 mg): 1 to 2 tablets P.O. at onset of headache or warning symptoms, followed by 1 tablet q 30 minutes, if necessary; may give up to 6 tablets per attack and 10 tab-

lets per week; or give ½ to 1 cafergot suppository P.R. Dihydroergotamine mesylate: 1 mg I.M. or I.V., repeated at 1-hour intervals to maximum of 3 mg I.M. or 2 mg I.V. (maximum weekly dose: 6 mg I.M. or I.V.) Ergotamine: one 2-mg tablet S.L. initially, then 1 to 2 mg q 30 minutes to maximum of 6 mg/day and 10 mg/week. Or 1 inhalation of ergotamine inhaler initially; if headache doesn't subside in 5 minutes, repeat 1 inhalation; may repeat inhalations at least 5 minutes apart to maximum of 6 inhalations in 24 hours or 15 inhalations weekly

Points to remember

- Ergot alkaloids are most effective when used during prodromal stage or at onset of headache.
- Urge patient to immediately report numbness or tingling in fingers or toes or red or violet blisters on hands or feet.
- Oral drugs may be ineffective during acute headache because of vomiting or impaired drug absorption.
- These drugs are contraindicated in pregnant patients.

methysergide maleate

Adult dosage

4 to 8 mg/day P.O. in divided doses given with meals

Points to remember

- Administer only during cluster headache. Don't use for acute migraine, vascular headache, or tension headache.
- Monitor patient closely; this drug may cause retroperitoneal and pleuropulmonary fibrosis and fibrous thickening of cardiac valves.
- To minimize GI upset, introduce drug gradually and give with food.
- This drug is contraindicated in pregnancy.

sumatriptan succinate

Adult dosage

6 mg S.C. (maximum recommended dosage: two 6-mg S.C. injections in 24 hours given at least 1 hour apart)

Points to remember

- Don't give I.V. because coronary vasospasm may occur.
- Use cautiously in patients at risk for coronary artery disease; serious or life-threatening arrhythmias occasionally occur.

For prophylaxis against headache

clonidine hydrochloride

Adult dosage

0.2 to 0.6 mg/day P.O. divided in three doses

Point to remember

- Don't stop therapy abruptly; taper dosage when discontinuing drug.

cyproheptadine hydrochloride
Adult dosage
12 to 20 mg/day P.O. divided in three or four doses, to maximum of 0.5 mg/kg/day
Point to remember
- Sedative effect disappears within 3 or 4 days.

propranolol hydrochloride
Adult dosage
80 to 240 mg P.O. t.i.d. or q.i.d.
Points to remember
- To increase drug absorption, give drug with meals.
- Don't stop therapy abruptly; taper dosage when discontinuing drug. ■

Meningitis

Antibiotic therapy for this life-threatening CNS infection must begin immediately after lumbar puncture. Common causative pathogens include *Streptococcus pneumoniae, Neisseria meningitidis,* and *Haemophilus influenzae.* Ideally, drug selection is based on results of culture and sensitivity testing. However, empiric therapy (described below) may be used.

third-generation cephalosporins
Adult dosage
Cefotaxime: 2 to 3 g I.V. q 6 hours
Ceftazidime: 2 to 4 g I.V. q 8 hours
Ceftriaxone: 2 g I.V. q 12 hours
Points to remember
- If methicillin-resistant *Staphylococcus aureus* is suspected, vancomycin should be added (intrathecal or intraventricular admnistration may be necessary).
- If gram-negative organism is suspected, gentamicin should be added (intrathecal or intraventricular administration may be necessary).
- An antipseudomonal penicillin may be substituted for third-generation cephalosporin if organism is susceptible.
- Ampicillin should be added if *Listeria monocytogenes* is suspected; usual dose is 2 g I.V. q 4 to 6 hours.
- Chloramphenicol is an alternative for patients who are allergic to penicillin or cephalosporins; usual dose is 4 to 6 g/day I.V. in four divided doses.
- In AIDS patients, opportunistic infections should be treated empirically. ■

Multiple sclerosis

No treatment can prevent multiple sclerosis (MS) from progressing. Patients may recover partially from acute exacerbations but may suffer relapses without warning.

MS management includes measures to reduce muscle spasticity, relieve urinary incontinence, and ease other dysfunctions. Baclofen or diazepam may be used to relieve spasticity and flexor spasms; physical therapy also plays an important role.

interferon beta-1b
Adult dosage
8 million IU (0.25 mg) S.C. every other day
Points to remember
- Drug is indicated for patients with relapsing, remitting MS.
- Inject immediately after reconstitution.
- Bedtime administration may minimize mild flulike symptoms that commonly occur.
- Before therapy starts and at periodic intervals, most doctors order the following laboratory tests: hemoglobin, CBC, platelet count, and blood chemistry profile (including liver function tests).

prednisone
Adult dosage
60 to 80 mg/day P.O. for 1 week; reduce dosage gradually over the next 2 or 3 weeks
Points to remember
- This drug may be used to hasten recovery from acute MS relapses; long-term therapy provides no benefit and doesn't prevent relapses.
- Prednisone therapy may follow methylprednisolone administration (1 g I.V. for 3 days). ■

Myasthenia gravis

The chief treatments for this disease are anticholinesterase drugs, immunosuppressants, thymectomy, and plasmapheresis. Aminoglycosides should be avoided because they may exacerbate myasthenia gravis.

▼FIRST-LINE DRUGS

anticholinesterase drugs
Adult dosage
Neostigmine: 7.5 to 30 mg P.O. q.i.d.
Pyridostigmine bromide: 60 mg P.O. three to five times daily
Points to remember
- Tailor dosage to patient's requirements throughout the day.
- Overdose may cause increased weakness.

immunosuppressants
Adult dosage
Azathioprine: 50 mg/day P.O.
Prednisone: 15 to 25 mg/day P.O.; increase by 5 mg/day at 2- to 3-day intervals until patient shows marked improvement or reaches dose of 50 mg/day; maintain this dose for 1 to 3 months, then grad-

ually switch to alternate-day regimen over 1 to 2 months

Points to remember

- Prednisone or another corticosteroid is indicated for patients who have undergone thymectomy and respond poorly to anticholinesterase drugs.
- Monitor patients on long-term prednisone therapy to prevent or relieve adverse effects.
- Azathioprine may enhance therapeutic effects of prednisone (or another glucocorticoid) and may permit reduction in prednisone dosage. ■

Parkinson's disease

Currently no drug cure for Parkinson's disease exists. A regimen of exercise and rest is the therapy of choice for patients with mild symptoms.

▼FIRST-LINE DRUGS

levodopa or levodopa-carbidopa

Adult dosage

100 mg P.O. t.i.d. initially (levodopa only); or (for combination product) one tablet containing 25 mg of carbidopa with 100 mg of levodopa P.O. b.i.d. initially, to maximum dosage of 200 mg of carbidopa with 800 mg of levodopa

Points to remember

- Although levodopa is the most effective drug for treating Parkinson's disease, its therapeutic effectiveness decreases with time.
- A "drug holiday" may restore drug efficacy, but symptoms may increase dramatically during this period. Usually, drug is tapered gradually, not discontinued abruptly.
- Combining levodopa with carbidopa decreases incidence of side effects and allows reduction in levodopa dosage.
- Patients requiring higher levodopa dosages should receive levodopa-carbidopa tablets containing 25 mg of carbidopa and 250 mg of levodopa.
- Increase dosage slowly over several weeks to minimize GI upset.
- Use caution when administering these drugs with antihypertensives, phenytoin, or antipsychotics and when giving them to patients with a history of glaucoma, MI, peptic ulcer disease, or urine retention.

amantadine hydrochloride

Adult dosage

100 mg P.O. b.i.d. to maximum of 400 mg/day

Points to remember

- Amantadine is an option for first-line therapy. However, many patients develop tolerance after 6 to 12 weeks.

- Amantadine may worsen edema, CHF, and seizures.
- Elderly patients and those with renal impairment may require lower dosages.
- To prevent acute worsening of symptoms, don't abruptly discontinue drug. Instead, decrease dosage gradually.

benztropine mesylate
Adult dosage
0.5 to 6 mg/day P.O.
Points to remember
- Benztropine is an option for first-line therapy. It may also be used in combination with levodopa.
- This drug is more effective against tremors and rigidity than against bradykinesia.
- Instruct patient to take drug with food to decrease GI upset.
- Advise patient to avoid alcoholic beverages and other CNS depressants.

bromocriptine mesylate
Adult dosage
1.25 mg P.O. once or twice daily initially; increase by 1.25 mg/day q 1 to 2 weeks until maximum effect is reached
Points to remember
- Bromocryptine usually is added to levodopa regimen when levodopa efficacy decreases or patient can't tolerate higher levodopa dosages.
- Dosages above 30 mg/day haven't been shown to increase efficacy.
- Use caution when administering to patients with hypertension.
- Disulfiram reaction may occur when drug is taken with alcohol.

pergolide mesylate
Adult dosage
0.05 mg/day P.O. for 2 days; then increase gradually by 0.1 to 0.15 mg/day q 3 days to maximum of 5 mg/day
Points to remember
- Pergolide usually is added to levodopa regimen when levodopa efficacy decreases or patient can't tolerate higher levodopa dosages.
- Administer with food to decrease nausea.
- Give drug at night to minimize dizziness.

selegiline hydrochloride
Adult dosage
5 mg/day P.O. taken at breakfast and lunch
Points to remember
- Selegiline is added to levodopa regimen when levodopa efficacy decreases or patient can't tolerate higher levodopa dosages.
- Most patients don't receive more than 10 mg/day.

trihexyphenidyl hydrochloride
Adult dosage
1 to 15 mg/day P.O.

Points to remember

- Trihexyphenidyl is an option for first-line therapy. It may also be used in combination with levodopa.
- This drug is more effective against tremors and rigidity than against bradykinesia.
- Instruct patient to take drug with food to decrease GI upset.
- Advise patient to avoid alcoholic beverages and other CNS depressants. ■

Status epilepticus

In this life-threatening condition, a patent airway must be maintained and the patient's head and tongue protected. If an artificial airway can't be inserted, the patient is placed on his side to prevent aspiration of secretions or saliva. An I.V. infusion of normal saline solution is begun. Because hypoglycemia may cause seizures, patients may receive 100 mg of thiamine and 50 ml of 50% dextrose by I.V. push.

Once the initial seizures are controlled with drugs, therapy focuses on preventing seizure recurrence by trying to determine, and then eliminate, their cause (such as electrolyte disorders, sepsis, tumors, and hypoxia).

benzodiazepines

Adult dosage

Diazepam: 10 mg I.V. (one-time dose) for acute management; 100 mg in 500 ml of D_5W (0.2 mg/ml) at 8 mg/hour for long-term control

Lorazepam: 0.1 to 0.15 mg/kg I.V. (up to 4 mg for 2 doses) for acute management

Points to remember

- Benzodiazepines are indicated for acute management of seizures. I.V. diazepam infusion may also be used for prolonged control of seizures. However, because lorazepam has longer duration of action, I.V. infusion is rarely necessary.
- Dilute lorazepam with an equal amount of normal saline solution before injection.
- Don't exceed infusion rate of 2 mg/minute.
- Withdrawal syndromes may occur in patients receiving these drugs for more than 2 weeks.

phenobarbital

Adult dosage

8 to 20 mg/kg I.V., no faster than 100 mg/minute; may divide in two to four doses given at 30-minute and 1-hour intervals

Points to remember

- Phenobarbital is used after acute treatment with benzodiazepines and in patients whose seizures are uncontrolled by (or who can't tolerate) phenytoin.

- Avoid extravasation.
- Dose-dependent sedative. Monitor patient's blood pressure and respiratory rate during administration.
- Phenobarbital may cause agitation, confusion, and depression in elderly patients.
- This drug is contraindicated in patients with a history of serious reaction to barbiturates (such as Stevens-Johnson syndrome, hives, or hepatotoxicity).

phenytoin
Adult dosage
18 to 20 mg/kg I.V. loading dose at 20 to 40 mg/minute (not to exceed 50 mg/minute); then 200 to 400 mg/day P.O. as maintenance dose
Points to remember
- Phenytoin is usually given for more prolonged seizure control after acute treatment with a benzodiazepine.
- It may be given through an I.V. line infusing normal saline solution, or it may be diluted in 100 to 500 ml of half-normal or normal saline solution. (Don't dilute with D_5W.) If diluted, prepare solution immediately before use, infuse no longer than 1 hour, and use a 0.45- to 0.22-micron in-line filter.
- Hypotension and arrhythmias may occur even at administration rates below 50 mg/minute. If they do, decrease infusion rate or temporarily stop infusion.
- In elderly patients, decrease maximum infusion rate to 25 mg/minute.
- Avoid extravasation, and don't give I.M. Drug's high pH may cause local irritation and skin sloughing.
- Loading dose may last up to 24 hours. Therapy may be continued with phenytoin or an alternative agent.
- Patients who have previously received this drug may receive smaller loading dose, depending on serum levels. However, in status epilepticus, don't withhold loading dose while awaiting serum drug levels.
- Drug is contraindicated in patients with a history of serious reaction to phenytoin (such as rash, hepatotoxicity, Stevens-Johnson syndrome, or toxic epidermal necrolysis). ■

Trigeminal neuralgia

Patients with this painful facial nerve disorder may require surgery or microvascular decompression if they don't respond to or can't tolerate drug therapy.

▼FIRST-LINE DRUG
carbamazepine
Adult dosage
100 mg/day P.O. initially; titrate to 200 mg q.i.d. as needed

Points to remember

- If patient is pain-free, adjust dosage periodically or withdraw drug.
- Patients who are allergic to TCAs may exhibit cross-sensitivity to carbamazepine.
- During long-term therapy, monitor CBC, platelet count, and serum carbamazepine levels.
- Advise patient to take drug in divided doses with food. Increasing dosage slowly over several weeks decreases GI upset.
- Some patients develop increased sensitivity to sunlight while taking this drug. Advise patient to avoid excessive sunlight and tanning booths and to use sunblock with SPF of 15 or higher.
- This drug is contraindicated in absence, myoclonic, or atonic seizures; heart block; blood dyscrasias; and bone marrow depression.
- Discontinue drug if patient develops rash.
- Elderly patients are more likely to suffer certain side effects, such as confusion, agitation, bradyarrhythmias, heart block, and syndrome of inappropriate antidiuretic hormone secretion.

phenytoin

Adult dosage

200 to 600 mg/day P.O.

Points to remember

- Phenytoin is an alternative drug for patients who can't tolerate carbamazepine.
- Divide dosages greater than 300 mg/day to maximize absorption.
- Increase total daily dosage gradually over several intervals, by no more than 100 mg/day.
- Phenytoin preparations aren't interchangeable. Tell patient not to change brands or generic preparations without consulting the doctor.
- Drug is contraindicated in patients with a history of serious reaction to phenytoin (such as rash, hepatotoxicity, Stevens-Johnson syndrome, or toxic epidermal necrolysis). ■

MUSCULOSKELETAL DISORDERS

Gout

Drug therapy for gout aims to reduce serum uric acid levels and relieve pain and inflammation. Patients should avoid obesity, fasting, excessive alcohol, and dehydration. They should also avoid hydrochlorothiazide, furosemide, low-dose aspirin, and nicotinic acid because these drugs may worsen hyperuricemia. Sudden reduction of serum uric acid levels may trigger gouty arthritis attacks; thus, gouty arthritis attacks and hyperuricemia must be treated separately.

▼FIRST-LINE DRUG

allopurinol

Adult dosage

100 mg/day P.O. for 1 week; increase dosage if serum uric acid level remains high

Points to remember

- This drug is used for long-term therapy.
- Daily doses of 200 to 300 mg may maintain normal serum uric acid level.
- Use cautiously in renal insufficiency.
- Allopurinol is contraindicated in asymptomatic hyperuricemia.

▼FIRST-LINE DRUG

indomethacin

Adult dosage

50 mg P.O. q 8 hours

Points to remember

- This agent is an NSAID; other NSAIDs may be substituted.
- Patients should continue to take this drug until symptoms resolve.

colchicine

Adult dosage

Acute attack: 0.5 to 0.6 mg P.O. q hour until pain subsides or until nausea or diarrhea occurs
Long-term prophylaxis: 0.6 mg P.O. b.i.d.

Points to remember

- Usual total dose is 4 to 8 mg.
- Colchicine is contraindicated in inflammatory bowel disease.

corticosteroids

Adult dosage

Methylprednisolone: 40 mg/day I.V.; decrease dosage over 7 days
Prednisone: 40 to 60 mg/day P.O.; decrease dosage over 7 days
Triamcinolone: 10 to 40 mg intra-articularly

Point to remember

- These drugs are reserved for acute attacks in patients who can't take oral NSAIDs.

uricosuric agents

Adult dosage

Probenecid: 0.5 g/day P.O.; increase gradually to 1 to 2 g/day
Sulfinpyrazone: 100 mg/day P.O.; increase gradually to 200 to 400 mg/day

Points to remember

- These agents are used for long-term therapy in patients with increasingly frequent or severe acute attacks of gout.
- They're not effective in patients with renal insufficiency.
- Patients should maintain daily urine output of 2,000 ml or more to minimize uric acid precipitation in urinary tract. ■

Osteoarthritis

Patients with this disease may require orthopedic measures to correct developmental anomalies, deformities, disparity in leg lengths, and severely damaged joint surfaces. To relieve pain, salicylates or NSAIDs and muscle relaxants (in low doses) may be given.

aspirin
Adult dosage
0.6 to 1 g (two to three 300-mg tablets) P.O. q.i.d. with meals and h.s.; then titrate dosage upward until desired response occurs
Points to remember
- Drug is used as an analgesic and anti-inflammatory agent.
- Instruct patient to take drug with meals and to take a mild antacid between meals to reduce GI distress.
- Tinnitus may indicate drug toxicity.

ibuprofen
Adult dosage
400 to 800 mg P.O. q.i.d.
Points to remember
- Drug is used as an analgesic and anti-inflammatory agent.
- Instruct patient to take drug with food or milk to reduce GI upset.
- Therapeutic effects may take up to 1 month to achieve.

naproxen
Adult dosage
250 mg P.O. b.i.d. to a maximum of 1,250 mg/day.
Points to remember
- Drug is used as an analgesic and anti-inflammatory agent.
- Avoid use with aspirin and alcohol. ■

Osteoporosis

Specific treatment varies with the underlying cause of osteoporosis. Hormone therapy is most commonly used. Many patients also take supplementary calcium salts that provide up to 1 g/day of calcium. Patients with malabsorption or osteomalacia may also need vitamin D (2,000 to 5,000 units/day). Instruct them to consume adequate dietary protein, calcium, and vitamin D.

▼FIRST-LINE DRUGS

estrogens
Adult dosage
Conjugated estrogens: 0.625 to 1.25 mg/day P.O.
Estradiol: 1 to 2 mg/day P.O.
Ethinyl estradiol: 0.02 to 0.05 mg/day P.O.

Point to remember
- Women with an intact uterus must take estrogen with progestin (medroxyprogesterone acetate) to reduce risk of endometrial cancer. Cycled regimen involves estrogen on calendar days 1 through 25 each month and medroxyprogesterone on calendar days 16 through 25.

calcitonin
Adult dosage
100 IU/day S.C.
Points to remember
- This drug must be given parenterally.
- Drug's efficacy is limited.

diphosphonates
Adult dosage
Etidronate disodium: 400 mg/day P.O. for 2 weeks q 3 months
Pamidronate disodium: 30 mg I.V. once q 3 months
Point to remember
- These drugs may cause electrolyte disturbances. ■

Paget's disease

Most patients with Paget's disease don't require treatment. Therapy is reserved for patients with persistent pain, neuronal compression, progressive deformities, heart failure, hypercalcemia, renal stones, or repeated fractures.

Mild pain may be controlled with NSAIDs, such as ibuprofen or indomethacin. Total hip replacement or osteotomy may be necessary for patients with deformities or fractures. To prevent or minimize hypercalcemia, maintain good hydration and help the patient ambulate after orthopedic procedures.

calcitonin
Adult dosage
Human: 500 mcg/day S.C.; may decrease to two to three times per week
Salmon: 50 to 100 IU S.C. two to three times per week
Points to remember
- This drug is indicated for patients with moderate to severe bone pain that's not controlled by NSAIDs.
- To minimize side effects, start at lower dosage, and then increase dosage gradually over 2 weeks. Also, give drug at bedtime.
- Use reconstituted solution within 6 hours.
- Protect the solution from light. Inspect for discoloration or particles before use.
- Over time, patient may show decreased response to salmon calcitonin.

etidronate disodium
Adult dosage
5 to 10 mg/kg/day P.O. (for no more than 6 months) or 11 to 20 mg/kg/day P.O. (for

no more than 3 months); if relapse occurs, treatment may be repeated in 3 to 12 months

Points to remember

- Drug is indicated for patients with moderate to severe pain or neural compression that's not controlled by NSAIDs.
- Drug effects may last up to 1 year after discontinuation.
- To maximize drug absorption, tell patient to take drug on empty stomach.
- Dividing daily dose may minimize nausea and vomiting.
- Advise patient not to take drug with milk or milk products, antacids, or mineral (calcium, magnesium, iron, or aluminum) supplements.
- Warn patient that drug may take 1 to 3 months to bring noticeable improvement.
- Patients with renal impairment may need decreased dosages.

NSAIDs (various)

Adult dosage

Ibuprofen: 400 to 800 mg P.O. t.i.d., not exceeding 3.2 g/day

Naproxen: 250 to 500 mg P.O. b.i.d., not exceeding 1.5 g/day

Piroxicam: 20 to 40 mg/day P.O.

Sulindac: 150 to 200 mg/day P.O.

Points to remember

- These drugs are useful for relieving mild pain.
- Give with food or antacids to minimize GI upset.
- Instruct patient to avoid alcoholic beverages.
- Don't administer to patients with aspirin sensitivity, bleeding disorders, active bleeding, or peptic ulcer disease. Use caution when administering to patients with a history of peptic ulcers or those receiving heparin, warfarin, or thrombolytic agents.

pamidronate disodium

Adult dosage

30 mg I.V. over 4 to 24 hours weekly for six doses

Points to remember

- Drug is indicated for patients with neural compression or moderate to severe pain that's not controlled by NSAIDs.
- Don't mix this drug with calcium-containing fluids, such as lactated Ringer's solution.
- Use caution when administering to elderly patients or those with renal or heart failure. Monitor serum electrolyte levels, and check for fluid overload. Lower dosages or slower administration rates may be necessary. ■

Tendinitis and bursitis

Treatment for these conditions includes resting the involved joint and avoiding joint trauma and overuse. A rotator cuff tear may require surgical repair if it doesn't respond to physical therapy and NSAIDs.

▼FIRST-LINE DRUGS

NSAIDs (various)

Adult dosage

Ibuprofen: 400 to 800 mg P.O. t.i.d., not exceeding 3.2 g/day
Naproxen: 250 to 500 mg P.O. b.i.d., not exceeding 1.5 g/day
Piroxicam: 20 to 40 mg/day P.O.
Sulindac: 150 to 200 mg/day P.O.

Points to remember

- Don't administer to patients with aspirin sensitivity, bleeding disorders, active bleeding, or peptic ulcer disease.
- To minimize GI upset, instruct patient to take these drugs with food or antacids or to use enteric-coated aspirin products.
- Instruct patient to avoid alcoholic beverages.
- Use caution when administering to patients with a history of peptic ulcers or those receiving heparin, warfarin, or thrombolytic agents.

betamethasone sodium phosphate

Adult dosage

1.5 to 12 mg intra-articularly or 6 mg intrabursally

Points to remember

- Betamethasone (or another corticosteroid) is used to treat bursitis and tendinitis that don't respond to NSAIDs.
- Dosage depends on joint size and location and degree of inflammation. For example, 1.5 to 3 mg may be given for tendons, 6 to 12 mg for larger joints, and 1.5 to 6 mg for smaller joints.
- Effects of injection should last 1 to 2 weeks; however, injection may be repeated as often as every 3 to 7 days.
- Before injection, 1% to 2% lidocaine may be mixed in syringe to minimize pain of injection. However, don't use preparations containing parabens or phenol.
- Use sterile technique to avoid infection.
- Local administration minimizes potential for systemic side effects. ■

G.I. DISORDERS

Cirrhosis

Irreversible cirrhosis usually results from chronic alcohol ingestion. Liver transplantation is the only definitive therapy. Drugs are used to manage the sequelae of cirrhosis, such as portal hypertension, varices, ascites, and hepatic encephalopathy. Correction of nutritional deficiencies, protein restriction, and alcohol avoidance are important adjunctive measures.

▼FIRST-LINE DRUG

spironolactone

Adult dosage

150 to 400 mg/day P.O. in divided doses

Points to remember

- Drug reduces ascites while preventing hypokalemia.
- The usual goal is to reduce the patient's weight by approximately 1 lb/day.
- Monitor patient's BUN and serum electrolyte levels.

furosemide

Adult dosage

40 to 240 mg/day P.O. or I.V. in single or divided doses

Points to remember

- This drug is used to treat ascites in patients who don't respond to spironolactone.
- Monitor patient's fluid status, serum electrolyte levels, blood pressure, BUN, and creatinine levels.
- This drug has a stronger diuretic effect than spironolactone.

lactulose

Adult dosage

30 to 45 ml P.O. t.i.d. or q.i.d. until diarrhea ensues; then reduce dosage to minimum required to produce two to four soft bowel movements daily

Points to remember

- Lactulose is used to treat portal-systemic encephalopathy.
- Drug can be diluted in water, fruit juice, or milk to disguise taste.
- When giving lactulose by nasogastric tube, dilute well to prevent vomiting.

vasopressin

Adult dosage

0.2 to 0.4 units/minute I.V. via peripheral vein

Points to remember

- This drug is used to constrict vessels in bleeding esophageal varices.
- It's often used in conjunction with balloon tamponade.
- Administer only in intensive care setting.
- Usually, drug effect is temporary and rebleeding recurs. ■

Corrosive esophagitis and stricture

Drug therapy, the first-line treatment for these disorders, aims to reduce gastric acidity and enhance GI motility. Adjunctive drug therapy includes antacids, especially alginic, acid-based products such as Gaviscon. Additional measures include avoiding cigarettes and alcohol, avoiding meals within 3 hours of bedtime, elevating the head of the bed, and losing weight. Resistant strictures usually must be manually dilated.

▼FIRST-LINE DRUGS

H_2-receptor antagonists

Adult dosage

Cimetidine: 300 to 600 mg/day P.O. q.i.d.; alternatively, 400 to 600 mg P.O. b.i.d.
Famotidine: 20 to 40 mg P.O. b.i.d.
Nizatidine: 150 to 300 mg P.O. b.i.d. to t.i.d.
Ranitidine hydrochloride: 150 to 300 mg P.O. b.i.d. to t.i.d.

Points to remember

- These drugs reduce acid production so that less acid is available for reflux into the esophagus.
- Instruct patient to take drug 1 hour before meals and at bedtime.
- Higher dosages are needed to treat reflux disease than to treat peptic ulcer disease.
- Symptom recurrence often precludes reduction in maintenance dosage.
- Reduce dosage in elderly patients and in those with renal dysfunction.
- Cimetidine is available generically at reduced cost.

▼FIRST-LINE DRUG

prilosec

Adult dosage

20 mg P.O. once or twice daily

Points to remember

- Drug reduces acid production so that less acid is available for reflux into the esophagus.
- It's prescribed for patients with acute symptoms; many patients are maintained with ranitidine, famotidine, or nizatidine therapy.
- Patients taking a single daily dose should take it 1 hour before bedtime; those taking two daily doses should take one dose 1 hour before breakfast and the other at bedtime.
- Recommended maximum period for continuous therapy is 8 weeks.

cisapride

Adult dosage

10 to 20 mg P.O. q.i.d.

Points to remember

- This is a second-line drug added to prilosec or H_2-receptor antagonist regimen.
- Start with 10 mg q.i.d., and increase dosage if necessary.
- Instruct patient to take drug at least 15 minutes before meals.
- Reduce dosage in renal and hepatic dysfunction.

- Use cautiously in patients with underlying heart disease; drug may precipitate torsades des pointes in susceptible patients.
- This drug isn't recommended for children under age 18. ■

Crohn's disease

Drug therapy, the primary treatment for this disease, is directed at reducing symptoms, not achieving a cure. Adjunctive treatments include nutritional support and surgery to correct intestinal obstructions, fistulas, or intractable hemorrhage.

▼FIRST-LINE DRUG

sulfasalazine

Adult dosage

1 g P.O. t.i.d. to q.i.d.

Points to remember

- Drug is used to reduce inflammation in the GI tract.
- Don't administer to patients with known sulfa allergy.
- Instruct patient to maintain adequate fluid intake.
- Titrate dosage gradually to improve patient's tolerance of GI effects.
- This drug is available generically at lower cost.

mesalamine (Asacol)

Adult dosage

0.8 to 2.4 g/day P.O. in three divided doses

Points to remember

- When the large intestine is the only disease site, Asacol, a delayed-released form of mesalamine that doesn't act until it reaches the large intestine, is preferred.
- This drug is a more expensive alternative to sulfasalazine; generally, it's used in patients who are allergic to or can't tolerate sulfasalazine.
- Mesalamine isn't approved by the FDA for use in Crohn's disease.
- Patient must swallow tablet whole.
- Reduce dosage in renal dysfunction.

mesalamine (Pentasa)

Adult dosage

1.5 to 4 g/day P.O. in four divided doses

Points to remember

- For more widespread disease involvement, Pentasa, which is released sooner than Asacol, is preferred.
- This drug is a more expensive alternative to sulfasalazine; generally, it's used in patients who are allergic to or cannot tolerate sulfasalazine.
- Mesalamine isn't approved by the FDA for use in Crohn's disease.
- Patients with hepatic or renal dysfunction may require dosage reductions.

methylprednisolone
Adult dosage
1 to 2 mg/kg I.V. in divided doses for acute episodes
Points to remember
- Drug reduces inflammation in GI tract.
- Patient may begin oral prednisone therapy as soon as diarrhea and bleeding subside.
- High-dose initial therapy may be used in acute disease exacerbations.
- If patient has received high doses (more than 7.5 mg/day) for more than 10 days, taper dosage slowly to prevent adrenal crisis and disease exacerbation.
- Drug may cause or aggravate gastritis, peripheral edema, confusion, depression, or hypertension.

metronidazole
Adult dosage
250 to 500 mg P.O. q.i.d.
Points to remember
- Exact mechanism of action is unknown, but drug is thought to reduce colonization of organisms and toxin buildup in intestines.
- Drug may be used as an alternative to sulfasalazine; in some patients, it's used in combination with that drug.

prednisone
Adult dosage
2.5 to 60 mg/day P.O. in single or divided doses
Points to remember
- Drug is used for its anti-inflammatory effect in maintenance management of severe episodes of Crohn's disease and to reduce flare-ups; it's usually given after I.V. therapy with methylprednisolone.
- If patient has received high doses (more than 7.5 mg/day) for more than 10 days, taper dosage slowly to prevent adrenal crisis and disease exacerbation.
- This drug may cause or aggravate gastritis, peripheral edema, confusion, depression, or hypertension.
- Long-term use may accelerate osteoporosis, cataract formation, or glaucoma. ■

Diverticular disease

Treatment of this disease depends on its severity. The goal is to reduce inflammation caused by infection and to prevent perforation, intestinal obstruction, and fistulas. Patients must eat a high-fiber diet and drink plenty of fluids. Although drugs aren't used to manage the disease itself, they may be prescribed to treat associated infection or as a preventive strategy in patients with diverticulosis.

ampicillin
Adult dosage
500 mg I.V. q 6 hours

Points to remember
- Drug treats diverticulitis by decreasing bacterial colonization in intestine and reducing the risk of perforation.
- It's used in combination with clear liquid diet in mild diverticulitis.

cefazolin
Adult dosage
1 g I.V. q 8 hours
Points to remember
- Drug treats diverticulitis by decreasing bacterial colonization in intestine and reducing the risk of perforation.
- It's used in patients who are allergic to ampicillin.

clindamycin
Adult dosage
300 to 900 mg I.V. t.i.d.
Points to remember
- Drug is used in combination with gentamicin and metronidazole to treat severe diverticulitis with or without perforation and subsequent peritonitis.
- It must be diluted before I.V. injection.
- If persistent diarrhea develops, drug should be stopped or patient monitored closely.

gentamicin
Adult dosage
60 to 100 mg I.V. q 8 hours
Points to remember
- This drug is used in combination with clindamycin and metronidazole in acutely ill patients with diverticulitis with or without perforation and subsequent peritonitis.
- Monitor patient's renal function closely.
- Reduce dosage in elderly patients and those with renal dysfunction.

metronidazole
Adult dosage
15 mg/kg I.V. as a loading dose, then 7.5 mg/kg I.V. q 6 hours
Points to remember
- This drug is used in combination with gentamicin and clindamycin to treat severe diverticulitis.
- Reduce dosage in liver dysfunction. ■

Gastritis

Besides general supportive measures, management of gastritis aims to prevent further episodes, treat associated disease, and eliminate exacerbating agents. Drug therapy may help prevent gastritis and aid healing of lesions.

▼**FIRST-LINE DRUGS**

antacids
Adult dosage
Aluminum or magnesium hydroxide: 30 ml P.O. q 1 to 6 hours
Points to remember
- Shake suspension.

- Give antacid at least 1 hour apart from other medications.
- Monitor for aluminum or magnesium toxicity in patients with renal impairment.

▼FIRST-LINE DRUGS
H_2-receptor antagonists
Adult dosage
Cimetidine: 400 mg P.O. b.i.d. or 300 mg I.V. q 6 hours
Famotidine: 20 mg P.O. or I.V. b.i.d.
Ranitidine: 150 mg P.O. b.i.d. or 50 mg I.V. q 8 hours
Point to remember
- Adjust dosage in renal dysfunction.

▼FIRST-LINE DRUG
sucralfate
Adult dosage
1 g P.O. q 6 hours
Point to remember
- Sucralfate may inhibit absorption of other drugs; administer other medications 2 hours before or after sucralfate. ■

Gastroenteritis

When caused by *Salmonella* organisms, gastroenteritis doesn't require therapy. Drug therapy is indicated when gastroenteritis progresses and involves other body systems.

For gastroenteritis caused by **Shigella**

▼FIRST-LINE DRUG
co-trimoxazole (sulfamethoxazole-trimethoprim)
Adult dosage
One double-strength tablet (160 mg trimethoprim and 800 mg sulfamethoxazole) P.O. b.i.d. for 5 days
Point to remember
- Don't administer to patients with sulfonamide hypersensitivity.

ampicillin
Adult dosage
500 mg P.O. q.i.d. for 5 days
Points to remember
- Adjust dosage in renal dysfunction.
- Don't administer to patients with penicillin hypersensitivity.

ciprofloxacin
Adult dosage
500 mg P.O. q 12 hours for 5 days
Points to remember
- Drug may increase the risk of theophylline toxicity in patients who are also receiving theophylline; monitor serum theophylline levels closely.
- Instruct patient to avoid taking antacids and to drink plenty of fluids during therapy.

***For gastroenteritis caused by* Campylobacter**

▼FIRST-LINE DRUG
ciprofloxacin
Adult dosage
500 mg P.O. q 12 hours for 5 days
Points to remember
- Drug may increase the risk of theophylline toxicity in patients who are also receiving theophylline; monitor serum theophylline levels closely.
- Instruct patient to avoid taking antacids and to drink plenty of fluids during therapy.

▼FIRST-LINE DRUG
erythromycin
Adult dosage
500 mg P.O. q.i.d. for 5 days
Point to remember
- Erythromycin inhibits metabolism of other drugs eliminated by liver; stay alert for drug interactions.

***For gastroenteritis caused by* Entamoeba histolytica**

▼FIRST-LINE DRUG
metronidazole
Adult dosage
750 mg P.O. t.i.d. for 5 to 10 days
Point to remember
- Inform patient that drug may cause metallic taste and reddish brown urine.

▼FIRST-LINE DRUG
iodoquinol
Adult dosage
630 to 650 mg P.O. t.i.d. for 20 days
Point to remember
- This drug is administered after metronidazole therapy; both drugs must be given as first-line agents in recommended sequence. ■

Hepatic encephalopathy

Withhold dietary protein during acute episodes of this degenerative disease. Avoid giving narcotics or sedatives that are metabolized or excreted by the liver. Drug therapy aims to reduce serum ammonia levels.

▼FIRST-LINE DRUG
lactulose
Adult dosage
20 to 30 g P.O. t.i.d. or q.i.d. or as retention enema (over 30 to 60 minutes) in 700 ml of normal saline solution or sorbitol
Point to remember
- Titrate dosage so that patient passes no more than two or three soft stools per day.

▼FIRST-LINE DRUG
metronidazole
Adult dosage
250 mg P.O. t.i.d.

Point to remember

- This drug may cause metallic taste and reddish brown urine.

▼FIRST-LINE DRUG

neomycin sulfate

Adult dosage

500 mg to 1 g P.O. q 6 hours for 5 to 7 days

Point to remember

- This drug may cause diarrhea or malabsorption.

vancomycin hydrochloride

Adult dosage

1 g P.O. b.i.d.

Point to remember

- Reconstituted solution remains stable for 2 weeks when refrigerated. ■

Hepatitis, viral

Viral hepatitis is classified as hepatitis A, B, C, D, or E. Hepatitis A and E are self-limiting and warrant supportive measures. Hepatitis B, C, and D may become chronic and fulminant; when acute, they're managed with supportive measures. Fulminant cases are life-threatening and require emergency liver transplantation. Vaccines and immune globulin are available for preexposure and postexposure prophylaxis against hepatitis A and B. Interferon has been used to eradicate chronic hepatitis B and C.

For chronic hepatitis B

interferon alfa-2b

Adult dosage

30 to 35 million IU I.M. or S.C. per week administered as 5 million IU I.M. or S.C. q day, or 10 million units I.M. or S.C. three times a week for 16 weeks

Points to remember

- Discontinue drug if patient doesn't respond after 16 weeks.
- This agent may cause a flulike syndrome, which becomes milder over time. Giving acetaminophen before each dose may help.

For chronic hepatitis C

interferon alfa-2b

Adult dosage

3 million IU I.M or S.C. three times a week for up to 6 months

Points to remember

- Discontinue drug if patient doesn't respond after 16 weeks.
- Drug may cause flulike syndrome, which becomes milder over time. Giving acetaminophen before each dose may help. ■

Irritable bowel syndrome

Patients with this disorder should avoid GI stimulants, such as caffeine-containing beverages. Anxiety-reducing measures, including regular exercise and periods of quiet time, may also prove helpful. Anticholinergic agents may control symptoms in some patients. Psychotherapy with antianxiety drugs or antidepressants may also help.

dicyclomine hydrochloride
Adult dosage
20 to 40 mg P.O. q.i.d.
Point to remember
- Dosage should be increased to 160 mg/day unless side effects occur. ■

Liver abscess

Patients with liver abscess typically receive antimicrobial agents (third-generation cephalosporins and metronidazole) that are effective against the causative organisms. Hepatic candidiasis commonly responds to amphotericin B given I.V. If the patient doesn't respond rapidly and adequately, the doctor typically performs needle or surgical drainage.

amphotericin B
Adult dosage
0.25 mg I.V./day initially, increased gradually as tolerance allows, but should not exceed total daily dosage of 1.5 mg/kg; therapy continues until total dose of 2 to 9 g is given
Points to remember
- Drug is indicated for hepatic candidiasis.
- Administer by slow I.V. infusion.
- Monitor for possible side effects, including fever, shaking chills, malaise, joint pain, hypokalemia, and renal tubular acidosis. ■

Pancreatitis

Acute pancreatitis is usually self-limiting, and most patients improve within 3 to 7 days. Treatment includes analgesics for pain and I.V. fluids to maintain intravascular volume. Fasting reduces pancreatic secretions (however, with prolonged fasting, the patient may require parenteral nutrition). After several days of bowel rest, a diet is usually resumed gradually, starting with clear liquids. Patients with mild to moderate pancreatitis also may receive nasogastric suction to decrease gastric contents in the duodenum.

Patients with chronic pain and malabsorption may require pancreatic enzymes. Anticholinergics and H_2-antagonists aren't indicated for acute pancreatitis; antibiotics aren't necessary unless infection is present. Surgery may be necessary to drain and remove necrotic tissue.

Intermittent attacks of chronic pancreatitis are treated the same as acute pancreatitis. Patients should avoid alcoholic beverages and fatty foods. Pancreatic duct obstruction or pseudocysts may warrant surgery.

pancreatic enzymes
Adult dosage
Pancrelipase: three to eight tablets or capsules taken with meals
Points to remember
- Pancreatic enzymes are used to treat chronic pain and malabsorption. They shouldn't be given for acute pancreatitis.
- Tell patient to take the drug before or with meals.
- Caution patient not to take pancreatic enzymes at the same time as iron supplements or antacids.
- Instruct patient not to chew or crush tablets or capsules.
- Tell patient not to change drug brands without consulting the doctor. ■

Peptic ulcer disease

Treatment of peptic ulcer disease includes nondrug therapy, such as stopping smoking, avoiding alcohol and caffeinated beverages, and discontinuing NSAIDs and glucocorticoids, if possible. Bland diets don't seem to help. Some patients may require treatment for acute GI bleeding.

Relapses of peptic ulcer disease are common and may be related to infection with Helicobacter pylori and cigarette smoking. Frequent relapses may warrant maintenance therapy with H_2-receptor antagonists, antibiotics, surgery, or a combination of these. To eradicate H. pylori, metronidazole may be given in conjunction with bismuth subsalicylate; tetracycline or amoxicillin may be added. Antacids may be given to decrease pain; however, their use as primary therapy is limited by side effects (such as diarrhea) and the need for frequent administration.

▼FIRST-LINE DRUGS

H_2-receptor antagonists
Adult dosage
Cimetidine: 400 to 1,200 mg/day P.O.
Famotidine: 20 to 40 mg/day P.O.

Ranitidine hydrochloride: 150 to 300 mg/day P.O.
Nizatidine: 150 to 300 mg/day P.O.

Points to remember

- These drugs are especially useful in milder disease.
- Various regimens may be used, depending on indication for therapy and the drug used.
- Initial therapy usually lasts 8 weeks. For maintenance, these drugs typically are given in single dose at bedtime.

bismuth subsalicylate

Adult dosage

525 mg P.O. q.i.d.

Points to remember

- This drug, given in combination with metronidazole, is first-line therapy for eradicating *H. pylori.*
- Use cautiously when administering to patients with salicylate sensitivity or bleeding disorders and to those receiving anticoagulants, heparin, or high-dose salicylate therapy.
- Warn patient that drug may turn stools black.
- Don't give this drug to pregnant women or to children with signs or symptoms of influenza or varicella.
- Emphasize importance of completing full course of therapy.

metronidazole

Adult dosage

250 mg P.O. t.i.d.

Points to remember

- This drug, given in combination with bismuth subsalicylate, is first-line therapy against *H. pylori.*
- Instruct patient to avoid alcoholic beverages during therapy.
- Don't give to patients taking warfarin or to women in first trimester of pregnancy.
- Patients with hepatic disease may need lower doses.
- Emphasize importance of completing full course of therapy.

misoprostol

Adult dosage

100 to 400 mcg P.O. q.i.d.

Points to remember

- This drug is used for long-term prevention of gastric ulcers caused by NSAIDs. It isn't indicated for short-term or long-term treatment of peptic ulcers.
- Misoprostol is absolutely contraindicated during pregnancy. Warn women of childbearing age to use an adequate form of contraception.

omeprazole

Adult dosage

10 to 20 mg/day P.O. for 4 to 8 weeks

Points to remember

- Omeprazole is an alternate first-line drug.
- Inform patient that capsule may be opened, if necessary, but that coated beads inside shouldn't be crushed.

- This drug isn't recommended for maintenance therapy because of risk of long-term achlorhydria.

sucralfate
Adult dosage
1 g P.O. q.i.d. 1 hour before meals and h.s.; or 2 g b.i.d. for 4 to 8 weeks of initial treatment
Points to remember
- This is an alternate first-line drug.
- Tell patient to take drug on empty stomach.
- If patient is receiving tube feedings, withhold feeding for 1 to 2 hours before and after sucralfate administration to prevent formation of gastric bezoars. Flush feeding tube with water before and after administration to prevent clogging.
- If needed, create suspension by placing one tablet in 20 to 30 ml of water. ■

Peritonitis

Supportive care for patients with peritonitis includes antibiotics, analgesics, and fluids. Initial antibiotic selection depends on the presumed infection source; the antibiotic regimen may be revised based on results of culture and sensitivity tests. Sometimes, combination therapy is necessary. Abdominal or pelvic abscesses or diverticula may require surgical intervention.

cephalosporins
Adult dosage
Cefotetan: 2 g I.V. q 12 hours
Cefoxitin: 2 g I.V. q 6 to 8 hours
Points to remember
- These drugs are prescribed for suspected gram-negative aerobic and anaerobic organisms.
- Use caution when administering these drugs to patients with a history of serious allergic reactions to cephalosporins or penicillins.
- Adjust dosage in renal dysfunction.
- Instruct patient to complete full course of antibiotic therapy.

clindamycin
Adult dosage
900 mg I.V. q 8 hours
Points to remember
- Clindamycin may be given as an alternative to metronidazole for suspected or isolated anaerobic organisms.
- Instruct patient to complete full course of antibiotic therapy.

gentamicin or tobramycin
Adult dosage
2 mg/kg I.V. initially, then 1.5 mg/kg q 8 hours; alternatively, total daily dose may be given q 12 to 24 hours

Points to remember
- These drugs are used to treat isolated or suspected gram-negative aerobic organisms.
- Reduce dosage in renal dysfunction.
- Instruct patient to complete full course of antibiotic therapy.

metronidazole
Adult dosage
500 mg I.V. q 6 hours for 7 to 10 days
Points to remember
- Drug is often prescribed when anaerobic organisms are the suspected cause of infection.
- Caution patient to avoid alcoholic beverages.
- Metronidazole is contraindicated in patients taking warfarin and during first trimester of pregnancy.
- Instruct patient to complete full course of therapy.
- Patients with hepatic disease may require lower dosages. ■

Pseudomembranous enterocolitis

During therapy for this inflammatory bowel disorder, discontinue unnecessary antibiotics or drugs that inhibit peristalsis, such as diphenoxylate. Some patients need fluid and electrolyte replacement. Relapses may occur after therapy from residual spores or failure to restore normal flora. Retreatment with the same drug or an alternative agent may be necessary.

▼FIRST-LINE DRUG
vancomycin hydrochloride
Adult dosage
125 mg P.O. q.i.d. for 7 to 10 days
Points to remember
- Drug is poorly absorbed from GI tract. Don't use in other systemic infections.
- Refrigerate drug after reconstitution. (It will remain stable for 14 days.)
- Emphasize need to complete full course of therapy.

cholestyramine
Adult dosage
4 g P.O. t.i.d. to q.i.d.
Points to remember
- This drug typically is prescribed for patients with mild disease.
- Instruct patient to mix drug in 2 oz (60 ml) of cold water or juice and then refill glass and drink again to make sure all medication has been taken.

metronidazole
Adult dosage
500 mg P.O. t.i.d. to q.i.d. for 7 to 10 days
Points to remember
- Metronidazole is an alternative drug.

- Drug is less expensive than vancomycin.
- Tell patient to avoid alcoholic beverages.
- Don't give to patients taking warfarin or to those in first trimester of pregnancy.
- Patients with hepatic disease may require lower dosages.
- Emphasize need to complete full course of therapy. ■

Ulcerative colitis

Supportive care for patients with this condition includes correcting fluid and electrolyte disorders. Severe anemia may warrant blood transfusions. Patients with severe disease typically receive parenteral or elemental enteral feedings to rest the bowel. Antidiarrheal agents, such as loperamide, diphenoxylate, and codeine, usually are avoided because they may cause toxic megacolon. A colectomy may be done in patients with severe disease who do not respond to medical therapy or who require long-term corticosteroid therapy. Patients with severe, chronic, debilitating disease may need psychiatric support and treatment for depression.

azathioprine
Adult dosage
1 to 2 mg/kg/day P.O.
Points to remember
- This drug may allow reduction in daily dosages of corticosteroids in patients requiring long-term corticosteroid therapy. It's not indicated for single-dose therapy.
- Administer in divided doses after meals to minimize GI upset.
- Reduce dosage in patients on concurrent allopurinol therapy and those with liver impairment.
- Monitor CBC weekly.
- Tell patient to avoid people with bacterial or viral infections and to avoid vaccinations containing live viruses.
- Warn patient that drug therapy may reactivate herpes zoster.
- Patients who are pregnant or breast-feeding should not take this drug.

corticosteroids
Adult dosage
45 to 60 mg/day P.O. of prednisone or its equivalent
Points to remember
- Patient should receive lowest dosage needed to control disease.
- After acute exacerbation of ulcerative colitis, dosage may be tapered over 2 to 3 months. Abrupt discontinuation after prolonged therapy may result in acute hypoadrenalism.
- Some patients continue to take lower doses (10 to 15

mg/day) on long-term basis to prevent relapses.
- To minimize adrenal suppression, give drug in the morning or every other day.

mesalamine
Adult dosage
4 g by retention enema nightly for 3 to 6 weeks
Points to remember
- This drug usually is prescribed for patients with mild distal proctocolitis. It also may given orally to patients who are allergic to sulfa drugs.
- Shake the suspension well before giving it.
- Recommend that patient empty bowel before administration and try to retain the enema all night.
- Alternate-night regimens are sometimes used.

sulfasalazine
Adult dosage
500 mg P.O. b.i.d. initially; increase by 500 mg/day to maximum of 4 to 6 g/day
Points to remember
- Sulfasalazine is indicated for mild to moderate acute ulcerative colitis and for prevention of relapses.
- Drug is contraindicated in patients with a history of G6PD deficiency, severe allergy to sulfa drugs, porphyria, or liver impairment.
- Tell patient to take drug with meals to decrease GI upset.
- Instruct patient to increase fluid intake to maintain urine output of 1,200 to 1,500 ml (about 1½ qt) daily.
- Advise patient to avoid excessive exposure to sunlight and to wear a sunblock with SPF of 15 or higher.
- Adjust dosage in renal dysfunction. ■

RENAL AND UROLOGIC DISORDERS

Glomerulonephritis, chronic

Treatment of chronic glomerulonephritis aims to prevent further disease progression (except in patients with end-stage disease). Managing hypertension and maintaining fluid and electrolyte balance are the mainstays of therapy.

For poststreptococcal-induced chronic glomerulonephritis, only supportive therapy is used, along with management of fluid overload and hypertension. For immunoglobulin G or A glomerulonephritis, corticosteroids, cytotoxic agents, or a combination may be used. Rapidly progressing glomerulonephritis may warrant corticosteroids, cytotoxic agents, and plasmapheresis.

For focal glomerulosclerosis, cytotoxic agents or

cyclosporine may be used. Patients with membranoproliferative glomerulonephritis may receive corticosteroids, anticoagulants, or dipyridamole. Membranous nephropathy and associated systemic lupus erythematosus commonly is treated with corticosteroids, cytotoxic agents, or cyclosporine.

cyclophosphamide
Adult dosage
2 mg/kg/day P.O. initially; then adjust dosage based on patient's WBC count and side effects
Points to remember
- Intermittent therapy may decrease side effects.
- Cytotoxic agents, such as azathioprine or chlorambucil, may be substituted.

cyclosporine
Adult dosage
5 mg/kg/day P.O. initially; then adjust dosage based on serum cyclosporine trough levels
Points to remember
- Administer at same time each day (bioavailability is highly variable).
- Toxicity is more likely to occur with trough levels above 500 ng/ml (RIA method).
- Nephrotoxicity and hypertension are common side effects; monitor serum creatinine and blood pressure.
- Once remission occurs, patient should be maintained on lowest effective dose.

prednisone
Adult dosage
Dosage and duration of therapy must be individualized; usual dosage ranges from 0.5 to 1 mg/kg/day P.O.
Points to remember
- Administer in morning.
- Decrease dosage as soon as possible to reduce risk of hypothalamic-pituitary-adrenal suppression but still maintain effective drug blood level.
- Lowest possible dose and shortest duration of therapy should be used.
- Other corticosteroids may be substituted. ■

Lower urinary tract infection

For lower urinary tract infection (UTI), antibiotic selection is based on results of culture and sensitivity testing. A 3-day drug regimen may be used for patients who meet the following criteria:
- signs or symptoms of lower UTI present for less than 7 days
- no signs or symptoms of pyelonephritis
- no history of recurrent UTIs
- no history of diabetes mellitus

- younger than age 65
- not pregnant
- not using a diaphragm.

Patients who don't meet these criteria should use a 7-day drug regimen.

▼FIRST-LINE DRUG
amoxicillin
Adult dosage
500 mg P.O. q 8 hours
Points to remember
- Don't give to patients with penicillin allergy.
- Drug is safe for use during pregnancy.

▼FIRST-LINE DRUG
ampicillin
Adult dosage
500 mg P.O. q 6 hours
Points to remember
- Don't give to patients with penicillin allergy.
- Drug is safe for use during pregnancy.

▼FIRST-LINE DRUG
co-trimoxazole (sulfamethoxazole-trimethoprim)
Adult dosage
One double-strength tablet (containing 800 mg sulfamethoxazole and 160 mg trimethoprim) P.O. q 12 hours
Points to remember
- This drug is contraindicated in pregnant patients.
- Trimethoprim may be given alone at dosage of 100 mg P.O. q 12 hours.

cephalexin
Adult dosage
500 mg P.O. q 6 hours
Point to remember
- This is a second-line drug.

ciprofloxacin
Adult dosage
250 mg P.O. q 12 hours
Points to remember
- This is an alternative drug.
- Drug is more expensive than other drugs used to treat lower UTIs.
- Other fluoroquinolones may be substituted.
- Ciprofloxacin is contraindicated in pregnancy.

nitrofurantoin
Adult dosage
100 mg P.O. q 6 hours
Point to remember
- This is an alternative drug. ■

Poststreptococcal glomerulonephritis, acute

This disease is usually reversible. The mainstay of therapy is managing hypertension and maintaining electrolyte and fluid balance. If cultures are positive for group A streptococci, antibiotics typically are used; however, they don't alter the disease course. Some patients may need temporary hemodialysis.

▼FIRST-LINE DRUG
penicillin G benzathine
Adult dosage
One-time dose of 1.2 million units I.M.
Points to remember
- Administer deep I.M. into upper outer quadrant of buttocks.
- Drug may cause pain at injection site.

▼FIRST-LINE DRUG
penicillin V potassium
Adult dose
250 mg P.O. q 8 hours for 10 days
Point to remember
- One-time dose of penicillin G benzathine may be preferable in patients unable or unwilling to comply with 10-day regimen.

erythromycin
Adult dosage
250 mg P.O. q 6 hours for 10 days
Point to remember
- This is an alternative drug for patients who are allergic to penicillin. ■

Pyelonephritis, acute

When acute pyelonephritis results from a hospital-acquired or relapsing infection, the causative organism is more likely to be resistant to antibiotics. Parenteral therapy is indicated for patients with vomiting or urosepsis; once the patient improves, oral therapy can be substituted. Usually, the total course of antibiotic therapy is 10 or 14 days. Antibiotic selection is based on results of culture and sensitivity testing. Empiric therapy is described below.

▼FIRST-LINE DRUG
ampicillin
Adult dosage
Parenteral: 1 g I.V. q 6 hours
Oral: 500 mg P.O. q 6 hours
Points to remember
- Common side effects include diarrhea and rash.
- Drug is safe for use during pregnancy.
- Amoxicillin 500 mg P.O. q 8 hours may be substituted for ampicillin.

▼FIRST-LINE DRUG
co-trimoxazole (sulfamethoxazole-trimethoprim)
Adult dosage
Parenteral: 80 mg (based on trimethoprim component) I.V. q 12 hours
Oral: One double-strength tablet (containing 800 mg sulfamethoxazole and 160 mg trimethoprim) P.O. q 12 hours
Point to remember
- This drug is contraindicated in pregnancy.

▼FIRST-LINE DRUG

gentamicin

Adult dosage

Dosage is based on patient's weight and renal function (loading dose of 1.8 to 2 mg/kg and maintenance dose of 1.3 to 1.5 mg/kg at intervals based on creatinine clearance)

Points to remember

- Aim for peak serum drug level of 4 to 5 mcg/ml.
- Aztreonam may be substituted if patient is at high risk for nephrotoxicity. (Usual aztreonam dosage: 500 mg I.V. q 8 to 12 hours.)

cefazolin sodium

Adult dosage

1 g I.V. q 8 hours

Points to remember

- This is a second-line drug.
- Drug isn't effective against all gram-negative organisms.
- Second- or third-generation cephalosporins may be substituted for more drug-resistant organisms.
- Cephalexin is an oral antibiotic with antimicrobial activity similar to that of cefazolin. After patient improves, he can be switched to oral cephalexin (500 mg q 6 hours).

ciprofloxacin

Adult dosage

Parenteral: 200 to 400 mg I.V. q 12 hours

Oral: 250 mg P.O. q 12 hours

Points to remember

- This is a second-line drug.
- Adjust dosage in renal dysfunction.
- Ciprofloxacin is contraindicated in pregnancy. ■

Renal calculi

Treatment of renal calculi varies with the type of calculi. For calcium oxalate calculi, therapy focuses on correcting the underlying cause, such as hyperparathyroidism, hypercalcemia, acidosis, or hyperoxaluria. Patients with idiopathic calcium oxalate calculi require hydration and dietary calcium restriction. Struvite calculi usually arise secondary to bacterial urinary infections; chronic antibiotics may partially dissolve these calculi, but some patients may require lithotripsy, renal pelvis irrigation with Renacidin, or surgery. Uric acid stones usually result from gout or chemotherapy for myeloproliferative disorders; treatment consists of administering fluids, alkalinizing the urine, and administering allopurinol.

▼FIRST-LINE DRUG

allopurinol

Adult dosage

Uric acid stones secondary to gout: 100 to 300 mg/day P.O.

Points to remember

- Give with meals to decrease GI upset.
- Instruct patient to maintain adequate fluid intake during therapy. Alkalizing or neutralizing urine helps prevent precipitation of uric acid calculi.
- Tell patient to avoid drinking alcoholic beverages in large amounts, which can increase uric acid levels.
- Discontinue drug at first sign of rash, which may indicate a severe hypersensitivity reaction.
- Decrease dosage in renal impairment. ■

Renal infarction and renal vein thrombosis

Acute therapy for these disorders involves anticoagulant or thrombolytic agents, surgery (such as thrombectomy or nephrectomy), and supportive care. Transient or persistent hypertension may follow renal infarction and should be treated. In chronic ischemic disease, surgical revascularization can preserve and improve renal function.

heparin

Adult dosage

70 to 100 units/kg (5,000 to 10,000 units) as I.V. bolus; then continuous I.V. infusion of 15 to 25 units/kg/ hour. Titrate dosage to keep activated partial thromboplastin time between 1.5 to 2 times the normal level.

Points to remember

- Drug is used for acute anticoagulation.
- Heparin therapy may be started after administration of thrombolytic agents.
- Therapy usually lasts 7 to 10 days.

thrombolytic agents

Adult dosage

Streptokinase: 250,000 units infused I.V. over 30 minutes, followed by 100,000 units/ hour for 24 to 72 hours
Urokinase: 4,400 units/kg infused I.V. over 30 minutes, followed by 4,400 units/kg/ hour for 12 hours

Points to remember

- Don't administer any other drugs through the same I.V. line used to administer streptokinase.
- These agents are contraindicated in aneurysm, active bleeding, brain tumor, cerebrovascular accident (CVA), uncontrolled hypertension, recent thoracic or neurologic surgery, and trauma.
- Avoid unnecessary movement of patient, I.M. injections, and invasive procedures.

warfarin sodium

Adult dosage

2 to 10 mg/day P.O.

Points to remember

- Drug is used to prevent pulmonary embolism; it's usually more effective in younger patients with acute renal vein thrombosis.
- Adjust dosage to maintain international normalized ratio between 2 and 3.
- Instruct patient to consume relatively stable intake of vitamin K.
- Give vitamin K_1 in case of warfarin overdose.
- Warfarin is contraindicated in recent lumbar puncture, trauma, childbirth or surgery and in severe liver or renal impairment, endocarditis, pregnancy, thrombocytopenia, severe uncontrolled hypertension, pericarditis, active bleeding, and CVA.
- Elderly patients may be more susceptible to bleeding during therapy.
- Advise patient to inform other health care professionals that he's on long-term warfarin therapy and to carry identification indicating such therapy. ■

Tubular necrosis, acute

Patients with this disorder should discontinue, if possible, any drugs that may contribute to renal impairment. Such drugs include acetaminophen, allopurinol, captopril, gentamicin, gold salts, methotrexate, and tobramycin. Supportive care measures include correcting ischemia (which may contribute to tubular necrosis) and correcting fluid and electrolyte disorders (which may arise secondary to acute renal failure). Loop diuretics may be necessary to improve urine output, increase the glomerular filtration rate, and treat edema.

loop diuretics

Adult dosage

Bumetanide: 1 mg I.V.; may repeat dose (no more than 1 mg/minute) q 2 to 3 hours p.r.n., to maximum daily dose of 10 mg

Furosemide: for edema, 20 to 80 mg I.V., and repeated q 6 to 8 hours p.r.n.; to increase urine output, 2 to 3 mg/kg I.V. and repeated p.r.n. to a maximum of 10 mg/kg, or by continuous I.V. infusion of 1 to 4 mg/minute and titrated according to patient's response to maintain urine output of at least 40 ml/hour

Points to remember

- Side effects include hypokalemia, orthostatic hypotension, and dehydration.
- Elderly patients are more susceptible to side effects. ■

ENDOCRINE DISORDERS

Acromegaly and gigantism

Surgery and radiation are the primary treatments; drug therapy is adjunctive.

bromocriptine mesylate
Adult dosage
1.25 to 2.5 mg/day P.O. h.s.; increase by same amount q 3 to 7 days (average daily effective dosage is 20 to 60 mg)
Points to remember
- This drug is a second-line alternative drug.
- Drug isn't uniformly effective.
- Monitor patient's blood pressure and watch for signs of peptic ulcer disease.
- Bromocriptine may cause cold-induced digital vasospasm; instruct patient to keep fingers warm.
- Reduce dosage in severe hepatic disease. ■

Adrenal hypofunction

Drugs are used as first-line therapy in this disease. Treatment focuses on replacing adrenal hormones (glucocorticoids and mineralocorticoids). The patient's weight, blood pressure, and serum electrolyte levels must be monitored periodically.

▼FIRST-LINE DRUG
cortisone
Adult dosage
12.5 to 50 mg/day P.O. in divided doses
Points to remember
- Alternatives include hydrocortisone and prednisone; when switching from one to the other, remember that 25 mg of cortisone is equipotent to 20 mg of hydrocortisone or 5 mg of prednisone.
- Cortisone may aggravate peptic ulcer disease.
- Administer with food or milk.

▼FIRST-LINE DRUG
fludrocortisone acetate
Adult dosage
0.05 to 0.1 mg/day P.O.
Points to remember
- Drug may aggravate CHF, hypertension, and hypokalemia.
- Instruct patient to consume 3 to 4 g of sodium daily. ■

Adrenogenital syndrome

This disorder results from abnormal activity of the adrenal cortex. Usually congenital, the condition may be acquired during adulthood from drug therapy or from a tumor that suppresses or stimulates the adrenal glands. Glucocorticoid administration inhibits excessive androgen production and stems virilization. Surgery is commonly required to correct abnormal genitalia.

fludrocortisone acetate
Pediatric dosage
0.05 to 0.10 mg/day P.O. in morning
Points to remember
- This drug is used in combination with hydrocortisone in patients with low serum sodium levels or elevated renin levels.
- Monitor blood pressure and serum potassium levels.

hydrocortisone
Pediatric dosage
20 to 25 mg/m^2/24 hours P.O. in two divided doses
Points to remember
- Dosage must be individualized based on patient's growth and hormone levels (which must be monitored).
- This therapy should continue indefinitely.
- Administer with food or antacid.
- Increase dosage during stress or infection. ■

Cushing's syndrome

This syndrome results from chronic and excessive production of corticotropin (primary Cushing's syndrome) or from administration of large doses of glucocorticoids for several weeks or longer (iatrogenic Cushing's syndrome). A pituitary gland tumor that triggers increased corticotropin secretion is the most common cause of the primary syndrome; surgery to remove the pituitary tumor is the definitive treatment. (If an adrenal gland tumor secretes excessive corticotropin, the adrenal tumor is removed.) Drug therapy aims to reduce adrenal cortisol secretion. For the iatrogenic syndrome, reducing the dosage of exogenous glucocorticoids or stopping the drug entirely is preferred. However, an underlying condition may preclude glucocorticoid withdrawal.

▼FIRST-LINE DRUG
ketoconazole
Adult dosage
400 to 500 mg P.O. b.i.d.
Points to remember
- Drug reduces corticotropin secretion by inhibiting synthesis of adrenal steroids and testosterone.
- Ketoconazole is approved for investigational use only in Cushing's syndrome.
- Ketoconazole may cause hepatotoxicity.

aminoglutethimide
Adult dosage
250 mg P.O. q.i.d.

Points to remember

- Drug is used in patients who can't tolerate ketoconazole.
- It's used only in combination with metyrapone.
- Aminoglutethimide is approved for investigational use only in Cushing's syndrome.
- Many patients have GI intolerance to this drug.
- Aminoglutethimide is rarely used for long-term therapy.

metyrapone

Adult dosage

500 mg P.O. q.i.d.

Points to remember

- This is a second-line drug.
- It's used in patients who can't tolerate ketoconazole.
- Drug is approved for investigational use only in Cushing's syndrome.
- Metyrapone is used only in combination with aminoglutethimide.
- Many patients have GI intolerance to this drug.
- Drug is expensive and is rarely used for long-term therapy.

mitotane

Adult dosage

3 to 6 g/day P.O. in divided doses

Points to remember

- More expensive and less well tolerated, mitotane is used as a third-line alternative to other drugs.
- Drug is approved for investigational use only in Cushing's syndrome.
- Drug carries an 80% response rate but a high recurrence rate after therapy stops.
- Adequate clinical response to this drug requires weeks to months of therapy. ■

Diabetes insipidus

In this disorder, drugs that may cause nephrogenic diabetes insipidus must be discontinued. Most patients require emergency treatment for hypertonic encephalopathy or maintenance therapy for polyuria. Replenishing body water while reducing elevated serum sodium level is the goal of treatment for hypertonic encephalopathy. Antidiuretic hormone replacement is the treatment of choice for the pituitary form of the disease.

▼FIRST-LINE DRUG

desmopressin acetate (DDAVP)

Adult dosage

10 to 40 mcg/day in one to three divided doses by nasal insufflation; alternatively, 2 to 4 mcg/day I.V. in two divided doses

Points to remember

- Drug is used as a synthetic hormone replacement for primary pituitary disease.

- Desmopressin is first-line therapy for pituitary diabetes insipidus, but it's not effective in nephrogenic diabetes insipidus.
- With nasal insufflation, drug must be administered correctly to make sure it reaches high in nasal cavity and does not go into the throat.
- Intranasal route is preferred unless nasal occlusion or irritation prohibits it.
- For I.V. infusion, dilute drug in 10 to 50 ml of normal saline solution, and infuse slowly over 15 to 30 minutes; monitor patient's blood pressure and pulse closely.

lypressin
Adult dosage
One to two sprays in one or both nostrils once or twice daily
Point to remember
- This drug is a second-line option in patients who don't respond to other treatments or who can't tolerate desmopressin.

chlorpropamide
Adult dosage
250 to 500 mg/day P.O.
Points to remember
- This is a third-line drug used for patients with some residual antidiuretic hormone production.
- Drug may cause hypoglycemia. ■

Diabetes mellitus

In this disorder, the goal of treatment is to control hyperglycemia and prevent long-term complications. Dietary management is the first-line treatment; drugs are used as second-line therapy. Insulin replacement and oral antidiabetic drugs are the major drugs used. Dietary management, weight reduction, and exercise may be effective alone or when used adjunctively with a drug regimen. Therapeutic measures and drug dosages are based on regular blood glucose measurements.

▼FIRST-LINE DRUG
glyburide
Adult dosage
2.5 to 30 mg P.O. once daily or in divided doses b.i.d.
Points to remember
- This is the oral antidiabetic drug of choice for many patients with non-insulin-dependent diabetes mellitus (Type II).
- Start with low dosage, and titrate upward gradually to control blood glucose level.
- Instruct patient to take drug 30 minutes before meals.
- Duration of action may be too long in elderly patients; drug is rarely recommended for them.

- Reduce dosage in hepatic and renal dysfunction.

glipizide
Adult dosage
2.5 to 40 mg P.O. once daily or in divided doses b.i.d.
Points to remember
- This drug is the alternative oral antidiabetic drug of choice for many patients with Type II diabetes.
- Start with low dosage, and increase gradually.
- Instruct patient to take drug 30 minutes before meals.
- Because its duration of action is slightly shorter than that of glyburide, glipizide may be safer for elderly patients.
- Reduce dosage in hepatic or renal dysfunction; proceed judiciously with dosage titration.

insulin
Adult dosage
S.C. or I.V. injection; dosage varies, based on blood glucose measurement before each dose
Points to remember
- Regular blood glucose monitoring is critical to dosage titration and blood glucose control.
- Human insulin is current treatment standard.
- Selection of dosage and regimen is highly individualized and may change daily.
- Most patients receive some combination of regular and longer-acting insulin to mimic normal insulin secretion patterns.
- Intensive blood glucose control helps to prevent or delay disease complications. ■

Diabetic ketoacidosis

Treatment for this acute, life-threatening condition must begin immediately after diagnosis. Therapeutic measures include administering insulin, replacing fluids and electrolytes, correcting precipitating disorders, and avoiding complications.

▼FIRST-LINE DRUG
insulin, human (regular)
Adult dosage
Highly variable; most commonly given by I.V. infusion
Points to remember
- Usually, priming dose of 10 to 20 units is administered I.V. first; then I.V. infusion begins.
- Regular insulin typically is diluted in normal saline solution.
- Only regular insulin is used for I.V. administration.
- Frequent blood glucose monitoring is necessary. ■

Hyperaldosteronism

Primary aldosteronism resulting from an adenoma usually calls for surgical excision. Other measures include restricting dietary sodium. Drug therapy aims to control hypertension and hypokalemia.

spironolactone
Adult dosage
25 to 100 mg P.O. q 8 hours
Points to remember
- This drug is used to control hypertension and hypokalemia.
- Spironolactone therapy succeeds in treating some patients for years; however, long-term therapy in men is usually limited by development of gynecomastia, decreased libido, and impotence. ■

Hyperthyroidism

Treatment of this disorder varies with its cause and severity and with the patient's age, clinical status, and desires. Surgery is usually preferred in children, pregnant women who respond poorly to low doses of thioureas, patients with large goiters, and those in whom thyroid cancer is suspected. Radioactive iodine may be administered to destroy overactive thyroid tissue. Drug therapy is used to relieve such symptoms as tachycardia, tremors, and diaphoresis.

propranolol hydrochloride
Adult dosage
20 mg P.O. q.i.d.
Points to remember
- This drug generally is used for symptomatic relief until hyperthyroidism resolves.
- Drug is a first-line treatment for thyroid storm.

thioureas
Adult dosage
Methimazole: 15 to 60 mg/day P.O., depending on disease severity (maximum daily dosage: 150 mg)
Propylthiouracil: 100 mg P.O. q 8 hours, to maximum of 300 mg q 8 hours
Points to remember
- Thioureas typically are given to children, young adults, and pregnant women as well as patients with small goiters.
- These drugs also are used to prepare hyperthyroid patients for surgery.
- Agranulocytosis is a rare but serious complication.
- Obtain WBC count before therapy and periodically during therapy.
- These drugs don't cause permanent thyroid damage. Patients treated with thioureas have lower rate of posttreatment hypothyroidism

(but higher rate of recurrent hyperthyroidism after 1 year or more of therapy) when compared with patients treated with radioactive iodine or surgery. ■

Hypopituitarism

Surgery or radiation therapy (or both) is used if hypopituitarism results from a pituitary gland tumor, the most common cause. The mainstay of drug therapy is lifelong replacement of hormones secreted by the target glands.

▼FIRST-LINE DRUGS

corticosteroids

Adult dosage

Dexamethasone: 0.25 mg/day P.O.
Hydrocortisone: 15 to 25 mg/day P.O. in divided doses
Prednisone: 5 to 7.5 mg/day P.O.

Points to remember

- Mineralocorticoids rarely are needed.
- The patient also must receive hydrocortisone during stressful periods.

▼FIRST-LINE DRUGS

sex hormones

Adult dosage

Conjugated estrogens (0.625 to 1.25 mg) or ethinyl estradiol (10 to 20 mcg) P.O. daily on days 1 through 25 of every month plus medroxyprogesterone acetate (5 mg/ day) P.O. on days 16 through 25
Testosterone enanthate or cypionate: 300 mg I.M. q 3 weeks

Points to remember

- For I.M. use, administer deep into gluteal muscle; do *not* inject I.V.
- Instruct patient receiving testosterone to notify doctor if vomiting, edema, priapism, or jaundice occurs.
- Instruct patient receiving estrogen or medroxyprogesterone to notify doctor of any leg pain, chest pain, abnormal vaginal bleeding, missed menstrual periods, breast lumps, severe headache, dizziness, or jaundice.

levothyroxine sodium (T_4)

Adult dosage

0.1 to 0.2 mg/day P.O.

Points to remember

- Use of this drug in panhypopituitarism is rare, except in patients receiving corticosteroids.
- Lack of adrenal function may make patients exceedingly sensitive to this drug. ■

Hypothyroidism

This is a readily treatable disease. Drug therapy aims to replace thyroid hormone.

▼FIRST LINE DRUG

levothyroxine sodium (T_4)

Dosage

Adults: 25 to 50 mcg/day P.O. for 1 week; increase by 25 mcg/day q 1 to 2 weeks to maximum of 100 to 150 mcg/day

Children under age 1: 25 to 50 mcg/day P.O.; increase to 50 mcg/day

Points to remember

- Levothyroxine provides stable and easily measurable serum concentrations for use in monitoring therapy.
- Levothyroxine allows physiologic regulation of extrathyroidal triiodothyronine (T_3) production. ■

Pheochromocytoma

Ideally, therapy for this disorder involves surgical tumor removal. Until surgery can be performed, medical therapy may be necessary to control hypertension. Postoperatively, monitor the patient for hypoglycemia and hypotension. Administering dextrose-containing fluids and plasma volume expanders helps to maintain urine output.

alpha-adrenergic blockers

Adult dosage

Phentolamine: in acute situations, 2 mg I.V. q 5 minutes to normalize blood pressure, or 500 mcg to 1 mg/minute I.V.

Phenoxybenzamine: in chronic disease, 10 mg P.O. initially; then titrate to 30 to 60 mg P.O. b.i.d to decrease blood pressure

Points to remember

- These drugs are used to control blood pressure.
- Administer these agents before initiating beta-blocker therapy to avoid exacerbating low blood pressure.

beta-adrenergic blockers

Adult dosage

Metoprolol: 100 to 400 mg/day P.O. divided in two doses

Nadolol: 20 to 40 mg/day P.O.

Propranolol: 10 to 20 mg/day P.O. divided in two doses

Points to remember

- These drugs are used to control hypertension and tachyarrhythmias. To avoid exacerbating hypertension, they are typically given only after patient has received phentolamine.
- These drugs may worsen asthma, COPD, diabetes, depression, peripheral vascular disease, Raynaud's disease, and CHF.
- Carefully check I.V. dosages, which may be substantially smaller than oral dosages of some of these drugs. ■

Protoporphyria

In this disorder, marked by increased fecal excretion of protoporphyrin, beta-carotene may be given to decrease photosensitivity. Topical sunscreens are rarely effective in reducing skin sensitivity.

beta-carotene
Adult dosage
30 to 300 mg/day P.O.
Points to remember
- Beta-carotene helps decrease the severity of photosensitivity reactions.
- Yellow skin discoloration is common after several weeks of therapy.
- Patients with renal or liver impairment may require lower dosages. ■

Simple goiter

When this condition is mild, it may not require treatment. Exogenous goitrogenic factors, such as calcium and fluorides in drinking water or excessive intake of cabbage, cauliflower, cassava, brussels sprouts, and turnips, should be identified and removed. If possible, discontinue drugs known to cause hypothyroidism, such as iodides, phenylbutazone, amiodarone, and lithium. Patients with goiter resulting from iodine deficiency (which is rare in areas where iodized salt is used) typically receive replacement iodine. Goiters that cause respiratory obstruction may be surgically removed.

levothyroxine (T_4)
Adult dosage
100 mcg/day P.O. initially; titrate by 50-mcg increments to maximum dosage of 150 to 200 mcg/day, as needed, to suppress thyroid-stimulating hormone (TSH) level below 0.1 mU/L.
Points to remember
- Levothyroxine suppresses TSH secretion and decreases goiter growth.
- This drug is contraindicated if goiter isn't suppressible with levothyroxine.
- Elderly patients and those with coronary artery disease require lower dosages and incremental increases to avoid angina exacerbation. ■

Thyroiditis

This disorder may result from a bacterial or viral infection. In AIDS patients, *Pneumocystis carinii* may cause thyroiditis. Bacterial infections can be treated by surgical thyroid removal as well as with antibiotics. Otherwise, the disease may be self-limiting. In mild cases, aspirin alone can be used to relieve fever and pain.

aspirin
Adult dosage
325 to 650 mg P.O. q 4 to 6 hours as needed
Points to remember
- Aspirin is usually prescribed for mild pain and fever.
- Don't give to patients with aspirin sensitivity, bleeding disorders, active bleeding, or peptic ulcer disease. Use caution when administering aspirin to patients with a history of peptic ulcers or those who are receiving heparin, warfarin, or thrombolytic agents.
- To minimize GI upset, advise patient to take aspirin with food or antacids and to avoid alcoholic beverages. Taking enteric-coated aspirin also may help. Patients at high risk for serious GI toxicity may take misoprostol concurrently.

prednisone
Adult dosage
20 to 40 mg/day P.O.
Points to remember
- Prednisone (or another glucocorticoid) typically is prescribed for severe symptoms not controlled by aspirin.
- Use lowest dosage possible. To minimize adrenal suppression, single daily dose should be given in morning or in alternate-day regimen.

propranolol hydrochloride
Adult dosage
40 to 120 mg/day P.O. in divided doses
Points to remember
- Propranolol hydrochloride (or another beta-adrenergic blocker) usually is prescribed to treat thyrotoxicosis symptoms, such as tachycardia, sweating, and tremor.
- These drugs may worsen asthma, COPD, diabetes, depression, peripheral vascular disease, Raynaud's disease, and CHF.
- Carefully check I.V. dosages, which may be substantially smaller than oral dosages. ■

Thyroid storm

During infection, which can precipitate thyroid storm, patients with this disorder should receive appropriate antibiotics. Other supportive measures include administering fluids to correct dehydration and giving vitamin B complex and glucocorticoids for hypoadrenalism. A hypothermia blanket may be necessary to control fever. Atrial fibrillation may be treated with digoxin; patients in shock may receive I.V. pressors.

dexamethasone
Adult dosage
2 mg P.O. or I.V. q 6 hours for 24 to 48 hours
Points to remember
- Dexamethasone (or another glucocorticoid) is used to inhibit hormone release and prevent hypoadrenalism.
- Regimens shorter than 7 days usually don't require tapering before therapy is stopped.

iodine preparations
Adult dosage
Iodine, strong solution (USP [Lugol's Solution]): 1 ml P.O. t.i.d.
Sodium iodine: 500 mg to 1 g I.V. q 12 hours
Sodium iopodate: 500 mg to 1 g/day P.O. or 3 g P.O. q 3rd day
Points to remember
- These drugs are used to decrease thyroid hormone release.
- Give first dose at least 1 hour after propylthiouracil.
- To avoid GI upset, administer in 8-oz (240-ml) glass of water or juice.
- Don't use strong iodine solution if it's yellowish brown. Crystallization can occur if solution is refrigerated. To resolve crystals, warm and shake solution gently.
- To dissolve sodium iopodate granules, place in 60 ml (2 oz) of water and stir vigorously.
- Patients with renal impairment may require lower dosages.

propranolol hydrochloride
Adult dosage
40 to 80 mg P.O. or 2 mg I.V. q 6 hours p.r.n.
Points to remember
- Propranolol (or another beta blocker) is used to treat thyroid storm symptoms, such as tachycardia, sweating, and tremor.
- Carefully check I.V. dosages, which may be substantially smaller than oral dosages.

propylthiouracil (PTU)
Adult dosage
100 mg P.O. q 2 hours or 200 to 400 mg P.O. q 4 hours; may decrease dosage after first few days as symptoms resolve
Points to remember
- This drug is used to decrease thyroid hormone production during pregnancy and lactation as well as to treat thyroid storm.
- In emergencies, when patient cannot swallow tablets, propylthiouracil may be given by nasogastric tube or by rectal suppository or enema. ■

FLUID AND ELECTROLYTE DISORDERS

Hypercalcemia

For asymptomatic patients, treatment for hypercalcemia consists of managing the underlying cause. Emergency treatment for symptomatic patients involves aggressive I.V. fluid replacement with normal saline solution, followed by diuresis with furosemide. Drug therapy aims to remove calcium.

▼FIRST-LINE DRUG

biphosphonates

Adult dosage

Etidronate sodium: 7.5 mg/kg/day I.V. over 2 or more hours for 3 consecutive days

Pamidronate disodium: 60 to 90 mg I.V. over 24 hours

Point to remember

- Pamidronate is more potent than etidronate.

calcitonin

Adult dosage

0.5 mg/day (human) or 100 to 400/day IU (salmon) S.C. or I.M.

Points to remember

- Calcitonin alone rarely lowers serum calcium level, but it may be added to etidronate.
- Repeated calcitonin therapy is rarely effective.

gallium nitrate

Adult dosage

100 to 200 mg/m²/day I.V. for 5 days, infused over 24 hours

Points to remember

- This drug may increase the BUN and serum creatinine levels.
- Ensure adequate hydration.

plicamycin

Adult dosage

25 mcg/kg I.V. for 3 to 4 days, infused over 4 to 6 hours; repeat at 1-week intervals p.r.n.

Point to remember

- Therapeutic effect may be delayed for 24 to 48 hours. ■

Hyperchloremia

Treatment of hyperchloremia focuses on correcting the underlying cause. Fluids are given to dilute circulating chloride. Some patients may require small doses of sodium bicarbonate.

sodium bicarbonate

Adult dosage

325 mg to 3 g up to four times daily

Points to remember

- One gram of sodium bicarbonate provides 11.9 mEq of sodium and 11.9 mEq of bicarbonate.
- Maximum daily intake is 16 g (200 mEq) in patients

under age 60 and 8 g (100 mEq) in those over age 60. ■

Hyperkalemia

Patients with this disorder require emergency treatment if they show signs of cardiac toxicity or muscular paralysis or if the serum potassium level exceeds 6.5 mEq/L. Patients with protracted renal insufficiency may need hemodialysis or peritoneal dialysis to remove potassium from the body. Drug therapy aims to remove potassium.

For emergency treatment

calcium
Adult dosage
Calcium chloride: 5% solution in 5 to 30 ml of I.V. solution p.r.n.
Calcium gluconate: 10% solution in 5 to 30 ml of I.V. solution p.r.n.
Point to remember
- Infuse slowly.

insulin
Adult dosage
5 to 10 units regular insulin plus 25 g of 50% glucose I.V. p.r.n.
Point to remember
- Effects may not occur for 30 to 60 minutes.

For nonemergency treatment

furosemide
Adult dosage
40 to 160 mg I.V. or P.O. p.r.n.
Point to remember
- This drug may be given in combination with sodium bicarbonate (0.5 to 3 mEq/kg/day).

sodium polystyrene sulfonate
Adult dosage
Oral: 15 to 30 g P.O. in 20% sorbitol p.r.n.
Rectal: 50 mg in 20% sorbitol p.r.n.
Point to remember
- Chilling oral suspension makes it more palatable; however, don't heat it because heat inactivates resin.

For emergency or nonemergency treatment

albuterol
Adult dosage
10 to 20 mg in 4 ml of normal saline solution by nebulizer over 10 minutes p.r.n.
Points to remember
- Drug distributes potassium into cells.
- Onset of action occurs within 15 to 30 minutes.

sodium bicarbonate
Adult dosage
I.V.: 44 to 88 mEq I.V. p.r.n.
Oral: 0.5 to 3 mEq/kg/day P.O.

Point to remember
- Avoid adding sodium bicarbonate to parenteral solutions containing calcium because precipitation may occur. ■

Hypermagnesemia

Treatment of this disorder aims to alleviate renal insufficiency. Hemodialysis or peritoneal dialysis may be indicated. Calcium salts act as an antagonist to magnesium.

calcium chloride
Adult dosage
500 mg I.V. p.r.n.
Points to remember
- Calcium antagonizes magnesium.
- Give by slow I.V. infusion.
- Monitor patient's ECG during I.V. calcium administration. ■

Hypernatremia

Treatment of this disorder involves correcting the cause of fluid loss and replacing water and electrolytes, as needed. However, reversing hypernatremia too quickly may lead to an osmotic imbalance, causing water to enter the brain cells. This, in turn, may result in cerebral edema and potentially severe neurologic impairment. For this reason, fluid therapy should be administered over 48 hours; a reasonable goal is to decrease the serum sodium level by 1 mEq/hour. For hypernatremia with hypovolemia, use normal saline solution; for hypernatremia with euvolia, use D_5W. ■

Hyperphosphatemia

The underlying cause of hyperphosphatemia must be treated. If the cause is renal failure, dialysis may be used to decrease the serum phosphate level. Drug therapy aims to bind serum phosphate or remove it from the body.

▼FIRST-LINE DRUG
aluminum hydroxide
Adult dosage
500 mg to 2 g P.O. b.i.d. to q.i.d.
Point to remember
- Stay alert for signs of aluminum toxicity.

▼FIRST-LINE DRUG
calcium carbonate
Adult dosage
0.5 to 1 g P.O. t.i.d. with meals
Point to remember
- Calcium carbonate may cause constipation. ■

Hypocalcemia

Severe, symptomatic hypocalcemia calls for I.V. calcium gluconate. Asymptomatic hypocalcemia warrants administration of oral calcium and vitamin D preparations.

vitamin D preparations
Adult dosage
Calcifediol: 20 to 200 mcg/day P.O.
Calcitriol: 0.25 to 5 mcg/day P.O.
Dihydrotachysterol: 0.2 to 1 mg/day P.O.
Ergocalciferol: 25,000 to 200,000 units/day P.O.
Points to remember
- Urge patient to swallow drug whole; warn him not to crush or chew it.
- Tell patient to notify doctor of any weakness, lethargy, headache, anorexia, nausea, vomiting, excessive urine output, or muscle or bone pain.

For asymptomatic hypocalcemia

▼FIRST-LINE DRUG
calcium carbonate
Adult dosage
250 to 500 mg P.O. q.i.d.
Point to remember
- Calcium carbonate contains 40% elemental calcium.

For severe, symptomatic hypocalcemia

▼FIRST-LINE DRUG
calcium gluconate
Adult dosage
93 to 186 mg I.V. over 10 to 15 minutes, then 10 to 15 mg/kg I.V. over 4 to 6 hours
Point to remember
- Keep in mind that 10% calcium gluconate solution contains 93 mg (4.7 mEq) of calcium per 10 ml. ■

Hypokalemia

Oral potassium is the safest therapy for patients with mild to moderate hypokalemia. Patients with severe hypokalemia and those who can't take oral potassium supplements usually require I.V. potassium replacement.

potassium chloride and potassium gluconate
Adult dosage
For patients with serum potassium levels above 2.5 mEq/L and no ECG abnormalities: 10 mEq/L/hour I.V. (concentration shouldn't exceed 40 mEq/L)
For severe hypokalemia: infuse I.V. at rate of up to 40 mEq/L/hour
Point to remember
- Monitor patient's ECG continuously. ■

Hypomagnesemia

Therapy includes I.V. fluids containing magnesium as chloride or sulfate. In severe hypomagnesemia, 240 to 1,200 mg/day (or 10 to 50 mmol/day) are given, followed by 120 mg/day (5 mmol/day) for maintenance.

▼FIRST-LINE DRUG

magnesium oxide

Adult dosage

250 to 500 mg P.O. b.i.d. to q.i.d.

Point to remember

- This agent replaces magnesium stores in chronic hypomagnesemia.

magnesium sulfate

Adult dosage

200 to 800 mg/day I.M. in four divided doses

Point to remember

- Monitor serum magnesium levels; adjust dosage to keep level below 2.5 mmol/L. ■

Hyponatremia

The underlying cause of hyponatremia must be corrected, and the patient's water intake should be limited to less than 1 or 2 liters/day. Drug therapy aims to restore normal serum sodium levels.

▼FIRST-LINE DRUG

saline solution with furosemide

Adult dosage

100 to 200 ml of 3% saline solution with 0.5 to 1 mg/kg of furosemide, given I.V. p.r.n.

Points to remember

- Therapy is indicated only for symptomatic patients.
- Measure urinary sodium and plasma sodium levels approximately every 4 hours.

demeclocycline

Adult dosage

300 to 600 mg P.O. b.i.d.

Points to remember

- This agent is useful in patients with syndrome of inappropriate antidiuretic hormone secretion who can't adhere to water restriction or who need additional therapy.
- Onset of action may take up to 1 week. ■

Hypophosphatemia

The best treatment for hypophosphatemia is prevention, including phosphate in replacement and maintenance fluids. Because the serum calcium level may fall rapidly with parenteral phosphate administration, oral replacement is preferred.

I.V. phosphates (such as sodium or potassium phosphate with phosphorus content of 93 mg/ml)
Adult dosage
2 to 7.5 mg/kg I.V. infused over 6 to 8 hours
Point to remember
- These agents are contraindicated in hypoparathyroidism, renal insufficiency, tissue damage and necrosis, and hypercalcemia.

oral phosphates
Adult dosage
250-mg phosphorus capsule or tablet (Neutra-Phos, K-Phos-Neutral, or Uro-KP-Neutral); or 125- or 250-mg phosphorus capsule or tablet (Neutra-Phos-K or K-Phos) q.i.d.
Point to remember
- These agents are contraindicated in hypoparathyroidism, renal insufficiency, tissue damage and necrosis, and hypercalcemia. ■

Metabolic acidosis

Treatment of metabolic acidosis aims to correct the cause. Supplemental sodium bicarbonate is indicated in hyperkalemia and certain forms of normal anion-gap acidosis. However, its use is controversial in increased anion-gap metabolic acidosis. Many patients tolerate the combination product Bicitra better than sodium bicarbonate.

Bicitra
Adult dosage
10 to 30 ml in 1 to 3 oz water t.i.d.
Point to remember
- Follow dose with more water. Monitor urine pH. ■

Metabolic alkalosis

Most patients can tolerate mild metabolic alkalosis. However, severe or symptomatic alkalosis requires urgent treatment. Therapy for saline-responsive metabolic alkalosis aims to correct the extracellular volume deficit. Therapy for saline-unresponsive metabolic alkalosis may include surgery to remove a mineralocorticoid-producing tumor and spironolactone to block aldosterone's effect.

acetazolamide
Adult dosage
250 to 500 mg I.V. q 4 to 6 hours
Point to remember
- This drug is indicated in pulmonary or cardiovascular status that precludes adequate volume replacement. ■

CHAPTER 17

ENSURING SAFETY FOR MATERNAL AND NEONATAL PATIENTS

GIVING DRUGS DURING LABOR AND DELIVERY

Learning about drug action in pregnant patients

Numerous pregnancy-related organic and physiologic changes can alter the absorption, distribution, metabolism, and excretion of a drug administered to a pregnant patient. The fetus also significantly influences drug distribution and disposition.

Absorption

During pregnancy, the tone and motility of the GI tract decrease, probably from an increased serum progesterone level and a decreased level of GI motilin (an intestinal hormone that increases intestinal motility). These effects prolong gastric emptying and intestinal transit times. Hydrochloric acid formation in the stomach also decreases. All these factors delay absorption of drugs that need an acidic environment or that are absorbed in the small intestine.

Absorption of drugs administered parenterally also may change during pregnancy. Because of peripheral vasodilation, drugs given subcutaneously, intramuscularly, or intradermally may be absorbed more rapidly.

Distribution

The physiologic changes during pregnancy also alter drug distribution. Interstitial and intracellular water both increase, as does blood volume (elevated nearly 45% by the end of gestation). These increases change the ratios of blood constituents that affect drug distribution. For example, the ratio of albumin to water decreases during pregnancy, altering protein-binding capacity.

During pregnancy, estrogen and progesterone levels rise, as do the levels of free fatty acids (triglycerides, cholesterol, and phospholipids) from increased fatty tissue metabolism. These effects are accompanied by increased competition for protein-binding sites. With fewer binding sites, a larger percentage of drug remains free to move to receptor sites or across the placenta.

Drug transport across the placental barrier

The term *placental barrier* can be misleading because it implies that the placenta protects the fetus from drug effects. In fact, many drugs ingested by a pregnant patient cross the placenta and reach the fetus. Although some drugs, such as heparin and insulin, don't cross the placenta, most do when they're administered at therapeutic levels.

Placental transport of substances to and from the fetus starts at approximately the 5th week of gestation. Later in pregnancy when the placenta thins, drugs with high lipid solubility or low protein-binding ability pass more easily through the placenta.

The fetus may affect drug distribution and disposition by fetal circulation, the binding of plasma and tissue proteins, and excretory activity.

Metabolism
Metabolically active, the placenta also can affect drug disposition. The placenta seems to be capable of several enzymatic reactions that can make a drug's metabolites less potent. Conversely, these reactions may produce a more potent and toxic metabolite, thereby increasing fetal danger. (See *Pregnancy risk categories*, page 680.)

Excretion
Numerous changes in the urinary system that occur during pregnancy can affect drug excretion. The glomerular filtration rate (GFR) and renal plasma flow increase early in pregnancy; the GFR continues to remain elevated until delivery. Because of the increased plasma flow, drugs that normally are excreted easily may be eliminated even more rapidly.

The fetus has slower drug clearance than the adult; drug concentration is greater in the fetus; and drugs stay longer in the fetus's tissue and blood than in the mother's. (For information on the effects of maternal drug therapy on a breast-feeding infant, see "Understanding Drug Therapy and Breast-feeding" later in this chapter.) ■

Giving terbutaline

Terbutaline sulfate is the drug of choice to inhibit uterine contractions by stimulating $beta_2$-adrenergic receptors in uterine smooth muscle. It's also used during labor to treat fetal distress that's precipitated by uterine activity.

S.C., oral, or I.V. administration
Give 0.25 to 0.5 mg of terbutaline S.C. every 20 to 60 minutes, or 5-mg tablets orally after preterm labor has stabilized. The drug can also be administered I.V. continuously via a subcutaneously placed terbutaline pump if contractions continue despite S.C. therapy.

ALERT

Pregnancy risk categories

Some drugs are riskier than others for the fetus of a pregnant patient. The FDA has established five categories (A, B, C, D, and X) that indicate a drug's potential for causing birth defects or fetal death.

A: Controlled studies show no risks to pregnant patients. Adequate studies in pregnant patients fail to show risks to the fetus.

B: There is no evidence of risk in humans. Either animal studies show risk and human studies do not; or, if no adequate human studies have been done, animal findings are negative.

C: Pregnancy risk is unknown and cannot be ruled out. Human studies are lacking, and animal studies either show fetal risk or are lacking. However, potential benefits of use in pregnant women may justify the potential risk.

D: Evidence of risk to the fetus exists. However, potential benefits of use in pregnant women may outweigh potential risks.

X: The drug is contraindicated in pregnancy. Studies in humans or animals show fetal risk that clearly outweighs any benefits of use in pregnant women.

Patients may use a terbutaline pump at home; if preterm labor stabilizes, they can progress gradually to oral administration.

Nursing considerations

- Maintain the patient in the left lateral position to minimize the risk of hypotension.
- Monitor the patient's vital signs including apical pulse and fetal heart tones before beginning the I.V. infusion, every 15 to 30 minutes during the infusion, and then every 4 hours during oral administration.
- Monitor the patient for side effects of terbutaline therapy, including tachycardia, hypotension, and arrhythmias.
- When terbutaline is ineffective, magnesium sulfate may be administered temporarily. After 24 hours, the magnesium sulfate I.V. infusion may be discontinued and terbutaline resumed. ■

Giving magnesium sulfate

Magnesium sulfate is used to prevent and control seizures in preeclamptic and eclamptic pregnant patients. It also may be used to treat preterm labor, although it's not approved by the FDA for this purpose.

A CNS depressant, magnesium sulfate has its effect at the peripheral neuromuscular junction. It also acts as a myometrial relaxant, thereby inhibiting uterine activity.

I.V. administration

To give magnesium sulfate I.V., prepare a loading dose of 4 to 6 g as a 10% solution in 250 ml of I.V. fluid; administer this rapidly over 15 to 30 minutes. Follow with a continuous I.V. infusion of 1 to 2 g per hour delivered by an infusion pump via the piggyback method. Piggyback the solution to the primary line at the connector closest to the patient.

Managing preterm labor

Magnesium sulfate may be used alone or as adjunctive therapy when an oral tocolytic, such as terbutaline, fails to inhibit labor. Maintenance doses of up to 3 g/hour may be given. After labor has been inhibited for 24 hours by I.V. magnesium sulfate, terbutaline may be administered.

Monitoring the patient

- When administering magnesium sulfate, be sure to monitor the patient's fluid intake and output hourly. Because magnesium sulfate is excreted by the kidneys, decreased fluid output leads to a buildup of the drug in the body. As a result, the patient may experience decreased respiratory rate and decreased deep tendon reflexes.
- Also monitor serum magnesium levels. Keep in mind that the therapeutic level ranges from 4 to 7 mEq/liter. Deep tendon reflexes are absent when the level is 10 mEq/L; respiratory failure occurs when the level is 12 to 15 mEq/L; and cardiac arrest may occur when it's 15 mEq/L or more.
- Check the patient's deep tendon reflexes hourly; these reflexes disappear before respiratory arrest occurs.
- Notify the doctor if the patient's respiratory rate drops below 12 breaths/minute, which may indicate respiratory depression.

Nursing considerations

- Minimize the patient's fluid intake; a preeclamptic patient can't tolerate a fluid overload because of renal impairment.

- Patients receiving this drug commonly complain of flushing, a sensation of warmth, and fatigue.
- A transient drop in blood pressure, caused by smooth-muscle vasodilation and relaxation, may occur during the 1st hour after magnesium sulfate administration.
- Uterine activity may decrease in the preeclamptic patient; labor augmentation may be necessary with oxytocin.
- Keep calcium gluconate, a magnesium sulfate antagonist, on hand in case of a magnesium sulfate overdose. Expect to administer 10 ml of a 10% solution (1 g) I.V. over 3 minutes.
- Pulmonary edema may occur with concomitant use of magnesium sulfate and corticosteroids.
- Neonates of patients who receive this drug may exhibit respiratory and motor depression. ■

Administering oxytocin safely

The hormone oxytocin stimulates the uterine smooth-muscle fibers to contract, thereby promoting cervical dilation. The doctor may order synthetic oxytocin (such as Pitocin or Syntocinon) to induce or augment labor or to control bleeding and enhance uterine contraction after the placenta is delivered.

Administer oxytocin I.V. during labor, using an infusion pump to help regulate the dosage (which will depend on uterine sensitivity) and to prevent uterine hyperstimulation (which may slow fetal blood flow). Additional nursing responsibilities include managing the infusion and monitoring maternal and fetal responses and possible complications.

Oxytocin may be given I.M. after delivery to prevent or control excessive bleeding.

Indications and contraindications

Oxytocin is indicated in pregnancy-induced hypertension, prolonged gestation, maternal diabetes, Rh sensitization, premature or prolonged rupture of membranes, incomplete or inevitable abortion, and evaluation of fetal distress after 31 weeks.

The drug is contraindicated in such conditions as placenta previa and diagnosed cephalopelvic disproportion. Administer the drug cautiously to a patient with an overdistended uterus or a history of cervical surgery, uterine surgery, or grand multiparity.

Gathering the equipment

Begin by gathering an administration set for a primary I.V. line, infusion pump and tubing, I.V. solution as ordered, external or internal fetal monitoring equipment, oxytocin, a 20G 1″ needle, label, and venipuncture equipment with an 18G over-the-needle catheter if the patient doesn't already have an I.V. line in place.

Note: Although you can administer oxytocin without using an electronic fetal monitor or an infusion pump, using a pump ensures maternal and fetal safety as well as accurate dosage and titration.

Preparing the solution

- When preparing the oxytocin solution, rotate the I.V. bag to disperse the drug throughout the solution, and label the I.V. container with the name of the medication.
- Then attach the infusion pump tubing to the I.V. container, and connect the tubing to the pump. Because infusion pump features vary, review the manufacturer's directions before proceeding.
- Next, attach the 20G 1″ needle to the piggyback tubing, and insert the needle into the primary I.V. line. Then set up the equipment for internal or external fetal monitoring.

Preparing the patient

- Explain the procedure to the patient, and provide privacy. Wash your hands. Describe the equipment, and forewarn the patient that she may feel a pinch from the venipuncture.
- Help the patient to a lateral-tilt position, and support her hip with a pillow.

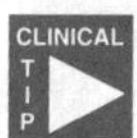

Don't let the patient lie supine; in this position, the gravid uterus presses on the great vessels, producing maternal hypotension, reducing uterine perfusion and, eventually, causing fetal hypoxia.

- Identify and record the fetal heart rate (FHR), and assess uterine contractions occurring in a 20-minute span to establish baseline fetal status and evaluate spontaneous uterine activity.

Starting the infusion

- Start the primary I.V. line, using an 18G over-the-needle catheter throughout labor and delivery. Use this line to deliver not only oxytocin but also fluids, blood, or other medications, as needed.
- Piggyback the oxytocin solution (metered by the infusion pump) to the primary I.V. line at the Y-injection site closest to the patient. Piggybacking maintains I.V. line patency (and preserves the line should you discontinue the oxytocin infusion). Be-

sides, using the Y-injection site nearest the venipuncture ensures that the primary line contains the lowest concentration of oxytocin if you must stop the infusion.

Giving the right dosage

- Start the oxytocin infusion, as ordered. The typical recommended labor-starting dosage ranges from 0.5 to 1 milliunit (mU)/minute. (The maximum dosage is 20 mU/minute.)
- Because oxytocin begins acting immediately, be prepared to start monitoring uterine contractions.

Increasing the infusion

- Increase the oxytocin infusion, as ordered. As a rule, each increase should range no more than 1 to 2 mU/minute, infused once every 15 to 30 minutes. When induced labor simulates normal labor (contractions occurring every 2 to 3 minutes and lasting 40 to 60 seconds) and cervical dilation progresses at least 1 cm/hour in first-stage, active-phase labor, you should stop increasing the dosage.
- Continue the infusion at the dosage and rate that maintain the activity closest to normal labor.

Monitoring contractions

- Before each increase in the oxytocin infusion, be sure to note the frequency and duration of contractions; palpate the uterus to identify contraction intensity; and assess maternal vital signs and FHR, rhythm, and variability. Doing so will ensure maternal and fetal safety and help you detect possible complications.
- If you're using an external fetal monitor, the uterine activity strip or grid should show contractions occurring every 2 to 3 minutes. The contractions should last for about 60 seconds and be followed by uterine relaxation.
- If you're using an internal fetal monitor, look for an optimal baseline value ranging from 5 to 15 mm Hg. Your aim is to verify uterine relaxation between contractions.
- Reposition the patient on her other side as needed, and continue assessing maternal and fetal responses to the oxytocin. For example, every 10 to 15 minutes, evaluate the FHR, rhythm, and variability; maternal response to increased contraction activity and subsequent discomfort; and maternal pulse rate and pattern, blood pressure, respiratory rate and quality, and uterine contractions.

Preventing hyperstimulation

- Review the infusion rate every 10 to 15 minutes to prevent uterine hyperstimulation. Signs of hyperstimulation include contractions occurring less than 2 minutes apart and lasting 90 seconds or longer, uterine pressure values that don't return to baseline between contractions, and intrauterine pressure that rises to more than 75 mm Hg.

- To reduce uterine irritability, try to increase uterine blood flow. Do this by changing the patient's position and increasing the infusion rate of the primary I.V. line. Don't exceed the maximum total infusion of 20 mU/minute.
- To manage hyperstimulation, discontinue the oxytocin infusion, administer oxygen, and notify the doctor.

Resuming the infusion after hyperstimulation resolves

Depending on maternal and fetal conditions, choose one of the following methods:

- Resume the infusion, beginning at 0.5 mU/minute; increase the dosage to 1 mU/minute every 15 minutes; and increase the rate as before.
- Resume the infusion at one-half of the last dosage given, and increase the rate as before.
- Resume the infusion at the dosage given before hyperstimulation signs occurred. Check your facility's policy and the doctor's order for the appropriate method.

Ensuring fluid balance

Monitor and record the patient's fluid intake and output. At rates of 16 mU/minute and more, oxytocin has an antidiuretic effect, so you may need to administer an electrolyte-containing I.V. solution, such as lactated Ringer's solution, to maintain electrolyte balance.

Charting maternal status

Record maternal response to contractions, blood pressure, pulse rate and pattern, and respiratory rate and quality on the patient's labor-progression chart. Also record FHR, rhythm, and variability; oxytocin infusion rate; and intake and output. Describe uterine activity as well.

Administering oxytocin after delivery

- After placental delivery, oxytocin may be given to decrease postpartum bleeding or uterine atony. As ordered, administer 10 to 40 units of oxytocin added to 1,000 ml of physiologic electrolyte solution. Infuse this solution at a rate titrated to produce the desired response.
- As an alternative, administer 10 units of oxytocin I.M. until you can establish the I.V. line. If the patient doesn't want an I.V. line, give her an

I.M. injection of 10 units of oxytocin.

Charting oxytocin administration

Record the amount of oxytocin given and the route — and, if added to the I.V. solution, the amount of solution in the I.V. bag at the time you added the pitocin. Also record uterine tone and height as well as the amount and character of lochia.

Watching for complications

- Oxytocin can cause uterine hyperstimulation that may progress to tetanic contractions, which last longer than 2 minutes. Other potential complications include fetal distress, abruptio placentae, and uterine rupture.
- Also watch for signs of oxytocin hypersensitivity, such as elevated blood pressure.
- Rarely, oxytocin leads to maternal seizures or coma due to water intoxication. ■

AVERTING NEONATAL HEALTH THREATS

Providing neonatal eye prophylaxis

Eye prophylaxis is an essential part of neonatal nursing care. Most states require administration of erythromycin 0.5% ophthalmic ointment to neonates to prevent ophthalmia neonatorum, a severe eye infection caused by *Neisseria gonorrhoeae* or *Chlamydia trachomatis.* This medication is used in all neonates — whether delivered vaginally or by cesarean section.

Administering erythromycin ointment

First, clean the neonate's eyes of mucus, blood, and meconium. Then, apply one strip of erythromycin ointment about ½″ to 1″ (1 to 2 cm) long in the lower conjunctival sac of each eye once within 1 hour after delivery.

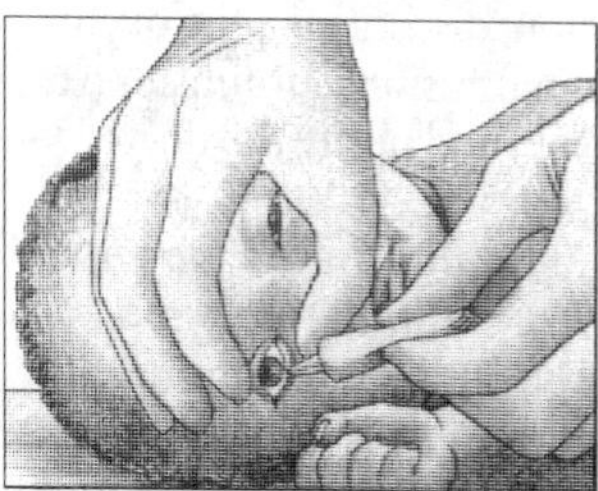

Don't irrigate the eyes after instillation. (Use a new tube of ointment for each neonate.) ■

Administering RhoGAM

RhoGAM is a concentrated solution of immune globulin that contains Rho(D) antibodies. I.M. injection of RhoGAM prevents an Rh-negative mother from producing active antibody responses and forming anti-$Rh_O(D)$ antibodies to Rh-positive fetal blood cells and endangering future Rh-positive infants.

Maternal immunization to the Rh antigen commonly results from transplacental hemorrhage during gestation or delivery. If unchecked during gestation, incompatible fetal and maternal blood can lead to hemolytic disease in the neonate.

Who should get RhoGAM?
RhoGAM is indicated for the Rh-negative woman after abortion, ectopic pregnancy, or delivery of a neonate having $Rh_O(D)$-positive or D_u-positive blood and Coombs' test-negative cord blood, accidental transfusion of Rh-positive blood, amniocentesis, abruptio placentae, or abdominal trauma. To prevent future maternal sensitization, RhoGAM should be administered within 72 hours.

During subsequent pregnancies, the Rh-negative woman must be screened to detect previous inadequate RhoGAM administration or low Rh-positive antibody titers.

Prophylactically administering RhoGAM at approximately 28 weeks' gestation can protect the fetus of the Rh-negative mother from unexpected sensitization.

The dosage is determined according to the fetal packed RBC volume that enters the mother's blood. A volume under 15 ml usually calls for one vial of RhoGAM; significant fetal-maternal hemorrhage calls for more than one vial if the fetal packed RBC volume exceeds 15 ml.

Preparing the injection
To administer RhoGAM, gather the following equipment, including a 3-ml syringe, a 22G 1½″ needle, a vial of RhoGAM, alcohol sponges, gloves, and agency-specific and patient identification forms (from the blood bank or laboratory).

Some facilities require that two nurses check the vial's identification numbers and sign the triplicate form that comes with the RhoGAM. Complete the form as indicated. Attach the appropriate copy to the patient's chart. Send the remaining two copies, along with the empty RhoGAM vial, to the laboratory or blood bank. Refer to your policy and procedures manual for details.

Preparing the patient
First, identify the patient. Then explain RhoGAM administration, and answer her questions. Give her an opportunity to voice any guilt or anxiety she may feel should she perceive her body as acting

against the fetus. If she refuses the injection, notify the doctor or nurse-midwife.

Giving the injection
Provide privacy, wash your hands, and put on gloves. Then withdraw the RhoGAM from the vial with the needle and syringe. Clean the gluteal injection site with an alcohol sponge, and administer RhoGAM intramuscularly.

Give the patient a card that identifies her Rh-negative status, and instruct her to carry it with her or keep it in a convenient location.

Watching for complications
After the injection, check for redness and soreness at the site. Complications of a single RhoGAM injection occur rarely and are usually mild and confined to the injection site. After multiple injections (given after Rh mismatch), complications may include fever, myalgia, lethargy, discomfort, splenomegaly, and hyperbilirubinemia.

Documenting the injection
Record the date, time, and site of the RhoGAM injection. (If applicable, note the patient's refusal to accept the injection.) Also document your patient teaching about RhoGAM. Note whether the patient received a card identifying her Rh-negative status. ■

Understanding drug therapy and breast-feeding

Because most drugs and chemicals ingested by the mother appear in breast milk, the doctor must weigh the risks and benefits of drug therapy before prescribing drugs for a breast-feeding patient.

Drug ingestion in the breast-feeding infant
Unlike the fetus, the infant cannot depend on the placenta for metabolism and excretion of drugs ingested by the mother. The amount of drug the infant ingests is affected by his sucking behavior, the amount of milk consumed per feeding, and breast-feeding frequency. The infant's low gastric acidity and slower absorption rate affect the amount of drug absorbed.

Changes in the infant's plasma-protein binding may alter drug concentration at receptor sites. Furthermore, drugs that are metabolized insufficiently and excreted by an immature neonatal system may accumulate, increasing the risk of toxicity. As a precaution, instruct your breast-feeding patient to check with the doctor before taking any drug. ■

CHAPTER 18

AVOIDING PROBLEMS IN PEDIATRIC PATIENTS

Tailoring drug therapy for pediatric patients

Building a rapport with pediatric patients

TAILORING DRUG THERAPY FOR PEDIATRIC PATIENTS

Learning about drug action in children

Providing pediatric drug therapy is challenging. Physiologic differences between children and adults, including those in vital organ maturity and body composition, strongly influence drug effectiveness. What's more, about 75% of all drugs currently lack full FDA approval for use in children.

A child's physiologic state, body composition, immature organ function, and other factors can affect the absorption, distribution, metabolism, and excretion of a drug.

Absorption

The route of drug administration affects its absorption.

Oral drugs

After a drug is administered orally, its absorption depends on the child's age, underlying disease, dosage form, and presence of other drugs or foods taken concurrently.

In a young child, gastric pH is higher or less acidic than in an adult. As the child grows, gastric pH decreases, acidity increases, and drug absorption is altered. The presence of milk and formula also can affect gastric pH and alter absorption. Therefore, most pediatric medications are administered when the child's stomach is empty.

Several other factors can influence drug absorption from the GI tract and make it less predictable and less efficient in a child under age 2. The child's short intestine as well as diarrhea can reduce the amount of time a drug is available for absorption. Reduced transit time through the GI tract also can decrease drug absorption.

Drugs given I.M. and S.C.

Absorption of I.M. drugs in infants may be unpredictable because of vasomotor instability and decreased muscle tone. Percutaneous absorption of S.C. medications in infants is greater because of an underdeveloped epidermal barrier and increased skin hydration.

Topical drugs

Children absorb topical drugs at about the same rate as adults, but they absorb such drugs more extensively because of their greater body-surface area relative to total body mass.

Distribution

A drug's dilution in the body affect its distribution. The higher percentage of total body water in neonates and infants dilutes water-soluble drugs, reducing their blood levels. Consequently, neonates and infants often require higher doses (in milligrams per kilogram) to achieve therapeutic blood drug levels.

Body composition also affects the distribution of fat-soluble drugs — but to a lesser degree than water-soluble ones. As the percentage of fat increases with age, so does the distribution of fat-soluble drugs. Therefore, the distribution of these drugs is more limited in children than in adults.

Neonatal drug distribution

In neonates, the immature liver also may affect drug distribution by decreasing the formation of plasma proteins; this, in turn, causes lower serum protein levels and higher fluid volume than occurs in an adult. That means there are fewer plasma proteins to which drugs may bind. Because only unbound, or free, drugs produce a pharmacologic effect, the neonate's decreased protein binding intensifies drug effects and may lead to toxicity.

Metabolism

In an infant, the immature liver may metabolize drugs inefficiently. As the liver matures during the 1st year of life, drug metabolism improves.

An infant with immature liver function or liver disease may require an altered dosage or a choice of therapeutic agent. Immature liver function increases the risk of toxicity with some drugs, such as chloramphenicol. When the liver fails to inactivate this drug, toxic levels can accumulate in the blood and cause *gray syndrome*, characterized by rapid respirations; ashen gray cyanosis; vomiting; loose, green stools; progressive abdominal distention; vasomotor collapse; and even death. Stopping the drug when symptoms appear can reverse this syndrome.

Drugs that require oxidation

Theophylline, caffeine, phenobarbital, phenytoin, and other drugs that require oxidation are metabolized more rapidly in children than in adults. The rate of metabolism for such drugs as aspirin and sulfonamides, which are catalyzed by microsomal or nonmicrosomal enzymes, can vary and may be genetically determined. These differences in metabolism can affect dosage requirements for a pediatric patient.

Excretion
Because most drug excretion occurs in the urine, the degree of renal development can affect drug excretion and dosage requirements for pediatric patients.

At birth, the kidneys are immature, renal excretion is slow, and drug dosages must be adjusted carefully. As the kidneys mature during the first few months, renal excretion of drugs increases, although the rate of increase is slow in a premature neonate.

Some drugs, such as nafcillin, are excreted by the biliary tract into the GI tract. In the first few days after birth, however, biliary blood flow is low, which can prolong drug effects. ■

Ensuring safe drug administration in children

Your skill in administering drugs is a key factor in ensuring accurate and safe drug delivery to children. To administer a drug with the least amount of discomfort, you must understand a child's physiologic and developmental vulnerabilities.

Young children don't understand their illness — or the reason why they need medication. Even if you try to reduce their fear of the unknown before administering a drug, such as by teaching them about the procedure and role-playing, many children will try to resist by kicking, screaming, and hitting.

To develop successful methods for administering drugs, enlist the aid of the parents (or caregivers). In some instances, you may even suggest that the parent give the drug, with your help and supervision.

Avoiding injury and reducing discomfort
Administering drugs safely and with little discomfort is your goal. An important part of the procedure is stabilizing the part of the body involved to avoid injury. However, trying to administer a drug to a struggling child can lead to unnecessary injury from a needle or cup.

Also, leaning on a child too hard or holding an arm or a leg with too much force is not only painful but frightening. What's more, it will only lead to increased resistance in future attempts.

Observing the five rights
To prevent injury to a child, you must also observe the "five rights" of drug administration: the right *name,* right *drug,* right *dose,* right *route,* and right *time.*

The pediatric patient also needs the right *dilution,* the right *volume in one site* for an

I.M. injection, and the right *rate* and right *dilution* for an I.V. infusion.

To make sure the child receives the correct drug, check his identification bracelet. Also check the medication administration record before and during drug preparation, just before administration, and when giving the drug. ■

Adjusting dosages for children

Although drug administration routes are the same for children and adults, safe dosage ranges can differ greatly.

Pediatric dosages differ from those for adults because a child's immature body systems may be unable to handle certain drugs. For example, a child has a much higher volume of total body water than an adult, and this affects drug distribution. The pharmacokinetics, pharmacodynamics, and pharmacotherapeutics of drugs also differ in children, necessitating special dosages.

Calculating dosages

To calculate pediatric drug dosages accurately, use the dosage per kilogram of body weight or body-surface area method. Other methods, based on the child's weight or age, are less accurate but may be used for rough estimates. Whichever method you use, remember that you are professionally and legally responsible for making sure that the prescribed pediatric dosage falls within the safe dosage range.

Kilogram of body weight method

Many pharmaceutical companies provide information about safe drug dosages for pediatric patients in milligrams per kilogram of body weight. Based on this information, you can determine the pediatric dosage by multiplying the child's body weight in kilograms by the milligrams of drug per kilogram. Most health care professionals consider this the most accurate method for determining pediatric drug dosages.

Here's an example of how to use this method: If the suggested pediatric dosage for a drug is 50 mg/kg/day, use the dosage per kilogram of body weight method to calculate how much of the drug to give an infant who weighs 20 lb (9 kg):

$$50 \text{ mg:kg} :: X \text{ mg:9 kg}$$

$$1 \text{ kg} \times X \text{ mg} = 50 \text{ mg} \times 9 \text{ kg}$$

$$X = \frac{50 \text{ mg} \times 9 \text{ kg}}{1 \text{ kg}}$$

$$X = 450 \text{ mg (daily dose)}$$

AVOIDING PROBLEMS IN PEDIATRIC PATIENTS

If 450 mg is to be given daily in three divided doses, follow these steps to decide how much to give every 8 hours:

$$X = \frac{450 \text{ mg daily}}{3}$$

Then X = 150 mg given every 8 hours.

Body surface area method

To calculate safe pediatric dosages by body surface area (BSA), plot the patient's height and weight on a nomogram to determine the BSA in square meters (m^2).

Next, multiply the child's BSA by the suggested pediatric dosage given in mg/m^2. The following equation shows how:

$$\text{Child's dose} = \frac{m^2 \text{ (child's BSA)} \times \text{(drug dose)}}{1 \text{ mg/m}^2}$$

This method is often used to calculate safe adult and pediatric dosages for antineoplastic drugs, such as methotrexate and cytarabine.

To calculate an approximate pediatric dose based on an adult dose, use the child's BSA in the following equation:

$$\text{Child's dose} = \frac{\text{Child's BSA} \times \text{average adult dose}}{\text{average adult BSA } (1.73\text{m}^2)}$$ ■

Administering oral medication to a child

When administering oral medication to a child, you may need to adjust your usual administration technique to the child's age, size, and developmental level. For example, for a young child, you may need to crush a tablet and mix it with a liquid for oral administration.

Avoiding dosage errors

- Start by checking the doctor's order for the prescribed medication, dosage, and route. Then compare the order with the drug label, check the expiration date, and review the patient's medication administration record for allergies.
- Next, carefully calculate the dosage, if necessary, and have another nurse verify it. Typically, you'll double-check dosages for potentially hazardous or lethal medications, such as insulin, heparin, digoxin, epinephrine, or narcotics. Check your facility's policy to learn which medications must be calculated and checked by two nurses.

Gathering equipment

Obtain the prescribed medication; plastic disposable syringe, plastic medicine dropper or spoon, or medication cup; and water, syrup, or jelly for tablets or fruit juice.

Giving medication to an infant

- Use a plastic syringe without a needle, or use a drug-specific medicine dropper to measure the dose. If the medication comes in tablet form, first crush the tablet (if appropriate), and mix it with water, syrup, or jelly. Then draw the mixture into the syringe or dropper.
- Pick up the infant, raising his head and shoulders or turning the head to one side to prevent aspiration. Hold the infant close to your body to help restrain him.
- Then, using your thumb, press down on the infant's chin to open the mouth. Slide the syringe or medicine dropper into the infant's mouth alongside the tongue. Then release the medication slowly to allow him time to swallow and to prevent choking. If appropriate, allow the infant to suck on the syringe while you expel the medication.

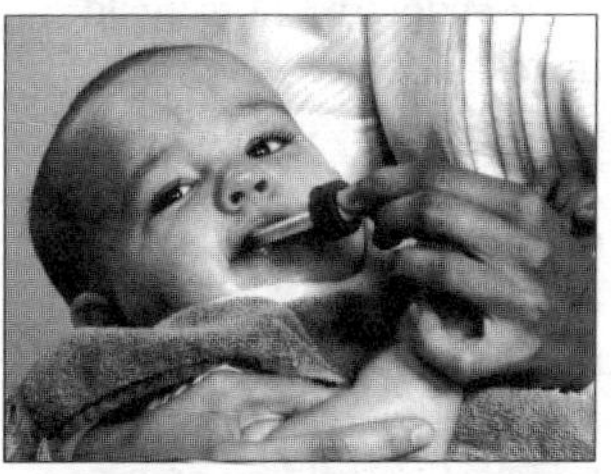

- If not contraindicated, give fruit juice after giving the medication.
- Then place a particularly small or inactive infant on his side to prevent aspiration. Let an active infant assume the position most comfortable for him to prevent agitation; avoid forcing him into a side-lying position, which could cause crying and vomiting.

Giving medication to a toddler

- Use a plastic disposable syringe or dropper to measure liquid medication. Then transfer the fluid to a medication cup (or leave it in the syringe or dropper).
- Elevate the toddler's head and shoulders, but don't lean the head back to prevent aspiration. If possible, ask the child to help hold the cup to enlist his cooperation. Otherwise, hold the cup to the toddler's lips, or use a syringe or a spoon to administer the liquid. Make sure the toddler ingests all the medication.

Giving medication to an older child

- If possible, let the child choose both the liquid in which to mix the medication and the beverage to drink after taking it.
- Also let the child choose where to take the medica-

tion, for example, sitting in bed or on a parent's lap.

- If the medication comes in tablet or capsule form, and if the child is old enough (between ages 4 and 6), teach him how to swallow solid medication. (If the child already knows how to do this, review the procedure out loud for safety's sake.) Tell the child to place the pill on the back of the tongue and to swallow it immediately by drinking water or juice. Focus most of your explanation on the water or juice to draw the child's attention away from the pill.
- Make sure the child drinks enough water or juice to keep the pill from lodging in the esophagus. Afterward, look inside the child's mouth to confirm that the pill was swallowed.
- If the child can't swallow the pill whole, crush it and mix it with water, syrup, or jelly. Or, after checking with the child's doctor, order the medication in liquid form.
- If possible, have a parent give prescribed oral medications while you supervise. ■

Giving nose drops to a child

To administer nose drops properly, adjust your technique to the patient's age.

Tips for infants

- Before giving nose drops to an infant, warm the medication by holding the closed bottle under warm water. Then wash your hands, and put on gloves.
- Position the infant on your arm so that his head tilts backward.
- Draw up the medication by squeezing the dropper's bulb until the correct dose fills the dropper.
- Open the infant's nostril, taking care to support his head. Next, instill the medication, and keep the infant's head tilted back for 5 minutes.

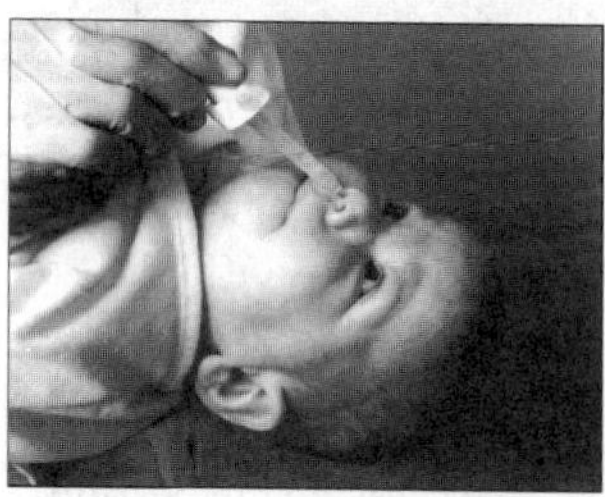

- Observe for signs of aspiration. If the infant begins to cough, help him into an upright sitting position, and gently pat his back until he clears his lungs.
- Then document drug administration.

Tips for older children

- To give nose drops to a child who's too large to hold in your arms, you'll need a pillow.
- Have the child lie on his back, and place the pillow

under his shoulders. Gently tilt his head back, supporting it between your forearm and body. Use your other arm to steady his position and, if necessary, to restrain his arms and hands.

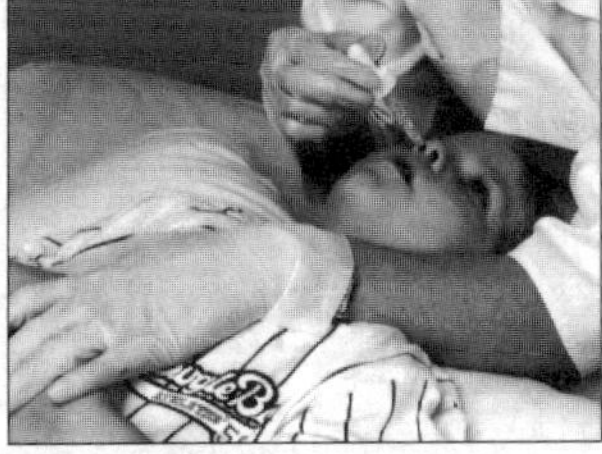

▪ Instill the medication, and keep the child's head tilted back for about 5 minutes. ■

Giving an injection to a child

When administering an injection to a child, consult the parents (or caregivers) for tips. They may be able to tell you which injection methods and approaches have succeeded in the past. However, avoid asking a parent to help with injections because the child may perceive his parent as the cause of pain.

Building rapport

Establish a trusting relationship with the child and parents so you can offer support and promote cooperation even when a medication causes discomfort.

If the child will receive one injection, allow him to choose from the appropriate sites. If the child must receive many injections, site rotation must follow a set pattern. Let the child play with a medication cup or syringe and pretend to give the medication to a doll or stuffed animal.

Be honest

When giving medication to an older child, be honest. Reassure the child that the discomfort will be brief. Emphasize that he must remain still to promote safety and minimize discomfort. Explain to the child and his parents that an assistant will help the child remain still, if necessary. Keep your explanations brief and simple.

Use distraction

To divert attention, have the child start counting just before the injection, and challenge him to try to reach 10 before you finish the injection. If the child cries, don't scold or allow the parents to scold.

Encourage parents to hold and comfort a younger child. Praise him for any act of cooperation while you give the injection. Apply an adhesive bandage to the injection site as a reward or badge.

Gathering equipment

Obtain the prescribed medication and a syringe and needle of the appropriate size.

Using S.C. injectors

Currently available for use by patients at home, S.C. injectors feature disposable needles or pressure jets to deliver doses of prescribed medications, such as short-acting insulin. Appropriate for use in children, these devices deliver medication safely and accurately.

The NovoPen, for instance, has disposable needles and replaceable cartridges. Preci-Jet, Vitajet, and Medi-Jector draw their medications from standard bottles. A pressure jet deposits the drug in subcutaneous tissue.

Although relatively expensive, these devices are easy to use. Studies show that jet-injected insulin is dispersed faster and absorbed more rapidly because it avoids the puddling effect common with needle delivery.

Needle injection

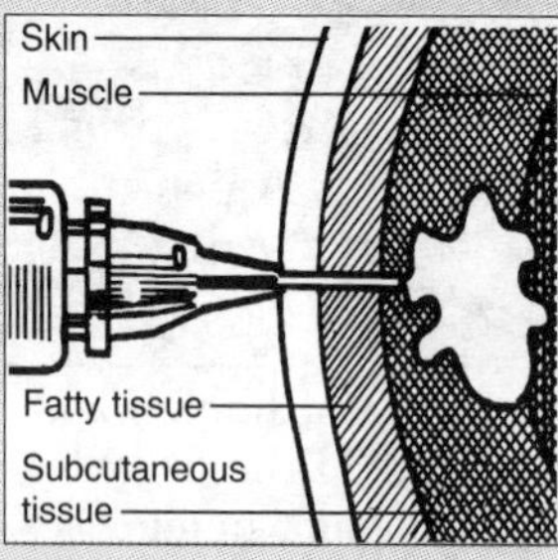

Pressure-jet injection

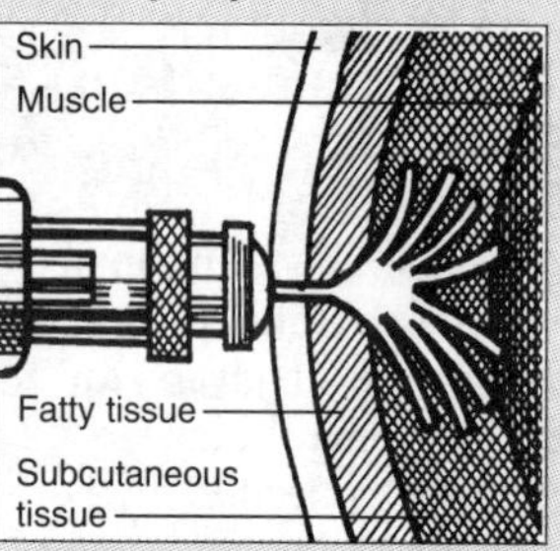

Typically, for I.M. injections in infants, you'll use a 25G ¾″ needle; in older children, a 23G 1″ needle. For S.C. injections, select a ¾″ or ½″ needle. (See *Using S.C. injectors.*) For intradermal medications, use a 27G ½″ needle. To administer viscous medications, select a larger-gauge needle.

You'll also need alcohol sponges or povidone-iodine solution, gloves, gauze pads, cold compresses, and an adhesive bandage.

Verifying identification

- Identify the child by comparing the name on his identification bracelet with the name on the medication administration record. If the child can talk and respond, ask him to state his name.
- Then explain the procedure to the child and parents in terms the child can under-

stand. Provide privacy, especially for an older child.

Giving an I.M. injection

- Choose the injection site based on the child's age and muscle mass. (See *Choosing I.M. injection sites in children,* pages 700 and 701.)
- Position the patient appropriately for the site chosen. Then locate key landmarks, for example, the posterior superior iliac spine and the greater trochanter. Have someone help you restrain an infant; gain an older child's cooperation first before you enlist his assistance.
- Put on gloves, and clean the injection site with an alcohol sponge or povidone-iodine solution. Wipe outward from the center in a circular motion to avoid contaminating the clean area.
- Grasp the tissue surrounding the site between your index finger and thumb to immobilize the site and to create a muscle mass for the injection.
- If you're using the vastus lateralis site, position the child by grasping the chosen leg firmly below the knee with your nondominant hand. Lean across the child's torso with your upper body, being careful not to put too much pressure on the child's chest (as shown at top of column two). With your dominant hand, give the injection.

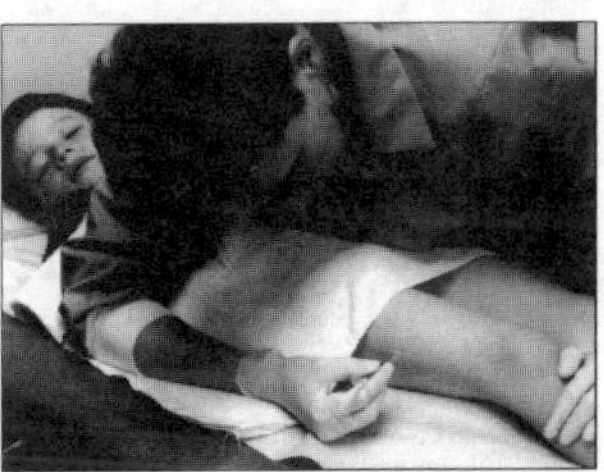

- Insert the needle quickly, using a darting motion. If you're using the ventrogluteal site, insert the needle at a 45-degree angle toward the knee.
- Aspirate the plunger to ensure that the needle isn't in a blood vessel. If no blood appears, inject the medication slowly so the muscle can distend to accommodate the volume.
- Then withdraw the needle, and gently massage the area with a gauze pad to stimulate circulation and enhance absorption. Avoid using an alcohol sponge, which could cause additional discomfort from stinging or burning. Be sure to praise the child, and provide comfort as necessary.

Giving a subcutaneous injection

- Choose one of these possible sites:
  - — middle third of the upper outer arm
  - — middle third of the upper outer thigh
  - — abdomen.
- Put on gloves and clean the injection site with an alcohol sponge or povidone-iodine solution according to the pa-

Choosing I.M. injection sites in children

When choosing the best site for a child's I.M. injection, consider the child's age, weight, and muscular development; the amount of subcutaneous fat over the injection site; the type of drug you're administering; and the drug's absorption rate.

Vastus lateralis and rectus femoris muscles
For a child under age 3, you'll typically use the vastus lateralis or rectus femoris muscle. Constituting the largest muscle mass in this age-group, these two muscles have few major blood vessels and nerves.

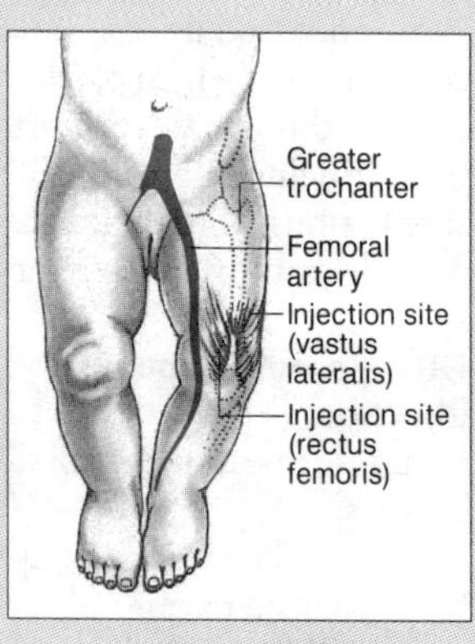

Ventrogluteal and dorsogluteal sites
For a child over age 3 who can walk, use the ventrogluteal and dorsogluteal sites. Like the vastus lateralis muscle, the ventrogluteal and dorsogluteal areas also have few major blood vessels and nerves. Before you select either site, however, make sure the child has been walking for at least 1 year to ensure sufficient muscle development.

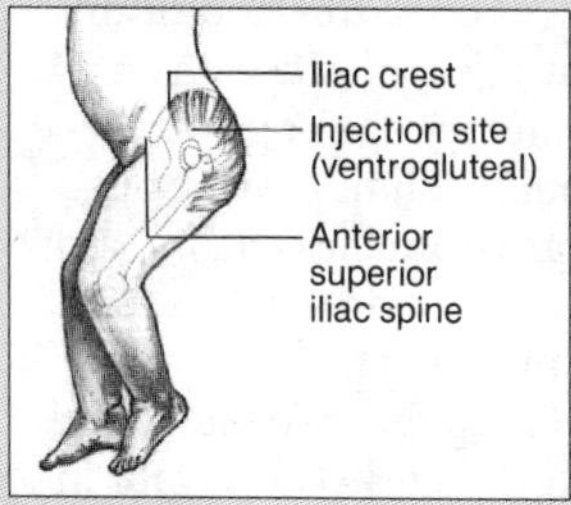

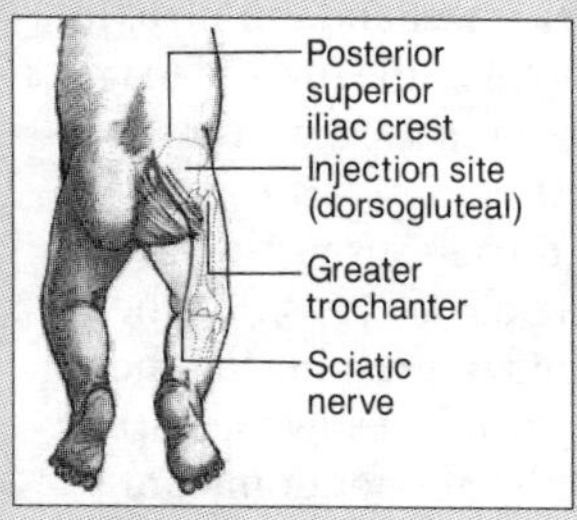

tient's needs and your facility's policy.

- Then pinch the tissue surrounding the site between your index finger and thumb to ensure injection into the subcutaneous tissue. Holding the needle at a 45- to 90-degree angle, quickly insert it into the tissue. Release your

Deltoid muscle
For a child older than 18 months who needs rapid drug action, consider using the deltoid muscle. Because blood flows faster in the deltoid than in other muscles, drug absorption should be faster.

But use this site cautiously. The deltoid muscle doesn't develop fully until adolescence. In a younger child, it's small and close to the radial nerve, which may be injured during needle insertion.

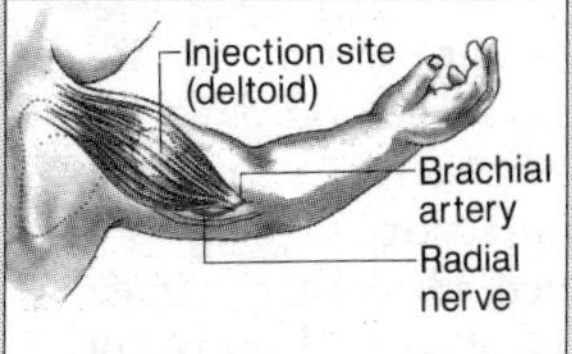

grasp on the tissue, and slowly inject the medication. Remove the needle quickly to decrease discomfort.

Easing discomfort
Unless contraindicated, gently massage the area to promote absorption. You may also apply a cold compress to the injection site to minimize pain.

Giving an intradermal injection
- Put on gloves, and pull the skin taut (the site of choice is the inner aspect of the forearm).
- Insert the needle, bevel up, at a 10- to 15-degree angle just beneath the outer skin layer.
- Slowly inject the medication, and watch for a bleb to appear. Quickly remove the needle, taking care to maintain the injection angle.
- If appropriate (for example, if the injection is given for allergy testing), draw a circle around the bleb, and don't massage the area, which will interfere with test results.

Watching for side effects
Carefully observe the child for a rash, pruritus, cough, or other signs.

Documenting administration
Record the medication, form, dose, date, time, route, and site of administration. Also record the effect of the medication, the patient's tolerance of the procedure, complications, nursing inter-

ventions, and any patient teaching.

Special considerations

- If you have any doubts about the medication dosage, consult the doctor who ordered the drug. Double-check information in a drug reference.
- Compile a list of emergency drugs, calculating the dosages according to the patient's weight. Post the list near the patient's bed for reference in an emergency. ■

Administering emergency drugs to children

Many emergency drugs used for adults require special dosage instructions when they're administered to children. Read what follows to learn about administering drugs for advanced life support to children.

Treating cardiac arrest

When giving epinephrine, calcium chloride, glucose, or sodium bicarbonate to a child, adjust the dosage as described below.

Epinephrine

By causing vasoconstriction, this drug elevates perfusion pressure during chest compression, improving oxygen delivery to the heart. Epinephrine also enhances myocardial contractions and stimulates spontaneous contractions.

For a child with bradycardia, give epinephrine as ordered in a dose of 0.01 mg/kg (1:10,000 solution) by the I.V. or intraosseous route. Or give it endotracheally in a dose of 0.1 mg/kg (1:1,000 solution).

For a child with asystole or ventricular fibrillation, the initial dose is 0.01 mg/kg (1:10,000 solution) by the I.V. or intraosseus route, followed by doses of 0.1 mg/kg (1:1,000 solution). Doses as high as 0.2 mg/kg may be effective.

Calcium chloride

Calcium chloride is essential for myocardial excitation-contraction coupling. As ordered, administer an initial dose of 10% calcium chloride (5 to 7 mg/kg) slowly through a central line access port to avoid causing vein sclerosis. Repeat the initial dose in 10 minutes, if necessary. However, before you give additional doses, the child's serum calcium level should be determined.

Administer calcium slowly to children, especially to those receiving digoxin, because this drug can cause cardiac arrhythmias. Keep in mind that calcium isn't recommended during initial resuscitation unless hypocalcemia is evident.

Glucose

Glucose is crucial for children because they can't store glycogen. In documented hypoglycemia or if the child doesn't respond to standard resuscitation measures and is considered at risk for hypoglycemia, the usual dose is 2 to 4 ml/kg by continuous I.V. infusion. Avoid giving glucose by I.V. bolus.

Sodium bicarbonate

Sodium bicarbonate is useful for treating documented, severe metabolic acidosis secondary to cardiac arrest. The recommended dose is 1 mEq/kg by the I.V. or intraosseus route or in a dose calculated by multiplying 0.3 by the kilograms of body weight by the base deficit. The dose may be repeated every 10 minutes. Flush the I.V. tubing between doses of sodium bicarbonate and calcium.

Treating heart rhythm disturbances

Adenosine, atropine, lidocaine, or bretylium may be given to a child to treat cardiac arrhythmias.

Adenosine

This is the drug of choice for treating supraventricular tachycardia. Because of its short half-life (10 seconds), adenosine causes relatively few side effects. The recommended pediatric dose is 0.1 mg/kg, administered by rapid I.V bolus. Higher doses may be needed for peripheral, rather than central venous, administration. If no therapeutic effect occurs, the dose may be doubled. The maximum single dose shouldn't exceed 12 mg.

Atropine sulfate

This drug is used to treat bradycardia accompanied by hypotension or poor perfusion. The initial pediatric dose is 0.02 mg/kg I.V.; the minimum dose is 0.1 mg. The maximum single dose is 0.5 mg I.V. in children and 1 mg I.V. in adolescents. This dose can be repeated in 5 minutes, to a maximum total dose of 1 mg I.V. in children and 2 mg I.V. in adolescents. The I.V. dose may be given intraosseously or endotracheally. Be aware that atropine administration may result in tachycardia.

Lidocaine

When giving this drug, you may repeat the initial pediatric dosage of 1 mg/kg I.V. every 5 minutes for 15 minutes. If ventricular fibrillation (VF) or PVCs persist, you may start an infusion of 20 to 50 mcg/kg/minute, if ordered. Be aware that excessive serum drug levels cause myocardial and circulatory depression as well as CNS effects, such as drowsiness and disorientation.

Bretylium

If defibrillation and lidocaine fail to correct VF, a rapid I.V. bolus of 5 mg/kg may be administered; this should be followed by defibrillation. If VF persists even after an additional defibrillation attempt, a dose of 10 mg/kg may be given.

Maintaining cardiac output

A child may receive dopamine or dobutamine to improve cardiac output.

Dopamine

Usually given by continuous I.V. infusion, this drug may be administered at a rate of 2 to 5 mcg/kg/minute. To improve blood pressure, perfusion, and urine output, you may increase the dosage to 20 mcg/kg/minute, if ordered.

Don't mix dopamine with sodium bicarbonate. Also, be aware that it may cause tachycardia and vasoconstriction.

Dobutamine

This drug usually is infused at a dosage of 2 to 20 mcg/kg/minute, titrated to the individual patient. It may cause tachycardia in high doses. ■

BUILDING A RAPPORT WITH PEDIATRIC PATIENTS

Teaching children about medication

Ingenuity is the key to teaching children about medication. Adjust your teaching style to fit the child's physical, emotional, and intellectual levels. Keep teaching sessions brief. Offer frequent praise and encouragement.

Teaching young children

Because children learn more easily through participation, help them grasp information by using play. Invite parents to join you, and later reinforce what you taught.

Allow time for the child to absorb information and ask questions. Meet with parents alone to give them more detailed information and answer their questions.

Teaching adolescents

At around age 12, adolescents' thought processes are similar to those of adults, so teach them much the same as you would grown-ups.

However, adolescents develop their identity in relation to their peers and in opposition to their parents. So teaching them with their parents present may be inappropriate. And don't assume that adolescents know more about their anatomy and physiology than they actually do. Use illustrations to reinforce what you teach.

Finally, be honest with adolescents. If their lifestyle will change because of their disease and medication regimen, prepare them for that change. They'll need your help to understand and develop ways to adapt to those changes whenever possible.

Helping a child cope with a medication routine

Facing a disease that requires medication for a long time can frighten children and their parents. As the child's primary nurse, you provide some continuity. You want parents to perceive you as a competent, concerned individual who assists them in their caregiver role. And you want the child to trust and accept you.

To build rapport, speak to both the child and parents during your initial interview. The older the child, the more information you can provide him; but even a very young child will want attention. Find out what the child likes to be called, and address him by that name.

Whatever the age, try to assess the child's emotional readiness. Keep in mind that children understand (and fear) much more than they can verbalize. A child's silence may indicate terror, not calm.

Understanding fears

Just what the child fears about the disease and medication regimen depends on his age and developmental level. For instance, a preschooler can worry about bodily injury and pain. In a school-age child, fears of pain and injury are compounded by the stress caused by loss of control and forced dependence on a mysterious medication routine.

An adolescent may also feel added stress and may worry that having to take medication will make him seem different than everyone else and "abnormal."

Eliciting fears

To determine what the child fears, ask him if he's had any experience with hospitals or knows anyone who has to take medication routinely, as he will. Listen to the emotional content of the response. Help minimize the child's loss of control and forced dependence by providing as many choices as possible.

Your patient teaching becomes particularly important when the child is facing a new routine, such as medication administration, for the first time. It also gives you a chance to build rapport.

Your youngest patients may present the greatest challenge. Many have active imaginations. Stress that having to take medication is not a punishment for their injury or illness.

Fighting fear with knowledge

You can reduce a young child's fears by describing both what will happen and the sensations the child will feel. Use puppets or dolls as teaching aids. By using a toy, you can demonstrate how the medication will be given. Also, let the child practice any procedures that require cooperation.

When teaching an older child, include more cognitive terms, but explain words not usually in a child's vocabulary. Choose words without double meanings; for instance, say "the medicine will help your body fight your disease" rather than "the medicine will cure your disease."

Telling the truth

One small lie can destroy days of work in developing trust. For example, telling the child that taking medication will prevent illness and his need to be in the hospital isn't helpful. If you can't answer a question truthfully, redirect or distract the child.

But make sure you address the question after you've had a chance to think through your response, and choose the right time to discuss both the question and your answer.

Remembering the parents

Try to schedule your teaching sessions for times that are conducive to learning and coping, such as after rest or play. Don't forget that the parents may have their own fears. Tell them how their emotional response may influence the child's response. Also, teach them some nondrug pain-relief techniques, such as distracting the child with games, lullabies, imagery, or massage.

Is there anything in the family situation that might affect the child's ability to adhere to the medication regimen? Observe how the parents interact with each other and with the child. Do they talk with or at the child? Are they oversolicitous? If parental spoiling threatens to slow the child's recovery, you should politely intervene.

For both the child and parents, a long-term medication routine can cause anxiety. Your preparation may not only set the stage for a smooth transition but also influence the child's lifelong attitudes about nursing care. ■

CHAPTER 19

MODIFYING THERAPY IN GERIATRIC PATIENTS

TAILORING DRUG THERAPY AND TEACHING IN GERIATRIC PATIENTS

Learning about drug action in geriatric patients

Aging is usually accompanied by a decline in organ function. Such a decline can affect drug distribution and clearance, among other things. A disease or chronic disorder can exacerbate this physiologic decline. Together, these factors can increase the risk of drug toxicity and side effects in geriatric patients. Be aware of these changes when administering medications to a geriatric patient and when observing for side effects.

Absorption

Absorption of drugs administered by the oral, intramuscular, or subcutaneous route is frequently altered in geriatric patients.

Impaired absorption of oral drugs may stem from mucosal atrophy, decreased gastric emptying, reduced splanchnic blood flow, duodenal diverticula, and decreased GI motility. Decreased gastric acid secretion and higher pH may affect ionization and absorption of some oral drugs.

Reduced blood flow to the GI tract and fewer cells available for absorption can delay drug absorption. However, because GI transit time is slowed, drugs remain in the system longer, enhancing absorption. The effects of aging cause slow absorption, but complete absorption is still possible.

Absorption of I.M. and S.C. injected drugs may be delayed from reduced blood flow and altered capillary wall permeability.

Distribution

Total body mass and body water decrease with age. These changes in body composition lead to a relative increase in body fat and a decrease in body water, which alters the distribution patterns for most drugs.

In a geriatric patient, a highly fat-soluble drug, such as diazepam, has an increased volume of distribution and a prolonged distribution phase, leading to a prolonged half-life and duration of action. A highly water-soluble drug, such as gentamicin, has a decreased volume of distribution; hence more of the drug remains in the bloodstream, increasing the risk of drug toxicity.

Aging also reduces plasma levels of albumin, a blood protein that binds with and transports many drugs. As a result, more unbound drug may circulate in the bloodstream. This increases the pharmacologic action of drugs that are protein-bound, heightening the risk of side effects and drug toxicity. Also, multiple drug regimens may compete for binding sites, and some drugs may be displaced, resulting in increased free serum concentration of those drugs.

Other factors that alter distribution

Drug distribution also may be altered by declining cardiac output, poor nutrition, extremes of body weight, dehydration, electrolyte and mineral imbalances, inactivity, and prolonged bed rest.

Perhaps the most significant factor is physical size; geriatric patients typically are smaller than younger patients. So if a geriatric patient receives the same drug dose as a younger patient, the geriatric patient's typically lower fluid volume can result in higher blood drug levels.

Metabolism

Alterations in drug metabolism increase the risk of drug accumulation and toxicity and may prolong a drug's half-life. Aging reduces the liver's ability to metabolize drugs, and liver disease may further compromise liver function. So may other diseases that reduce hepatic blood flow, such as CHF.

Drug metabolism by the liver depends primarily on two processes: hepatic blood flow and metabolic enzyme action. Because aging reduces blood flow to the liver, less drug is delivered for metabolism to inactive compounds.

Two major phases

Hepatic enzymes metabolize drugs in two major phases. Aging, diminished liver mass, and altered nutritional status reduce the efficiency of both phases. However, phase I reactions (oxidation, reduction, or hydrolysis of drug molecules) are affected more than phase II reactions (coupling of the drug or its metabolite with an acid to produce an inactive compound). Aging leads to different clinical effects, depending on whether a drug is metabolized in phase I, phase II, or both.

Excretion

With aging, glomerular filtration and tubular secretion decline progressively. Also, dehydration and cardiovascular and renal disease may impair renal function. Keep in mind that a geriatric patient has a smaller renal reserve than a younger patient, even if BUN and serum creatinine levels appear normal.

Increased risk of toxicity
The kidneys excrete many drugs. In a geriatric patient who's receiving drugs that are not metabolized, watch for signs and symptoms of toxicity because drug clearance and excretion may be delayed.

Drug interactions and side effects
Response to drug therapy is determined by individual variables, such as drug history, body mass, and physiologic and psychological status. Older adults commonly suffer multiple diseases that require therapy with multiple medications (polypharmacy). This increases the risk of drug interactions and side effects.

Also, older adults may obtain prescriptions from different doctors. And they may use nonprescription drugs without informing the doctor and may share drugs with others. ■

Altering tablets and capsules

When caring for a geriatric patient, you may crush tablets or capsules so the patient can swallow them more easily. But first find out whether a liquid preparation of the same drug is available. If not, determine whether crushing will affect the drug's action, and follow these guidelines.

Which forms shouldn't be altered
Avoid crushing sustained-release (extended-release or controlled-release) drugs. However, some of these drugs can be scored and broken. Also avoid crushing capsules that contain tiny beads of medication. You may empty the beads into a beverage, pudding, or applesauce.

Don't crush or score enteric-coated tablets, which usually appear shiny or candy-coated, because they are designed to prevent GI upset.

Finally, avoid altering buccal and sublingual tablets.

Crushing tablets
If you need to crush a tablet, try to use a chewable form, which is easier to crush. Then, using a mortar and pestle or a pill crusher, press the tablet between two spoons, or place it in a small plastic bag and crush it with a rolling pin. Once the tablet is crushed, give the patient a drink to wet the esophagus. Unless contraindicated, mix the medication with 1 tsp or 1 tbs of pureed fruit or pudding.

Breaking tablets
If you need to break a tablet, use one that is scored. Use an instrument that can't cause injury, such as a spatula.

If a tablet isn't scored, it should be crushed, weighed,

and dispensed by the pharmacist. Also follow this procedure when breaking a tablet into smaller pieces than the score allows or when giving part of a capsule. ■

Modifying I.M. injections

Remember the physical changes that accompany aging, and choose your equipment, site, and technique accordingly.

Choosing the right needle
Because a geriatric patient usually has less subcutaneous tissue and less muscle mass than a younger patient, especially in the buttocks and upper arms, use a shorter needle than you would for a younger adult.

Selecting a site
Also keep in mind that a geriatric patient typically has more fat around the hips, abdomen, and thighs. This makes the vastus lateralis muscle and ventrogluteal site (gluteus medius and minimus, but not gluteus maximus muscles) the primary injection sites.

You should be able to palpate the muscle in these areas easily. However, if the patient is extremely thin, gently pinch the muscle to elevate it and to avoid putting the needle completely through it (which would affect drug absorption and distribution).

Note: Never give an I.M. injection in an immobile limb because of poor drug absorption and the risk of a sterile abscess at the injection site.

Checking your technique
To avoid inserting the needle in a blood vessel, pull back on the plunger, and look for blood before injecting the drug. Because of age-related vascular changes, geriatric patients are at greater risk for hematomas. To stop bleeding after an I.M. injection, apply direct pressure over the puncture site for a longer time than usual.

Gently massage the injection site to aid drug absorption and distribution. However, avoid site massage with any drugs given by the Z-track injection technique, such as iron dextran. ■

Recognizing side effects in geriatric patients

Geriatric patients are especially susceptible to drug side effects, such as urticaria and rashes, impotence, incontinence, and GI upset. (See *How aging increases the risk of side effects,* page 712.) The side effects described below are serious; you need to

How aging increases the risk of side effects

The physiologic changes of aging make geriatric patients more susceptible to drug-induced illnesses and side effects than younger adults. Other conditions common to many geriatric patients also increase the risk of side effects.

To help prevent these problems or detect them early, check the patient's history for the following risk factors:

- altered mental status
- patient is a woman
- small build
- financial problems
- frail health
- poor nutritional status
- patient lives alone
- history of previous side effects
- history of allergies
- multiple chronic illnesses
- renal failure
- treatment by several doctors
- polypharmacy or complex medication regimens.

know how to recognize them and intervene when appropriate.

Altered mental status

Agitation or confusion may follow use of anticholinergics, diuretics, antihypertensives, and antidepressants. Paradoxically, antidepressant drugs may cause depression.

Anorexia

This is a warning sign of toxicity — especially toxicity caused by digitalis glycosides such as digoxin. That's why the doctor usually prescribes a very low initial dose.

Blood disorders

If the patient takes an anticoagulant, watch for signs of easy bruising or bleeding, such as excessive bleeding after brushing his teeth. Such signs may signal thrombocytopenia or blood dyscrasias. Other drugs that may cause bruising or bleeding include antineoplastics, such as methotrexate; antibiotics, such as nitrofurantoin; and anticonvulsants, such as valproic acid and phenytoin. Tell your patient to report easy bruising to the doctor immediately.

Dehydration

If your patient is taking a diuretic, stay alert for dehydration and electrolyte imbalance. Monitor blood levels of the drug, and give potassium supplements, as ordered.

Many drugs, such as anticholinergics, cause dry mouth; suggest sucking on sugarless candy for relief.

Orthostatic hypotension

Marked by light-headedness or faintness and unsteady footing, orthostatic hypotension can be caused by sedatives, antidepressants, antihypertensives, or antipsychotics. Warn the patient not to sit up or get out of bed too quickly and to call for help in walking if dizziness or faintness occurs. Report orthostatic hypotension to the doctor, who may reevaluate the patient's drug therapy.

Tardive dyskinesia

This disorder is characterized by abnormal tongue movements, lip pursing, grimacing, blinking, and gyrating motions of the face and extremities. It may be triggered by psychotropic drugs, such as haloperidol or chlorpromazine. ■

Adjusting your teaching for geriatric patients

The abilities and needs of geriatric patients may differ from those of younger patients. If you tailor your style of teaching to fit geriatric patients' learning, motivational, and social differences, teaching them can be rewarding.

Understanding the effects of aging

Aging affects intellectual ability, sensory perception, and psychomotor function in various ways.

Loss in mental capacity

A person's intellectual ability changes with age. Most of us think of intellectual decline when we think of aging, but we're only half right. People have two kinds of intelligence: fluid and crystallized.

Fluid intelligence enables us to perceive relationships, to reason, and to perform abstract thinking. As degenerative changes occur, fluid intelligence declines, causing changes ranging from slowed processing time to test anxiety.

Crystallized intelligence is the wisdom we absorb during our lives: vocabulary and general information, understanding of social situations, math reasoning, and the ability to evaluate experiences. Because this kind of intelligence increases with age, you can enhance geriatric patients' learning ability by:
- using concrete examples
- asking them what they know about their medication before you begin.

Slowed processing time. Geriatric patients need more time to process and react to information, especially when learning about the relationship between a drug and its action. Adapt your teaching by avoiding long lists of directions.

To prevent misunderstandings, label each medication bottle, and then divide your instructions into discrete messages, waiting for the patient to respond to each one. Here's an example:

Nurse: Avoid taking this medication with antacids.

Patient: Does that mean I shouldn't take my heartburn medicine with the medication in the bottle labeled "Don't take with antacids"?

Nurse: That's right.

Stimulus persistence or "after image." Geriatric patients sometimes confuse the word or symbol you've just taught with the word or symbol you're introducing — for example, hypoglycemia and hyperglycemia. Again, wait for a response before introducing a new concept or definition. And when appropriate, use common lay terms, such as "high blood sugar" or "low blood sugar."

Decreased short-term memory. Give geriatric patients more time to comprehend what you've said, and repeat your demonstrations. Also, devise clues to help them remember information. Older people are especially anxious about making mistakes on tests, so they may need extra time to answer questions.

Hearing loss

A patient who routinely fails to respond to you or who responds inappropriately may have trouble hearing.

The ability to discriminate high-frequency sounds diminishes around age 50 and declines greatly after age 65. Severe impairment could make the patient feel isolated, suspicious, or even paranoid.

If the patient speaks loudly or tilts his head when listening, assess him for deafness. Check the ears for excessive cerumen, a common, reversible cause of hearing loss.

During teaching sessions, make sure a patient with a chronic hearing problem uses a hearing aid, if he has one. Face the patient when you talk. Speak slowly, clearly, and in a normal tone. Don't raise your voice.

If a patient has suffered a loss in hearing, provide written material to reinforce your oral instructions.

Vision loss

Cataracts and presbyopia prevent many older people from reading the small print on medication containers or glossy labels. Diabetic retinopathy and macular degeneration also cause vision problems. Yellowing of the ocular lens produces color distortion.

The drugs your patient is taking might affect his vision. For example, phenylbutazone, an anti-inflammatory drug, may cause blurred vision.

Impaired vision could prevent your patient from learning from videos, closed-circuit TV, or filmstrips. He may not be able to read written instructions or handle equipment such as medication syringes.

When teaching, make sure the patient has access to eyeglasses, contact lenses, or other devices, such as a magnifying glass. Use large teaching aids with oversized print.

Colors used in patient-teaching aids must be easily distinguished and have contrast to help the patient differentiate between print and background. Make sure that reading lights are bright but diffused and properly placed.

Loss in flexibility and fine motor skills

Aging causes gradual loss of muscle strength and endurance. This can limit flexibility and prevent your patient from completing tasks that require fine motor skills.

In fact, many older people can't turn a dial or knob. Check for such limitations before giving the patient a videocassette, a tape recorder, or an audiocassette for self-paced learning, or before demonstrating how to perform a procedure.

Loss of flexibility and fine motor skills may also impede the patient's ability to open medication containers or to handle or pick up pills. Instruct patients to ask for non–childproof medication containers if they have no children in their households.

Fostering motivation

- Conduct teaching sessions when the patient is alert and ready to learn. Make an appointment, and keep sessions brief. Make sure that he hasn't just taken medication that will impair his concentration. Break down the skills into steps, and teach just a few at each session.
- Avoid teaching sessions after activities that may sap the patient's energy. Find out if he has other immediate concerns, and try to address them.
- Be supportive. Positive reinforcement increases your patient's confidence about taking medication.
- Find out the activities and lifestyle that the patient wants to maintain after returning home. This will help you present information in a way that seems important to him.
- List the nursing diagnoses your teaching can correct. Identify these problems, and ask if the patient wants to overcome them. Explain the

relationship between the prescribed medication and the patient's desire to overcome health problems.

- If your patient doesn't see himself as having a role in his own health care (instead believing that the locus of control lies with the doctor), tell him that the doctor feels that the medication will help him.
- List health habits that will help keep the patient well. Explain how the things you're teaching will help achieve this goal.

Gaining the patient's confidence

Some older people adapt to their conditions so well that they don't consider them problems and don't want to learn about them.

Convincing a geriatric patient that you're teaching him something useful is only half the motivation battle. You may also have to convince him that the methods you're teaching are in his best interest. Here are some tips that will make this job easier.

- Ask the patient about his sleeping, eating, and other health habits.
- List the patient's health beliefs that will reinforce or hinder your teaching. Discuss these beliefs before you teach something new.
- Ask the patient what he knows about a technique or health care tip before you explain it.

Enlisting family support

Include the patient's family in teaching sessions (with the patient's permission, of course), and enlist their support.

Let family members see and understand the need for the patient to act in his own behalf. This can help prevent family members from taking over later because they feel they are better able to manage the patient's drug administration.

Overcoming other obstacles

Lack of other resources can also sabotage a teaching plan. For example, can the patient afford the prescribed medication? If not, will an agency help? Does the patient have transportation to the pharmacy and the doctor's office? If not, will a transportation service or family member help? Get answers to all these questions before you teach the geriatric patient. ■

INDEX

Note: i refers to an illustration; *t* refers to a table.